PLAY THERAPY

CREATIVE ARTS AND PLAY THERAPY

Cathy A. Malchiodi and David A. Crenshaw
Series Editors

This series highlights action-oriented therapeutic approaches that utilize art, music, dance/movement, drama, play, and related modalities. Emphasizing current best practices and research, experienced practitioners show how creative arts and play therapies can be integrated into overall treatment for individuals of all ages. Books in the series provide richly illustrated guidelines and techniques for addressing trauma, attachment problems, and other psychological difficulties, as well as for supporting resilience and self-regulation.

Creative Arts and Play Therapy for Attachment Problems
Cathy A. Malchiodi and David A. Crenshaw, Editors

Play Therapy: A Comprehensive Guide to Theory and Practice
David A. Crenshaw and Anne L. Stewart, Editors

Creative Interventions with Traumatized Children, Second Edition
Cathy A. Malchiodi, Editor

Music Therapy Handbook
Barbara L. Wheeler, Editor

Play Therapy

A COMPREHENSIVE GUIDE TO THEORY AND PRACTICE

EDITED BY

David A. Crenshaw
Anne L. Stewart

Foreword by Stuart Brown

THE GUILFORD PRESS
New York   London

© 2015 The Guilford Press
A Division of Guilford Publications, Inc.
370 Seventh Avenue, Suite 1200, New York, NY 10001
www.guilford.com

Paperback edition 2016

Printed in the United States of America

This book is printed on acid-free paper.

Last digit is print number: 9   8   7   6

The authors have checked with sources believed to be reliable in their efforts to
provide information that is complete and generally in accord with the standards
of practice that are accepted at the time of publication. However, in view of the
possibility of human error or changes in behavioral, mental health, or medical
sciences, neither the authors, nor the editors and publisher, nor any other party who
has been involved in the preparation or publication of this work warrants that the
information contained herein is in every respect accurate or complete, and they are
not responsible for any errors or omissions or the results obtained from the use of
such information. Readers are encouraged to confirm the information contained in
this book with other sources.

Library of Congress Cataloging-in-Publication Data

Play therapy (Crenshaw)
  Play therapy : a comprehensive guide to theory and practice / edited by David A.
Crenshaw and Anne L. Stewart.
     p. ; cm.—(Creative arts and play therapy)
  Includes bibliographical references and index.
  ISBN 978-1-4625-1750-3 (hardcover : alk. paper)
  ISBN 978-1-4625-2644-4 (paperback : alk. paper)
  I. Crenshaw, David A., editor.   II. Stewart, Anne L., 1951 November 25– editor.
III. Title.   IV. Series: Creative arts and play therapy.
  [DNLM: 1. Play Therapy—methods. 2. Child. WS 350.4]
  RJ505.P6
  618.92′891653—dc23
                                                                2014010771

About the Editors

David A. Crenshaw, PhD, ABPP, RPT-S, is Clinical Director of the Children's Home of Poughkeepsie, New York, and Adjunct Visiting Assistant Professor at Teachers College, Columbia University. He is a Board Certified Clinical Psychologist by the American Board of Professional Psychology, a Fellow of the American Psychological Association and of its Division of Child and Adolescent Psychology, and a Registered Play Therapist–Supervisor by the Association for Play Therapy. Dr. Crenshaw is Past President of the Hudson Valley Psychological Association, which honored him with its Lifetime Achievement Award, and of the New York Association for Play Therapy. He served on the editorial board of the *International Journal of Play Therapy*; taught graduate play therapy courses at Johns Hopkins University; and has published numerous journal articles, book chapters, and books on child therapy, child abuse and trauma, and resilience in children. Dr. Crenshaw is a frequent presenter at statewide and national conferences on play therapy.

Anne L. Stewart, PhD, RPT-S, is Professor of Graduate Psychology at James Madison University, where she teaches, supervises, and conducts play therapy each week. She has written and presented internationally about crisis intervention, attachment, supervision, military families, improvisation, and resilience. She is Founder and President of the Virginia Association for Play Therapy, Chair of the National Foundation for Play Therapy, and an editorial board member of the *International Journal of Play Therapy*. Dr. Stewart is a recipient of the Distinguished Service Award from the Association for Play Therapy and the Outstanding Faculty Award from the State Council of Higher Education for Virginia.

Contributors

Jeffrey S. Ashby, PhD, ABPP, College of Education, Georgia State University, Atlanta, Georgia

Bonnie Badenoch, PhD, LMFT, Nurturing the Heart, Vancouver, Washington

Steven Baron, PsyD, private practice, Bellmore, New York

Helen E. Benedict, PhD, RPT-S, Department of Psychology and Neuroscience, Baylor University, Waco, Texas

Phyllis B. Booth, MA, LPC, LMFT, RPT-S, The Theraplay Institute, Chicago, Illinois

Sue C. Bratton, PhD, LPC, RPT-S, Center for Play Therapy, University of North Texas, Denton, Texas

Stuart Brown, MD, National Institute for Play, Carmel Valley, California

Heather McTaggart Bryan, LPC, RPT, Gil Institute for Trauma Recovery and Education, Fairfax, Virginia

Angela M. Cavett, PhD, LP, RPT-S, Beacon Behavioral Health Services and Training Center, West Fargo, North Dakota

Peggy L. Ceballos, PhD, LPC, RPT-S, Department of Counseling, University of North Carolina at Charlotte, Charlotte, North Carolina

Kathleen McKinney Clark, MA, LPC, private practice, Alpharetta, Georgia

David A. Crenshaw, PhD, ABPP, RPT-S, Children's Home of Poughkeepsie, Poughkeepsie, New York

Greg Czyszczon, EdS, LPC, Harrisonburg Center for Relational Health, Harrisonburg, Virginia

Eric Dafoe, MA, Center for Play Therapy, University of North Texas, Denton, Texas

Lennis G. Echterling, PhD, Department of Graduate Psychology, James Madison University, Harrisonburg, Virginia

Tracie Faa-Thompson, MSW, Turn About Pegasus, Northumberland, United Kingdom

Diane Frey, PhD, RPT-S, Department of Counseling, Wright State University, and private practice, Dayton, Ohio

Brijin Johnson Gardner, MSW, LSCSW, RPT-S, Operation Breakthrough, Parkville, Missouri

Eliana Gil, PhD, LMFT, RPT-S, ATR, Gil Institute for Trauma Recovery and Education, Fairfax, Virginia

Myriam Goldin, LCSW, RPT-S, Gil Institute for Trauma Recovery and Education, Fairfax, Virginia

Louise F. Guerney, PhD, RPT-S, National Institute of Relationship Enhancement, Bethesda, Maryland

Christopher Hill, MS, MA, Clinical and School Psychology Doctoral Program, James Madison University, Harrisonburg, Virginia

Kevin B. Hull, PhD, LPC, Hull and Associates, Lakeland, Florida

Heidi Gerard Kaduson, PhD, RPT-S, Play Therapy Training Institute, Monroe Township, New Jersey

Sueann Kenney-Noziska, MSW, LISW, LCSW, RPT-S, Play Therapy Corner, Las Cruces, New Mexico

Theresa Kestly, PhD, RPT-S, Sandtray Training Institute of New Mexico, Corrales, New Mexico

Elizabeth Konrath, LPC, RPT, Gil Institute for Trauma Recovery and Education, Fairfax, Virginia

Terry Kottman, PhD, LMFT, RPT-S, The Encouragement Zone, Cedar Falls, Iowa

Garry L. Landreth, EdD, LPC, RPT-S, Center for Play Therapy, University of North Texas, Denton, Texas

J. P. Lilly, MS, LSCW, RPT-S, private practice, Provo, Utah

Liana Lowenstein, MSW, RSW, CPT-S, private practice, Toronto, Ontario, Canada

Dianne Koontz Lowman, EdD, Harrisonburg Center for Relational Health, Harrisonburg, Virginia

Lauren E. Maltby, PhD, Department of Psychiatry, Harbor–UCLA Medical Center, Torrance, California

Joyce C. Mills, PhD, RPT-S, The Story Play Center, Scottsdale, Arizona

Claudio Mochi, RP, RPT-S, Association of Play Therapy of Italy, Rome, Italy

John B. Mordock, PhD, ABPP, private practice, Poughkepsie, New York

Kristie Opiola, MA, Center for Play Therapy, University of North Texas, Denton, Texas

Sarah C. Patton, PsyD, Psychology Service, North Florida/South Georgia Veterans Health System, Gainesville, Florida

Mary Anne Peabody, EdD, LCSW, RPT-S, Social and Behavioral Sciences Program, Lewiston–Auburn College, University of Southern Maine, Brunswick, Maine

Phyllis Post, PhD, LPC-S, NCSC, RPT-S, Department of Counseling, Special Education, and Child Development, University of North Carolina at Charlotte, Charlotte, North Carolina

Dee C. Ray, PhD, LPC-S, RPT-S, Department of Counseling and Higher Education, University of North Texas, Denton, Texas

Scott Riviere, MS, LPC, RPT-S, Kids Interactive Discovery Zone (K.I.D.Z.),
Lake Charles, Louisiana

John W. Seymour, PhD, LMFT, RPT-S, Department of Counseling and Student Personnel,
Minnesota State University, Mankato, Mankato, Minnesota

Jennifer Shaw, PsyD, Gil Institute for Trauma Recovery and Education, Fairfax, Virginia

Angela I. Sheely-Moore, PhD, NCC, Department of Counseling and Educational Leadership,
Montclair State University, Montclair, New Jersey

Janine Shelby, PhD, RPT-S, Department of Psychiatry, Harbor–UCLA Medical Center,
Torrance, California

William Steele, PsyD, MSW, National Institute for Trauma and Loss in Children,
Clinton Township, Michigan

Anne L. Stewart, PhD, RPT-S, Department of Graduate Psychology,
James Madison University, Harrisonburg, Virginia

Debbie C. Sturm, PhD, LPC, Department of Graduate Psychology, James Madison University,
Harrisonburg, Virginia

Kathleen S. Tillman, PhD, Department of Counseling Psychology and Community Services,
University of North Dakota, Grand Forks, North Dakota

Jessica Anne Umhoefer, PsyD, NCSP, Department of Graduate Psychology,
James Madison University, Harrisonburg, Virginia; Fairfax County Public Schools,
Alexandria, Virginia

Risë VanFleet, PhD, RPT-S, CDBC, The Playful Pooch Program, Family Enhancement
and Play Therapy Center, Boiling Springs, Pennsylvania

William Whelan, PsyD, Virginia Child and Family Attachment Center, University of Virginia,
Charlottesville, Virginia

Marlo L.-R. Winstead, LSCSW, LCSW, RPT-S, Department of Social Work,
University of Kansas, Kansas City, Kansas

Foreword

Accessing the richness of *Play Therapy: A Comprehensive Guide to Theory and Practice* allows the reader-practitioner to dive deeply into the transformative power of play itself. Each chapter acknowledges play as a force of nature, captured in its essence and refined through the comprehensive skill, broad scholarship, and multiple foci of accomplished authors and editors. The result of this immersion is inspiration and deepened professional identity for the practitioner, and healing mercies for those who become safe and playful through its applications. Guided, chapter by chapter, through this volume's varied and verdant landscapes, the reader emerges with a treasure of theoretical and philosophical grounding plus solid clinical guidance for greater professional excellence. No small accomplishment.

The diverse inclusions in Part I, Play Therapy Theories and Approaches, provide a personal narrative and professional identity for the play therapist—a necessary anchor in a windswept theoretical sea. What has evolved within responsible therapeutic domains allows varied approaches and numerous theoretical foundations—client-centered, Jungian, psychoanalytic, Adlerian, cognitive-behavioral, or attachment-based—to become united by their reliance on play. The experience of play itself is the transformative magic, but it does require grounding on the part of the therapist.

Let's look more fully at the shared source of healing in the chapters: play. What is it that most profoundly *engages* us with ourselves and the world?

Play.

It takes us out of time's arrow, allows us to exist in a separate "state" of being from all others, and when it occurs, is a self-organizing phenomenon driven by intrinsic motivation, with myriad patterns and forms, but still a process of *being* and *doing* something just for its own sake. And the prerequisites for discovering or rediscovering its bounties when it has been missed or lost are in-depth professional wisdom and diagnostic and clinical skill. By guiding a client into experiencing it more fully, play grants gifts that endure well beyond the immediate experience itself—one boon from this truly comprehensive guide.

What is the world without healthy authentic play? Or a better question might be, what is it that healthy play bestows, that its absence or deprivation reveals as missing? The capacity for joy, freedom to explore the possible, detection and enactment of one's unique talents, safety in intimacy, and an optimistic hopeful approach to life and the future are among play's blessings and benefits. Bringing these life-giving qualities through play therapy in the settings and play-needy conditions described in Part II, Clinical Applications of Play Therapy, provides avenues for clients to become *fully human*. Without access to play, this human birthright is just not possible to enjoy. Fulfilling this deficit has direct personal emotional rewards that enliven the practitioner's professional identity and help to assure a more balanced life for therapist and client alike—another boon from the bounty of this guide.

For the well-versed player, life in all its challenges can be experienced as a complex playground. For the play deprived, life is too often seen as a battleground. Becoming more fully grounded in providing this foundational humanitarian outreach gives greater meaning and purpose to a noble professional life. And what is perhaps unique to the play therapist-practitioner is that this "work" is fun—yes, *fun!* So the benefits for professional and client are legion.

A broad overview of play behavior in animals and humans, tracing its evolutionary trajectories and supported by a flood of recent neuroscientific play-based discoveries, reveals play behavior as a fundamental survival drive. Housed in subcortical circuitry, the universally innate biological roots that drive play behavior require environmentally appropriate signaling (the many languages of play) to activate and sustain this primal drive. The elaboration and continuing crafting of body and mind, though most urgently needed in childhood, nonetheless persist throughout the human life cycle.

In order for professionals to serve as role models and mentors, they must be authentic players in their own personal lives. So skill in learning and living through life's complexities—the subtlety of play signaling, the free access within oneself, the bodily and gestural dance of nonverbal play languages—adds veracity and emotional grounding that transcend linear cognitive limitations. Yes, it is possible to bring personally crafted lived-out-in-life art into the science of play therapeutics. This art needs to be practiced and honed in life beyond the clinical playroom.

In Part III, Research and Practice Guidelines in Play Therapy, esteemed authors focus on what it takes to practice competently, joyfully, and in an attuned manner. A unique contribution of this book is its evident appreciation for the science and art of play and the emergent field of epigenesis. In studies indicating that environmental playfulness (at least in playful rats) turns on latent prefrontal cortical genes awaiting the right signal, animal play researchers are demonstrating in playful laboratory animals what human clinicians surmise is occurring in effective and transformative play therapy settings—namely, that new cerebral connections that "help craft the social brain" are specifically sparked into action by active play experiences. Clinicians sense that bringing play into *action* creates new cerebral "maps" with emotional regulation as an adjunctive benefit. This new animal-based knowledge is adding more and more depth and importance to affirming play as a lifetime necessity for adaptability and individual flexibility.

There is plenty of nourishment in this volume to establish it as a fresh and revelatory "bible" of play therapy, guiding the therapist to new and more effective personal and professional rewards.

STUART BROWN, MD

Contents

PLAY THERAPY

PLAY THERAPY

PART I

Play Therapy Theories and Approaches

INTRODUCTION

Long before Virginia Axline wrote the book *Dibbs: In Search of Self* (1964), which captured the imagination of aspiring and practicing play therapists around the world, play therapy was practiced within the four walls of child psychoanalysts' offices in Europe and the United States. Among the early child analysts was Freud's daughter, Anna Freud, and some of this rich history is contained in John B. Mordock's chapter on psychodynamic play therapy (Chapter 5). Axline's book was one of the influential works that led to the differentiation of play therapy as a separate field of its own, with its own practitioners, but, of course, within the larger context of child therapy and child therapists—some of whom, particularly those who chose not to work with preschool children, did not view themselves as practicing play therapy. Many child psychiatrists to this day receive little or no training in play therapy. Virginia Axline, Clark Moustakas, and Garry Landreth (see Dee C. Ray and Garry L. Landreth, Chapter 1) developed child-centered play therapy (CCPT) based on the person-centered theory of Carl Rogers. The University of North Texas, where Garry Landreth taught for many years, is still the largest training center for play therapists in the world, with emphasis placed on CCPT.

The object relations (attachment-based) approach to play therapy is eloquently presented and detailed by Sarah C. Patton and Helen E. Benedict in Chapter 2. Helen Benedict is one of the most respected

1

scholars and researchers in the play therapy field, most deservedly so. Terry Kottman and Jeffrey S. Ashby, in Chapter 3, present the tenets and key features of Adlerian play therapy. Although he describes himself as the "mechanic" of Jungian theory, J. P. Lilly shares a quite readable but masterful exposition of Jungian analytical play therapy (Chapter 4). Angela M. Cavett presents cognitive-behavioral play therapy in a scholarly but reader-friendly style (Chapter 6). These key theories with deep historical roots are followed by a diverse group of play therapy approaches.

The integrative approach to play therapy that, in our mind, is akin to the prescriptive approach made well known by Charles Schaefer is well illustrated by Eliana Gil and her colleagues at the Gil Institute for Trauma Recovery and Education in Chapter 7. Chapters by leaders in the play field follow on attachment-based play therapy in Chapter 8 (William Whelan and Anne L. Stewart); filial play therapy in Chapter 9 (Sue Bratton); Theraplay in Chapter 10 (Phyllis B. Booth and Marlo L.-R. Winstead); sandtray therapy in Chapter 11 (Theresa Kestly); StoryPlay therapy in Chapter 12 (Joyce C. Mills); family play therapy in Chapter 13 (Greg Czyszczon, Scott Riviere, Diane Koontz Lowman, and Anne L. Stewart); and in Chapter 14 an exciting chapter on a relatively new play therapy approach: animal-assisted play therapy (Risë VanFleet and Tracie Faa-Thompson).

The play therapy field continues to benefit from the strong foundation constructed by innovative thinkers, inspiring leaders who further developed theories and approaches to work with hurting children. A new generation of play therapists, some whose work appears in this book, continues to think deeply and creatively about the healing process with children and families.

REFERENCE

Axline, V. (1964). *Dibbs: In search of self.* Boston: Houghton Mifflin.

CHAPTER 1

Child-Centered Play Therapy

Dee C. Ray
Garry L. Landreth

The relationship is the therapy; it is not preparation for therapy or behavioral change.
—GARRY L. LANDRETH (2012, p. 82)

Child-centered play therapy (CCPT) is predicated on the belief that the relationship between therapist and child is the primary healing factor for children who are experiencing difficulties arising from contextual, developmental, and internal struggles. CCPT recognizes play as the child's developmentally appropriate language, a common principle among most schools of play therapy. However, CCPT is set apart from other play therapy approaches by its focus on the relationship and environment as sources to health and functioning. Landreth (2012) defined play therapy as "a dynamic interpersonal relationship between a child (or person of any age) and a therapist trained in play therapy procedures who provides selected play materials and facilitates the development of a safe relationship for the child (or person of any age) to fully express and explore self (feelings, thoughts, experiences, and behaviors) through play, the child's natural medium of communication, for optimal growth and development" (p. 11). It is

through the therapist's understanding and acceptance of the child's world, as well as the child's receptivity of these factors, that unleashes the child's potential to move toward self-enhancing ways of being.

CCPT was developed in the 1940s, distinguishing it as one of the longest-standing mental health interventions used today. Virginia Axline (1947) operationalized person-centered theory (Rogers, 1951) through the structure of CCPT, offering a method of working with children that was consistent with person-centered principles. Axline referred to this approach as *nondirective play therapy*, which was later termed *child-centered play therapy* by therapists in the United States. In the years since the introduction of CCPT, 62 outcome studies have explored its effectiveness, presenting evidence that CCPT is a viable and effective intervention for children (Ray, 2011). Currently, CCPT is recognized as the most widely practiced approach to play therapy in the United States (Lambert et al., 2005), and the approach has earned a strong international reputation (see West, 1996; Wilson, Kendrick, & Ryan, 1992). CCPT is operationalized in several volumes of literature, all in agreement on its basic tenets and structure (Axline, 1947; Cochran, Nordling, & Cochran, 2010; Landreth, 2012; Ray, 2011; VanFleet, Sywulak, & Sniscak, 2010).

Theoretical Constructs

Person-centered theory, upon which CCPT is based, was elegantly presented by Carl Rogers (1951, pp. 481–533) in 19 propositions, summarized in nine points below.

The person is viewed as:

1. Being the best determiner of a personal reality. The person's perceptual field is "reality."
2. Behaving as an organized whole.
3. Striving toward independence, maturity, and enhancement of self.
4. Behaving in a goal-directed manner in an effort to satisfy needs.
5. Being behaviorally influenced by feelings that affect rationality.
6. Behaving in ways that are consistent with the self-concept.
7. Not owning behavior that is inconsistent with the self-concept.
8. Responding to threat by becoming behaviorally rigid.
9. Admitting into awareness experiences that are inconsistent with the self if the self is free from threat.

Through these propositions, Rogers sought to explain the self-actualizing nature of the person and personality development; the roles of emotions, thoughts, and behaviors; and the development, or lack thereof, of self-enhancing ways of being. These propositions provide the rationale for the use of CCPT and serve as a guide for play therapists in understanding and facilitating the change process in children (Ray, Sullivan, & Carlson, 2012). The propositions emphasize that each person is the center of his or her own perceived phenomenological field, meaning that each person's perception of experience represents reality for that individual. Personal phenomenological experience, which encompasses the perception and integration of experiences from the phenomenological field into perceptions of self, guides the growth and development of the self. All organisms seek to actualize, maintain, and enhance the self.

A child's construct of self arises through interactions with others in the perceptual field throughout development. As interactions take place, a child comes to evaluate self-worth based on the perceived expectations and acceptance of others. These perceived conditions of worth are eventually integrated into the developing self, so that subsequent experiences represent the child's internalized representations of how he or she is valued. Thus, the personal valuing process may or may not contribute to optimal growth, depending on how internalized representations of experiences of being valued relate to the self-construct. Behavior is directly consistent with the view of self and the valuing process, whether or not it is within the awareness of the person. Behavior is seen as an attempt to maintain the organism and fulfill needs, depending on the perceived expectations of the environment, and the emotion accompanying behavior is seen as dependent on the perceived need for behavior. Hence, a person will behave and emotionally respond in a way that is consistent with the view of self, even if the view of self does not facilitate the optimal growth of the individual (Ray et al., 2012).

The self-structure is formed and continues to develop in relation to the child's experiences with others and the environment. Functionality is enhanced when a child integrates these experiences congruently with the self. Experiences that are incongruent with the self and denied integration can be perceived as threats to self, even if those experiences are potentially enhancing to the organism. When provided with a nonthreatening environment, a person can examine experiences in a nonjudgmental way and integrate them into a self-structure that is respectful of the intrinsic direction of the organism. Because of the self-actualizing and relational nature of the person, a congruent self-structure results in a person's desire and ability to enhance relationships with others.

Specific to play therapy, it is important to bring these person-centered principles to life when conceptualizing children. We attempt to describe the process in simpler terms. A child is born into the world viewing interactions in a unique and personal way that is apart from reality or others' perceptions. The child will move holistically toward what is most enhancing for the self-organism. A sense of self is established through interactions with significant others and the child's perceptions of those interactions. A child's interactions result in an attitude of self-worth that is influenced by a perceived sense of acceptance by and expectations of others. If a child feels unworthy or unaccepted for certain aspects of self, barriers to self-acceptance arise in turn. Because the organism is holistic in movement, a child's feelings and behaviors will be consistent. More concretely, if a child feels unaccepting of self or unaccepted by others, feelings and behaviors will be more negative and less self-enhancing. In describing maladjustment in children, Axline (1947) wrote: "The individual's behavior is not consistent with the inner concept of the self which the individual has created in his attempt to achieve complete self-realization. The further apart the behavior and the concept, the greater the degree of maladjustment" (p. 14).

This view of development has fundamental implications for the process of CCPT. First, the child can be trusted to move toward self-enhancing ways of being when provided with facilitative relationships and environment. Second, the best way to understand a child's behaviors and emotions is to understand how the child views his or her world. Third, the child's relationships with others within the environment are a crucial influence on the child's view of self and others. And finally, when the therapist can provide, and a child can perceive, an environment and relationship accepting of the child's internal world, the child will move toward self-enhancing integration and functionality.

Therapeutic Process

Because the therapeutic process of CCPT derives from the developmental theory of person-centered propositions, it can be concluded that the therapeutic relationship offered by the therapist is the essential feature of the intervention. The therapist's ability to provide a relationship and environment conducive for the child's growth is the primary concern of therapy. The practice of CCPT is particularly concerned with the removal of any threat to self-structure so that a child can explore experiences that are consistent or inconsistent with self, leading to integration into the revised self-structure (Ray, 2011). The removal of threats is the basis for the key person-centered stance of nondirectivity provided by the therapist to acknowledge the child's right to autonomy and belief in the child's constructive nature (Wilkins, 2010). Nondirectivity is an attitude that promotes the child's self-sufficiency by not guiding his or her goals or therapeutic content. The nondirective therapist is an active, engaged participant in the counseling process.

Landreth (2012) acknowledged that "a powerful force exists within every child that strives continuously for self-actualization. This inherent striving is toward independence, maturity, and self-direction. The child's mind and conscious thoughts are not what direct her behavior to areas of emotional need; rather, it is the child's natural striving toward inner balance that takes the child to where she needs to be" (p. 62). Therapy is focused on the child, not the problem of the child. When provided with a facilitative environment, the child will spontaneously move toward self-enhancement. Therefore, the therapist's role is to support the child in this movement, help remove barriers in the child's contextual world, and be present in the relationship for change to occur.

According to Rogers (1957), certain conditions are necessary to work toward constructive personality change, which he defined as "change in the personality structure of the individual, at both surface and deeper levels, in a direction which clinicians would agree means greater integration, less internal conflict, more energy utilizable for effective living; change in behavior away from behaviors generally regarded as immature and toward behaviors regarded as mature" (p. 95). Rogers identified six necessary and sufficient conditions for therapeutic change: (1) two persons are in psychological contact; (2) the first person (client) is in a state of incongruence; (3) the second person (therapist) is congruent in the relationship; (4) therapist experiences unconditional positive regard for client; (5) therapist experiences an empathic understanding of the client's internal frame of reference and attempts to communicate this experience to the client; and (6) communication to the client of the therapist's empathic understanding and unconditional positive regard is achieved to at least a minimal degree (Rogers, 1957).

Ray (2011) applied the person-centered conditions to CCPT, examining the details of how they are enacted in the play therapy process. In the first condition, the therapist and child must be in psychological contact, or in simpler terms, in a relationship. In this relationship, both the therapist and child must be in each other's awareness, allowing the other to enter the phenomenological field. Secondly, the child must be in a state of incongruence, which may be demonstrated through anxiety or vulnerability. Children will often exhibit incongruence through problematic behaviors that indicate an inability to function successfully within their environments; in other words, there is an incongruence between the self and the self's way of relating to the world. The following three *therapist attitudinal conditions* (Bozarth, 1998)—therapist congruence, unconditional positive regard (UPR), and empathic understanding (EU)—are the responsibilities of the therapist. These therapist attitudinal conditions provide an environment that promotes the actualizing tendency accessible within all persons, including children.

Therapist congruence is marked by the therapist's ability to feel free to be him- or herself within the therapeutic relationship and to experience congruence between experience and awareness of self (Rogers, 1957). Congruence involves a combination of the therapist's self-awareness, acceptance of such awareness, and appropriate expression of awareness to the child. The therapist must be congruent if he or she is to authentically express UPR and EU to the child. If the play therapist is not authentic, the child's perception of UPR and EU will be limited (Ray, 2011).

UPR is a warm acceptance of all aspects of the client's experience, without judgment or evaluation (Rogers, 1957). Additionally, UPR is a therapist-felt condition in which the therapist experiences a feeling of trust in the child's ability to move toward actualization. Landreth (2012) asserted: "The relationship provides consistent acceptance of the child, which is necessary for the development of enough inner freedom and security in the child for her to express herself in self-enhancing ways" (p. 83). UPR serves as the curative factor in CCPT, a natural antidote to the conditions of worth taken on by the child during development (Bozarth, 1998).

The final therapist attitudinal condition is the provision of EU by entering the child's world as if it were his or her own without losing a sense of self as the therapist (Ray, 2011). EU is intertwined with the concept of UPR, as empathy can be considered a vehicle for its expression (Bozarth, 2001). When a therapist enters the world of the child, there is an underlying message that the child's world is a valuable one in which the therapist has the utmost respect for the child's experience and abilities (Ray, 2011).

In order for personality change to occur, the final condition must be met: That is, the child must perceive the therapist's UPR and EU to at least a minimal level. The therapist has very little control over whether a child is able to perceive the conditions as offered by him or her; hence, this condition lies within the internal world of the child. Generally, if a therapist is able to achieve the prior conditions, a child will perceive the UPR and EU and engage in the therapeutic process of change. Yet, the achievement of this condition is nevertheless based on the child's receptivity to the therapist and the environment.

Goals and Objectives

Contrary to many popular beliefs about CCPT, we assert that the child-centered approach operates with certain goals in mind. Yet, the nature of CCPT goals is somewhat different from other approaches, in that CCPT goals center on the therapist's responsibility in the process and outcome. The goal of CCPT is to establish conditions so that the child can experience growth and integration, leading toward the child's chosen path to healthier functioning. Ray (2011) suggested that the effective CCPT therapist uses self and environment in such a way as to facilitate the child's active and innate processes for enhancement. She further stated: "When the therapist provides an environment that is non-threatening and sends a message of empowerment to the client, the client will emerge with a structure that is self-enhancing as well as positively influential on relationships" (p. 56). In CCPT, the child chooses goals for change, not the therapist or the parent. Because behaviors and emotions are manifested in attempts to

meet the needs of the internal world of the child, it is only the child who can decide what needs to change for healthier functioning. For young children, these decisions are not a cognitive process but rather a function of their innate process of moving toward independence, maturity, and enhancement of self when experiencing a psychologically safe and accepting relationship. When facilitating CCPT, the therapist undertakes the considerable commitment of sharing the self, moving into the child's world, and fully engaging in the communication of understanding to the child for the purpose of providing a relationship that releases the child's potential for change.

When the goal of relationship has been met in CCPT, some outcomes seem evident and were noted by Landreth (2012, pp. 84–85) as objectives for helping facilitate growth in the person of the child. The child will:

1. Develop a more positive self-concept.
2. Assume greater self-responsibility.
3. Become more self-directing.
4. Become more self-accepting.
5. Become more self-reliant.
6. Engage in self-determined decision making.
7. Experience a feeling of control.
8. Become sensitive to the process of coping.
9. Develop an internal source of evaluation.
10. Become more trusting of self. (pp. 84–85)

These objectives are focused on the child as a person, with the belief that as the child expresses and allows experiences within his or her awareness, the self becomes stronger and moves toward self-actualization.

Structure

Axline (1947, pp. 73–74) offered guidelines in the structure of CCPT for enacting the conditions that facilitate change. These guidelines helped define the nature of CCPT and the role of the therapist, and serve to direct practice. They are referred to as the "eight basic principles" and are paraphrased below:

1. The therapist develops a warm, friendly relationship with the child as soon as possible.
2. The therapist accepts the child exactly as is, not wishing that the child were different in some way.
3. The therapist establishes a feeling of permissiveness in the relationship so that the child can fully express thoughts and feelings.
4. The therapist is attuned to the child's feelings and reflects those back to the child to help him or her gain insight into behavior.
5. The therapist respects the child's ability to solve problems, leaving the responsibility to make choices to the child.
6. The therapist does not direct the child's behavior or conversation but rather follows the child.
7. The therapist does not attempt to rush therapy, recognizing the gradual nature of the therapeutic process.
8. The therapist sets only those limits that anchor the child to reality or make the child aware of responsibilities in the relationship.

These basic principles guide the CCPT process and can be seen as concrete steps to build a therapeutic relationship with a child and create an environment described in person-centered theory as facilitative of growth. If the therapist embraces Axline's principles, CCPT will be grounded in a person-centered approach to therapy. In order to provide more detailed direction for the therapist's role in CCPT, Axline (1947), Ginott (1961), Landreth (2012), and Ray (2011) listed specific types of responses that are reflective of CCPT guidelines. These response categories include reflect-

ing feelings (e.g., "You feel sad"), reflecting content (e.g., "You had a fight with your friend"), tracking behavior (e.g., "You're moving that over there"), facilitating decision making (e.g., "You can decide"), facilitating creativity (e.g., "That can be whatever you want"), encouraging (e.g., "You worked hard"), facilitating relationship ("You want me to know that you care about me"), and limit setting (e.g., "I'm not for hitting"). The responses are intended to demonstrate concrete ways of providing therapeutic conditions: For example, reflections demonstrate EU, just as facilitating decision making and creativity demonstrate UPR. However, Ray (2011) cautioned, "It should be the goal of every play therapist to move beyond the concrete skills, progressing to an abstract way of working in which the play therapist provides responses that convey the necessary conditions in a genuine and personal way" (p. 89).

Limit setting is utilized as necessary when the child might be a threat to self, others, or the room. Sweeney and Landreth (2011) cited several reasons for setting limits in the playroom: Limits (1) define the boundaries of the therapeutic relationship; (2) provide security and safety for the child, both physically and emotionally; (3) demonstrate the therapist's intent to provide safety for the child; (4) anchor the session in reality; (5) allow the therapist to maintain a positive and accepting attitude toward the child; (6) allow the child to express negative feelings without causing harm and experiencing the subsequent fear of retaliation; (7) offer stability and consistency; (8) promote and enhance the child's sense of self-responsibility and self-control; (9) promote catharsis through symbolic channels; (10) protect the play therapy room and materials; and (11) provide for the maintenance of legal, ethical, and professional standards.

Landreth (2012) offered a three-step therapeutic limit-setting model based on the acronym ACT: Acknowledge the feeling, Communicate the limit, Target an alternative. In applying ACT, the therapist first and foremost seeks to understand and communicate understanding of the child's intent by acknowledging his or her feeling (e.g., "You're mad at me"). Secondly, the therapist sets a clear and definitive limit (e.g., "I'm not for pinching"). Finally, the therapist provides an alternative to allow the child appropriate expression of the feeling (e.g., "You can pinch the doll"). Limit setting allows the child to perceive the playroom as a safe environment. As Axline (1947) noted, limits are typically set only when needed, in order to offer a child a permissive environment that allows for as much exploration and expression as possible, while also allowing the child to initiate enhancing self-regulation processes.

Notably, the description of play therapist responses excludes the use of directive skills or techniques such as questioning, play direction, or analysis. Landreth (2012) addressed the use of questioning by observing that questions force verbal expression, convey a lack of understanding, and place the therapist in control of the child's process. The purpose of play therapy is to provide a child with a nonverbal language from which to communicate in order to developmentally meet the child at the appropriate level. Asking questions, directing play, and providing interpretive statements place the child in the adult's world of verbal expression, as well as pressure the child to operate in relation to the therapist's goals. Furthermore, when a therapist responds to a child in an effort to move the child toward the therapist's goals, understanding of the child's world is impeded. From a child-centered perspective, these directive responses interfere with the child's movement toward self-enhancement and undermine the purpose and process of therapy.

Playroom and Materials

CCPT is conducted in a playroom supplied with carefully selected toys that encourage the expression of a wide range of feelings by a child. The playroom sends the message that all parts of the child are accepted in this environment (Ray et al., 2012). Although Landreth (2012) recommended that play therapy be conducted in a room measuring 12 feet by 15 feet, smaller or larger rooms can be used. Smaller rooms should ensure that there is enough space for the toys and open space for the child to move. Larger rooms can be sectioned off with curtains or shelves to limit the size of the playroom so that it is not overwhelming to the child. Landreth also suggested that therapists can sometimes choose to organize a "tote bag playroom"—a mobile for therapists who are not stationed in one setting. Materials for the playroom include toys, craft materials, paints, easel, puppet theater, sandbox, and child furniture.

Landreth (2012) proposed three categories of toys: real-life toys to help play out actual experiences, acting-out/aggressive toys to express intense emotions, and toys for creative expression and emotional release to allow for unstructured and expressive play. Typically, structured games such as board games and cards are not used in a CCPT playroom because they inhibit expression and promote competition; videogames are also not recommended for the same reasons. Toys are selected to promote expression and relationship, and each toy should serve a purpose in the playroom. Ray (2011) suggested that toys should be selected in accord with answers to the following questions: (1) What therapeutic purpose will this toy serve for children who use this room? (2) How will this toy help children express themselves? (3) How will this toy help me build a relationship with children? When toys meet a therapeutic purpose, help children express themselves, and help build the relationship between therapist and child, they can be considered valuable to the playroom (Ray, 2011).

Role of the Parent

Landreth (2012) referred to parents as *partners* in the play therapy process. Research has shown that play therapy has greater effects when parents are involved (Bratton, Ray, Rhine, & Jones, 2005). Both Ray (2011) and Sweeney and Landreth (2011) noted the legal rights of parents as the guardians and essentially the identified clients in the eyes of the law, emphasizing that their consent is required to provide services to a child. As the primary caretakers, parents are the most important figures in a child's life. Their presence or absence in a child's life influences development and emotional stability (Ray, 2011). Just as the goal of the CCPT therapist is to provide a facilitative relationship with the child, the relationship with parents is also vitally important. A play therapist seeks to develop relationships with parents in which they feel accepted, understood, and safe.

Ray (2011) suggested that play therapists operate with the following attitudes when working with parents. (1) Play therapists should respect the parent's role as the most important relationship in the child's life and the parent's knowledge of the child. Even the most neglectful of parents often possess intimate knowledge of the child and his or her development, and this knowledge is needed by the play therapist to enhance the effectiveness of the new therapeutic relationship. (2) Play therapists should hold affection for the parent as a person. When parents feel that the play therapist cares for them, they are more likely to engage in the therapeutic process. (3) Play therapists should have patience with parents; parents work at their own paces, and different parents work differently. (4) Play therapists should maintain a clear focus on the child as the client. All interactions between play therapist and parent are initiated to facilitate growth in the child. The focus on the child as client helps the therapist realize limitations when working with the parents, such as a parent who is in need of personal counseling or is unmotivated to make changes. (5) Finally, play therapists should convey a sense of their own expertise. When play therapists exhibit knowledge and experience regarding children and play therapy, parents are more likely to feel safe enough to share their vulnerabilities and concerns. From the CCPT perspective, expertise is revealed through knowledge of development, typical child behavior, and the teaching of parenting skills when appropriate. Expertise is not demonstrated through lecture, advice giving, or attempts to direct parents.

In the CCPT individual therapy model, children are the clients and parents are systemic partners. Therapists typically involve parents through consultations with them that are held every three to five sessions. The purposes of parent consultations include providing support, teaching knowledge or skills, and monitoring progress as perceived by parents. Children with complicated contextual problems or who are in crisis may require more frequent parent consultations. Lack of parent consultations may lead to lack of parent involvement and engagement in the process, and even premature termination of therapy. The goal of parent consultation is aligned with the CCPT goal of relationship with the child. The therapist seeks to intervene in the child's environment to identify and facilitate the removal of barriers that impede the child's growth. Often, parent consultations in CCPT focus on building the relationship between parent and child through planning experiences and providing skills that help the parent better understand the child and that facilitate a positive relationship between the two.

In filial therapy, one intervention that evolved from the CCPT approach, the therapist provides an educational intervention to enhance the parent–child relationship by teaching CCPT skills used in play sessions between parent and child. Filial therapy may be indicated when the child's difficulties seem linked to the parent–child relationship and the parent is able to focus on providing a facilitative environment for the child. Landreth and Bratton (2006) described a 10-session model of filial therapy that has demonstrated evidence of effectiveness.

Although parent involvement is desired in CCPT, it is not required for effectiveness. Axline (1947) was the first to highlight that children in therapy are able to make changes in their behaviors and ways of being in the world without the participation of parents. Bratton and colleagues (2005) supported this claim by reporting large effect sizes for play therapy outcomes without parent involvement. The belief in the power of the child to make changes even when the environment does not contribute to the change effort is yet another unique aspect of CCPT. However, it is widely agreed that a child is better able to embark on internal and external changes with the support of positive parental relationships.

Research Support

CCPT may have the longest history of research of any psychological intervention. In the earliest identified study, Dulsky (1942) attempted to study the relationship between intellect and emotional problems. He inadvertently established the effect of nondirective play therapy, matching the description of CCPT, which was to significantly improve social and emotional adjustments, but no improvement was shown on intellect. Early play therapy research was marked by flaws in design, such as a lack of control or comparison group, random assignment, detailed description of participants, and detailed description of intervention. In the last several decades, concerted efforts to investigate CCPT with the most rigorous methods have resulted in positive empirical support. Ray (2011) reviewed CCPT studies and found a total of 62 studies, conducted from 1940 to 2010, showing positive outcomes for CCPT. Of the 62 studies, 29 were categorized as experimental, employing a pre–post randomized control group design. Additionally,

CCPT research increased since 2000, with the identification of 19 studies in CCPT across the first decade of the millennium and the highest number in any one decade since the beginning of CCPT research in 1940. This finding is consistent with Elliott, Greenberg, Watson, Timulak, and Friere's (2013) observation of a revival in person-centered therapy research with adults as a recent development. Research results demonstrated positive effects for issues related to multiculturalism, externalizing/disruptive behaviors, attention-deficit/hyperactivity disorder (ADHD), internalizing problems, anxiety, depression, self-concept/self-esteem, social behavior, parent–teacher relationship, sexual abuse/trauma, homelessness, identified disability/medical condition, academic achievement/intelligence, and speech–language skills.

Clinical Case Example

Anita, in kindergarten, was referred to play therapy by her teacher and mother for different reasons. Anita's mother was concerned that Anita, who was raised in a mostly Spanish-speaking household, stopped speaking Spanish 2 months prior to referral and refused to speak Spanish even when prompted. Anita's mother was concerned because she only spoke Spanish, so she and Anita were no longer able to communicate. She felt that Anita was being deliberately defiant in refusing to speak Spanish. Anita's teacher referred Anita because Anita no longer spoke at all in the classroom. During the first month of school, Anita was happy, engaged, and participated actively in class. Anita's teacher explained that in the past 2 months, Anita had stopped interacting with her or other children; that Anita, who spoke English fluently, refused to talk in either Spanish or English; and that Anita no longer completed any of her school work, giving up quickly when she was challenged. The teacher shared great emotional concern for Anita in talking about her with the therapist: "I just don't know what's happened. She was such a happy girl, and now she just seems so withdrawn and sad."

The therapist met with both Anita's mother and teacher to listen to their concerns and tell them about play therapy. Because neither the mother nor teacher seemed to know the root of Anita's change, the therapist explained that she would meet with Anita in CCPT to allow Anita the opportunity to express herself in a nonverbal way. The therapist further explained that a nonverbal intervention seemed most in order for Anita so that she could express herself without words, through play, within the context of a safe relationship.

Play sessions were held in a school classroom where the therapist had set up a play area. The play area included a variation of toys set on shelves and organized according to real-life, aggressive, and expressive categories. Large shelves separated the play area from other parts of the classroom. The therapist first met Anita at the door of her classroom and introduced herself, "Hi, I'm Dee." Anita smiled weakly and looked down at the ground. The therapist held out her hand and said, "It's time for us to go to the playroom." Although she looked scared, Anita took the therapist's hand willingly and walked to the playroom. The therapist introduced the playroom. Commentary on dyadic interactions appears in brackets.

THERAPIST: Anita, in here is the playroom; you can play with the toys in lots of the ways you like. We will come here every Tuesday and Thursday.

ANITA: (*Smiles and stands in the middle of the room, holding on to her jacket and twisting her body nervously. She begins to look around the room without moving.*)

THERAPIST: You're looking around. You're just not sure about this place. [Attempts to reflect Anita's anxious movements.]

ANITA: (*Looks at the therapist and smiles.*)

THERAPIST: You kinda like it in here. [Notices Anita's slight relaxation when smile occurs.]

ANITA: (*Smiles and points at the Barbie doll on a shelf.*)

THERAPIST: Oh, you like her. [Respects Anita's choice to not verbalize and continues to follow her nonverbal communication to convey acceptance of Anita's way of communicating.]

ANITA: (*Nods her head vigorously in agreement that she likes the Barbie as she continues to stare at it.*)

THERAPIST: Looks like you really like her and want to play with her.

ANITA: (*Looks at the therapist as if to ask if it is okay to play.*)

THERAPIST: In here, you can decide what toys to play with. [This response returns responsibility to Anita, giving her the choice to play or not to play. She gets to decide.]

ANITA: (*Moves toward Barbie, picks it up, and begins to stroke her hair.*)

THERAPIST: You're checking her out, seeing what she's like.

ANITA: (*Turns toward the therapist and smiles, then begins to go through the Barbie clothes.*)

THERAPIST: Looks like you're seeing what she has and what you like. [This response is intended to recognize the importance of what Anita likes and values.]

ANITA: (*Tries to take skirt off Barbie to put on a new one; the skirt does not come off easily; Anita quickly gives up and puts the Barbie down.*)

THERAPIST: You chose not to change her. It was too hard.

ANITA: (*Does not look at the therapist; moves to painting easel.*)

THERAPIST: You decided to do something else.

ANITA: (*Paints a few strokes and then tries to move the paper; the paper is resistant and she gives up and moves to the kitchen.*)

THERAPIST: That seemed really hard. You're going to do something else.

Throughout the first session, Anita tried and gave up on several play activities. The kitchen cabinet door was a little resistant, and she moved to the puppet theater. A puppet she wanted was a little too high and she moved to the cash register. She could not figure out how to open the cash register and then she tried on hats for dress up. Each time there was slight difficulty to what she wanted to do, she gave up and went to something else. She never expressed frustration, as might be expected, but withdrew from the situation. While she engaged in this play behavior, she continued to interact nonverbally with the therapist, smiling and nodding when the therapist reflected her accurately. She never spoke. Throughout the play session, the therapist attempted to understand Anita's intentions in her play, recognize her shifts when she gave up without judging her, and provide a warm acceptance of Anita.

For the second session, the therapist came to the classroom doorway and Anita immediately smiled, popped up, ran to the therapist, and held out her hand. As they walked down the hall, Anita said, "You Ms. Dee?" The therapist responded, "Yes, I'm Dee. You can call me Dee. You seem excited today." Anita responded with a big smile and vigorous nod. After entering the playroom, Anita immediately began to engage in the same play behaviors, stopping each time she encountered any type of resistance. One noticeable difference was that Anita talked to the therapist throughout the session. She mostly talked about her clothes, the therapist's clothes, and clothes in the playroom, all subjects unrelated to whatever she was playing. An excerpt from this session follows.

ANITA: (*Walks over to the therapist and touches her necklace.*) I like your necklace.

THERAPIST: You wanted to see it up close.

ANITA: (*as she's holding it*) Yes, it's very pretty. My mother has one like this.

THERAPIST: This one reminds you of your mother.

ANITA: (*Moves to the paint easel; when she encounters resistance again with the paper, she moves to the kitchen.*) Do you like my shoes?

THERAPIST: It looks like you decided to do something else. That made you think about your shoes.

ANITA: They're pink.

THERAPIST: Looks like you like your pink shoes; you wanted me to notice them.

During this session and several thereafter, the routine was very similar. Anita continued to give up on play activities but engaged the therapist more and more. The therapist attempted to accept and return Anita's overtures for the relationship while also balancing reflections of what was happening in her play. Once a pattern was established, the therapist reflected deeper-level observations such as, "When things get hard, you move to something else"; "When it's tough, you don't like to do that"; and "Sometimes it just seems like things are tougher than they should be, so it's hard to keep trying." Deeper-level reflections indicated that the therapist understood how things seemed in Anita's internal world. The therapist resisted the temptation to urge Anita to keep trying and not give up. The therapist accepted that Anita saw even the simplest of tasks as very difficult and leaned on the relationship with the therapist to gain a sense of being okay. A change occurred in the fifth play session.

ANITA: (*Tries to open the kitchen cabinet door and gives up when it is resistant; looks*

around the kitchen for the first time and real-
izes she can put her hand through a hole in
the back of the kitchen cabinet.)

THERAPIST: You figured out a whole other way to get in the kitchen.

ANITA: (*Fills up all the bowls and plates with sand.*) I'm making you breakfast. It's a special recipe that my mom does. It's going to take me a long time. You have to wait. (*Uses all of her playtime to fill up every container to the very edge in a very careful way.*)

THERAPIST: (*Gave 5-minute warning, which Anita ignored.*) Anita, our time is up for today.

ANITA: Noooo, I'm almost done. You have to eat. Just wait.

THERAPIST: You really want me to eat what you've made, but our time is up for today. You can give it to me next Tuesday. [Uses the ACT limit-setting model to help Anita learn to work within contextual limitations.]

ANITA: No, no, *no.* (*Sounds very defiant.*)

THERAPIST: You really aren't ready to go, but our time is up for today.

ANITA: (*Turns her back toward the therapist while continuing to fill up containers.*) I'm not going.

THERAPIST: You want to choose to stay, but our time is up for today. You can come back next week.

ANITA: Okay, but you have to eat next time.

THERAPIST: You want to make sure I eat what you've made next time.

This interaction represented a change in Anita's play and in the expression of her will. For the first time, she used her creativity to problem-solve, and she also displayed a defiant side of herself that her mother had described but that had not been seen by the teacher or therapist up to this point. Her expression of will indicated progress because she exhibited the strength to speak out for what she wanted. In CCPT, this type

of expression is valued and accepted (and must be balanced with the need to work within limits of maintaining psychological and physical safety).

In subsequent sessions, Anita began to tap into her creativity and revisit each of the play challenges she had previously encountered. She kept working with Barbie's clothes until she could change them. She worked on the easel until she could get the paper off, and she jumped to get the puppet that she could not reach easily. For her last feat, she conquered the opening of the kitchen cabinet door. All of these challenges were conducted while also creating elaborate meals for the therapist. An excerpt from these exchanges follows.

ANITA: I'm going to make you something to eat that will be the best thing you've ever tasted.

THERAPIST: You really want to do something for me.

ANITA: It's going to make you feel better.

THERAPIST: I'm important to you. You want me to feel good.

ANITA: Yes, and this will do it.

As Anita nurtured the therapist more and more, she demonstrated greater strength in approaching her difficult tasks. In the 12th session, Anita began to do schoolwork during the session. She wrote words and sentences on the easel, as well as math problems. She spent time talking them through and trying to figure them out. Interestingly, Anita never asked for help from the therapist; she wanted to do things on her own.

In consultation with the teacher, the play therapist learned that Anita's initial behaviors in the playroom mirrored her classroom behaviors. Early in the school year, Anita engaged enthusiastically in activities but after a few weeks, she began to withdraw. The teacher reported that she would try each activity for a very short time and then give up when the activity became difficult for her. It became apparent that Anita had been intimidated by her schoolwork and most likely further overwhelmed by all of the academic expectations while also being in an environment that was new to her. It is likely that her reaction was to withdraw out of a sense of helplessness. Her defiance with her mother appeared to be a way to regain control over her environment, communicating in a language that her mother did not understand. The relationship between Anita and her mother was a safe one for Anita and hence the most likely place for her to assert her will to work through her sense of inadequacy.

The therapist encouraged Anita's teacher and mother to support her in this transition by understanding and reflecting her feelings. In parent consultation (using a translator), the therapist sought to understand the mother's frustration and sense of "losing" her daughter. The therapist helped the mother to see that Anita needed to develop skills to deal with her high level of anxiety regarding her own competence. As Anita's mother experienced the therapist's efforts to strengthen her relationship with her daughter, she became more open to suggestions, such as reflecting Anita's feelings and offering encouraging statements. In teacher consultation, the therapist provided the teacher with examples of reflecting and encouraging statements, such as "You weren't sure if you could do it, but you tried anyway," and "You're worried you won't do it right, but you're still trying." These statements gave the teacher a concrete way to help Anita when she was struggling without pressuring her to do her work "right."

In the environment of CCPT, Anita was able to figure out how to approach these challenges and to see herself as successful, especially with the support of a therapeutic partner in play therapy. At 5 years old, Anita was fully and naturally equipped to tackle her environmental problems when provided with a relationship and environment that allowed her to release her poten-tial to do so. By the 15th session, just over 7 weeks, both Anita's teacher and mother reported that Anita was now fully engaged at home and school, speaking and responding in both Spanish and English.

Conclusion

CCPT is marked by trust in the innate tendency present in all children to move toward growth-enhancing self-structure, emotions, and behaviors. Each child is a person that experiences the world in a unique way and is fully capable of enacting change in self and in relationship to others. When children are placed in certain environments or perceive the environment as threatening, behaviors and emotions will emerge accordingly to protect a rigid view of self and impede movement toward self-enhancing ways of being. In CCPT, the therapist's role is to create an environment that removes barriers to growth and to provide a relationship within which the child can access his or her own self-actualizing tendency.

The practice of play therapy requires many different resources, including a space, some furniture, and a variation of toys. The use of toys and play allows children to express themselves in a natural and developmentally appropriate way. But no resource in the play therapy room is more essential than the play therapist (Ray, 2011), the central provider of the environment to the child as well as to parents and other caretakers. The person of the play therapist is the most essential therapeutic tool in CCPT. Although CCPT relies on the relationship between therapist and child as the key therapeutic factor for change, it is the play therapist who initiates that relationship and maintains an environment that nurtures the relationship. When a child experiences a warm, accepting, understanding, and genuine relationship within a permissive environment conducive to self-expression, the child is able to determine the direction for therapeutic change and work toward internal and external behaviors and emotions that enhance his or her daily life experiences and relationships with others.

REFERENCES

Axline, V. (1947). *Play therapy*. New York: Ballantine.

Bozarth, J. (1998). *Person-centered therapy: A revolutionary paradigm*. Ross-on-Wye, UK: PCCS Books.

Bozarth, J. (2001). An addendum to beyond reflection: Emergent modes of empathy. In S. Haugh & T. Merry (Eds.), *Empathy: Rogers' therapeutic conditions–evolution, theory and practice* (Vol. 2, pp. 144–154). Ross-on-Wye, UK: PCCS Books.

Bratton, S., Ray, D., Rhine, T., & Jones, L. (2005). The efficacy of play therapy with children: A meta-analytic review of treatment outcome. *Professional Psychology: Research and Practice*, *36*(4), 376–390.

Cochran, N., Nordling, W., & Cochran, J. (2010). *Child-centered play therapy: A practical guide to developing therapeutic relationship with children*. Hoboken, NJ: Wiley.

Dulsky, S. (1942). Affect and intellect: An experimental study. *Journal of General Psychology*, *27*, 199–220.

Elliott, R., Greenberg, L., Watson, J., Timulak, L., & Friere, E. (2013). Research on humanistic-experiential psychotherapies. In M. Lambert (Ed.), *Bergin and Garfield's handbook of psychotherapy and behavior change* (pp. 495–538). Hoboken, NJ: Wiley.

Ginott, H. (1961). *Group psychotherapy with children*. New York: McGraw-Hill.

Lambert, S., LeBlanc, M., Mullen, J., Ray, D., Baggerly, J., White, J., et al. (2005). Learning more about those who play in session: The national play therapy in counseling practices project. *Journal of Counseling and Development*, *85*, 42–46.

Landreth, G. (2012). *Play therapy: The art of the relationship* (3rd ed.). New York: Routledge.

Landreth, G., & Bratton, S. (2006). *Child–parent relationship therapy (CPRT): A 10-session filial therapy model*. New York: Routledge.

Ray, D. (2011). *Advanced play therapy: Essential conditions, knowledge, and skills for child practice*. New York: Routledge.

Ray, D., Sullivan, J., & Carlson, S. (2012). Relational intervention: Child-centered play therapy with children on the autism spectrum. In L. Gallo-Lopez & L. Rubin (Eds.), *Play-based interventions for children and adolescents on the autism spectrum* (pp. 159–175). New York: Routledge.

Rogers, C. (1951). *Client-centered therapy: Its current practice, implications and theory*. Boston: Houghton Mifflin.

Rogers, C. (1957). The necessary and sufficient conditions of therapeutic personality change. *Journal of Consulting Psychology*, *21*(2), 95–103.

Sweeney, D., & Landreth, G. (2011). Child-centered play therapy. In C. Schaefer (Ed.), *Foundations of play therapy* (2nd ed., pp. 129–152). Hoboken, NJ: Wiley.

VanFleet, R., Sywulak, A. E., & Sniscak, C. C. (2010). *Child-centered play therapy*. New York: Guilford Press.

West, J. (1996). *Child centred play therapy* (2nd ed.). London: Hodder Arnold.

Wilkins, P. (2010). *Person-centred therapy: 100 key points*. London: Routledge.

Wilson, K., Kendrick, P., & Ryan, V. (1992). *Play therapy: A nondirective approach for children and adolescents*. London: Bailliere Tindall.

CHAPTER 2

Object Relations and Attachment-Based Play Therapy

Sarah C. Patton
Helen E. Benedict

Object relations/attachment-based play therapy is an integrative, multidimensional approach informed by object relations theories (Bowlby, 1988; Winnicott, 1965), research on children's thematic play (Benedict, 1997; Benedict & Grigoryev, 1995; Benedict & Hastings, 2002), neurobiological attachment literature (Schore, 2010), and a neurodevelopmental trauma framework (Perry, 2006). This experiential, relationally focused approach remediates disturbed object relations and trauma-related symptomatology in a manner and sequence that acknowledges their neurobiological underpinnings and reflects the hierarchical, experience-dependent nature of neurodevelopment (Perry, 2001). As such, this play approach is ideal for young children who have suffered attachment trauma such as sexual abuse, neglect, exposure to caregiver drug use, and/or abandonment during the critical developmental window of their early years. The object relations therapist intervenes via the therapeutic relationship by engaging the child in sensory-focused, "primary process" play (Gaskill & Perry, 2012; Schore, 1994),

and right-hemisphere, intersubjective, attuned, empathic transactions. Additionally, the therapist enters the child's unique representational world through thematic play, issuing metaphorical invitations to modify maladaptive working models.

The national incidence of children at risk for maltreatment likely approaches 3 million (U.S. Department of Health and Human Services, 2011), leading researchers to conclude that maltreatment is "our most important public health challenge" (van der Kolk, 2005, p. 401). Developmental neuroscientists have amassed a mountain of evidence indicating that early attachment trauma, especially when chronic, derails healthy neurodevelopment, literally programming the brain in a devastatingly dysfunctional manner (Perry, 2008). Maltreated children often exhibit manifold symptoms that are fundamentally neuropsychiatric in nature, such as impulsivity, poor emotional regulation, hypervigilance, irritability, aggression, inattention, and recklessness (van der Kolk, 2005). Fostering aberrant neurodevelopment and neurobiological functioning, interpersonal trauma may yield pervasive emotional, relational, social, cognitive, and health problems across the lifespan (Anda et al., 2006). Therefore, contemporary object relations play therapists must address dysfunction at the "micro" (i.e., neurobiological) level if they are to successfully intervene at the "macro" (i.e., relational) level (Perry, 2006).

Object relations play therapy is maximally effective when situated within a comprehensive treatment plan that provides sufficient therapeutic repetitions to facilitate meaningful changes (Gaskill & Perry, 2012; Perry, 2006). Children who have undergone attachment trauma often manifest symptoms that originate in lower brain areas (brainstem, diencephalon). Remediating these areas requires repetitive, patterned sensory input exceeding that which is provided by weekly psychotherapy (Perry, 2006). Comprehensive treatment may include parent–child dyadic work, occupational therapy, music or movement classes, and/or therapeutic educational programming. There are often substantial obstacles in implementing child–parent therapy with traumatized children, including severe caregiver mental illness and repeated placement changes. An attachment-focused individual therapy is particularly useful as a supplement or precursor to dyadic work if the child's primary attachment figures are unavailable or not psychologically ready to engage in therapy with their child. Although this chapter focuses primarily on the individual play therapy modality, it is vitally important that a child's whole system of care engage with treatment.

Historical Background

Play therapy emerged nearly 80 years ago and is now a well-established modality for the psychological treatment of children. Early play therapy was rooted in the psychodynamic approaches of Anna Freud and Melanie Klein and the nondirective approach of Virginia Axline (see Benedict,

2003). Theoretical developments within psychodynamic traditions have moved in the direction of object relations with an emphasis on early relationships. At the same time, object relations approaches have increasingly incorporated findings from neuroscience, especially the role of relational experience in early brain development (Shore, 2001, 2003, 2009, 2010). Benedict and colleagues (2006), elaborating on this emerging psychodynamic framework, incorporated thematic play into object relations play therapy. Benedict's (2004) research revealed that children's play reflects readily discernible themes (e.g., safety, nurturance) as well as affects (e.g., sadness, jealousy) and interactive patterns (e.g., good guy–bad guy) that can be reliably identified by sensitive clinicians. Through thematic play, a child's representational world comes alive in the here and now, manifesting the child's internalized relational models, as well as beliefs and feelings regarding self and others.

Theoretical Formulations

The theoretical foundation of object relations/attachment-based play therapy has become increasingly interdisciplinary, evolving from a primarily psychological to a neuropsychobiological framework. The deepest roots of this play therapy approach lie in the theoretical formulations of British object relations theorists John Bowlby (1988) and Donald Winnicott (1965, 1971a, 1971b) as well as Margaret Mahler's developmental theory (Mahler & Purer, 1968). Object relations theories converge on several key assumptions. First, significant relationships constitute the primary motivational impetus of human development (Glickhauf-Hughes & Wells, 1977). Second, infants and attachment figures co-create interactive patterns that infants subconsciously extrapolate into cognitive–affective blueprints called "internal working models" (Bowlby, 1988). These templates reflect beliefs and emotions regarding the self, others, and the self in relation to others. Internal working models reciprocally interact with ongoing interpersonal transactions, guiding habitual ways of perceiving and relating to significant others, oneself, and the world, while being shaped by ongoing relationships in return (Bowlby, 1988; Siegel, 1999). Therefore, object relations theorists ascribe enormous significance to a child's earliest attachment relationships, in which internal working models first arise.

This model inherits five psychological concepts from Winnicott (1971a) of the British object relations school: the false self, good-enough mothering, holding environment, attunement, and transitional object. The *false self* emerges when a child, in seeking approval, becomes disconnected from his or her authentic self through excessive compliance with caregivers. *Good-enough mothering* occurs in a caregiving environment that provides acceptance and fulfillment of needs while also protecting the child from impingement (Abram, 1996). A *holding environment* is the re-creation of this caregiving environment within the therapeutic relationship. Finally, *attunement* occurs whenever a caregiver accurately interprets a child's needs, and consistently, sensitively meets those needs. Fairburn's (1952) concept of *obstinate attachment*, which illuminates a child's paradoxical attachment to an abusive or neglectful caregiver, also informs this model.

Object relations theories reflect differing perspectives regarding how "an individual's mental representations of self and others become enduring psychic structures" (Glickauf-Hughes & Wells, 1997, p. 18). John Bowlby (1988), of the British object relations school, forecasted the "rapprochement" (Schore, 2010) between psychology and the biological sciences, characterizing development as a repetitive, interactive process between a child's genetic potential and the caregiving environment. Attachment theory, which Bowlby (1958) developed in concert with his research associate, Mary

Ainsworth, is now considered the most comprehensive, integrative model of psychological development (Hughes, 2009). In addition to shaping internal working models, the attachment relationship provides a "secure base" (Ainsworth, 1963) from which the child can explore, and a "safe haven" (Bowlby, 1988) to which a child runs in times of distress. These concepts contain both psychological and biological elements, as they reflect the dynamic relationships among a child's attachment, fear, and exploratory systems (Cassidy, 2008). The attachment system maintains proximity to caregivers via attachment behaviors (crying, approaching caregiver) and dampens the exploratory system when activated beyond a certain threshold. When the caregiver is comfortably nearby and perceived as available, the infant's attachment system quiets, promoting exploration (i.e., secure base). During times of distress, the fear and attachment systems are both activated, decreasing exploration and prompting the child to seek proximity to the caregiver (i.e., safe haven) (Ainsworth, 1963; Bowlby, 1988; Cassidy, 2008).

Contemporary developmental neuroscience literature loudly echoes the theoretical underpinnings of attachment theory. This research offers a paradigm-shifting (Schore, 2009), intricate depiction of how parent–infant interactions orchestrate neurodevelopment, thus merging psychological and biological constructs. Empirical data strongly confirm that optimal brain development simply cannot occur without a "growth-facilitating" attachment relationship (Schore, 2001). A secure attachment bond develops when a mother–infant dyad establishes emotionally significant, synchronized, predictable patterns of auditory-prosodic, visual-facial, and tactile-gestural communications (Schore, 2009). Infants demonstrate an innate relational expectancy, as evidenced by the distance of their optimal visual focus and their preference for attending to facial configurations (Sigelman & Rider, 2005). Even newborns seek intimate transactions with attach-ment figures and demonstrate awareness of their mother's subjective state (i.e., inter-subjectivity) (Trevarthen & Aitken, 2001). A mother instinctively utilizes "motherese" to convey emotional nuances and motives in a physiological, preverbal manner. Trev-arthen and Aitken (2001) write: "The dy-namic narrative envelopes of a mother's utterances, their pitch contours, and other dynamic qualities, have been identified as necessary alimentation for the infant's developing self-awareness and conscious agency" (p. 8). This preverbal contact cre-ates a "primary level of intermental com-munication" (Trevarthen & Aitken, 2001, p. 4), an essential foundation for secure attachment.

Careful scientific examination of the "protoconversations" (Bateson, 1971) of mother and infant reveal that they are highly complex, bidirectional (Lavelli & Fogel, 2013), and feature elements of adult conversation such as mutually con-tingent communication (Trevarthen & Aitken, 2001). Infants calibrate quickly to their mother's manner of engagement; by 2 months, infants exhibit decreased re-sponsiveness to the sounds and smiles of strangers whose interactive pattern differs from that of the infant's mother (Bigelow & Rochat, 2006). This response difference suggests an emerging relational template (i.e., working model) that is bodily based and preconscious. According to Schore's (2009) neurobiological attachment model, an infant develops regulatory capabilities through these synchronous, emotionally laden "protoconversations." An infant is born without the ability to independently modulate overly high or low arousal states; therefore, the caregiver's coregulating function is vital. Schore asserts: "Secure attachment depends not on the mother's psychobiological attunement with the in-fant's cognition or behavior, but rather on her regulation of the infant's internal states of arousal, the energetic dimension of the child's affective state" (2010, p. 20).

Coregulation involves a caregiver accu-rately "reading" the infant's nonverbal af-fective communications and adjusting his or her somatosensory signals to restore equilibrium (Schore, 1994). Schore (2009) underscores the importance of a caregiver mirroring the infant's "vitality affects" (Stern, 1985), which involves matching the energetic dimension of the infant's affect and modulating it back to equilibrium. Normative "ruptures" in the dyadic rela-tionship are inevitable, easily repaired, and actually growth-inducing for the infant's autonomous regulatory capacities (Schore, 2010). Misattunements, when quickly, sen-sitively corrected, provide opportunities for "interactive repair," which increase the infant's resilience and support the infant's internalization of the dyadic regulatory process (Schore, 2009).

Schore (2010) avows that coregulating dyadic exchanges transpire between the right hemispheres of both mother and in-fant, forging neural connections between the infant's subcortical, bodily based affec-tive states with conscious emotional states in higher brain regions of the right hemi-sphere. These circuits are vital to emotional processing, empathy, and development of the self. Because the right hemisphere and adjoining limbic system rapidly develop during the infant's first year of life (Schore, 1994), early attachment relationships have profound, long-term implications. An in-fant's emotional exchanges with attachment figures establish right-hemisphere cortical–subcortical networks that are stored in im-plicit procedural memory. These bodily based, subconscious encodings represent internal working models of relationships founded in "procedural expectations" (see Cortina & Liotti, 2007; Schore, 2010) of at-tachment figures' availability. These prever-bal models are right-, not left-brain domi-nant, and they guide a child's interpersonal patterns and habitual responses to stress long before a child consciously holds a negative belief system (left brain) regarding caregivers (Schore, 2010).

Major Constructs

Perry's (2006) six principles of neurodevelopment are extraordinarily relevant to conceptualization and treatment in attachment-focused play therapy. According to Perry, the brain is organized in a hierarchical manner, with external and internal sensory input initially entering lower, primitive, nonconscious brain areas (brainstem, diencephalon). The sensory input precipitates "neural patterns of activity" that can travel to higher brain regions (limbic, cortical) through connective neural networks. Perry asserts that the brain stores patterns of neural activity in its memory and is capable of linking stored patterns to danger. As new neural activity travels into higher brain regions, it is compared against the brain's stored templates. If a match is made, the child's "alarm system" may be activated, initiating "a wave a neuronal activity in key brainstem and diencephalic nuclei, which include neurons containing a variety of neurotransmitters" (Perry, 2006, p. 31). Of paramount importance, this alarm system activation occurs before reaching the limbic and cortical regions—that is, outside of conscious awareness (Perry, 2008). This suggests a nonconscious, bodily based component to a child's object relations.

Perry's principles indicate that the brain develops sequentially during specific periods, and in order of increasing complexity. Additionally, Perry asserts that the brain organizes in an "experience-dependent" manner that reflects the child's environment. The four major regions of the brain, ordered according to increasing complexity, are the brainstem, diencephalon, limbic system, and cortex (Perry, 2006). The brainstem develops most actively between 0 and 9 months and serves a critical role in the regulation of arousal, sleep, blood pressure, heart rate, body temperature, and fear states. Developing most actively between 6 months and 2 years, the diencephalon serves a critical role in controlling fine motor skills, promoting sensory integration, controlling motor functioning, and facilitating flexibility in relational exchanges. The limbic system most actively develops between the ages of 1 and 4 years and is critical to a child's ability to regulate emotions, interpret nonverbal information, experience empathy for others, feel a sense of social connectedness, and tolerate distress and differences. The cortex is the highest, most complex brain region, developing most actively between the ages of 3 and 6 years. The cortex is involved in abstract cognitive processing and integration of social–emotional information. A child's capacity to think abstractly, exhibit creativity, respect others, and form a spiritual or moral framework is contingent upon cortical functioning (Perry, 2006, 2008).

The timing of attachment trauma and the quality and quantity of incoming sensory input during critical developmental windows have profound implications (Perry, 2006). Children are born with undifferentiated neural brain systems that must be prompted by environmental and internal signals (neurotransmitters, neurohormones) to organize to their potential (Perry, 2001). A child's early experiences, particularly relational ones, direct molecular activators that literally program neural development in a manner that is adaptive for the child's environment. If incoming sensory input is inadequate, or creates pandemonium, a child's neural organization will reflect similar disarray (Gaskill & Perry, 2012). Adverse developmental experiences that compromise lower brain region organization are particularly devastating, as they automatically compromise higher brain region functioning as well. Crucial monoamine neural networks project from the brainstem and diencephalon into the more complex areas of the brain (Perry, 2008); therefore, higher levels of brain functioning are contingent upon lower areas.

Also foundational to this approach is the idea that play is a vital, essential component in healthy attachment and in a child's social, cognitive, and language development

(Cicchetti & Valentino, 2006, pp. 152–153). Through playful exchanges such as kissing noses, blowing on a tummy, and singing nonsense words, a parent–infant dyad shares moments of intersubjectivity (Trevarthen, Aitken, Vandekerckhove, Delafield-Butt, & Nagy, 2006, pp. 65–126) and positive affective states characterized by playful joy. This shared exuberance promotes affect regulation and secure attachment (Trevarthen et al., 2006, pp. 112–113). Play is complex, primal (Brown & Vaughan, 2009), and understood to be "the intrinsic, neurological process intended to program the child's brain" (Gaskill & Perry, 2012). Play is ideally suited for organizing the low brain regions, because it heavily involves preverbal, sensory communication such as eye contact, facial expressions, pitch, rhythm, movement, and touch (Gaskill & Perry, 2012; Schore, 1994). These elements are helpful to incorporate into an attachment-focused intervention to engage the nonverbal, low brain regions, particularly of the right hemisphere.

Lastly, Perry's (2006) description of the arousal continuum informs this model. As a child perceives threat, his or her internal state will move from the lower end (calm) to extreme arousal state (terror). For each of the five arousal states (calm, arousal attention, alarm, fear, terror), a certain brain region becomes dominant. For example, if a child's internal state is "alarm," his or her limbic/midbrain brain region will take control, limiting cortex-mediated functions such as reasoning and abstract thinking. If terrorized, a child's functioning is primarily mediated by the brainstem, and may appear regressed and chaotic (Perry, 2006).

Conceptualization of Psychopathology

Based on neurobiological (Schore, 2010) and neurodevelopmental principles (Perry, 2006), we know that attachment trauma exerts both psychological and biological effects, having complex immediate and long-term implications for child development. Neglectful and/or abusive caregiving environments, as discussed earlier, can derail neural organization, resulting in disorganization or neural atrophy. Low brain dysfunction profoundly impairs emotion regulation, attention, impulse control, cognition, and memory (Perry, 2008). The empirical evidence suggests that many children who experience "developmentally adverse interpersonal trauma" (DAIT; Ford, 2005) develop complex symptom pictures that extend beyond the three symptom domains of posttraumatic stress disorder (PTSD). This has led to van der Kolk's (2005) proposed diagnosis of developmental trauma disorder, which encapsulates trauma-related problems in cognitive, biological, and relational domains.

In the moment, traumatic experiences precipitate a fight or flight response, activating the sympathetic nervous system and generating intense emotions (van der Kolk, 1994). Increased adrenergic activity manifests physiologically (increased heart rate, blood pressure, anxiety, respiration, and sweating) (van der Kolk, 2006). Alarm system activation dampens brain regions responsible for verbal communication, memory, and integration of sensory input (van der Kolk, 1994). When frightened, a child's lower brain regions become dominant, inhibiting cortical regions that are readily overwhelmed and poorly equipped to restrain intense affect (Gaskill & Perry, 2012; Lehrer, 2009; van der Kolk, 2006). This cortical inhibition leaves a child vulnerable to emotional and relational instability and impedes learning and exploration.

Chronic interpersonal trauma precipitates prolonged periods of hyperarousal that may cumulatively shift a child's baseline physiological arousal upward, sensitize the stress response system, and increase alarm system reactivity (Perry, 2006). Drawing from Bowlby's formulations regarding the dynamics between the attachment and fear system, a young child who is chronically vigilant will engage in fewer exploratory behaviors of lower quality, resulting in reduced learning experiences (Bowlby, 1988; Cassidy, 2008). Drawing from neurodevelopmental principles (Perry, 2006), chronic trauma may establish an engrained, subcortical pairing of certain sensory cues with autonomic fear responses, causing the child to be repeatedly triggered by seemingly innocuous stimuli (e.g., a song, smell, frown) that his or her brain associates with danger. Because the triggering occurs rapidly in lower brain regions, before neural signals reach limbic and cortical regions, the child has no conscious awareness or understanding of this response.

Drawing from Schore's (2010) neurobiological attachment model, early relational trauma can profoundly disrupt the organization and functioning of neural networks in the right hemisphere, particularly within the orbitofrontal cortex, as well as its connections to the limbic system. Schore considers this region to be "the locus of Bowlby's attachment system," as it represents "the brain's most complex affect and stress regulatory system" (Schore, 2011, p. 80). According to this model, severe attachment trauma may ultimately give rise to habitual dissociative responses to stress, profound disruptions in a child's sense of self, and possibly severe psychological disorders in adulthood related to severe dissociation (e.g., dissociative identity disorder, borderline personality disorder) (Schore, 2010). According to Schore (2001, 2010), dissociation follows a prolonged sympathetic-dominant hyperarousal in which a child is chronically hypervigilant and overwhelmed. In extreme cases of interpersonal trauma (combined with an underlying constitutional vulnerability), some children transition from sympathetic-dominant (hyperarousal) into a parasympathetic-dominant response (dissociation). Dissociation is understood to be psychologically and biologically protective, sheltering the brain from neurotoxic, hypermetabolic output, which nevertheless leaves the child with inadequate resources

to sustain growth in the right hemisphere (Schore, 2010).

Severe examples of attachment trauma include "grossly pathological care" such as neglect, sexual abuse, and exposure to parental drug use (American Psychiatric Association, 1994). More subtle examples of relational trauma, such as maternal depression, also undermine development. Infants of depressed mothers show less responsiveness to human voices and faces (Field, Diego, Hernandez-Reif, & Ascencio, 2009), whereas 3-month-old infants of highly attuned mothers exhibit increased smiling, cooing, and gazing at their mothers (Legerstee & Varghese, 2001). An infant's temperament, illness, or sensory integration issues may also interfere with secure attachment. In addition, constitutional factors, such as basal physiological levels, may determine the infant's level of vulnerability to relational trauma, as these differentially predict developmental outcomes related to harsh caregiving (Sturge-Apple, Davies, Martin, Cicchetti, & Hentges, 2012).

Attachment trauma may lead a child to manifest maladaptive, readily identifiable emotional and behavioral patterns with caregivers. These patterns coalesce into categories of insecure attachment, failure to attach (Ainsworth, Blehar, Waters, & Wall, 1978; Schuder & Lyons-Ruth, 2004), and, at worst, disorganized attachment in which a child has no clear attachment strategy. Disorganized, "type D" attachment (Main & Solomon, 1986) is often seen in extremely pathological caregiving environments in which the caregiver precipitates extreme fear in the child. This fear creates an unbearable, paradoxical situation for the child, who is simultaneously compelled to seek proximity to the caregiver for protection, and to flee from the attachment figure who represents a source of terror. This leaves the child with no workable coping strategy (Schore, 2001).

Insecure attachment involves a disruption in the child's ability to use the attachment figure as a secure base and/or safe haven. Zeanah and Boris's (2000) categorical framework of attachment problems includes disrupted attachment disorders, secure base distortions, and disorders of nonattachment. Disorders of nonattachment involve children who appear not to have formed an attachment to a preferred caregiver. These children have difficulty expressing and regulating emotion, and in cooperating with others seeking comfort. Within the secure base distortion category, there are four subtypes: self-endangerment, clinging-inhibited, hypercompliance, and role reversal. These subtypes reflect an attachment figure's failure to serve as a secure base for the child's exploration of the world, and as a safe haven to which the child may turn for comfort (Cooper, Hoffman, Powell, & Marvin, 2005). The third category of disrupted attachment includes children whose initial attachment relationship was disrupted, sometimes permanently, by the caregiver's imprisonment, death, or abandonment of the child.

Techniques and Goals

According to this model, interventions must be situated within a deeply safe, meaningful relationship context with a therapist who is attuned and well-regulated emotionally. The techniques of object relations play therapy flow naturally from its theoretical foundations. The primary vehicles of intervention are the therapist's secure base relationship with the child, brainstem-focused calming activities, and thematic play invitations situated within a safe, empathic interpersonal context. The therapist facilitates the types of accepting, curious, empathic, and playful transactions (Hughes, 2009) that were distorted or infrequent during early development. There is a particular emphasis on the therapist's internal stance toward the child, capacity to modulate his or her own affect, and ability to empathize deeply with the child. Based on Schore's (2010) research, these elements are unconsciously conveyed

through somatosensory communications such as tone of voice, facial expressions, bodily posture, and eye contact.

The therapist achieves this attuned relationship through deliberately creating an environment that includes acceptance of the child, empathy, and moments of intersubjective attunement. As part of this basic therapeutic stance, the therapist provides constancy, both in his or her self-presentation and in the playroom. The latter can be accomplished by introducing new materials with preparation, having predictable places for materials in the playroom, and by providing children with a place (e.g., a plastic bin) where they can safely keep their "play in progress" until the next session. In addition, safety, both psychological and physical, must be assured. For example, the only limits in the playroom are safety limits, which are reiterated to the child whenever there is a threat to safety. Finally, the therapist needs to be able to comfortably relinquish control except for safety limits. This can be seen in the therapist's acquiescence to the child's demands and in provision of a child-friendly clock (an analog clock with stickers at the numbers) so the child can know the time remaining in the session (e.g., "We have to stop when the long hand gets to the elephant").

The second essential feature of the therapist's stance is the approach to regulation of the child. The therapist needs to act as a coregulator of the child's emotions and behavior because traumatized children have difficulties with self-regulation. This is done in various ways, including reflecting feelings and helping children know how the therapist recognizes their feelings so that they can thereby know their own feelings. The therapist also helps regulate the child by matching vitality affect (Hughes, 2009) and then either gently reducing overly aroused affect and behavior or, in the case where the child is shut down, gently engaging and arousing the child. Coregulation also involves shifting the child's response to threats to safety by helping reduce hypervigilance and enhancing self-soothing. Neurodevelopmental activities of the type recommended by Perry (2006) can be helpful here. Such activities need to be patterned, rhythmic, and repetitive, and can include art and music activities as well as rocking (i.e., having a rocking chair in the playroom).

Thematic Play

Play therapy researchers (Benedict, 1997, 2004; Benedict & Hastings, 2002; Benedict, Hastings, Ato, Carson, & Nash, 1998) have discovered that children enact a multitude of readily perceptible themes, with unique characters and conclusions that potentially reflect idiosyncratic meanings. Examples include family themes (e.g., nurturance, separation, reunion), safety themes (e.g., rescue and danger), and aggressive themes (e.g., good guy–bad guy, death play, aggressor–victim). A safety theme might be a boy trapped inside a collapsing building, with (upon the therapist's gentle invitation) ambulances and fire trucks quickly dispatched to retrieve him from the rubble. An aggressive theme could be a shark viciously attacking underwater divers and sinking their vessels. In the safe context of the playroom, the child's representational world is outwardly enacted in the here and now without unduly overwhelming his or her regulatory capacities. With distressing material externalized, the child is afforded sufficient psychological distance to convey, process, and resolve troubling memories, beliefs, and feelings. Trauma recovery, according to Gil (2003), can be expedited by externalization and projection.

Thematic play also allows the child an opportunity to indirectly test the therapist's capacity to tolerate, accept, and empathically modulate unbearable emotions. Although the therapist may readily discern the relevance of play themes to the child's real-life circumstances, overt interpretations are not necessary, and may even be overwhelming for the child if precipitously issued. Instead, the therapist intervenes indirectly by entering the child's representational world and communicating to the child within the metaphor, often through invitations (Gil, 1991). The person of the therapist often takes residence in some element of the metaphor, conveying empathy or offering solutions. At other times, the therapist's play character embodies unbearable elements of the child's experience, expressing perceptions and emotions in a way the child cannot do overtly.

Play therapy researchers avow that comprehensively assessing a child's play involves not only recognizing its themes, but also identifying recurrent affects and interpersonal patterns (Benedict, 2004; Benedict et al., 1998). Sensitive clinicians can reliably identify affects such as sadness, jealousy, and anger, as well as relational transactions such as protecting, controlling, helping, and sharing. These elements reveal the child's internal working models of self and other as well as the child's perception of relationships between self and other. With this understanding, the therapist can issue child-responsive invitations through play to challenge and modify maladaptive object relations. Thematic play provides a rich picture of the child's relationships, emotions, and experiences, and creates an arena for remediating disturbed working models and traumatic memories in a developmentally sensitive format.

Therapeutic invitations in play consist of various verbalizations and actions on the part of the therapist that gently offer the child a new direction for the play or a new understanding of feelings or actions. For example, a child playing out a very aggressive character killing other characters might prompt the therapist to invite the child to protect one of the remaining characters. It is *invitational* because it is offered tentatively with the therapist's full understanding that any response by the child, including ignoring the invitation, is acceptable. By the use of invitations, the therapist can challenge maladaptive internal working models and, by responding differently than would be expected by the child's internal working model, alter relational templates and change cognitive understanding of both self and other. Invitations can also be employed in the service of helping the traumatized child create a coherent attachment and self-narrative. This can be accomplished by shifting implicit trauma memories to cognitively mediated explicit memories of the trauma and by defusing triggers for those memories. Finally, storytelling and art activities can help the child know and feel safe knowing his or her own stories.

Clinical Case Example

Henry was 3 years old when he exuberantly careened into a community mental health clinic for treatment, his maternal grandmother frantically following. His developmental history featured probable prenatal drug exposure, attachment disruption, and interpersonal trauma in the context of maternal substance abuse. These traumas were best characterized as "ambient," a sad reality for Henry that evaded encapsulation into a single event. Henry's biological parents were acquaintances who conceived Henry during a period of extensive drug use. After suggesting an abortion, Henry's father disappeared. Having severed ties with parents, Henry's mother felt disheartened, overwhelmed, and acutely alone during her pregnancy. During Henry's infancy, his mother's drug use severely impaired her capacity for nurturing, attuned, intersubjective exchanges. The poor quality and infrequency of dyadic emotional communication compromised the development of Henry's "right brain systems that process visual-facial, auditory-prosodic, and tactile-gestural affective communications" (Schore, 2009, p. 194). Essential "empathic mirroring" (Kohut, 1971) was limited. Thus, Henry's developing limbic system, central to the processing of emotional meaning, re-

ceived inadequate input (following Dapretto et al., 2006; Schore, 2009).

Further compounding his adversities, Henry was chronically either under- or overstimulated, alternately neglected or frightened into hyperarousal during his mother's heavy drug use. He could not comfortably settle into a predictable communication pattern and pace, as healthy infants do; his mother's facial expressions, tone of voice, and vocal rhythms deviated drastically, which confused and scared him. Henry's prolonged dysregulation, lack of a coregulating figure, and altered neurobiological circuits left him overly sensitive to fear cues and vulnerable to intense emotions. Henry was abandoned at the maternal grandmother's home before his first birthday. A year later, his mother resurfaced to retrieve him; however, she brought Henry back a few weeks afterward without explanation. Henry seemed traumatized by the reunion and separation, exhibiting hyperactivity, prolonged tearfulness, vigilance, aggression, and recklessness. These symptoms persisted and worsened over time, precipitating his referral for psychological treatment.

Henry's therapist, Gabriella, conceptualized his symptoms using an attachment and neurodevelopmental trauma framework. Henry's attachment presentation was interpreted as a disrupted attachment with features of secure base distortion, particularly self-endangerment and hypervigilance (Zeanah & Boris, 2000). Henry appeared to hold pervasively negative internal working models of self, others, and relationships, and was unable to elicit or accept nurturing. He exhibited an intense need to control and distance caregivers, either acting aggressively or venturing off unsafely. Thus, Henry was unable to effectively use an attachment figure as either a "safe haven" or a "secure base" (Bowlby, 1988). Henry's developmental history suggested brainstem-level dysfunction, an overly sensitive stress response system, and poor right-hemisphere development necessary for affect regulation and healthy attachment/affiliation. He struggled with transitions between tasks, became easily upset, and exhibited impulsivity.

Gabriella focused the initial phase of therapy on establishing a secure base relationship with Henry and addressing his lower brain dysfunction. Without brainstem remediation, Henry would be unable to benefit from symbolic play or verbal interventions targeting limbic and cortical regions (Gaskill & Perry, 2012). Gabriella began engaging Henry in sensory-focused activities such as working with clay, playing with sand, singing, breathing activities, and painting. She coordinated with Henry's grandmother and preschool teacher so that relaxation activities, therapeutic massage, and music were incorporated into Henry's routines. In the early stages of therapy, Henry was fiercely independent, controlling, aggressive, and self-endangering. He positioned himself precariously atop tables, attempted steep climbs up shelving, hit himself with toys, and ran about recklessly. He irritably, sometimes aggressively, resisted Gabriella when she took actions to ensure their safety. Gabriella established safety by consistently setting limits and remaining regulated herself. Additionally, she demonstrated attunement by reflecting and affirming Henry's emotional expressions, drawing connections between his bodily expressions and affect (e.g., "I can hear how mad you are by your loud voice," "Seems like your body hurts when you have sad feelings"). Gabriella matched his affect vitality using her tone of voice, body language, and vocal volume, and she expressed empathy for how mad he felt when she kept him safe.

By incorporating a therapeutic stance of playfulness, acceptance, curiosity, and empathy (PACE; Hughes, 2009), using eye contact, vocal inflection, and body language, Gabriella invited safe bodily expressions of emotion, which helped Henry to modulate his arousal. She also established a predictable routine with Henry, such as offering a snack prior to the session and setting a timer to alert him that 10 minutes remained in the session. In addition, Gabriella and Henry established special routines that created states of intersubjectivity and shared positive emotions. For example, Gabriella and Henry often scampered to the window upon hearing a passing train. Gabriella served as a coregulating figure, using her voice, body language, and facial expressions to mirror Henry's excitement, share in his intense emotion, and then help him to modulate arousal. Henry's affect often spilled beyond the bounds of what he could regulate; therefore, after matching Henry's enthusiasm, Gabriella would guide him back to baseline by introducing a downregulating activity such as sandplay or painting.

As Henry became more regulated and relaxed, thematic play became a central part of his therapy. Henry's play contained strong themes of aggression, brokenness, and repair. Henry often perceived toys as irreversibly destroyed (e.g., "This doesn't work!") or dangerous, becoming acutely frightened, for example, by "the angry man" (a male puppet), as well as by a play sword. Henry exhibited a pattern of acting aggressively using toys that he initially perceived as threatening. For example, he donned a "scary" mask and charged forcefully toward Gabriella. Even Henry's snack time became an occasion of aggression, as he depicted his animal crackers fighting and hissing at one another. Henry's sandtray play contained alligators biting off arms and snakes fighting each other. Also, on a few occasions, he caught Gabriella off guard during quiet moments, yelling "BAM!" to scare her before bursting into laughter. These elements reflected his intense anxiety in trusting others and his negative internal relational templates of caregivers as threatening, controlling, unpredictable, and aggressive.

Henry's play characters always opposed or controlled Gabriella's figures. For example, Henry established a play "store" at which Gabriella's characters could never afford items. He assigned his character to be the sheriff who caught Gabriella's "bad" people. He also assigned himself a shark figure that sank Gabriella's people, who could not escape despite their best efforts. Henry's play themes reflected negative beliefs regarding relationships, as the majority of the relational dynamics in his play enactments were controlling or oppositional. Henry also exhibited a pervasively negative view of self; he once forbade Gabriella from using his name, and later expressed dislike when he saw himself in the mirror: "I hate me." When his mother gave birth to a second child during the middle phase of therapy, Henry slid back into aggressive and anxious states. He was incredibly ambivalent about showing Gabriella the baby pictures that he brought to therapy. He controlled her access to these photos, setting up a store at which she was unable to purchase the photos despite repeated efforts. Gabriella utilized invitations and reflections within Henry's metaphor to address his negative object relations by labeling the characters' emotions, inviting repairs of "broken" items, or suggesting rescuing or collaborative tasks between characters.

Henry began playing the hide-and-seek game with Gabriella, though frequently controlled this activity by coming out of hiding early. It seemed as though he didn't trust her constancy or availability. Gabriella created a sense of constancy for Henry by saving traces of his play in her office: "Is there anything that you want me to keep safe?" Henry began eliciting nurturing, though often in a testing manner, such as pretending to be stuck behind a table, and then laughing and coming out as Gabriella approached. Henry also began initiating nurturing play; however, he assigned Gabriella the role of the vulnerable patient and himself, the medical professional. She followed Henry's lead, verbalizing the underlying emotional needs that Henry could not yet accept or articulate for himself. Gabriella also verbalized emotions of fear during instances in which Henry was physically or verbally aggressive toward her, thus indirectly validating Henry's feelings, dis-

confirming his internal working model of others as emotionally unsafe, and modeling emotional competency.

As therapy progressed, Henry became more accepting of safety limits, nurturance, and collaborative invitations. His play became less controlling and increasingly featured a cooperative stance among characters. Central to Gabriella's work was her own self-awareness, her ability to remain regulated, and her capacity to empathically reflect Henry's strong emotions. At times Gabriella monitored her own emotions, for example, noticing that Henry's aggressive behaviors induced some anxiety and frustration. She worked through these normative responses with a trusted senior colleague, reflected upon their significance, and prepared for sessions by practicing deep breathing for a few minutes before Henry's arrival.

Conclusion

Object relations and attachment-based play therapy is a multifaceted, integrative approach for young children who have experienced attachment trauma during their early years. This approach draws from object relations theories, particularly attachment theory, and research on children's thematic play, as well as Perry's (2006) neurodevelopmental principles and Schore's (2009) neurobiological model of attachment. The therapist begins addressing the child's negative internalized relational models and trauma-related symptoms through creating a secure-base therapeutic relationship with the child that features attunement, intersubjectivity, coregulation, and empathy. The therapist utilizes sensory-focused play activities such as sandplay and finger painting to address dysfunction in lower areas of the brain, and involves the child's caretakers in establishing similar activities at home and school (Gaskill & Perry, 2012). The therapist enters the child's representational world of thematic play and utilizes playful, metaphorical invitations to modify the child's negative working models. Although the theoretical foundations and major constructs of this approach have strong empirical support, further research is needed to establish an empirical base for the effectiveness of the approach with young children who have experienced attachment trauma.

REFERENCES

Abram, J. (1996). *The language of Winnicott: A dictionary and guide to understanding his work.* Northvale, NJ: Aronson.

Ainsworth, M. D. S. (1963). The development of infant–mother interaction among the Ganda. In B. M. Foss (Ed.), *Determinants of infant behavior* (Vol. 2, pp. 67–112). New York: Wiley.

Ainsworth, M. D. S., Blehar, M. C., Waters, E., & Wall, S. (1978). *Patterns of attachment: A psychological study of the strange situation.* Hillsdale, NJ: Erlbaum.

American Psychiatric Association. (1994). *Diagnostic and statistical manual of mental disorders* (4th ed.). Washington, DC: Author.

Anda, R. F., Felitti, V. J., Bremner, J. D., Walker, J. D., Whitfield, C., Perry, B. D., et al. (2006). The enduring effects of abuse and related adverse experiences in childhood: A convergence of neurobiology and epidemiology. *European Archives of Psychiatry and Clinical Neuroscience, 256*(3), 174–186.

Bateson, M. C. (1971). The interpersonal context of infant vocalization. *Quarterly Progress Report of the Research Laboratory of Electronics, 100,* 170–176.

Benedict, H. E. (1997, September 12). *Thematic play therapy and attachment disorders.* Workshop presented at Southwest Missouri State University, Springfield.

Benedict, H. E. (2003). Object relations/thematic play therapy. In C. E. Schaefer (Ed.), *Foundations of play therapy* (pp. 281–305). New York: Wiley.

Benedict, H. E. (2004, October). *Using play themes in play assessment and for understanding play therapy process.* Preconference workshop presented at the 21st annual Association for Play Therapy International Conference, Denver, CO.

Benedict, H. E., & Grigoryev, P. (1995, October).

Practical applications of object relations theory to play therapy techniques. Workshop presented at 12th annual Association for Play Therapy International Conference, San Francisco.

Benedict, H. E., & Hastings, L. (2002). Object relations play therapy. In J. Magnavita (Ed.), *Comprehensive handbook of psychotherapy: Psychodynamic/object relations* (Vol. 1, pp. 47–80). New York: Wiley.

Benedict, H. E., Hastings, L., Ato, G., Carson, M., & Nash, M. (1998). *Revised Benedict play therapy theme code and interpersonal relationship code.* Unpublished working paper, Baylor University, Waco, TX.

Bigelow, A. E., & Rochat, P. (2006). Two-month-old infants' sensitivity to social contingency in mother–infant and stranger–infant interaction. *Infancy, 9,* 313–325.

Bowlby, J. (1958). The nature of the child's tie to his mother. *International Journal of Psycho-Analysis, 39,* 350–373.

Bowlby, J. (1988). *A secure base: Parent–child attachment and healthy human development.* New York: Basic Books.

Brown, S., & Vaughan, C. (2009). *Play: How it shapes the brain, opens the imagination, and invigorates the soul.* New York: Avery/Penguin.

Cassidy, J. (2008). The nature of the child's ties. In P. R. Shaver & J. Cassidy (Eds.), *Handbook of attachment* (2nd ed., pp. 3–22). New York: Guilford Press.

Cicchetti, D., & Valentino, K. (2006). An ecological transactional perspective on child maltreatment: Failure of the average expectable environment and its influence on child development. In D. Cicchetti & D. J. Cohen (Eds.), *Developmental psychopathology: Vol. 3. Risk, disorder, and adaptation* (2nd ed., pp. 146–148). New York: Wiley.

Cooper, G., Hoffman, K., Powell, B., & Marvin, R. (2005). The Circle of Security intervention: Differential diagnosis and differential treatment. In L. J. Berlin, Y. Ziv, L. Amaya-Jackson, & M. T. Greenberg (Eds.), *Enhancing early attachments: Theory, research, intervention, and policy* (pp. 127–151). New York: Guilford Press.

Cortina, M., & Liotti, G. (2007). New approaches to understanding unconscious processes: Implicit and explicit memory systems. *International Forum of Psychoanalysis, 16*(4), 204–212.

Dapretto, M., Davies, M. S., Pfeifer, J. H., Scott,

A. A., Sigman, M., Bookheimer, S. Y., et al. (2006). Understanding emotions in others: Mirror neuron dysfunction in children with autism spectrum disorders. *Nature Neuroscience, 9,* 28–30.

Fairburn, W. R. D. (1952). *An object-relations theory of the personality.* New York: Basic Books.

Field, T., Diego, M., Hernandez-Reif, M., & Ascencio, A. (2009). Prenatal dysthymia versus major depression effects on early mother–infant interactions: A brief report. *Infant Behavior and Development, 32*(1), 129–131.

Ford, J. D. (2005). Treatment implications of altered neurobiology, affect regulation and information processing following child maltreatment. *Psychiatric Annals, 35,* 410–419.

Gaskill, R., & Perry, B. (2012). Child sexual abuse, traumatic experiences, and their impact on the developing brain. In P. Goodyear-Brown (Ed.), *Handbook of child sexual abuse: Identification, assessment, and treatment* (pp. 29–48). Hoboken, NJ: Wiley.

Gil, E. (1991). *The healing power of play: Working with abused children.* New York: Guilford Press.

Gil, E. (2003). Art and play therapy with sexually abused children. In C. A. Malchiodi (Ed.), *Handbook of art therapy* (pp. 152–166). New York: Guilford Press.

Glickhauf-Hughes, C., & Wells, M. (1997). *Object relations psychotherapy: An individualized and interactive approach to diagnosis and treatment.* New York: Aronson.

Hughes, D. (2009). *Attachment-focused parenting.* New York: Norton.

Kohut, H. (1971). *The analysis of the self.* New York: International Universities Press.

Lavelli, M., & Fogel, A. (2013). Interdyad differences in early mother–infant face-to-face communication: Real-time dynamics and developmental pathways. *Developmental Psychology, 49*(12), 2257–2271.

Legerstee, M., & Varghese, J. (2001). The role of maternal affect mirroring on social expectancies in three-month-old infants. *Child Development, 72*(5), 1301–1313.

Lehrer, J. (2009). *How we decide.* Boston: Mariner Books.

Mahler, M. S., & Purer, M. (1968). *On human symbiosis and the vicissitudes of individuation.* New York: International Universities Press.

Main, M., & Solomon, J. (1986). Discovery of a new, insecure disorganized/disoriented attachment pattern. In T. B. Brazelton & M. W. Yogman (Eds.), *Affect development in infancy* (pp. 95–124). Norwood, NJ: Ablex.

Perry, B. D. (2001). The neuroarcheology of childhood maltreatment: The neurodevelopmental costs of adverse childhood events. In K. Franey, R. Geffner, & R. Falconer (Eds.), *The cost of maltreatment: Who pays?: We all do* (pp. 15–37). San Diego, CA: Family Violence and Sexual Assault Institute.

Perry, B. D. (2006). Applying the principles of neurodevelopment to clinical work with maltreated and traumatized children: The neurosequential model of therapeutics. In N. B. Webb (Ed.), *Working with traumatized youth in child welfare* (pp. 27–52). New York: Guilford Press.

Perry, B. D. (2008). Child maltreatment: The role of abuse and neglect in developmental psychopathology. In T. P. Beauchaine & S. P. Hinshaw (Eds.), *Textbook of child and adolescent psychopathology* (pp. 93–128). New York: Wiley.

Schore, A. N. (1994). *Affect regulation and the origin of the self: The neurobiology of emotional development.* Hillsdale, NJ: Erlbaum.

Schore, A. N. (2001). The effects of early relational trauma on right brain development, affect regulation, and infant mental health. *Infant Mental Health Journal, 22*(1–2), 201–269.

Schore, A. N. (2003). Early relational trauma, disorganized attachment, and the development of a predisposition to violence. In M. F. Solomon & D. J. Siegel (Eds.), *Healing trauma: Attachment, mind, body, and brain* (pp. 107–167). New York: Norton.

Schore, A. N. (2009). Relational trauma and the developing right brain: An interface of psychoanalytic self psychology and neuroscience. In W. J. Coburn & N. VanDerHeide (Eds.), *Self and systems: Explorations in contemporary self psychology* (pp. 189–203). Boston: Wiley-Blackwell.

Schore, A. N. (2010). Relational trauma and the developing right brain: The neurobiology of broken attachment bonds. In T. Baradon (Ed.), *Relational trauma in infancy* (pp. 19–47). London: Routledge.

Schore, A. N. (2011). The right brain implicit self lies at the core of psychoanalysis. *Psychoanalytic Dialogues: The International Journal of Relational Perspectives, 21*(1), 75–100.

Schuder, M. R., & Lyons-Ruth, K. (2004). "Hidden trauma" in infancy: Attachment, fearful arousal, and early dysfunction of the stress response system. In J. D. Osofsky (Ed.), *Young children and trauma: Intervention and treatment* (pp. 69–104). New York: Guilford Press.

Siegel, D. (1999). *The developing mind: Toward a neurobiology of interpersonal experience.* New York: Guilford Press.

Sigelman, C. K., & Rider, E. A. (2005). *Lifespan human development* (5th ed.). Belmont, CA: Wadsworth.

Stern, D. N. (1985). *The interpersonal world of the infant: A view from psychoanalysis and developmental psychology.* New York: Basic Books.

Sturge-Apple, M. L., Davies, P. T., Martin, M. J., Cicchetti, D., & Hentges, R. (2012). An examination of the impact of harsh parenting contexts on children's adaptation within an evolutionary framework. *Developmental Psychology, 48*(3), 791–805.

Trevarthan, C., & Aitkan, K. J. (2001). Infant intersubjectivity: Research, theory, and clinical applications. *Journal of Child Psychology and Psychiatry, 42*(1), 3–48.

Trevarthen, C., Aitken, K. J., Vandekerckhove, M., Delafield-Butt, J., & Nagy, E. (2006). Collaborative regulations of vitality in early childhood: Stress in intimate relationships and postnatal psychopathology. In D. Cicchetti & D. J. Cohen (Eds.), *Developmental psychopathology: Vol 2. Developmental neuroscience* (2nd ed., pp. 65–126). Hoboken, NJ: Wiley.

U.S. Department of Health and Human Services. (2011). *Child maltreatment 2011: Reports from the states to the National Child Abuse and Neglect Data System.* Washington, DC: Children's Bureau, Agency for Children and Families.

van der Kolk, B. (1994). The body keeps score: Memory and the evolving psychobiology of posttraumatic stress. Traumapages. Retrieved from *www.traumapages.com/a/vanderk4.php.*

van der Kolk, B. (2005). Developmental trauma disorder. *Psychiatric Annals, 35*(5), 401–408.

van der Kolk, B. (2006). Clinical implications of neuroscience research in PTSD. *Annals of the New York Academy of Science, 1071*(4), 277–293.

Winnicott, D. W. (1965). *The maturational processes and the facilitating environment: Studies in the theory of emotional development.* New York: International Universities Press.

Winnicott, D. W. (1971a). *Playing and reality.* London: Tavistock.

Winnicott, D. W. (1971b). *Therapeutic consultations in child psychiatry.* New York: Basic Books.

Zeanah, C. H., Jr., & Boris, N. W. (2000). Disturbances and disorders of attachment in early childhood. In C. H. Zeanah, Jr. (Ed.), *Handbook of infant mental health* (2nd ed., pp. 353–368). New York: Guilford Press.

CHAPTER 3

Adlerian Play Therapy

Terry Kottman
Jeffrey S. Ashby

Adlerian play therapy (AdPT) is an approach to play therapy based on the tenets of what Alfred Adler called *individual psychology* (Ansbacher & Ansbacher, 1956). The Adlerian play therapist uses a combination of directive and nondirective techniques to assist children with a variety of presenting problems. In the process of AdPT, the therapist assists children in developing and practicing new perceptions, attitudes, and behaviors (Kottman, 2003; Watts, 2006). The theoretical tenets of individual psychology offer a guide to aid the therapist in the conceptualization of client issues and subsequent treatment planning. The process of AdPT unfolds in four phases: (1) an initial relationship building phase, (2) a phase devoted to an exploration of client lifestyles, (3) a phase designed to help clients develop insight into their lifestyles, and (4) a final phase in which the play therapist facilitates client reorientation and reeducation. AdPT allows for play therapists to intervene in a manner that fits their personality and interpersonal approach. As a result, play therapists using AdPT can relax and use their natural style (e.g., some

emphasizing more directive interventions, others less directive, some utilizing lots of humor and silliness, some less) while still conceptualizing client issues from a coherent and consistent framework and moving toward related theoretical treatment goals.

Like most other play therapy approaches described in this text, AdPT is a comprehensive system of play therapy intervention described in considerable depth in other places (e.g., Kottman, 2003, 2009, 2011a). Thus, the purpose of this chapter is to give readers a perspective on how Adlerian play therapists understand clients and their families, and how they systematically intervene to facilitate well-being. We discuss the theoretical underpinnings of the theory, including the major constructs of Adlerian theory and the theoretical formulation used in client conceptualization. Because the goals of the therapeutic process and the roles of the therapist, child, and parents vary in the different phases of therapy, we describe each of these elements in the context of the four phases. Therapists use different strategies and techniques depending on the phase of play therapy, so this section of the chapter is also organized according to the phases. The clinical case study is intended to give readers a sense of what AdPT looks like in practice.

Description of the Approach

Major Constructs of Adlerian Theory

There is nothing so practical as a good theory.
—KURT LEWIN (1951, p. 169)

Although this epigram concisely addressing the usefulness of relating theory to practice may be overused, it applies extremely well to individual psychology. In the development of his theory and in its application, Adler was primarily interested in the practicality of the theory, going so far as to describe his approach as a "psychology of use" (Ansbacher & Ansbacher, 1956, p. 204). The practice of AdPT rests on several of Adler's primary theoretical tenets (Kottman, 2003) and constructs, described below.

People Are Self-Determining and Creative

We make choices about our behaviors, thoughts, feelings, and attitudes continually, and each of us is, as a result of this choosing, unique, special, and different from every other person (Adler, 1931/1958; Kottman, 2003). The Adlerian play therapist believes that all of us, as individuals, are affected by our environment and heredity, but we are not determined by either of them. In AdPT, the therapist emphasizes that clients have free will and can move toward more intentionality in the choices they make and the impact they have on their own lives and the lives of others.

People Perceive Reality Subjectively

The Adlerian play therapist takes a phenomenological view, assuming that subjectivity influences not only our perceptions and interpretations of experience, but our emotions and behavior as well (Adler, 1931/1958; Kottman, 2003). It is essential in the process of AdPT that the therapist consider the different perspectives of the child client, the child's parent(s), teacher(s), and any other individuals who interact with the child, all with an eye toward helping them understand and respect each other's perspectives.

Human Behavior Is Purposive and Goal-Directed

Each of us has a purpose directing every choice we make and every action we take (Dreikurs & Soltz, 1964; Kottman, 2003; Mosak & Maniacci, 2010; Sweeney, 2009). It is essential to remember, however, that in many cases, the goals of our behavior are outside of our awareness—so although there is a purpose to our behavior, we may not know what it is. In AdPT, the therapist helps clients learn to recognize the goals of their behavior and to shift their patterns and begin to make new choices so they are striving toward constructive, rather than destructive, goals.

People Have a Need to Belong and to Feel a Connection with Others

In Adlerian theory, the development of the need is referred to as *social interest* (Ansbacher & Ansbacher, 1956; Kottman, 2003). As a consequence of this tenet, the Adlerian play therapist seeks to understand clients in the social context in which they are embedded: the family, school, neighborhood, and so forth. As a means to establish that they belong, children observe the interactions of others—first in their families, then later with peers and at school—to determine ways to fit and to gain significance (Kottman, 2003). Although they are excellent observers, children sometimes come to erroneous conclusions about the "best" way to gain a sense of belonging. These erroneous conclusions may lead to them struggling, resulting in a referral for play therapy. The Adlerian play therapist helps children to develop their social interest: to learn new, more socially appropriate ways of gaining a sense of belonging and significance.

People Have a Tendency toward Feeling Inferior to Others

Although feelings of inferiority are common, resulting from the discrepancy between self-ideal and self-perception, the way in which individuals deal with these feelings can have important consequences, leading to either discouragement or inspiration (Ansbacher & Ansbacher, 1956; Kottman, 2003; Mosak & Maniacci, 2010). Those individuals who choose to be discouraged by feelings of inferiority often give up trying or overcompensate, leading to intrapersonal and interpersonal difficulties. The Adlerian play therapist helps clients to explore where their feelings of inferiority originated and gain adaptive coping strategies.

Lifestyle

As one of the most important conceptual lenses through which Adlerian play therapists generally seek to understand their clients (Kottman, 2003), the construct of lifestyle is comprised of a person's beliefs about self, others, and the world, and includes the behaviors based on those beliefs (Carlson, Watts, & Maniacci, 2005; Sweeney, 2009). Children form their style of life by the age of 8 by observing interactions and reactions, evaluating self-worth, and judging the best ways to belong and gain significance. Although they are acute observers, children do not always interpret accurately, leading them to develop mistaken beliefs and private logic. *Private logic* is the reasoning created by individuals that is consistent with their lifestyle—that is, their particular set of beliefs about self, others, and the world.

Maladjustment as Discouragement

The Adlerian play therapist generally believes the best way to understand maladjustment is in terms of discouragement (Carlson et al., 2005; Kottman, 2003; Sweeney, 2009). Discouragement may be related to poor social interest, which would result in an impaired sense of connectedness to other people and an impoverished feeling of belonging and community. Discouragement can also result when people are overwhelmed by, or overcompensating for, their feelings of inferiority (Eckstein & Kern, 2009). Finally, clients may experience maladjustment because of mistaken beliefs about self, others, and the world, or because of private logic that is interrupting their ability to function fully. The overarching goal of the Adlerian play therapist is to understand a client's style of life so that the therapist can facilitate the client's self-understanding and help him or her shift lifestyle beliefs and behavior toward greater functionality and adjustment.

Theoretical Formulation

In seeking to understand clients, the Adlerian play therapist uses a process of theoretical formulation called a *lifestyle assessment*. Although the bulk of the information gathering about lifestyles happens in the second phase of play therapy—exploration of the client's lifestyle—the Adlerian play therapist begins this process at the point of initial contact. Because lifestyle is the foundation of the theoretical formulation, the play therapist explores a number of important aspects of the client's lifestyle, including assets, functioning at life tasks, goals of misbehavior, "Crucial Cs" (discussed shortly), personality priorities, lifestyle convictions, and private logic (Kottman, 2003, 2009, 2011a). Since family constellation and family atmosphere play a pivotal role in the development of the client's lifestyle, the therapist also explores the impact of growing up in this particular family as well. Because

AdPT includes a parent consultation component (and a teacher consultation component when appropriate), the therapist simultaneously explores the same aspects of the lifestyles of the significant adults in a child's life as well.

Assets

Adlerian therapy is strength-based whenever possible. Since Adlerian therapists believe that discouragement is the primary source of struggling for clients, it is important to gather information about the assets (emotional, behavior, attitudinal) of clients and of other people in their lives as a vehicle for countering discouragement.

Life Tasks

Another theoretical formulation Adlerians use is a template of the five life tasks: work, love, friendship, spirituality/meaning of existence, and self (Mosak & Maniacci, 1999). "The tasks of life provide a useful overview as to how the client is currently functioning in the core issues confronting everyone" (Eckstein & Baruth, 1996, p. 116). The Adlerian play therapist examines how children are doing in each of these five areas to help determine which of the areas are strengths and which need external support or help for optimal functioning. In children, the life task of work would be assessed in terms of their functioning at school or preschool; the life task of love, their relationships with other family members; the friendship task would be peer relationships; the spiritual/ existential task would consist of their attitudes toward and relationship with some kind of higher being; and the task of self would involve the development of a sense of self-worth and self-efficacy.

Goals of Misbehavior

When children are discouraged, they often exhibit inappropriate behavior. According to Dreikur and Soltz (1964), there are four possible goals of misbehavior: gaining attention, power, or revenge and proving inadequacy. Because the intervention strategies of the Adlerian play therapist are goal-specific, it is important to determine the goal or goals of children's misbehavior. Recognizing and responding appropriately to the specific goal is also an essential skill to teach in parent and/or teacher consultation.

Crucial Cs

Another important area of theoretical formulation in exploring client lifestyles is the Crucial Cs (Lew & Bettner, 1996, 2000). Lew and Bettner (2000) developed the concept of the Crucial Cs to describe aspects of resiliency that distinguish children who are prepared to be successful in life and develop strong relationships from those who struggle. Lew and Bettner noted that successful children have four beliefs that serve as behavioral guides and determining principles in perception, attitude, and behavior. These beliefs are the certainty of "Being connected to others, feeling a sense of community; being capable of taking care of oneself; being valued by others, knowing that one counts and makes a difference; and having courage" (Lew & Bettner, 2000, p. 3). When children have the internal resources provided by the Crucial Cs (connection, capability, counting, and courage), they are resilient, resourceful, productive, and happy, prepared to cope successfully with challenges.

Children who have a solid sense of belonging have confidence in their own ability to form relationships, making and maintaining friends at school and in the neighborhood with little if any difficulty. In play therapy, they easily build rapport with the therapist and behave confidently in the playroom. Children who feel *capable* believe that they can take care of themselves. They are grounded in their own competence and confident in their ability to do things in the playroom and outside; they have a strong sense of self-efficacy at school and home. Children who believe that they *count* know they are worthy of love and attention, know that they have meaning and value without having to do something special to earn it. Without being arrogant, they have a sense of assurance that others recognize they are valuable and important. Children who have *courage* believe that they can face life and take psychological risks even in situations when there is not a guarantee of success. They feel hopeful, confident, and equal to others. They are willing to take the risk of trying new things.

In AdPT, the therapist assesses each of these areas (Kottman, 2003) as a means for building on strengths and remediating possible deficits. For Crucial Cs in which a client is weak, the therapist develops play therapy strategies and helps foster parenting strategies designed to strengthen them. For more well-developed Crucial Cs, the therapist emphasizes that the child can capitalize on them as assets. In parent–teacher consultation, the Adlerian play therapist also conceptualizes the Crucial Cs of the important adults in children's lives, working with them to improve the ones that are weak and capitalize on the ones that are strong (Kottman & Dougherty, 2014).

Personality Priorities

Another important aspect of the theoretical formulation of clients' lifestyles is identifying personality priorities (Kefir, 1981). *Personality priority* is the organizational principle for people's pattern of behavior and their reactions to interpersonal situations. It is based on beliefs about how to best acquire belonging, significance, and a sense of mastery. Combining the work of Kefir, Pew (1976), and others, Kottman (2003) identified four priorities: pleasing, comfort, control, and superiority. Children whose personality priority is to please others gain their sense of belonging and mastery by attempting to keep others happy. These children may lack confidence in their

self-worth and, as a result, strive to gain acceptance and approval through meeting others' needs. Children whose personality priority is comfort seek pleasure and ease. They are motivated to avoid stress, expectations, and responsibility and, as a result, may underachieve, have difficulty getting things done, and feel undervalued by others.

Kottman (2003) noted that the last two priorities, control and superiority, could both be split into two subcategories. For example, those with control as a priority might be committed to either control of self or control of others and everything. Children with control as a personality priority seek to gain significance and a sense of belonging by maintaining personal control or showing that others cannot control them. These children feel uncomfortable in situations in which they perceive they do not have control, and they work diligently to avoid feeling out of control. Children with this priority may be prone to anxiety and frustration, and they may have difficulty with spontaneity and intimacy.

Finally, children whose personality priority is superiority gain a sense of belonging and identity by striving for perfection and achievement in all they do. Similar to control as a personality priority, superiority can be divided into two subcategories: achieving, interested in personal accomplishment and mastery without the need to compare to others; or outdoing, prone to measuring their self-worth by comparing their performance to that of others. Children with superiority personality priorities typically devote considerable energy to accomplishment in order to be noticed and accepted by others. As a result, they may struggle with perfectionism and a sense of meaninglessness and futility. Kottman (2003) has noted that people have a primary and sometimes a secondary personality priority that is an organizing pattern for coping with situations and relationships. In consultation with important adults, the Adlerian play therapist assesses personality priorities and uses them as a means of custom designing suggestions and interventions (Kottman & Dougherty, 2014).

Family Constellation and Family Atmosphere

Pivotal to understanding the lifestyle of the client is an understanding of the family constellation and atmosphere. Adler (1931/1958) noted the impact of family constellation and birth order. More recent Adlerian theorists (Dreikurs & Soltz, 1964; Eckstein & Kern, 2009; Mosak & Maniacci, 1999) and researchers (e.g., Campbell, White, & Stewart, 1991; Eckstein et al., 2010; Stewart, Stewart, & Campbell, 2001) have emphasized psychological birth order rather than ordinal position in the family. Adlerians contend that the family context is the earliest place where individuals seek to belong. As a result, being an oldest, middle, youngest, or only child has an impact on lifestyle development. Similarly, the family atmosphere—the general affect or tone of the family—interacts with family constellation to impact lifestyle. Family atmosphere is created through an alchemy of parental characteristics: attitudes toward the children, discipline philosophies, lifestyles, family values, family atmosphere of their own family of origin, the marital relationship, parenting skills, assets, and any personal problems or life circumstances that might reduce their ability to provide warmth, respect, and structure for the children (Kottman, 2003). For instance, financial pressures or parental health issues can interact with family constellation to have a differential impact on family members. Understanding these issues of family constellation and atmosphere can help the therapist gain understanding of the client's lifestyle. In AdPT, the therapist seeks to develop an understanding of children by asking the question, "What is it like to be this particular child in this particular family at this particular moment in time? How has being this child in this family affected the child's patterns of thinking, feeling, and behaving?"

Basic Convictions and Mistaken Beliefs

From their individual experience and interpretation of an amalgam of all of these factors (assets, functioning at life tasks, goals of misbehavior, Crucial Cs, personality priorities, family constellation, and family atmosphere), children develop basic convictions about self, others, and the world, and they act as if their convictions were true and real (Kottman, 2003). In order to crystalize an understanding of the child's lifestyle, the Adlerian play therapist develops tentative hypotheses about how child clients (and parents and/or teachers) would finish the following sentence stems:

"I am . . . /I must be . . . /I should be . . ."
"Others are . . . /others must be . . . /others should . . ."
"The world is . . . /life is . . . /life must be . . ."
"Based on these convictions, I must/ should . . ."

As we have said, children are excellent observers who may have some distorted interpretations; they act as if their beliefs about self, others, and the world were true; and they often rely on confirmation bias to support their beliefs, getting into situations that prove again what they already believe. It is the task of the play therapist, in hypothesizing answers to the questions above, to determine which of the child's basic convictions about self, others, and the world are mistaken. In Adlerian formulations, a mistaken belief is a discouraged, self-defeating belief whose correction or readjustment would benefit the client. Once these mistaken beliefs have been identified, the Adlerian therapist helps the client gain insight by bringing these self-defeating patterns in thinking, feeling, and behaving into awareness and challenging them to adopt new, more adaptive ways of seeing self, others, and the world, and acting as if those new beliefs were true.

Goals of the Therapeutic Process and Role of the Therapist, Child, and Parents

In the service of moving the client from discouragement to empowerment, the Adlerian play therapist has several overarching therapeutic goals. The process of therapy is designed to (1) help the client gain an awareness of, and an insight into, his or her lifestyle; (2) change mistaken beliefs about self, others, and the world; (3) shift toward more positive goals of behavior; (4) replace destructive patterns for belonging and feeling significant with constructive patterns; (5) increase the client's social interest, the sense of connectedness with others; (6) adopt positive methods for coping with inferiority feelings; (7) recognize and capitalize on the client's assets; and (8) develop self-enhancing choices in the client toward increasingly positive attitudes, feelings, and behaviors (Kottman, 2003, 2009).

AdPT is comprised of four phases:

1. Building an egalitarian relationship.
2. Exploring the child's lifestyle.
3. Helping the client gain insight into lifestyle.
4. Providing reorientation/reeducation.

These are not always discrete, sequential stages of therapy, with clear and identifiable transitions. For instance, while building an egalitarian relationship (first phase), the therapist is typically also gathering initial impressions and developing early hypotheses about the client's lifestyle (second phase); and certainly helping the client gain insight into lifestyle (third phase) can also serve in reorienting/reeducating the client (fourth phase).

Each of the four phases has its own goal (Kottman, 2003, 2009; Kottman, Bryant, Alexander, & Kroger, 2008). The therapeutic goal of the first phase of AdPT is building egalitarian, empathic relationships—with the child client and with his or her parents (Kottman, 2003, 2009). In some cases, the therapist may also work on creating connections with additional family members; and if the child is struggling at school, the therapist will probably want to make a connection with the child's teacher as well.

In the second phase, the play therapist explores the lifestyles of the child and the other people who have an impact on the child. During this phase, the play therapist works to develop hypotheses about the child's beliefs, goals, emotions, attitudes, and motives, as well as those of his or her parents, not to mention (when appropriate) teachers, siblings, and other family members. It is also important to consider the interaction between the child's lifestyle and the lifestyles of these significant others. This is so that, in the third phase, the play therapist can help all of the interested parties gain insight into their own lifestyles, mistaken beliefs, and self-defeating behaviors and goals. The therapist also strives to help the adults in the child's life to understand the child better, to become more empathic, and to understand the interaction between their own lifestyles and that of the child. As the client develops insight, therapy moves into the fourth phase, where the goal is to help the client apply newfound understandings and encouraging perspectives, converting insight into action with attitudinal, cognitive, emotional, and behavioral changes.

"Through the process of Adlerian play therapy, the role of the therapist is that of partner, encourager, and teacher with children, parents, teachers and siblings" (Kottman, 2011a, p. 97). Adlerian play therapists believe that the family *system*, comprised of the child, his or her parents, and other family members, is the actual client, rather than the child alone. Consistent with this view, AdPT considers the child, the parents, and siblings as partners in therapy. Consequently, Adlerian play therapists are hopeful that all members of the system will be interested in gaining insight and making changes, and that they will be willing to actively participate in the process of therapy. We also believe that family members are the experts on their lives, so we rely on them to share information about how things work in the family.

Throughout the four phases of AdPT, the roles of the people involved in the therapeutic process often shift within the partnership framework. In the first phase, the Adlerian play therapist is relatively non-directive with the child. After establishing that "sometimes in here I get to be the boss and sometimes you get to be the boss," the therapist encourages the child to make many of the decisions in the playroom as a way of creating a partnership of teamwork and cooperation (Kottman, 2003, 2011a). The role of the child is to play, to learn to trust the play therapist, to fully engage in connection with this trustworthy adult, and to learn to share power in the spirit of partnership. With the adults in the child's life, the role of the therapist is to establish a trusting and honest connection by listening and providing encouragement and understanding. The role of the parents (and teachers) is to open up about what is going on in their family (or their classroom) and provide honest information about the presenting problem, family dynamics, and any past intervention strategies that have—or have not—worked.

During the second phase, the play therapist's role is much more active and directive, with the therapist asking questions and asking the child to tell stories, draw, do puppet shows, make sandtrays, play in the dollhouse or kitchen area, and engage in interactive games. The role of the child is to cooperate with this process, engaging playfully with the activities suggested by the therapist, and initiating other play. Meeting with parents and teachers, the therapist is active and directive, soliciting information about the adults' perceptions of the child's lifestyle, their own lifestyles, and the interaction between the two. In order to make

the best use of this process, the expectation of these significant adults is that they are forthcoming, cooperative, and honest. During this process, the therapist acts as a detective, trying to ferret out details of the clients' experience that might be clues to their lifestyles and developing a lifestyle conceptualization for each of the involved parties. Based on these conceptualizations, the therapist devises a treatment plan that guides the rest of the therapeutic process.

In the third phase, the play therapist continues in an active and directive role, in this case, in the service of helping the child and parents and teachers gain insight into their own and one another's lifestyles. Making interpretive comments and developing therapeutic metaphors, the therapist holds up a mirror for clients so that they can begin to capitalize on their strengths and recognize maladaptive patterns in their thinking, feelings, and behaving. The role of the child is to be open to this feedback from the therapist, and to be willing to consider alternative beliefs, goals, thoughts, attitudes, and behaviors. Similar to the child's role, parents and teachers should be willing to consider new ways of thinking about the child and their relationship, and be open to making changes in their own interactional patterns.

The therapist's role in the fourth phase, combining both nondirective and directive components, is focused on providing encouragement for progress and teaching skills. In the nondirective component the therapist observes the child's play and makes comments on effort, progress, and assets, and encourages the child's movement in a positive direction. It is important that the therapist use a similar strategy to encourage parents and teachers in making changes. The more directive component is the active teaching of skills with both the child and adults. The role of the child client in this phase involves a willingness to use the play for learning new skills, including anger management, friendship, negotiation, and so forth; and the role of the adults consists of acquiring and experimenting with new strategies for interacting with the child.

Strategies and Techniques

Not surprisingly, each phase of AdPT has a different set of strategies and techniques. In the first phase, these strategies are similar to the nondirective relationship-building techniques used in many different approaches to play therapy, combined with several techniques unique to AdPT (Kottman, 2011b). These relationship-building skills continue throughout the process, whereas other, more directive and uniquely Adlerian strategies are added in the other three phases.

Building an Egalitarian Relationship

The initial task in the process of AdPT is building an egalitarian relationship with the child. In order to do so, the play therapist tracks behavior, restates content, returns responsibility to the child, and reflects feelings—all techniques consistent with many other play therapy approaches (Kottman, 2011b). One of the ways the Adlerian play therapist builds relationships with clients is by using their metaphors. The Adlerian play therapist takes pains to use the language of the metaphor and participate in metaphorical play. The therapist might also use the whisper technique to acknowledge the metaphorical nature of the play. The whisper technique is simply a stage whisper used to ask the client about the therapist's role or next action in the sequence of play (e.g., "What should I do now?"). This technique honors the metaphor in the play and lets the therapist participate when the client wants and in ways consistent with the client's plan or agenda for the metaphor. In addition to these nearly universal play therapy techniques, there are a number of more distinctive interventions used by the Adlerian play therapist.

One somewhat distinctive aspect of AdPT is the allowance—even the suggestion—that the therapist engage in the interaction authentically and actively. To this end, the Adlerian play therapist interacts actively with the child, cooperating in playful activity, giving explanations, and asking and answering questions when it is appropriate.

Another distinctive aspect of AdPT is the intentional use of encouragement in the therapeutic process. In contrast to praise, *encouragement* is an acknowledgment of the child's progress and effort rather than of the result or product. Such an acknowledgment shows trust, confidence, and acceptance of the child. Both in this beginning phase and throughout the process of therapy, the Adlerian play therapist rarely does anything for clients that they could do themselves. Encouragement is a way to clearly communicate to clients that they can do things for themselves, learn to do things for themselves, or, in rare situations, cooperate with the therapist in finding a solution or doing things together (Kottman, 2003).

The Adlerian play therapist sets limits in a unique four-step process (Kottman, 2003). In the first step, the therapist states limits in a nonjudgmental manner using the phrase, "It is against the playroom rules to . . . [whatever the child might be about to do that violates a limit]." This is said in a calm but firm voice. The second step involves reflecting any feelings the child might be exhibiting and making a guess about the purpose of the child's behavior (e.g., "You are mad. I am guessing that you are trying to show me that I can't tell you what to do"; or "Could it be that you want to see how I react if you pour the sand on the floor?"). For the third step, the therapist engages the child in generating alternatives that would not violate the rules of the playroom by saying something like, "I bet we could figure out something you could pour the sand into that wouldn't be against the playroom rules." At the end of this step, the therapist and the child have come to a consensus about a behavior that both parties agree is appropriate in the playroom. In many cases, this is the last step that is necessary. Since the child has been involved in coming up with an acceptable alternative, he or she seldom continues the proscribed behavior. Every once in a while, the child makes the decision to repeat the disallowed behavior. When this happens, the therapist must implement the fourth step, which involves engaging the child in developing a logical consequence for abrogating the agreement set in Step 3. During this process, the therapist comes to an agreement with the child about those consequences and follows through with whatever consequences have been determined.

One other distinctive aspect of the AdPT approach is that the client and therapist clean up the playroom together at the end of the session (Kottman, 2003, 2011b). Although not a rigid requirement of AdPT, cleaning up the room together allows for the therapist and client to cooperate in completing a necessary task (someone must clean up eventually). This cooperation can help build the relationship and begin to build social interest in the client.

Exploring Clients' Lifestyles

The second phase of AdPT is exploring the client's lifestyle and the lifestyle of the other significant people in the client's life. In this phase of therapy, the therapist is involved in the process of gathering information that will allow him or her to propose tentative hypotheses about the client's lifestyle and then test those hypotheses with additional data. The Adlerian play therapist may initially attempt to understand the client's context by considering the client's family constellation and family atmosphere. The therapist also begins to consider hypotheses in a number of areas, including functioning at life tasks, assets, the goals of behavior and misbehavior, personality priorities, Crucial Cs, lifestyle convictions, and mistaken beliefs. In order to gather information as a vehicle for

developing the lifestyle conceptualization, the Adlerian play therapist asks questions of the child, parents, and teachers (Kottman, 2003). These questions are designed to gather information about the child: the presenting problem; relationships with peers; family dynamics; problem-solving strategies; how the child fits into the family, the classroom, and the neighborhood; and a myriad of other factors. The therapist may also use directive art techniques (e.g., family drawings, classroom drawings, self-portraits), sandtray techniques, play strategies (e.g., board games, interactive adventure techniques, movement and dance strategies), and early recollections to gather information about lifestyles of the child, the parents, and other involved individuals (Ashby, Kottman, & DeGraaf, 2008; Kottman, 2003, 2011b; Kottman, Ashby, & DeGraaf, 2001).

Sometimes the Adlerian play therapist observes the child's play, his or her interactions with others, or parents' actions and relationships as vehicles for gathering information about personality priorities, goals of misbehavior, and Crucial Cs. The following is an example of one Adlerian strategy in which the therapist observes behavior and interactions in the second phase of play therapy as a method of gaining an understanding of clients. As the therapist observes the child and others in the child's life, he or she assesses their personality priorities by internally asking a series of questions, starting with, "What is the person trying to avoid?" The person with a comfort personality priority is trying to avoid stress, responsibility, and expectations. A second question would be, "What is this person striving to achieve?" The person with a pleasing personality priority, for instance, is trying to meet the needs of others and keep everyone happy. A third question is, "What are the client's assets, or what does he or she do well?" The person with a control personality priority is often a good leader, for example, assertive, organized, and responsible. Finally, in order to assess the personality priority of a client, a play therapist can ask, "What is the price the client pays for the way he or she interacts with others?" The person with a superiority personality priority may feel overwhelmed and overinvolved. Internally asking these questions while interacting with the child, talking with teachers and parents, and observing the child's play can assist in identifying personality priorities.

To determine the goal of a particular misbehavior, the Adlerian play therapist asks the following questions:

What is the child's misbehavior?

How does the child feel when he or she exhibits the misbehavior?

What is underneath the child's misbehavior?

What need does the child have that is not being met?

How does the parent or other adult feel when the child exhibits the misbehavior?

What does the parent or other adult do in response to the misbehavior?

What does the child do in response to any disciplinary or corrective action taken by the parent or other adult?

A child who exhibits misbehavior designed to get attention feels as though he or she does not matter when not getting attention. The child's misbehavior could include bothering others, showing off, creating minor mischief, acting the class or family clown, saying "I can't," being anxious or lazy, or other similar behaviors. Underneath the child's misbehavior is an attempt to get attention by any means possible. All of us need and want attention, and if we cannot get attention in positive ways, we shift into the mode of getting attention in negative ways. Parents or other adults, when encountering misbehavior aimed at getting attention, usually feel irritated or annoyed and ask the child to stop the misbehavior. When a child striving for attention is corrected, he or she usually stops for a short time, only to resume the attention-seeking behavior after a brief interval.

Children whose goal is power feel that they only count when dominating or making sure that others do what they want them to do. They also want to communicate, "You cannot control me." They may argue, contradict, throw tantrums, be dishonest, be defiant, get into power struggles, be disrespectful, be stubborn, disobey, do little or no work, or exhibit passive–aggressive tendencies. Underneath the power-directed misbehavior is usually a feeling of being out of control or unsafe when someone else is in control. These children need to have some age-appropriate control of their lives, along with structure, routine, and rules with predictable consequences for noncompliance. When parents or other adults encounter this behavior, they tend to get angry, feeling challenged, threatened, or provoked. After some kind of corrective response from an adult, children who are striving for power tend to escalate, working harder to dominate others or show that others cannot control them.

A child who is seeking revenge has almost always been hurt in some way by others in his or her life and is aiming to make sure that no one else can have a chance to repeat an abusive or neglectful scenario. These children feel that other people are dangerous and that they must push others away to stay safe. Their need for safety has not been met by the significant adults in their lives and they do not trust the safety of their environments. Underneath this behavior is a desire to make a preemptive strike to prevent being vulnerable and/or a belief that relationships involve the infliction of pain and suffering. Behaviors may include malicious or violent outbursts or attacks, being cruel or hurtful to others (either verbally or physically), stealing, acting like a bully, making threats, and using withholding to wound others. When parents or other adults encounter these behaviors, they may feel hurt, they may desire payback against the child, or they may withdraw from the relationship in order to protect themselves. When this child experiences discipline or consequences, he or she tends to "up the ante" on his or her revenge-seeking behaviors.

Children who are striving to prove that they are inadequate believe that they cannot do anything right, so they decide that they will not try to do anything at all. Underneath their determination to demonstrate their incompetence is the belief that they are not capable, and they don't count. The important adults in their lives have not adequately fostered these two Crucial Cs, and the result is a sense of disconnection and a failure of courage. These children simply do not try—in school, at home, in life—and they give up easily, are often depressed, and may be suicidal. Adults, when interacting with them, feel discouraged, helpless, and hopeless. These children get criticized for being underachieving, but seldom get punished because they do not actively do much. When they feel judged or criticized, they become even more discouraged and shut down even more radically.

There are similar processes for assessing each of the Crucial Cs, the life tasks, lifestyle convictions, and mistaken beliefs. Throughout the second phase, the play therapist considers the child's behavior, asks questions, and uses direct play therapy techniques to gather information to systematically conceptualize the child and the adults in the child's life and to create a treatment plan for intervention in the third and fourth phases of the process.

Helping Clients Gain Insight into Their Lifestyles

During the third phase of AdPT, the therapist is again active and directive in the playroom, using a tentative hypothesis format to metacommunicate about patterns and themes connected to his or her theoretical formulation of the lifestyles of the involved parties (Kottman, 2003, 2011a). The play therapist makes interpretive guesses about the child's functioning at life tasks, his or her assets, the goals of behavior and misbehavior, personality priorities and Crucial Cs, as well as family dynamics, relationship patterns, problem-solving strategies, and any other aspects of the child's lifestyle that might be outside of the child's awareness and/or might be getting in the way of optimal functioning. In this phase, the Adlerian play therapist metacommunicates about single events/behaviors, about the meaning of specific events/behaviors, about patterns within or across sessions, and/or about lifestyle themes. The therapist also shares hypotheses about the fact that the child acts as if his or her mistaken beliefs are true. Pointing out patterns in which a client is acting in ways that are self-defeating because of mistaken beliefs is called "spitting in the client's soup" and is a particularly Adlerian technique (Kottman, 2003; Sweeney, 2009).

Metacommunication and spitting in the soup are the primary tools for helping parents and teachers gain insight into the child's lifestyle, into their own lifestyles, and into the interaction between the child's lifestyle and their own lifestyles. During this phase, the play therapist also uses didactic teaching to help parents and teachers learn about lifestyle components such as personality priorities and Crucial Cs. The play therapist also tries to reframe the child's behavior and help the adults in the child's life to appreciate the child's assets and the underlying dynamics of the goals of the misbehavior.

The other primary tool during the third phase of AdPT is designing and delivering therapeutic metaphors. Using a variety of delivery formats (e.g., puppet shows, dollhouse play, making books, drawing or painting, telling stories), the play therapist develops a story that has some relationship to a situation, problem, or relationship in the child's life. The therapist includes a protagonist who represents the child and characters that represent others in the child's life (allies, resource people, and antagonists). The process is designed to give the child suggestions about possible new ways to deal with problems, or to help the child learn new skills or gain a more positive perspective on difficult situations. If the therapist is intimidated by the prospect of having to generate an original story, he or she can use good children's literature to create a bibliotherapy intervention. Adlerian play therapists also use an adapted version of mutual storytelling (Gardner, 1993; Kottman, 2003, 2011b), creative characters (Brooks, 1981; Kottman, 2003, 2011b), and shared stories as vehicles for communicating stories and therapeutic metaphors to help the child gain insight into his or her lifestyle. The therapist may even use storytelling with parents and teachers, telling metaphorical stories about other adults who have experienced similar situations and how they handled them.

The Adlerian play therapist also uses directive art techniques, sandtrays, role playing, immediacy, confrontation, and humor in the third phase of counseling, both with child clients and with parents and teachers. During this third phase, the therapist may also invite other family members or classmates of the child to participate in play sessions.

Reorienting and Reeducating Clients

In the fourth phase of AdPT, the emphasis is on teaching skills to child clients and their parents, teachers, and family members. The therapist uses play as a vehicle to help the child generate alternative, appropriate behaviors and attitudes, teach the child new behaviors and attitudes, and help the child practice those new behaviors and attitudes, including their application outside the playroom. Focusing on shifts in thinking, feeling, and behaving, the therapist uses art, sandtrays, storytelling, role-playing, and adventure therapy activities (Ashby et al., 2008; Kottman, 2003; Kottman et al., 2001) to work with the child on learning skills for effectively solving problems; building better

relationships; optimizing assets; enhancing Crucial Cs; functioning optimally at all five life tasks; shifting to more appropriate behavioral goals; manifesting the constructive aspects of personality priorities rather than the negative aspects; and substituting positive convictions about self, others, and the world for mistaken beliefs. The child may also need help in learning basic skills for managing anger, making and maintaining friends, being appropriately assertive, dealing with frustration, regulating emotions, and so forth. Encouragement related to effort and progress helps to cement the learning that has occurred throughout the therapeutic process.

With parents and other significant adults, the Adlerian play therapist uses these same tools to actively teach Adlerian concepts such as Crucial Cs, personality priorities, and goals of misbehavior. He or she works with parents and teachers to help them become better at fostering the Crucial Cs and developing the positive aspects of children's personality priorities. These adults learn to use encouragement, natural and logical consequences, and limited choices in dealing with children. They engage in conversations about problem ownership and paying attention to children's needs. The therapist encourages them to look at how their own issues might be interfering with their ability to be fully present with children; and if these problems are significant, the play therapist may refer parents for marital counseling, personal counseling, or family therapy as a more appropriate and efficacious venue for change.

Research Support

To date, the effectiveness of AdPT has not been systematically investigated. However, there is some recent evidence for its efficacy in school settings. For instance, Meany-Walen, Bratton, and Kottman (2014) found that AdPT was effective in reducing elementary school students' disruptive behaviors. In addition, Rosselet and Stauffer (2013) reported that, in a case study example with a gifted adolescent, AdPT techniques combined with role-playing games facilitated increased psychosocial development.

Clinical Case Example

In this purely hypothetical case study (not drawn from actual clinical material), Karen is a 6-year-old African American female in first grade in a public elementary school. She lives with her mother and stepfather (of 2 years). Karen has one younger sibling, a half-brother, Darius, who is 6 months old and whose biological father is Karen's stepfather. Karen does not have a relationship with her biological father. Karen's mother referred her for play therapy because of recent withdrawal and social isolation at school and home. "She just came home from Grandma's different. . . ."

In an initial consultation with Karen's parents, the therapist learns that Karen had been living with her maternal grandmother in another state over the summer before returning home to begin school. Since her return home, Karen has been withdrawn, engaging in only limited social interaction at school, in contrast to her experience in kindergarten. Karen appears to have an average to above-average IQ and was an early reader, a skill she practiced with her grandmother over the summer.

In the first phase of AdPT, the therapist works to develop an egalitarian relationship with Karen. By sharing leadership in the playroom, the Adlerian play therapist can invite Karen into play, as well as cooperate with her in any play in which Karen would like the therapist to be included. While the therapist is working to build an egalitarian relationship, he or she is also beginning to assess Karen's lifestyle, personality priority, functioning in life tasks, Crucial Cs, etc. In this initial phase and throughout the AdPT process, the therapist consults with parents

and other important adults (e.g., teachers). In assessing Karen's lifestyle, the therapist is likely to first consider the assets and strengths on which Karen can build (e.g., her intelligence). The therapist might also assess Karen's Crucial Cs, personality priorities, and private logic to discover how she has developed a style to fit into the world and gain a sense of belonging. The therapist can then test initial hypotheses by gathering more information through further observation, interactive play, and ongoing parental and teacher consultation.

In Karen's case, the therapist might have an initial hypothesis that Karen doesn't feel she counts. Given the recent changes in her family constellation, including the arrival of her new sibling, shifts in family atmosphere, her mother's marriage and the arrival of a stepfather, and the shift from being the center of attention at her grandmother's back to sharing attention and focus at home, Karen may not feel an adequate sense of belonging and significance. In the second phase of AdPT, the therapist will use a variety of techniques, depending on the child, the developing lifestyle assessment of the child, and the personal style of the therapist, to fully explore the client's lifestyle, testing this and other initial hypotheses.

In the third and fourth phases of AdPT with Karen, the therapist will work to facilitate Karen's understanding and insight into her lifestyle, build on her assets, and help her practice and generalize new ways of thinking and behaving. In the service of these goals, the Adlerian play therapist is limited in intervention only by imagination and time. For instance, the therapist may use metaphor, bibilotherapy, puppets, formal games, sandplay, etc. The one caveat is that the Adlerian play therapist uses the techniques in ways consistent with a treatment plan based on the client's lifestyle assessment and sources of discouragement. In the case of Karen, the therapist might well use techniques to foster her Crucial Cs, particularly the degree to which she counts.

The therapist might also work to shift Karen's mistaken beliefs about her ability to fit in her family, her school, and the world.

Conclusion

AdPT is a method of integrating the concepts and techniques of individual psychology with play therapy. Through four phases of therapy, the Adlerian play therapist seeks to establish a relationship with the client, explore the client's lifestyle, help the client gain insight into his or her lifestyle, and reorient and reeducate the client. AdPT offers several unique ways to conceptualize children and the important adults in their lives: through assessment of their goals of misbehavior, the Crucial Cs, and personality priorities. In the practice of AdPT, play therapists can utilize a wide variety of play therapy strategies and techniques, while still staying theoretically grounded and practicing with a natural style that allows therapists to be themselves.

REFERENCES

Adler, A. (1958). *What life should mean to you* (A. Porter, Ed.). New York: Prestige. (Original work published 1931)

Ansbacher, H., & Ansbacher, R. (Eds.). (1956). *The individual psychology of Alfred Adler: A systematic presentation in selections from his writings.* New York: Harper & Row.

Ashby, J., Kottman, T., & DeGraaf, D. (2008). *Active intervention for kids and teens.* Alexandria, VA: American Counseling Association.

Brooks, R. (1981). Creative characters: A technique in child therapy. *Psychotherapy, 18,* 131–139.

Campbell, L., White, J., & Stewart, A. (1991). The relationship of psychological birth order to actual birth order. *Individual Psychology: Journal of Adlerian Theory, Research, and Practice, 47*(3), 380–391.

Carlson, J., Watts, R., & Maniacci, M. (2005). *Adlerian therapy: Theory and practice.* Washington, DC: American Psychological Association.

Dreikurs, R., & Soltz, V. (1964). *Children: The challenge.* New York: Hawthorn/Dutton.

Eckstein, D., Aycock, K. J., Sperber, M. A., McDonald, J., Van Wiesner, V., III, Watts, R. E., et al. (2010). A review of 200 birth-order studies: Lifestyle characteristics. *Journal of Individual Psychology, 66*(4), 408–434.

Eckstein, D., & Baruth, L. (1996). *Theory and practice of life-style assessment.* Dubuque, IA: Kendall Hunt.

Eckstein, D., & Kern, R. (2009). *Psychological fingerprints* (6th ed.). Dubuque, IA: Kendall Hunt.

Gardner, R. (1993). *Storytelling in psychotherapy with children.* Northvale, NJ: Aronson.

Kefir, N. (1981). Impasse/priority therapy. In R. Corsini (Ed.), *Handbook of innovative psychotherapies* (pp. 400–415). New York: Wiley.

Kottman, T. (2003). *Partners in play: An Adlerian approach to play therapy* (2nd ed.). Alexandria, VA: American Counseling Association.

Kottman, T. (2009). Adlerian play therapy. In K. O'Connor & L. Braverman (Eds.), *Play therapy theory and practice: Comparing theories and techniques* (2nd ed., pp. 237–282). New York: Wiley.

Kottman, T. (2011a). Adlerian play therapy. In C. Schaefer (Ed.), *Foundations of play therapy* (2nd ed., pp. 87–104). New York: Wiley.

Kottman, T. (2011b). *Play therapy: Basics and beyond* (2nd ed.). Alexandria, VA: American Counseling Association.

Kottman, T., Ashby, J., & DeGraaf, D. (2001). *Adventures in guidance: How to integrate fun into your guidance program.* Alexandria, VA: American Counseling Association.

Kottman, T., Bryant, J., Alexander, J., & Kroger, S. (2008). Partners in the schools: Adlerian school counseling. In A. Vernon & T. Kottman (Eds.), *Counseling theories: Practical applications with children and adolescents in school settings* (pp. 47–84). Denver, CO: Love.

Kottman, T., & Dougherty, A. M. (2014). *Casebook of psychological consultation and collaboration in school and community settings* (6th ed.). Belmont, CA: Brooks/Cole.

Lew, A., & Bettner, B. L. (1996). *Responsibility in the classroom.* Newton Center, MA: Connexions.

Lew, A., & Bettner, B. L. (2000). *A parent's guide to motivating children.* Newton Center, MA: Connexions.

Lewin, K. (1951). *Field theory in social science: Selected theoretical papers* (D. Cartwright, Ed.). New York: Harper & Row.

Meany-Walen, K. K., Bratton, S. C., & Kottman, T. (2014). Effects of Adlerian play therapy on reducing students' disruptive behaviors. *Journal of Counseling and Development, 92,* 47–56.

Mosak, H., & Maniacci, M. (1999). *A primer of Adlerian psychology: The analytic–behavioral–cognitive psychology of Alfred Adler.* New York: Routledge.

Mosak, H., & Maniacci, M. (2010). Adlerian psychology. In R. Corsini & D. Wedding (Eds.), *Current psychotherapies* (9th ed., pp. 67–112). Belmont, CA: Brooks/Cole.

Pew, W. (1976). The number one priority. In *Monograph of the International Association of Individual Psychology* (pp. 1–24). Munich, Germany: International Association of Individual Psychology.

Rosselet, J., & Stauffer, S. D. (2013). Using group role-playing games with gifted children and adolescents: A psychosocial intervention model. *International Journal of Play Therapy, 22,* 173–192.

Stewart, A. E., Stewart, E. A., & Campbell, L. F. (2001). The relationship of psychological birth order to the family atmosphere and to personality. *Journal of Individual Psychology, 57*(4), 363–387.

Sweeney, T. (2009). *Adlerian counseling and psychotherapy: A practitioner's approach* (5th ed.). New York: Routledge.

Watts, R. (2006). Play therapy. In J. Carlson, R. E. Watts, & M. Maniacci (Eds.), *Adlerian therapy: Theory and practice* (pp. 227–249). Washington, DC: American Psychological Association.

CHAPTER 4

Jungian Analytical Play Therapy

J. P. Lilly

To date there have been two very excellent chapters authored by Craig Peery (2003) and Eric Green (2009) that are similar in content to the one that I was asked to write for this text. Being personally acquainted with both Peery and Green, having presented with both of them, and being very familiar with their writings, the request for me to write this chapter was rather daunting. Both of these men are brilliant in their understanding and presentation of Jungian analytical play therapy (JAPT). I have referred to them in my presentations as high-grade engineers, and I have always viewed my talents in this field much like the mechanic who keeps the wheels rolling. In accepting this challenge, I squarely placed myself in front of the mirror and asked myself what I could contribute that would not simply replicate the powerful writings of these two men, but that would actually augment our collective mission to increase the understanding of JAPT among general play therapy clinicians who might not be well acquainted with this theoretical approach. After some internal wrestling, I was able to clearly see that my contribution to this theoretical approach was grounded in delivering a very practical application of JAPT.

As the self-proclaimed "lead mechanic" of JAPT, I have been utilizing the basic tenets of this approach for more than 24 years. During that time, I have seen and experienced many successes and failures. Out of each success and failure, I learned more and more about the practical application of this theory. However, as I have stated in my presentations over the years, theory without practical application is philosophy, and practical application without a theoretical foundation is *dangerous*—for both the clients we serve and the therapists treating them. It is my desire to create therapeutically responsible corners and structure for the application of JAPT. It is also my desire to utilize my thousands of hours "in the saddle" to assist clinicians from all theoretical backgrounds to see and understand the applicability of a delicate and complicated theoretical approach.

Jungian analytical psychology is not an easy method. It is difficult to understand for a number of reasons. One, Jung made up a number of his own terms in defining psychological phenomena. Two, Jung's approach deepened and morphed over the years of his writings. Three, this theoretical approach is concerned with the psychological well-being of the therapist as well as the "unstable" nature of the client. Four, this approach is heavily rooted in phenomena that we cannot quantify, and even the thought of an "objective psyche" is enough to scare most clinicians from this approach. However, if one is willing to brave the depths of this approach and embrace its theoretical principles for their heuristic value, there is another world that opens up with which to help children more fully and profoundly—and that world is the unconscious.

JAPT is not rooted in technique. It does not accept the notion that, simply because children come through the door with a cluster of symptoms that can be easily pigeonholed into a diagnosis, treatment should be dictated by some didactic treatment protocol. This approach does not ascribe to the dictates of "treatment protocol," but rather receives every child into the therapeutic world as a unique individual who has and is processing his or her life in a unique and personally meaningful way. Our goal is not to systematize treatment modalities, but to champion the individual freedom of all children who cross the threshold of safety into our play therapy rooms. We seek to awaken the healer within them to ensure that their healing is genuine and authentic—not the product of an outside agent. Our goal is a true transformational healing, not an elimination of a cluster of symptoms. The reduction and elimination of symptoms are natural results of transformational healing.

This chapter assists readers in understanding how a practitioner of JAPT would view and assess a child who is presented for treatment. I introduce a model that I have been using for more than a decade in understanding the "process" of dysfunction occurring in a child; I address the issues that keep a child stuck in his or her dysfunction and the process by which the clinician can unlock the doors to healing. I also address a few of the key psychological dynamics of Jungian analytical theory (see also Green, 2009; Peery, 2003) to assist the reader in more easily understanding the process by which children heal utilizing this theoretical approach.

Description of the Approach

The foundation of JAPT begins with the structure of the psyche. The word that Jung used for psyche was the German word *seele*, which does not translate equally into English. Jung's (1971) definition encompassed the "totality of all psychic processes, conscious as well as unconscious" (para. 797). Although simplistic in definition, for our purposes I use the word *psyche* to encompass both conscious and unconscious structures.

Jung's view of the conscious mind was similar to that of Freud. Both viewed consciousness as acted upon both by the unconscious and by the world at large. Freud gave us the "ego" as that part of the psychological structure that mediates between societal mores and norms (superego) and the instinctual sexual impulses of the unconscious (id). Jung's view of the ego was much more complex, with the ego having both a collective and personal quality. He used the term "collective consciousness" to represent the collective (or the "many") of society, community, and culture that defines for us (the individual) what is normal, customary, and acceptable. Jung theorized that one of man's greatest challenges in each person's life is that of "individuation," whereby one becomes truly one's truest self by individuating from both the collective consciousness and the collective unconscious. Both Freud and Jung viewed the role of the ego as mediating between the conscious and unconscious minds; however, Jung's theoretical structure did not accept the view that the ego was the center of the personality. According to Jung, the ego was not capable of identifying personality by itself; it needed another component to become whole, and that was the *Self* (capitalized to differentiate it from the conscious self). This meant that there had to be a level of connectedness between the ego and the Self in order for the personality to be whole. This relationship between the ego and the Self was later named by Edward Edinger (1972/1992) as the "ego–self axis," whereby there is an interchange of both conscious and unconscious energy. Jung (1958) referred to this dynamic exchange in analogical terms: "[the] ego stands to the Self as the moved to the mover, or as object to subject" (CW 11, para. 391). This interconnection between the ego and the Self is critical in understanding the methodology of the JAPT therapist. It is our belief that when ego defenses become too impermeable, the Self has no ability to influence the ego, and the child has no "inner direction" by which he might recover, adapt, or live in harmony with Self. Edinger illustrated this process by showing that a child with thick ego defenses is detached from the Self and prone to "outbursts and snapping" (1972/1992, p. 5). He also noted that when there are no ego defenses, the child can be "uncontrollable and hyperactive" (p. 5). One of the primary tasks of the JAPT therapist is to create an environment that facilitates the restoration of a healthy ego–Self axis in the child. The methodology by which we accomplish this is illustrated later in this chapter.

Similarities and Differences between Jung and Freud

Jung's view of the unconscious was similar to Freud's in referencing material that was inaccessible to the ego. They also both viewed the unconscious as having different layers of depth to it, with Freud using the term *preconscious* to describe the part of the unconscious that is just outside of consciousness and that contains material that could be easily retrieved with little to no effort (e.g., a telephone number or street address). Jung also believed in different strata to the unconscious. However, that is where the similarities between the two theorists ended. Jung did not view the unconscious solely as a repository of instinctual and sexual im-

pulses, forgotten and repressed material, and personal experiences. Jung rejected the Lockean notion of the psyche as simply a *tabula rasa* onto which experiences are etched from the inception of life onward. Instead Jung forwarded the theoretical position that the unconscious is a source of powerful psychological activity and that it has an objective quality to it. As with the conscious mind, the unconscious has both collective and personal components. Jung called the "layer" of the unconscious that holds the memories and experiences specific to an individual that are either repressed or forgotten the "personal unconscious." This layer rests upon the deeper part of the psyche, called the "collective unconscious," the storehouse of the patterns or "archetypes" of humanity's lived experiences across millennia. The collective unconscious operates independently from the ego, and its method of communication is not conscious to the ego but is manifested through archetypes, images, metaphors, symbols, and fantasies. Due to the content of material embedded in the collective unconscious, Jung considered it to be more significant than the personal unconscious. Jung also considered the collective unconscious to be the source of ultimate psychic power, psychological wholeness, and inner transformation.

One more layer of the unconscious that needs to be included here is the "archaic ego." This is the part of the unconscious that has an instinctual function in service of survival. It was postulated that this part of the unconscious is responsible for early-emerging survival skills demonstrated in babies, such as gripping onto things and suckling. Green (as cited in Kalsched, 1996) postulated that this "inner space" of the archaic ego might also be the seat of dissociation. It is generally thought that this part of the psyche, having served its function for early survival, becomes dormant and unnecessary once the ego begins to adapt to life, but it is an interesting thought to view dissociation as a survival function of the archaic ego in the unconscious.

The Collective Unconscious

Jung's view of the collective unconscious is a central focus for the JAPT therapist because he or she views the play therapy room as a collection of archetypal potentials. Toys, games, and art supplies that convey symbols, metaphors, and images of the collective unconscious welcome the healer archetype to become actively engaged with the child's ego. These healing archetypal activities can be seen in the toys that children select and in the themes they enact with those toys. We select toys that carry the images of the hero, the villain, the great mother, the trickster, and other symbols that embody the archetypes that shape all our lives. Attending to the toys with which the child plays and then how that symbolic image is put into play becomes our roadmap to deepening our understanding of the child and facilitating his or her healing. Our objective is to provide a forum in which unconscious properties of the collective unconscious can emerge and take an active role in the healing process of the wounded child. We fully trust that the collective unconscious, under the right conditions, will become active in the child's ego and direct him or her on the path needed to heal from the damage he or she has suffered.

Archetypes of the Unconscious

According to Jung, archetypes are inherited parts of the psyche. He originally referred to these archetypes as primordial images, but later (in 1917) shifted to the term *archetypes*, which refer to unconscious "blueprints" or templates that are manifested across great cultures and personal lives. Archetypes also generally come in pairs of opposites, so, for example, as counterpart for the villain, there is the hero; for the mother, there is the father; for good, there is evil; and for the destroyer, there is the healer. Jung identified the central organizing archetype of the unconscious as the Self or the "God within." The Self is that which

we were destined to become. Its counterpart is the Shadow, or all that is true about us that we don't want anyone else to know.

Deintegration in the Healing Process

At birth the ego and the Self are coalesced, but as the ego begins its journey into life in the real world, the relationship between the ego and Self becomes fragmented. This fragmentation is not a break between the ego and the Self, but indeed becomes the process by which ego strength is formed. This process of developing ego strength continues as the ego encounters something in the world that is new or unfamiliar, such as a new rule or a new concept. This newness produces "deintegration" (Fordham, 1973) in the ego because the ego holds no previous knowledge or experience with what has been encountered. The ego then assesses the situation and, relying on previously obtained scripts and schemas, "assimilates" old patterns of behavior in order to "reintegrate" and achieve a level of homeostasis (Ault, 1977). If no previous scripts and schemas exist, the ego must create a new way of managing the situation by "accommodating" new behaviors in order to regain homeostasis and facilitate reintegration or not. This process of breaking down and building up again is the means by which ego strength is developed. Naturally the more scripts and schemas we have available to us, the less our egos deintegrate. Children have weaker ego strength by virtue of not having had the time to gather myriad adaptive scripts and schemas, therefore their egos are more fragile and susceptible to situations that cause deintegration.

Complex and Protocomplex

The experiences and material that are more than the ego can effectively manage to reintegrate are often repressed and form a "protocomplex" (Peery, 2003). Protocomplexes respond as fully developed "complexes" do and are seen as behaviors (symptoms) accompanied by very powerful emotions. These emotions are attached to an archetypal core and are often "triggered" by situations that are similar dynamically to the events that caused the material to be repressed. The central difference between a protocomplex and a fully developed complex is the depth to which the material is repressed. A protocomplex is not as deeply repressed unconsciously and is therefore more accessible to the ego, and the manifestation of it is not as intense (but is likely more frequent) as with fully developed complexes.

Because the language of the collective unconscious is comprised of symbols, images, archetypes, and metaphors, it can only be fully understood through outward manifestations that require interpretation—predominantly from an outside source. This interpretive function becomes one of the central roles for the JAPT therapist. The manner in which we complete this task is explained more fully later in this chapter; however, it needs to be mentioned here to stress the point that a practitioner of JAPT must become familiar with the language of the unconscious in order to be able to fully understand the child he or she is treating.

This fundamental understanding guides the JAPT therapist to respond in a manner that facilitates healing in the child. The other two roles of the JAPT therapist are as witness and container. These roles are more fully explained below, when discussing the concept of *temenos*.

Figure 4.1 illustrates the process by which a protocomplex or complex is formed. In the illustration, the large orb represents the unconscious. The ego, represented by the smaller orb, is separating itself from the unconscious to move into the outer world. At a given time, an intrusive event occurs that causes the ego to "deintegrate" or break down. The result of this deintegration can be seen in behavioral changes, cognitive shifts, and emotional unsettledness—what we call symptoms. The ego is moved toward reintegration and draws upon its prior behavioral, cognitive, and emotional experiences of learning to restore equilibrium to itself and create a state of reintegration. Piaget described this cognitively as "disequilibration" and hypothesized that the brain would move in one of two different directions to resolve this state of imbalance. One of the ways that this was done was through "assimilation," wherein

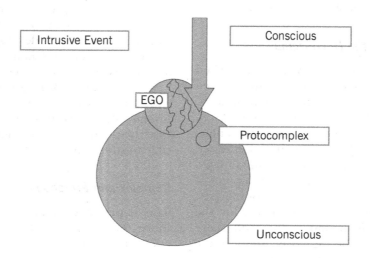

FIGURE 4.1. The protocomplex model.

the brain applies previously learned scripts and schemas to the new experience. Children do this behaviorally and emotionally as well. For example, a child might hold a script of attending a birthday party that was a pleasant experience. This behavioral experience carries with it both an affective and cognitive response. If it was a pleasant experience, the child, in being invited to a birthday party, would have an accompanying pleasant affective response. The other way that the brain functions to restore equilibrium is via "accommodation," whereby the brain opens up to new information on how to manage the situation. Accommodation requires more ego strength as it requires enough tolerance and resiliency to allow the development of new scripts and schemas. Children also accommodate behaviorally and emotionally in order to achieve "reintegration" and normal ego functioning. For example, take the child who is going to the doctor for a vaccination shot. His previous experience with shots has been that the shots are painful and unpleasant. The child's older brother tells him that if he simply holds his breath and blows out his cheeks as big as possible, the shot won't hurt as much. The child accommodates a new behavior with "hope" (different affect than fear) that it will not be as unpleasant as his previous experience.

There are times, however, when the child does not possess the experience, life scripts and schemas, and ego strength to engage the source of deintegration. When the ego is overwhelmed by the experience (either behaviorally, cognitively, or emotionally), the material is repressed into the unconscious. This repressed material has the potential to form into a protocomplex or a fully developed complex. The critical element determining whether or not the material can be engaged is the ego strength of the child. If sufficient support is given to the child, he or she can openly engage the experience/material and create ways to restore ego integration.

My Model

I created my model, shown in Figure 4.2, nearly two decades ago out of necessity. I was unsuccessful in my lobbying efforts to get some of the "engineers" to create one, so I created one that made sense to me. This model has proven to be more versatile than I had originally intended, and I was very pleased when it was used by Kevin O'Connor to forward his behavioral approach to play therapy. The purpose of this model is to illustrate how the JAPT therapist views the process of how a child becomes "damaged" and in need of treatment, to explain why the child is not healing on his or her own, and to introduce the role of play therapy in the healing process. I have had great success in using my model to educate parents on the issues of psychological damage to their children, why their children are "stuck," and the healing process of play.

The model (from left to right in Figure 4.2) represents both the response of a healthy child not in need of treatment and one of an unhealthy child in need of treatment. The model starts with the introduction of a new, unfamiliar, or traumatic event. In the most basic form in this life, we do three things: We think, we feel, and we act. (One could make an argument that we relate, and that there is a spiritual component to our experience here, but for the sake of simplicity, I chose to only list these three aspects of the human experience.) When these new or unfamiliar events occur, deintegration occurs across the three aspects of the human experience. I borrowed Bandura's (1969) terminology to describe behavioral deintegration, Piaget's (Berk, 1989) term to represent cognitive deintegration, and I made up the term to describe emotional deintegration. These deintegrating features in the three different areas are *deterioration* for behavioral deintegration, *disequilibration* for cognitive deintegration, and *decompensation* for emotional deintegration.

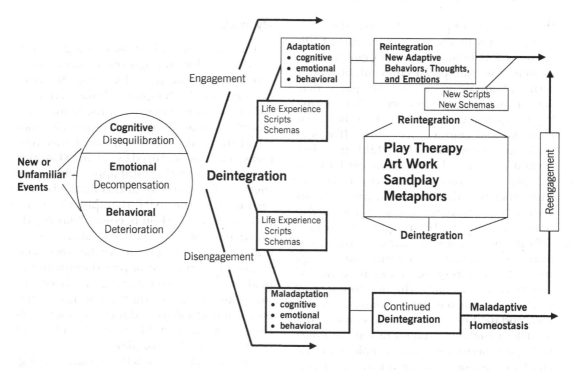

FIGURE 4.2. My model of play therapy.

At the time this deintegration occurs, the ego has to assess its state of readiness to engage the event. Engagement, in my model, indicates a conscious awareness of the event/material and an inherent ability to confront it. This engagement requires a level of ego strength proportional to the level of deintegration of the event. Ego strength is built through previous life experiences, learned scripts and schemas, and the safety and support to which the child has access in his or her environment. In the process of engagement the ego can adapt through assimilation or accommodation on all three levels of the human experience. The result is the formation of new behavioral, cognitive, and emotional scripts and schemas. These lead to the reintegration of the ego and the restoration of equilibrium.

Let's take the example of a child who comes from a healthy environment and is abused by a stranger in a park one day when walking home from school. Because her ego strength is sufficient to confront this event on all three levels of the human experience, she begins to adapt in a healthy way to the trauma. Her adaptation on all three levels would look like the following: (1) healthy behavioral adaption—"I won't go into the park alone again" or "When I go through the park, I am taking Ripper [the family Rottweiler] with me"; (2) healthy cognitive adaptation—"It was not my fault," or "I'm not dirty," or "I am not for treating that way"; and (3) healthy emotional adaptation—"I was scared," or "I'm angry about what happened," or "I hate that person." These healthy adaptations are specific in relation to the event that occurred and are therefore useful in restoring the child to a normal level of ego integration.

Conversely, the children we usually encounter in our practices are not experiencing healthy ego adaptation and their egos are actively working to repress the material/event. This avoidant energy, or dynamic, I have chosen to call *disengagement*—meaning that the child's ego is actively working to repress the material or to disengage from it. The ego knows intuitively whether it possesses the strength to adapt to the overwhelming power of the event. This disengagement gives rise to what I have termed *maladaptation*. Using the same example with the sexually abused little girl, the problematic process might proceed as follows: The child's behavioral maladaptation might take the form of acting out sexually with other children, bullying other children, or refusing to go outside of the home. Cognitive maladaptation would sound something like "It never happened," "It was my fault," or "I deserved it." Emotional maladaptation would be experienced as "I liked it," "I want to be with that person again," or emotional numbing. Naturally, this is not an exhaustive list of the many different forms of maladaptation, but it gives a general feel for how maladaptation keeps the child's ego from engaging material that needs to be engaged in order for the Self to effectively help in the healing process. It is key to remember that the function of disengagement is to avoid confrontation with the event and its effects upon the ego. Maladaptation assuages the disturbing emotions of the protocomplex and forming complex, but, due to its disengaging influence, it is impossible for any healthy adaptation to occur. This is usually when the parents become aware that there is a problem with their child and come through our doors for help.

It is assumed by the JAPT therapist that the child has exhausted all of his or her conscious abilities to resolve the overwhelming material. It is our understanding that the child is not actively pursuing a maladaptive course because something new was learned or because something new was conditioned in him or her. We reject this notion because of our understanding of the structure of the psyche and the presence of the Self in the child. It is our deeply founded belief that our job at the time the child enters our room is to assist him or her in safely engaging the overwhelming material, activating the self-healer from within, and allowing the Self to make contact with the ego and express the healing process through the use of the symbols we have assembled in the play therapy room. It should also be noted that we do not always know what the healer archetype will look like for the child or how it will appear. This is why Green so accurately described one of the qualities of the JAPT therapist as "patient observers" (Green, 2009).

A note about symptoms is appropriate here. The JAPT therapist is ever grateful for the presence of symptoms, which are viewed as a maladaptive means to disengage with an event or material that is overwhelming the ego. Interestingly, the symptoms usually carry a "confirmational" or "compensatory" dynamic that is usually tied to the protocomplex or budding complex. An example of this would be the young boy who has been physically abused who starts punching other children on the playground at recess. If he had experienced helplessness and powerlessness during his abuse, and those feelings returned as part of the repressed material he had not consciously engaged, punching another child would be a "compensatory" act to reempower himself. Or, conversely, the boy continues to put himself in situations in which he keeps getting beat up. This behavior "confirms" the experience the child had with the abuser and was stimulated by his need to try and overcome his feelings of powerlessness. This socially inappropriate behavior temporarily assuages the feelings of inadequacy and powerlessness but, because the behavior does not lead toward the engagement, no resolution is reached. Symptoms are dynamically connected to the protocomplex or complex of the child and, with some careful analysis, one can see the connection between the conscious acts and the underlying dynamics repressed in the unconscious.

The next step in the model for the struggling child is the introduction to play therapy. This is the place where engagement with events and disturbing material can and does take place. JAPT therapists are keenly aware that the child has exhausted all conscious means to resolve the deintegration of the disturbing event. The child simply does not have the ego strength, for whatever reason, to engage the material and is working very hard at not engaging it. We know this because the child is experiencing and demonstrating symptoms that are beyond his or her ability to control. Play therapy begins in the play therapy room and with creating *temenos* in the room and in the relationship between the child and the therapist.

Therapeutic Safety

Temenos was a word used by the early Greeks to define the sacred precinct within which God's presence could be felt. Jung used the word to describe the therapeutic safety that must exist in order for a client to consciously approach repressed or complex material. The term is used here to describe the safety of the play therapy room and of the therapeutic relationship between the child and the therapist. *Temenos* is first created by providing a safe, contained, private room in which the child can access the richness of the archetypal language of symbol. Peery (2003) does an excellent job in describing the physical attributes of a play therapy room—size, flooring material, separation from other therapy offices and from the waiting room where parents are waiting, access to the outdoors, and having a dedicated play therapy room—so I won't repeat his suggestions here.

I will add a few other points concerning the play therapy room, however. All of the toys do need to be accessible to the child and openly displayed. The toys should be carefully selected for their capacity to elicit symbolic representations of archetypal material. Since archetypal material is held in dyadic pairs (e.g., hero–villain; rescuer–destroyer; killer–healer), it is important to

balance the toys that hold these symbolic representations. Green (2009) makes a very important point in addressing the issue of the symbolic properties of the toys. He indicates that because children are drawn, deeply and intensely, to the symbolic embodiment of archetypal material, it is necessary, as time is expiring for the session, to "reground" them before they leave. To this end it is important to have toys and materials that are grounding for children as well, meaning that there are things that they encounter in everyday life outside of the play therapy room. These would be considered "real-life toys" that Garry Landreth describes eloquently in his book *Play Therapy: The Art of the Relationship* (2002). (Landreth also has a useful list of toys on pages 144–145.) Byron and Carol Norton (1997) provide some excellent guidance in selecting toys for the play therapy room, standard interpretations of toys (Appendix B), interpretation of environments (Appendix C), and interpretation of animals (Appendix D), in their text. (Landreth and the Nortons are excellent teachers of theory and practical application of play therapy, and they have been giants in the field instructing young play therapists in creating fantastic play therapy rooms for the effective treatment of children.)

The bottom line for JAPT therapists is to create a play therapy room that is balanced in both the symbolic and the practical domains. In addition to the archetypal potential that exists in the properties of the toys, JAPT therapists consider their own relationship and response to the toys so that these can be monitored during a session. Because we are dealing with symbols, it is easy for JAPT therapists to also get lost in the energy of the toy and not even be aware of it. Occasionally, I have one of my colleagues come in and critique the symbolic value of my room. On one of those occasions my good friend Craig Peery entered the room carrying a rubbery octopus and indicated to me that my room had become too masculine. Good catch, Peery! We also need to be aware that our relationship with the toys can and does change over time, and that we too are in a constant state of evolution.

Another dynamic to monitor that adds security and safety in the play therapy room is the arrangement of the toys. This critical aspect of creating *temenos* is addressed by Peery (2003). Green (2009) also addresses the issue of moving from consciousness into the unconscious, and back out again. Another critical element to consider is whether or not the toys cover the range of cognitive development for the children we are treating. One of the easiest ways to note regression in a child is when he or she begins playing with material from an earlier cognitive developmental stage. I like to order my toys with the least cognitive development on the bottom, and then progressively work my way upward. On my bottom shelves are blocks, balls, toys of motion, and toys without demands of talking or sophisticated manipulation. Landreth (2002) notes clear considerations when selecting toys for the play therapy room: "Toys and materials should be carefully selected for (a) the contribution they make to the accomplishment of the objectives of play therapy and (b) the extent to which they are consistent with the rationale for play therapy" (pp. 133–134). For JAPT therapists, the objectives are to allow for the outward manifestation of archetypal material (play) directed by the Self and to facilitate "reconciling the polarities" between the conscious ego and the unconscious Self.

The next aspect of creating and maintaining *temenos* is the relationship between the child and the therapist. Peery (2003) addresses this area in his chapter on "The Role of the Therapist." From the very beginning the therapist strives to create an atmosphere of acceptance, safety, and comfort for the child. The initial task of the JAPT therapist is to create this environment by establishing the relationship with the child. Axline's (1947) eight basic principles are applicable here in guiding the JAPT therapist's

responses to the child. The focus is on the child. Questions are not asked except for clarification and the child is made to feel at the center of the relationship world. This is obviously a marked shift for any child, and one that is often met with some element of surprise. By providing this environment for the child, a crucial element occurs from the JAPT perspective—that of ego inflation.

Role of Ego Inflation

Edinger (1972/1992) has a magnificent treatise of ego inflation in his book *Ego and Archetype*. His references in the first chapter are to the healthy child and the fear that the child's ego will become overinflated and carry the child into danger. Peery (2003) referred to the myth of Theseus and compared the child–therapist relationship to Ariadne's thread, which led Theseus out of the labyrinth where he had killed the minotaur. Later on in his life, however, due to his repeated successes in overcoming many trials, Theseus succumbed to ego inflation. He accompanied his friend Pirithous into Hades to demand that Hades release his wife, Persephone, to Pirithous so that they could be married. The two were bound to a bench by vipers "forever." Prometheus suffered a similar fate in stealing fire from the gods, ending up bound to a rock to have his liver eaten out on a daily basis. The myths are filled with examples of ego inflation gone wrong. This inflation usually occurred when a "mortal" ventured into the world of the "gods" to try and claim that to which they had no claim. A parallel can be drawn here with the Self as representing what is "godlike," whereas mortality represents the ego.

The children we treat are not suffering from ego inflation, and if they are, it is a maladaptation caused by overwhelming material they are actively working to repress. Ego inflation is a necessary component by which children engage the consciously "unengageable." Children must be able to act out the hero, superhero, the police, the good guys, overpowering the bad guy, the bully, etc., in order to inflate themselves sufficiently to confront that which needs to be confronted. The JAPT therapist combines the use of the relationship, along with the rich collection of archetypal potential (toys), to effectively facilitate the necessary inflation for engagement. It is our belief that providing these critical elements will activate the Self and healer within children, and they will be guided through the journey of healing as the therapist performs the critical roles of interpreter (when necessary), witness, and container for the material that is expressed in play therapy.

Unique Features of JAPT

One of the unique components of JAPT is that we use a wide variety of techniques from different theoretical positions to create and maintain *temenos* in the play therapy room. Chaotic play that alienates and disengages ego from Self in the play therapy room does little to assist in resolution and healing. In a chaotic environment there cannot be any development of new, healthy scripts and schemas, so it is often necessary to use behavioral interventions to restore some order in the room. A JAPT therapist might also employ some relaxation or guided imagery for a child suffering with overwhelming anxiety, or offer cognitive explanations to reduce the cognitive dissonance that exists when a child encounters something new or unfamiliar. Knowing when to step forward and disrupt the independent path of the child is a difficult skill for the clinician to learn, but one that is absolutely necessary to maintain the *temenos* of the play therapy room and the relationship.

Another unique feature of the JAPT therapist is the use of Self in the process of play therapy. We allow children to use us as a play companion, an interpreter at times, a witness to their work, and a container for the powerful emotions that come forward from a protocomplex or complex issue.

Children often need our support and use us as critical parts of their play to complete the tasks necessary for their healing. For example: A disempowered, deflated child enters the play therapy room and, as he or she becomes inflated, there arises a need in him or her to dominate the relationship. The child might put us in "jail" or "talk down to us" as means of expressing this inflated state and internally compensate for feeling weak. The child might express the same dynamic as a need to be dominated, communicating to the therapist what it was like to be overpowered and wounded. In either case, the child has a need to have the active participation of another safe human being to fully experience the dynamic being forwarded by unconscious energy.

Much of the time, the JAPT therapist is an active but patient observer of the process by which unconscious material is engaged. In accomplishing this, it is important for the JAPT therapist to "pace" with the child, meaning that it is our task to stay with the child behaviorally, cognitively, and emotionally. We work to match the behavioral energy of children. Their demonstrative expressions of behavior guide us in knowing how to respond, and it is our job to match what children produce. Any discrepancy between the behavioral level of the child and that of the therapist puts the child at risk of being led by the therapist. We also work on the cognitive level of children. We try very hard to communicate with them in developmentally appropriate language, and to use the words that they use for objects. Finally, we rise and fall with the emotions of the child, but we don't extend beyond the child's present level of emotional range. Any extension of the current range of affect is leading the child, and we strenuously attempt to avoid that. Pacing with children on all three levels of their experience in the play therapy room creates and maintains *temenos* and facilitates the engagement process.

By the time the child comes into the play therapy room, the JAPT therapist has a pretty good understanding of his or her issues. This understanding emerges from a very thorough assessment (covered later in this chapter) of the child's multigenerational system, the child's current level of adaptive functioning, and a comprehensive understanding of any events or issues that may have given rise to the child's maladaptive behavior. So, when a child first enters the play therapy room, the JAPT therapist is very attentive to which symbolic objects the child engages and how these objects are put into a comprehensive theme. The child acting out the play is often unaware of what he or she is doing, and it is the JAPT therapist's task to strengthen the child's understanding of what is happening. This "deepening" of the play therapy experience, which is a key dynamic of this theoretical method, is always accomplished by staying in the metaphor that the child has presented and making comments that are directly tied to the dynamic being presented in the form of a "soft hypothesis." The hypothesis is *soft* because our understanding might be wrong, and we are prepared for that eventuality.

For example, let's suppose that a child who has been physically abused comes for therapy. We know that the abuse has stopped and the child is working to overcome its effects. We have a good idea as to how the child is processing the abuse by her symptoms. If the child is acting out aggressively, we can hypothesize that she is compensating for her feelings of inadequacy and powerlessness. If the child is withdrawn and dropping out socially, we can hypothesize that she is fearful and that the feelings of abuse are being transferred onto the world in which she lives. If she presents with no symptoms at all, we can hypothesize that the child has engaged with the abuse and is on a healing path. Naturally, we would see adaptive behavior created by the child in this healing process. For the sake of the following example, let us posit that the child comes from an unhealthy environment, but now lives in a healthy one.

During a play therapy session, let's suppose the child decides to play with two animals. One of the animals is a domesticated one, say a dog, and the other is clearly a predator animal, a T-rex perhaps. The child begins to engage the animals in battle, with the T-rex destroying the dog. A suitable comment for testing a "soft hypothesis" that the dog represents the child and the T-rex represents her abuser might be, "It didn't look like there was anything that the dog could have done to stop that mean T-rex." This comment represents and empathizes with the child's feelings of powerlessness when she was abused, and deepens the behavioral activity to a cognitive and emotional level. If the therapist is wrong, the child will correct the therapist as long as the *temenos* in the relationship has been established.

Conversely, if the child has the dog destroy the T-rex, indicating a compensatory dynamic, and an appropriate comment might be, "Wow, that dog is really tough and amazing to be able to beat up that thing that's so much bigger than him." Again, the comment emphasizes the compensatory dynamic of the smaller, weaker object beating up the bigger, stronger object. The comment also empathizes with the child's compensatory play. This is "witnessing" the play from an analytical perspective.

Interpretation is one step beyond witnessing, and this advanced technique requires the use of emotional language and an understanding of the child's complex. Using the same T-rex example, the JAPT therapist might state, "I'll bet that bigger guy was surprised at just how powerful that little one was," or "That dog must feel so proud of himself to be able to stop such a big, strong thing like that." The interpretation solidifies and summarizes the play theme for the child in language that she can understand easily, and it facilitates contact between the unconscious act and conscious understanding, leading to what Green (2009) has termed "meaningful integration." This technique requires the JAPT therapist to understand the play theme in reference to the complex issue. Such an understanding allows the JAPT therapist to see and interpret the play theme of the child in a number of different ways. A good analytical attitude of the JAPT therapist would be to hold at least two to three different hypotheses regarding the play theme of a child. This "deeper" work creates therapeutic resonance on both a conscious and unconscious level between the therapist and the child, creating a very fertile ground from which amazing creativity can and does take place. Where the internal, unconscious energy of the child meets the child's play is the sacred place we call *healing*.

Conscious contact with the complex is always accompanied by highly charged emotions. It is the natural way that complexes are engaged, and it is the intensity of the emotions that help the JAPT therapist understand that contact has been made. Green (2009) refers to this intense energy as the child's "rage," and it is the JAPT therapist's task to contain, reverence, and—most importantly—not be disturbed by that energy. Maintaining this steadiness requires JAPT therapists to be keenly aware of their issues, both resolved and unresolved, from their past. Intense complex energy can very likely trigger an emotional response from the therapist, and it is imperative that the therapist be able to handle the intensity and depth of that emotion without disengaging from it or stopping it altogether.

Another unique feature of JAPT is that the therapist is considered to be part of the play therapy environment. I have already mentioned that the JAPT therapist acts as a witness (patient observer) and an interpreter. The other unique role of the JAPT therapist is that of "container." This is a unique role of the JAPT therapist and addresses the effective use of countertransference. It is the belief of this approach that the naughty word *countertransference* can have a positive effect on the treatment of children. In the play therapy experience, not only is the therapist active in contain-

ing the energy of the child's complex, but the JAPT therapist is also willing to take on the emotional burden of the child when the child is willing to hand it to him or her. This means that the child trusts the relationship with the therapist to the extent that he or she is willing to have the therapist emotionally feel his or her intense emotions. This experience may be unpleasant for the therapist but highly liberating for the child. In order to be able to experience this "handing off" of emotion from the child to the therapist, the therapist must be aligned with the child on an emotional level and then maintain the integrity of the therapeutic container—which is the therapist him- or herself. Naturally this requires the therapist to know what issues are his or hers, and which belong to the child. It is critical for the JAPT therapist to have undergone, or be undergoing, his or her own analysis to prevent any unresolved personal issues from intruding into the play therapy of a child.

Clinical Case Example in Supervision

An example of this containment process can be illustrated from a supervision I was doing with a talented play therapist. She had been working with an 8-year-old boy who had been physically abused by his father. He had been removed from the home, and he was now living in a healthy environment, but his behavior had deteriorated and he was violent and mean toward other family members. The therapist had met with him on several occasions and had done an excellent job of creating a *temenos* for this boy; as a consequence he felt the freedom to pursue his healing journey. The therapist described a recurring theme in the play therapy room in which the boy would "tie [her] up" to her chair and then advance closer and closer to her, swinging a sword at her face, getting much too close for the therapist's comfort. Her inclination was to shut the play theme down, but she knew that something bigger was happening than his terrorizing her, so she fought off the intense feelings and went with the play. This play therapist had some history of abuse in her distant past, and I asked her what she was feeling when the boy was advancing closer and closer to her. She admitted that she had some extreme feelings of fear. She described her interpretation and feedback to the child as amplifying his feelings of power and strength. She replied to his sword swinging advances toward her with, "Wow, you are so powerful and strong. I am helpless here." She felt that she had reached an impasse with this boy because he was stuck on this behavioral fugue.

I encouraged her to share her intense feelings of fear with the boy during the next session. It was my theoretical belief that this boy was handing over his deep feelings of fear to the therapist, but, without her verbalizing it to him, he was unsure that she was fully able to empathize with his experience. The next session began as the others, and pretty soon the therapist was tied to the chair and the boy began advancing toward her with the sword. As he began moving toward her again, she spoke to him: "I am so afraid right now. I feel so powerless to stop you from what you are doing, and I am afraid." The boy stopped immediately and looked deeply into the eyes of the therapist, who then uttered in a moment of therapeutic genius, "I understand." This is the deepest level of empathy that we can share with children. It transcends understanding to actually feel what children are trying so desperately to communicate. In this way, by being willing to carry the emotional burden, we have the ability not only to fully witness what the child's experience was like but also to share that experience in the sanctity of the play itself.

Interpreting, Witnessing, and Containing

This technique brings up the next issue regarding *temenos*, and that is the manner in which feedback is given to the child. From the JAPT perspective feedback can be given in a number of ways. Initially, at the beginning stages of therapy, it is very common for the JAPT therapist to "track" children's behavior in the play therapy room, exactly the way that is taught by child-centered play therapy. This consists of providing a running dialogue, with the therapist describing the child's play to the child as it unfolds. Landreth (2002) writes that these "tracking responses communicate the therapist's involvement and help the child feel the therapist is participating with him" (p. 212). The emphasis is on the child and what he or she is doing. Comments such as "You found what you were looking for" or "You knew just what to do with that" are common in this early stage of therapy. Tracking is a cautious approach that facilitates the development of *temenos* in the play therapy room. Other features of tracking responses include the previously mentioned "pacing" the child's level of emotion; personalizing the responses to the child, often calling him or her by name; not asking questions other than for clarification; and centering the feedback on the child.

The next level of feedback, regarding the child's cognitions, is considered the next level of depth for the child and is more intrusive to the psyche than tracking. Comments typical of this level of feedback include "You're just not sure what that does," or "That thing didn't do what you wanted it to do," or "That thing turned out to be different than what you thought." The objective of this level of feedback is to identify the cognitive process occurring in the child at any given point in the process of play. Giving the child information about his or her own processes creates a deeper resonance with the child and enhances the development of trust between the child and the therapist. Moving from tracking to this level of feedback is risky because it exposes something more about the child than he or she might be expecting. Given that JAPT therapists works from the position of soft hypotheses, we are prepared to be corrected or ignored on any level of feedback.

The most intrusive and personal level of feedback the JAPT therapist uses is that of affect identification. As noted by Peery (2003), "emotions are seen by the analytical therapist as deep-level communications from the patient's psyche, and they are considered to be profound and meaningful communication" (p. 37). This level of feedback deals with the most exposed parts of the children we treat, and needs to be considered as the most sacred and tender of psychological phenomena. It is most effective to remain in the metaphor or theme that the child has introduced when giving feedback on this level. This feedback might sound something like "That one seemed *so* angry with that other one," or "That one seems very sad to me." However, when the play is just between the child and the therapist, the therapist can respond directly to the child about his or her feelings. This might sound like "You seem really mad at me right now," or "You look really sad right now."

The language of the soft hypothesis is very nonconfrontational, and just that— *soft*. The JAPT therapist uses language that leaves room for the child to deny, escape, or avoid the therapeutic response. This language might include "I'm just not sure

about that thing over there," or "That one *seems* hurt, or sad," or "I'm wondering about that thing right there." The child maintains control of what to do with the feedback, and depending on the level of ego strength at the time, he or she is free to confront, ignore, or avoid the response altogether. The therapeutic response, however, is placed in the psychological field nonetheless and is available to the child from this point onward, whether he or she picks up on it or not.

Countertransference

The basis for giving effective therapeutic responses is rooted in the unconscious and conscious relationship between the child and the therapist. Figure 4.3 depicts a healthy therapeutic relationship between the therapist and the child. The lines drawn in the illustration indicate the active dynamic that takes place between the child and the therapist on both a conscious and unconscious level.

The conscious egos are differing in size because the therapist has had much more experience in ego development by virtue of age; the child's ego is smaller because it has not had the same amount of time to develop. The unconscious spheres of both the therapist and the child are the same

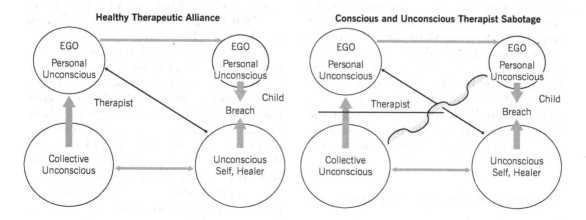

FIGURE 4.3. Healthy (left) and unhealthy (right) models.

size to represent all that is contained in the unconscious. This theoretical approach recognizes no difference in the capacity of the unconscious for either the therapist or the child. The archetypes of Self and healer are added to the unconscious field of the child to underscore their presence in the unconscious of the child. The "collective" was added to the unconscious of the therapist to illustrate the resources available to any therapist stepping into a play therapy setting with a child.

I have chosen to use the word *breach* to describe what happens between the child's ego and unconscious due to the consciously overwhelming nature of events that occurred in the child's young life. With the subsequent development of ego defenses, the Self and healer archetypes have no directive value to the ego. The ego–Self axis has been compromised to the extent that the Self is "contained" within the unconscious, with no power to create a meaningful integration of healing. It is also possible that the ego–Self axis can become so permeable that a large number of archetypes, both constructive and destructive, have access to and influence over the child's ego. However, due to a lack of organizational properties in the ego, it is unable to use the unconscious material to achieve a state of integration specific to the event that took place. Without the ability to effectively influence the ego, or if the ego lacks the strength to effectively filter and organize archetypal material, the Self does not serve a healing function.

The therapist, on the other hand, has access to the rich archetypal material of the unconscious and can recognize it in the child. The two-directional arrow between the unconscious of the therapist and the unconscious of the child represents the unconscious connection between the therapist and the child. There is an energetic exchange of psychic energy on this level that can be felt by both. Because this exchange is unconscious, the JAPT therapist looks for palpable manifestations of it in

him- or herself. Feelings are manifestations of this unconscious connection, and JAPT therapists are sensitive to what they are feeling in the process of being with a child in the play therapy experience. An example might be to feel a dislike for a child when no behavioral activities have taken place. Another example would be to find oneself actually feeling sexual energy in working with a child who has been sexually abused. Again, nothing has occurred in the play therapy room of a sexual nature, but the feelings are there. It is important for JAPT therapists to recognize these feelings as part of this unconscious connection with the child.

The child may experience this connection with the therapist as anxiety, fear, or nervousness if the therapist is new to the field or not very confident of his or her abilities to be helpful. The child may also experience unresolved psychological issues from the therapist, and, in rare cases, the child actually does the caretaking for the therapist. I have witnessed this in supervising some cases. In one case in particular, the child was presenting with some severe symptoms of sexual abuse. The child began working through some of these issues with a younger play therapist who had not done any work on her own sexual abuse, and the play behavior triggered a reaction in the play therapist. The child stopped what she was doing and said to the play therapist that they "could do something different now."

The unidirectional line between the child's unconscious to the conscious ego of the therapist represents the unconscious material that children bring forward in therapy. The JAPT therapist recognizes the healer in the play even though the child hasn't achieved a meaningful integration of the unconscious material. The therapist now has the opportunity to assist in mediating the "transcendent function" (Jung, 1960, para. 121) of the symbolic representation of archetypal material. This is done by first recognizing the play's symbolic representation of the unconscious. The JAPT therapist next understands the "meaning" of the play as it is connected to the complex and then communicates the information to the child, using the metaphor as the structure onto which he or she can deepen and amplify the meaning of the material.

Clinical Case Example

Let me reference a young boy I worked with many years ago as an example of this process. This boy was 5 years of age when he was brought into therapy. He'd had a tremendously abusive past, including being raped, physically abused, and burned with cigarettes. His symptoms were consistent with those of a victim complex and, additionally, he had started demonstrating sexually reactive behaviors toward his siblings, indicating a sexual complex tied in with being a victim. His work was about creating safety in the first few sessions until, at the end of one session, he took a predator animal from the shelf and placed it in the garbage can. He had me exit the room in front of him so that he could do this behavior without my seeing it. I caught a glimpse of it over my shoulder, and when I was cleaning up the room, I saw the T-rex in the trash. I knew that his ego was strengthening and that he was preparing for a confrontation with his "predators."

The confrontation happened in the next session; his attack was accompanied by intense complex energy as he was killing his predators. He worked methodically and purposefully, killing more and more of the predators and dumping them in the trash. I was able to feel his anxiety in performing this heroic task, and I verbalized to him my feelings of anxiety associated with his journey. He acknowledged my comment with only a look, but he knew that I understood his emotions. When his task was completed and he had killed all of the predators, I recognized the trash can as not only the repository of the dead predators from his life, but also as the container for them. I verbalized

to him, "They can't come back and hurt us anymore" (I used the word *us* because he had deputized me in the killing of the predators). He responded like a delighted 5-year-old and quipped "Yup."

This young boy's journey had metaphorically placed him in front of his abusers. He undertook the hero's journey, like Hercules or Jason, and confronted them with courage and all of the magical power his inflated ego could muster. "We" took that journey together and conquered the evil in his life. My part in bringing the unconscious into consciousness was to interpret the "container" and the properties of the container as the holder of garbage and as something from which things did not return. "We" were safe from the return of those evil predators; it was something that I saw, interpreted, and then expressed to my young, courageous friend. This is the task of the JAPT therapist when unconscious material manifests itself: to assist the child to consciously understand it, and in this case, understand it more fully.

Naturally the therapeutic relationship is in jeopardy if the unconscious material of the child triggers unresolved, disturbing material in the unconscious of the therapist. The therapist, without any conscious understanding, starts "guiding" the session out of the direction of the child's lead. Rarely, but it does occur, the therapist might even use the child to work through his own issues. The JAPT therapist has to always be vigilant in assessing his or her own psychological state during the course of a session to ensure that this kind of therapeutic sabotage does not occur. The JAPT therapist recognizes that any time we begin dealing with unconscious material, either our own or another person's, we run the risk of getting lost in our own unconscious material. The responsible JAPT therapist is familiar with his or her unconscious issues and, through participating in his or her own analysis, is able to achieve an understanding of that material as it manifests through emotional responses. Knowing where one ends and the client begins is a major task for the JAPT therapist.

William James is said to have referred to the use of symbolism in psychology as a "most dangerous method" (Kerr, 1994). However, when JAPT therapists understand the language of the unconscious (symbols, images, metaphors), they can create a safe, inviting environment, a *temenos*. Unconscious material can then be safely engaged and the process of transformation initiated. As the child's unconscious material emerges, the JAPT therapist remains aware of, and contains, his or her own psychological issues in order to not contaminate the child's work. By effectively tracking his or her own process during the child's therapy, the JAPT therapist is able to follow the process and effectively use countertransference to amplify and assist the child's inner archetypal healer in the healthy transformation from complex material to resolved material. By venturing deep into the unconscious of each child, respecting that each child is uniquely different in his or her healing process, the JAPT therapist facilitates healing for the child not only in the behavioral, cognitive, and emotional parts of life, but also unconscious healing as well.

REFERENCES

Ault, R. (1977). *Children's cognitive development, Piaget's theory, and the process approach.* New York: Oxford University Press.

Axline, V. (1947). *Play therapy: The inner dynamics of childhood.* Cambridge, MA: Houghton Mifflin.

Bandura, A. (1969). *Principles of behavior modification.* New York: Holt, Rinehart, & Winston.

Berk, L. (1989). *Child development.* Boston: Allyn & Bacon.

Edinger, E. (1992). *Ego and archetype: Individuation and the religious function of the psyche.* Boston: Shambhala. (Original work published 1972)

Fordham, M. (1973). Maturation of ego and self in infancy. In M. Fordham, R. Gordon, J. Hubback, K. Lambert, & M. Williams (Eds.), *The library of analytical psychology: Analytical psychology and modern science* (Vol. 1, pp. 82–94). London: Heinemann.

Green, E. (2009). Jungian analytical play therapy. In K. J. O'Conner & L. M. Braverman (Eds.), *Play therapy theory and practice: Comparing theories and techniques* (2nd ed., pp. 100–139). Hoboken, NJ: Wiley.

Jung, C. G. (1960). The structure and dynamics of the psyche. In *Collected works* (Vol. 8). Princeton, NJ: Princeton University Press.

Jung, C. G. (1958). *Collected works of C. G. Jung* (Vol. 11). Princeton, NJ: Princeton University Press

Jung, C. G. (1968). Psychology and alchemy. In *Collected works* (Vol. 12). Princeton, NJ: Princeton University Press

Jung, C. G. (1971). *The collected works of C. G. Jung.* Princeton, NJ: Princeton University Press.

Kalshed, D. (1996). *The inner world of trauma: Archetypal defenses of the personal spirit.* New York: Routledge.

Kerr, J. (1994). *A most dangerous method: The story of Freud, Jung and Sabina Spielrein.* London: Sinclair Stevenson.

Landreth, G. (2002). *Play therapy: The art of the relationship* (2nd ed.). New York: Brunner-Routledge.

Norton, B., & Norton, C. (1997). *Reaching children through play therapy: An experiential approach.* Denver, CO: Publishing Cooperative.

Peery, C. (2003). Jungian analytical play therapy. In C. Schaefer (Ed.), *Foundations of play therapy* (3rd ed., pp. 14–54). Hoboken, NJ: Wiley.

CHAPTER 5

Psychodynamic Play Therapy

John B. Mordock

The term *psychodynamic* has come to mean the interplay of forces or influences within the mind. In contrast to the behavioral therapist, who connects behaviors to observable antecedents and consequences, the psychodynamic therapist considers the reasons for behavior as more complex than what is revealed by observable behaviors. Children have a meaningful mental life, a mind with feelings that can become unbalanced, conflicted, and intruded upon by noxious thoughts. In the simplest of terms, the psychodynamic play therapist examines how children's feelings lead them to display certain troublesome behaviors that are considered symptomatic of deeper, underlying problems.

Major Assumptions

Psychodynamic play therapy is based on four fundamental assumptions: (1) symptoms have meaning; (2) children's problems arise from internalized unconscious conflicts, failure to successfully assimilate overwhelming experiences, and failure to cope with developmental deficits, all of which they reveal in their play; (3) children's play is symbolic, a projection of their inner feel-

ings onto play materials in efforts to obtain mastery over both present and past experiences (their symbolic play provides the camouflage and distance needed for emotional control and psychological safety); and (4) transference-based thoughts characterize much of children's behavior, displayed both in therapy sessions and elsewhere.

Goals of Psychodynamic Play Therapy

The goals of psychodynamic play therapy are typically more ambitious than those of other approaches. The goals are not just to diminish symptoms or to decrease suffering (by quelling anxiety and related bodily symptoms), but to enhance the more fundamental aspects of children's functioning, especially the way they cope with developmental challenges. Efforts are directed at removing obstacles to healthy psychosocial development and moving development to higher levels after it has been arrested (halted or fixated) or when it has regressed, following an external trauma or internal conflict. Psychodynamic play therapy attempts to restructure the personality as a whole, doing so by helping children to develop more mature defenses against anxiety; by clarifying their misperceptions and cognitive distortions; by reconstructing their screen and repressed memories; by revealing the influence of unfulfilled expectations, thwarted intentions, or undelivered communications; and by exploring fantasies and unrealistic wishes.

Specific aims are to strengthen relationships with caretakers, increase the capacity for sound judgment making (improved reality testing), reduce excessive and unrealistic self-preoccupation, increase understanding of the feeling world, increase understanding of choices and consequences, fortify weak defenses and ease rigid defenses against experiencing overwhelming anxiety, strengthen adaptive skills, and increase understanding of self.

Psychodynamic play therapy can soften an overly harsh conscience in children with primitive superegos, sometimes displayed in self-punishing behaviors, such as accident proneness, picking fights with stronger children, and self-mutilation. It can help children to better integrate aspects of their personalities, much like Gestalt therapists attempt to create a better functioning whole. Promoting their resiliency and adaptability, psychodynamic play therapy can help detached children connect more to themselves and to others; it can help inhibited children become more spontaneous, lively, and carefree; impulsive children more controlled, reflective, and responsible; and narcissistic children, less susceptible to wounded self-esteem and the accompanying reactive rage. It can even reduce predisposed children's vulnerability to psychotic and borderline functioning, especially when they are under stress (see Ekstein, 1966).

More specifically, goals include lifting depression; resolving complicated grief; overcoming the effects of trauma; facilitating better adjustment to life events, such as death and divorce; coping better with illness and complying with medical treatment; mastering phobias; improving attention, leading to better learning in school; and better management of personal anger

and aggression. It can also assist children who have real and significant limitations, such as learning disabilities or physical handicaps, to come to terms with who they are and to develop more adaptive, compensating, and self-accepting ways to function.

The psychodynamic play therapist strives to "therapeutically hold" the child (Winnicott, 1971). Like a mother holding her baby, the therapist "holds" the child—not physically, but psychologically, absorbing the overwhelming anxiety and distress that the child cannot bear alone without displaying symptomatic behavior. The therapist confirms the child's experience, fostering the child's trust in his or her own perceptions and feelings, leading to the development of a more genuine sense of self, a keystone of psychological health.

Difference from Psychoanalytic Play Therapy

Readers familiar with psychoanalytic concepts might wonder why this chapter isn't entitled, "Psychoanalytic Play Therapy." Although the goals of psychodynamic and psychoanalytic play therapy do not differ (see Bromfield, 1992, 2007; Lee, 1997), many psychodynamic play therapists do not accept all of the tenets of psychoanalytic theory, especially the thesis that personality develops out of libidinal influences, although if the term *libidinal* is used in its broadest sense to include love as well as sexuality, then the lack of unconditional love in children's lives is clearly a root cause of many with serious difficulties.

As initially conceptualized by Sigmund Freud and his early followers, psychoanalytic theory views personality development as a dynamic, multifaceted process based on the concept of infantile sexuality, with its sequence of libidinal phases characterized by distinct instinctual drives and their related energies. Psychoanalysts believe that behavior is motivated by the expression of these drives and their object cathexes (the investment of mental and/or emotional energy in a person, object, or idea). These libidinal or psychosexual phases are oral, anal, phallic, latency, and genital.[1] Although psychoanalysts believe that personality continues to change and adapt, they hold the view that if a traumatic neurosis occurs during the first 6 years of life, especially the failure to resolve the Oedipus complex, it will create the regressions, fixations, and exaggerated defensive maneuvers viewed by others as symptoms.

I have been involved in the treatment of countless numbers of neglected and abused children, especially those in day and residential treatment centers, who behave like much younger children. Although their chronological age falls within the latency phase, their development has been arrested at levels far below this relatively calm stage of development, in which children typically devote considerable energy to academic achievement and to calming hobbies, such as those that involve collecting, sorting, and organizing materials. Because their energies are directed at meeting needs that weren't met when they were younger (see Abraham Maslow's [1954] need hierarchy theory), these troubled children have little energy left for academic pursuits or for developing age-appropriate friendships.

Some of the latency-age, troubled children I have treated display almost no frustration tolerance and act like impulsive infants, demanding constant adult attention and reassurance. They typically have insatiable appetites, especially for sweets; steal and hoard food, even food that has been discarded; respond only to concrete rewards when asked to achieve something; and constantly suck on the baby bottle found in some of the play therapy rooms or wrap themselves up in blankets and assume the fetal position. Their behavior and attitudes suggest fixation at Freud's oral phase of psychosexual development.

Those children who are slightly more advanced have more variable self-control, but they both defy and cling to caretakers and have wide mood swings. They can be pre-occupied with anal cursing, flaunting their buttocks and "mooning" others, pulling down other children's pants or smacking them on the rear end, gulping air in order to pass gas, creating "fart" sounds in a variety of ways, smelling and nose picking (often eating their phlegm), stuffing toilets, playing sadistic tricks on peers, playing aggressively, and engaging in anal masturbation. When highly anxious, they may smear their feces and torture small animals. Unlike regressed psychotic children, however, they try to hide these activities from adult caretakers. If exposed to finger paints, clay, or a sandbox in a play therapy room, the paints are smeared together until they become brown, the clay molded into simulated feces (which the therapist is sometimes asked to eat), and the sand wetted until the therapist has to limit this behavior.

More advanced children will control their behavior for a preferred adult, but are easily aroused by anything they perceive as sexual. Because of their sexual preoccupations, they confuse affectionate with sexual behavior (making it difficult for caretakers to relate to them), fondle their genitals excessively, engage in sex play with peers (sometimes sexually molesting them), and display agitated and excited behavior that makes concentration difficult during calm activities. When extremely anxious, they may set fires. In therapy, they are highly agitated when given the freedom to select play activities, and they display seductive behavior toward the therapist regardless of his or her sex.

I have worked with young girls who struggled with the Electra complex, displaying seductive behavior toward both their fathers and myself. One precocious 11-year-old often wore her dead mother's clothes and high heels and strutted seductively around the house, a scene she also re-created in play therapy after placement in residential treatment. Her perplexed father neither encouraged nor supported these behaviors, but her troubles were complicated by her younger brother's death.

She had neglected to watch over him as her father backed their car out of the garage, and he was run over and killed. Because of considerable jealous anger (once grabbing another child's drawing and tearing it up as she stormed out of the playroom cursing the therapist), I wanted to explore whether she purposively neglected her duties in order to have her father all to herself, but after her seductive behaviors diminished, she was discharged before I could address this issue.

Working with children with arrested (fixated) and regressed behavior (treatment planning needs to clarify whether a child's primitive behavior is arrested or regressed, as the plans differ for both conditions) has given me a healthy respect for many tenets of psychoanalytic theory, but like Edith Weigert, an early Freudian, I do not accept without reservation all of Freud's tenets. Weigert said (in an interview with Holmes, 2010, p. 20):

> I am not entirely convinced of the universality of incestuous attachments as seen in the Oedipus complex. Nevertheless, sexual desires for a parent or a sibling as well as the desire of a rival's death could surface in the life of a child who does not grow up in the security of a sympathetic surrounding.

Many psychodynamic play therapists don't believe that the pleasure principle is the primary motivating force in life or that libidinal needs are more important in development than are other needs. The troubled child who directs little energy toward academic mastery is, in his or her own way, trying to achieve other goals that conflict with those of caretaking adults. One predelinquent boy once told me, "Since I can't be good, I might as well be the 'baddest' boy I can be." Because I believe that the needs discussed in the next section better explain deviant child development than do those emphasized in classical Freudian theory, I prefer the term *psychodynamic* play therapy over *psychoanalytic* play therapy.

Theory and Approach

My therapeutic practices, as well as those of many psychodynamic play therapists, are based more on the tenets of ego psychology than on classic psychoanalytic theory. Important are the contributions of Alfred Adler (1964) on the development of social interest; Anna Freud (1937) on the development of defenses; Heinz Kohut (1971) on self psychology; John Bowlby (1988) on attachment and loss; Margaret Mahler (1969) on separation and individuation; Donald Winnicott (1965, 1971) on the "holding environment," the use of "transitional objects," the "good-enough mother," and the sense of self; Karen Horney's (1945) 10 basic needs; Erik Erikson's (1950) eight stages of psychosocial development; Abraham Maslow's (1954) need hierarchy theory; and those demonstrating the positive influences of corrective emotional experiences (Alexander & French, 1946; Alpert, 1957; Rank & MacNaughton, 1956; Werner & Kaplan, 1973).

The needs identified by Horney (1945) that apply to children are *affection and approval* (pleasing others and being liked by them); *power* (the ability to bend wills and achieve control over others); *social recognition* (gaining prestige and the limelight); *personal admiration* (for both inner and outer qualities to be valued); *personal achievement*; *self sufficiency*; *independence*; and *perfection*. When children feel unlovable, powerless, unworthy, unsuccessful, inadequate, overly dependent, flawed, or any combination of the above, they typically adopt exaggerated and inappropriate behaviors in attempts to change these feelings.

Horney (1945) also states that another basic need is the need to *exploit others* (to get the better of them, to manipulate them, fostering the belief that people are there simply to be used). Although this need is displayed by lots of troubled children, early psychoanalyst Alfred Adler (1964), who significantly departed from Freudian thinking, would not see this need as a basic one, but as one resulting from failure to develop *social interest*: a striving for superiority at the expense of others instead of on behalf of others.

Erikson (1950), first a teacher in a school for disturbed children and later a psychoanalytic play therapist, formulated his concepts following his clinical experience. In his first stage, *hope*, corresponding to Freud's oral phase, children's concerns are dominated by issues of *trust versus mistrust*. In his second stage, *will*, corresponding to the anal stage, children are concerned with issues of *autonomy versus shame and doubt*. In his third stage, *purpose*, children are preoccupied with issues of *initiative versus guilt*. In his fourth stage, *competence*, corresponding with the latency stage, children become engaged by issues involving *industry versus inferiority* (psychoanalyst Alfred Adler based his theory of personality development on the latter issues).

Many of the themes revealed in the play of troubled children include those of a need for nurturance; control, dominance, and power; experiences of abandonment and/or rejection; separation and loss; shame and guilt; threat; and healing and caring for wounded and broken things (Crenshaw & Mordock, 2005a). Many psychodynamic play therapists believe that the theories of Erikson, Horney, and Maslow shed more light on reasons for these themes than do those of Freud and his early followers.

The Role of Cognitive Development

Children at different phases, or stages, of development conceive of events differently, and psychodynamic play therapists develop their treatment plans accordingly. Children younger than 4 or 5 often fail to distinguish between thoughts and actions. If a boy wished something would happen and it did, he may believe his wish caused the occurrence of the desired event. Angry at another child, a girl may wish her dead. If the child actually dies, the girl may feel responsible for the death. A child can also think that his or her actions caused a related event. A boy may believe that playing with his genitals led to his sexual abuse by an adult that followed the play, especially when the perpetrator blames him for his "sexual" overtures, which many perpetrators do.

Adult rape victims often regress to this level of thinking, believing they did something that resulted in their rape or something they could have done to avoid it. These attitudes, as well as other misconceptions and cognitive distortions that adult rape victims often display, need to be addressed in therapy. Adults, with the help of nonjudgmental and empathic interviewers, can express some of their irrational beliefs to others, but young children typically cannot, so the play therapy must be designed to help reveal them. Similarly, a young child's view of sexuality, different at different stages of development, may affect the child's response, not only to sexual abuse, but also to other traumatic events as well.

Time concepts are also poorly developed in young children. Play therapy sessions with victims of disasters often reveal their incorrect perceptions of time, time sequences, and time duration, all factors that need to be addressed in therapy. If a child pulled on the ropes of a tent and an hour later the tent collapses and the child is trapped inside, the child may believe the earlier actions caused the tent's collapse. As a result, the child may be traumatized by the tent's collapse, whereas the other children trapped in darkness under the tent were merely frightened. Simply exposing this child to structured tent play, relaxation training, and *in vivo* desensitization (cognitive-behavioral techniques) will have less impact on the child's posttraumatic symptoms than will efforts to address the predisposing factor.

Young children view their parents as perfect, as omnipotent. When traumatized by an event, young children can become angry at their parents for failing to protect them, as well as angry at themselves for being unworthy of protection—perhaps they did something bad that resulted in their parent's failure to protect them. Perhaps they expected more protection than usual because of past illnesses or injuries. A cornerstone of psychodynamic play therapy is addressing the idiosyncratic meanings children give to incidents.

All of the different play therapies described in this handbook hold the view that children's play is often more than simply play. On occasion, it's the child's way of mastering situations. Often the play is conflict free, but just as often it's an attempt to master situations that have aroused anxiety.

The girl who repeatedly places a doll in a box and prays over it after a grandparent's death is trying to master the anxiety aroused by the death and funeral. If the girl has the continued support of others, this "funeral play" will diminish over time. In contrast, if she keeps repeating the play and its repetition interferes with completion of important developmental tasks, then the repetitive play has not resulted in mastery of the anxiety connected with the grandparent's death and she may develop other symptoms and be referred for treatment. Perhaps the girl felt that she contributed in some way to the grandparent's death. Although concerned adults can easily relate the burial play to the grandparent's death, the *precipitating* cause of the reaction, they cannot easily identify the child's thoughts, the *predisposing* cause, that made the grandparent's death more traumatic to the child than to her siblings. Another example is a girl whose friends stopped playing with her because she'd only play "school," was always the "teacher," and ordered her playmates around. Eventually she refused to get on the school bus, displaying a full-blown school phobia. Neither the precipitating nor predisposing factors were known, but it was clear that school avoidance lowered her overwhelming anxiety.

In other cases, the relation between the traumatizing event and the repetitive play is unknown. An example is a child who refuses to ride the school bus and when forced to do so tries to jump out the bus windows. It may take some time for both the child and his or her caretakers to connect this seemingly bizarre behavior with a traumatizing precipitating event. Perhaps the child was abused on a bus or other large vehicle. Without therapeutic intervention, the precipitating event may never be identified. And even when the precipitating event is known, other children exposed to the same event may have displayed no such behavior, suggesting that some predisposing factors resulted in the child reacting differently than his or her peers. Identification of both *precipitating* and *predisposing* causes is one of the chief differences of psychodynamic play therapy from some of the other therapies presented in this volume.

The Role of Interpretations

One popular misconception about psychodynamic play therapists is that they rely exclusively upon the development of insight to effect change; that they always interpret for children the meanings of their symbolic play. Historically, the concept of interpretation comes from psychoanalysis, in which psychotherapy focuses on unmasking clients' unconscious motivations and making them aware of how these motivations produce their symptomatic behaviors. Early British play therapist Melanie Klein (1932/1984) saw children's play as the equivalent of adult free associations and therefore made interpretations directly to children's unconscious wishes. Nevertheless, few American psychotherapists follow her approach. Her chief contribution was not her methods (called *wild analysis* by others), but her focus on the young child's experiences of abandonment, envy, and rage—concepts no less relevant today.

Most of the psychodynamic play therapists who make timely interpretations to children are influenced by the work of Anna Freud. Her methods (1928) were more measured than Klein's and, unlike Klein, she emphasized the interpretation of defensive behavior because a focus on unconscious wishes typically raised her clients' anxieties and overwhelmed them.

Many play therapists believe that communicating the meanings of their play to troubled children increases their awareness of their internal conflicts. By understanding why they behave in certain ways, they become free to choose, or to learn, more adaptive ways to manage their anxiety. Nevertheless, this belief is an oversimplification. In another publication, David Crenshaw and I (Crenshaw & Mordock, 2005a) devoted two chapters, totaling 27 printed pages, to discussing the role of interpretations in treatment. Interpretations are subdivided into two major categories: those that the therapist uses to help children understand feelings are called *empathic* interpretations and those that address defenses and hidden motives are called *dynamic* interpretations.

Empathic interpretations are further subdivided into *attention* statements, *reductive* statements, and *situational* statements—all efforts to help children understand universal feelings, individual feelings, personal conflicts, and the behavior and motives of others. The most basic attention statements are running comments about the child's silent play, such as "The man and woman are fighting. . . . The woman runs away. . . . The boy hides under the bed." Melvin Lewis (1974) gives an example of how one attention statement (that no female figure ever occurred in the child's aggressive play) led to a boy's recognition that he had displaced his unreasonable anger at his mother onto his father, the safer figure.

Reductive statements are made to identify the disparate behavioral patterns that children have never noticed about themselves, such as, "You only seem to get angry at me following a home visit." An example of a situational statement, used only when children are aware of their feelings, is, "Every time you ask me for things that you know I can't give you, you get angry at

me for denying you." Even when using empathic interpretations, many children need intermediate steps, such as making the statements indirectly through some other hypothetical child or within the context of the play, such as, for example, "Lots of bunnies might feel sad about that," "Alligator puppet seems angry," or "Chicken doesn't want to share with Bunny!"

Dynamic interpretations provide explanations of defenses (including the contents of defensive fantasies), transferences and displacements, and drives and wishes (including the contents of dreams, fantasies, and bodily sensations). Some simple illustrative comments are "When the baby doll gets anxious, she tries to hide it behind anger," "You make me the bad guy when I'm really not," and "Brown Bunny would like Gray Bunny to notice him." Dynamic interpretations are used only with children who possess considerable ego strength and, for this reason, they may never be used in the treatment of some troubled children. When a child has reached a developmental level where it is appropriate to interpret the suspected meanings revealed in play, the defenses the child uses to prevent the expression of hidden wishes and anxieties are always interpreted before the actual wishes and anxieties are examined.

Interpretations proceed in a step-by-step progression, with the line between affective education and therapy often blurred. First, the child learns that common elements exist in a series of events (attention statements); second, the child realizes that he or she displays specific behaviors in certain situations (reductive statements); third, the child learns that a specific behavior is manifested in a specific situation, such as a boy in a competitive situation where rivalry is expected (situational statements); fourth, in the preceding example, the boy learns that his rivalrous feelings are not conscious ones but ones replaced by defensive behavior, such as avoiding competition (interpretation of the defense of avoidance); fifth, the boy learns how the defense (avoiding competition) helps him to avoid humiliation and loss of self-esteem; and sixth, the boy learns how this behavior originated in response to certain events in his early life ("earlier similar situations") and encompasses reactions and tendencies that could be grouped under the heading of "rivalry with an unsupportive, demeaning father."

Unfortunately, many therapists, overwhelmed with a child's confusing play, often interpret the wrong things at the wrong time and with the wrong words. Considerable tact is required when interpreting the defenses of troubled children, even when made within a metaphorical statement. Children experience attempts to analyze their defenses as attacks on the self. Even sympathetic exploration can be perceived as implied criticism. In addition, disturbed children have considerable difficulty both tolerating ambivalence and accepting their own hostile wishes or fantasies. Interpretations should always be tentatively worded in the form of questions that leave room for doubt, and they should also convey that it's all right to have the feeling that is interpreted. Conveying this implication requires careful wording. Included in the two chapters on interpretation in Crenshaw and Mordock (2005a) are numerous examples of poorly worded interpretations contrasted with those that are ego supportive.

Although clarifications and interpretations are useful techniques, they are not made simply to help children gain an intellectual understanding of their problems. Intellectual understanding plays a relatively small part in most treatment successes. Hermine von Hug-Hellmuth, the second female member of the Vienna Psychoanalytic Society, was the first psychoanalyst to formally treat children with both talk and play. In 1920 she wrote: "The analysis both of the child and of the adult has the same end and object; namely, the restoration of the psyche to health and equilibrium which have been endangered through influences known and unknown" (p. 287), but she believed that conscious insight was not a requisite to a child's finding relief and help through play.

In psychodynamic child therapy, the goal is rarely insight into the roots of a conflict. Rather "insight" is revealed as a shift in the child's attitude of mind, a decrease in the need to project feelings and anxieties, which eventually leads to an increased capacity for self-understanding and results from the internalization of an insightful, or insight-seeking, therapist. In essence, what the child experiences is what the philosopher Bertrand Russell (1917) called "knowledge by experience" as opposed to "knowledge by description."

Another popular misconception about psychodynamic play therapy is the belief that, similar to adult psychoanalysis, the therapist actively promotes the communication of transference wishes and fantasies and interprets their meanings to the child, thereby enabling the child to develop an understanding and tolerance for these feelings. Psychodynamic play therapists understand that children often respond to them as a parent figure, or another significant adult, and project early experiences, feelings, and thoughts onto them, but they rarely interpret the wishes revealed in the transference. For example, physically abused children rarely strike their parents, more often displacing their anger onto siblings, peers, or animals, but some try to strike the therapist, who must limit such actions in order not to reinforce maladaptive retaliation behavior. Rather than interpreting this behavior, "You hit me like you wish you could hit your parents who hurt you," the therapist helps the child display anger in more appropriate ways, an ego supportive technique. The therapist might start out with, "You can't hit me, but you can hit the dummy" (action play); move to drawing a face, taping it onto the dummy, and then hitting it (delayed-action play) and encouraging the child to duplicate these actions; then move to expressing anger in doll play (play action); then to drawing or psychodramatic play with miniature people, accompanied by verbalizations (symbolic play); and perhaps, finally, to direct verbal expression (see Ekstein, 1966).

Helping children's play move from action play to symbolic play is an ego-supportive technique, which, by itself, is curative because it helps children develop better defenses against anxiety (distancing and more adaptive displacement) and utilize reenactment play to master feelings. Much more on this topic appears in Mordock and Crenshaw (2005a, 2005b).

Many psychodynamic play therapists credit their approach to relationship building to the work of humanist Clark Moustakas (1953, 1997) who describes the type of therapist–child relationship needed to make therapy a growth experience: one of close attention and attunement to the child's changing feelings. His stages start with children expressing generally negative feelings and as they are expressed, they diminish in intensity, resulting in the emergence of more positive feelings. In other words, transference feelings, and their accompanying projected images, diminish over time without necessarily requiring their interpretation and, as a result, children begin to respond to the adults in their lives less as "earlier similars" (Van Ornum & Mordock, 1983) and more as persons in their own right.

Psychodynamic play therapists also realize that many disturbed children progress slowly and rarely in a linear fashion. A step forward is often followed by a step backward, or by long periods with no noticeable growth. Like the ancient Chinese philosopher Lao-tzu, who founded Taoism, they realize that, "Even the longest journey must begin where you stand" (Chan, 1963).

There are many cases in the clinical literature that demonstrate the helpfulness of interpreting the neurotic child's defenses and then, when these interpretations are accepted, interpreting the underlying age–phase wishes that have gotten the child into trouble. Nevertheless, such activities are not part and parcel of the initial treatment plans designed to foster the development of many troubled children.

Introducing Structure

Another misconception about psychodynamic play therapy is that, like client-centered play therapy, the child's lead is always followed. Unfortunately, many children's actions in the playroom can lead nowhere! Often children actively avoid or lack meaningful play and fail to interact with the therapist in any meaningful way. The play can be solitary and repetitive, resulting in the therapist's feeling shut out, or it can become so aggressive that limits have to be constantly set (see Crenshaw & Mordock, 2005a). The avoidance or the aggressive play can be endless. In such cases, therapists need to take an active role in expanding the play and making it more emotionally significant. Initially, the play might reflect the child's struggles with flexibility or even with transference feelings, and characters can be introduced to engage the child while bringing these difficulties into focus.

As a result, the psychodynamic therapist, much like the cognitive-behavioral play therapist, often plays an active role in structuring the play therapy sessions by introducing play materials designed to reach certain goals, such as stimulating conflict-related play (see Crenshaw, 2006, 2008; Crenshaw & Mordock, 2005).

Unlike the approach of well-known play therapist Haim Ginott (1961), who simply watched children play and then commented on it, the therapist becomes a full participant whose engagement with children is an integral part of the play created. One of the first psychodynamic play therapists to actively play with children was David Levy (1938), who would introduce play materials that he thought would reveal the child's concerns. He called his approach "Release Therapy." Gove Hambidge (1955) expanded on his work by introducing many make-believe situations in play therapy and coined the term "Structured Play Therapy."

The format of the approach was to establish rapport, rec-reate the stress-evoking situation, and play out the situation, followed by free play to calm the child and reduce any leftover anxieties.

Strengthening Adaptive Skills and Developing Defenses

Rather than relying on interpretations to effect change, the psychodynamic therapist's treatment plan more often involves strengthening children's adaptive skills by helping them find better ways to express pent-up feelings and to develop more mature defenses against anxiety. These efforts are often called *ego-supportive* ones, and they, too, are discussed in detail in Crenshaw and Mordock (2005a, 2005b) and in Mordock (1997, 2001).

Considerable time is devoted to helping children give up their rigid use of primitive defense mechanisms, such as displacement and projection, and adopt more mature ones, such as undoing and sublimation. Sometimes they do so by introducing into the child's spontaneous play a more mature defense a child could use. For example, a child plays out a chaotic scene where everyone is injured, and the therapist introduces a toy ambulance to take the injured to the hospital (undoing). Other times structured activities can be introduced that emphasize the use of more mature defenses.

Asking Questions

Unlike client-centered therapists, psychodynamic therapists will often ask the child open-ended questions as therapy progresses, most often within the metaphor of the child's play rather than directly, often asked by an ignorant interrogator, such as a stupid-looking hand puppet. This approach allows the child to answer metaphorically rather than literally, important not only because many troubled children need the psychological distance it provides, but also because they cannot articulate their con-fused thoughts into words. Others have limited vocabularies, making it difficult to express verbally many of the issues and difficulties they face. Examples of questions within the metaphor of structured play activities appear in many publications by psychodynamic therapists, and some have even developed specific sets of questions to ask following specific play activities (e.g., see Crenshaw, 2006).

Therapeutic work in psychodynamic play therapy takes place on several levels. For example, a therapist who asked a boy feeling-related questions after observing his hostile interchanges between puppets might notice slight changes in the puppets' interchanges in future play activities, even though the boy never answered the questions directly. Continued efforts along these lines helps the boy identify and label his actual feelings, verbalize these feelings, engage in further problem-solving, take the better perspective of another, manage conflict better, and perhaps become more self-assertive rather than timid or aggressive.

Working with Caretakers

Psychodynamic play therapists use the information they gain from understanding children's play to help parents and teachers become aware of children's emotional issues and to give them positive ways to deal with their problem behaviors. In fact, it's often changes in caretaker actions toward children that enable them to change rather than the actions of the therapist in the playroom. For example, a 3-year-old girl was referred to an outpatient clinic for displaying nighttime terrors. In the first play session, she created play scenes of "monsters with different-colored hair." Her mother, a prostitute, loved her child; when the therapist asked in a nonjudgmental manner if she could change the arrangement of her customers' visits so her daughter had no contact with them, she did so and the girl's nightmares stopped. Although the therapist would have preferred a healthier living environment for the girl, the therapist knew that many unhealthy influences cannot be changed by therapeutic interventions.

Another example reveals the serendipitous result of one play session. A 7-year-old boy was simply told by the male therapist in his first therapy session, "It's all right to play with the toys in the room." He did so without revealing much of anything in his play with miniature toys and people. During his play, the therapist made only attention statements.

The therapist received a phone call the following day from the boy's irate mother asking him why he had asked her son questions about his absent father. The therapist reassured her that he had not asked her son questions of any kind. He then introduced the notion that because he was an older male who simply played with the boy, perhaps it stimulated him to ask her these questions. She said she didn't want to answer them because her ex was a "bad man" and her son should know nothing about him. The therapist suggested that she could at least clarify that it was nothing her son did that made his father leave and to emphasize any positive traits her ex had, no matter how insignificant they had been to her, such as good looks, good at his job, job stability, or any skills or athletic prowess he possessed. She wasn't sure she'd follow this advice and said that she wasn't bringing him back to therapy. Nevertheless, feedback several weeks later from school staff indicated that the boy was no longer symptomatic.

Current Status

There has been a significant decline in the use of psychodynamic treatment approaches over the last 40 years, not only in children's treatment but also in adult treatment. The fields of psychiatry and psychiatric nursing, enamored with a quick-fix philosophy, currently place considerable emphasis on the use of psychotropic drugs in the treatment of both adults and chil-

dren. Psychologists still receive training in psychotherapy, but the vast majority of psychology departments in universities across the country are enamored with approaches based on learning theories. Unlike psychodynamic concepts that were initially developed primarily by physicians, learning theory approaches were developed primarily by psychologists.

Academic psychologists also reject the system of hypothetical constructs created by psychodynamic theorists to interpret the behaviors they observe, considering the constructs as metaphysical, or as resulting from speculative philosophy, rather than from science. They believe the hypothetical constructs to be far-fetched, if not fanciful, and therefore unable to be tested under laboratory conditions. Nevertheless, psychodynamic theories, especially Freudian theory, have been subject to more scientific appraisal than any other psychological theory. For example, 35 years ago Fisher and Greenberg (1977) examined over 2,000 individual studies and were impressed with how often the results supported Freud's theories. They concluded: "We have actually not been able to find a single systematic psychological theory that has been as frequently evaluated scientifically as have Freud's concepts" (p. 396). This view could be also expressed today (see Shedler, 2010).

Clinical Case Example

Elsewhere I have discussed interview goals in psychodynamic play therapy, as well as presented numerous concrete case examples of psychodynamic therapeutic interventions, especially examples of those employed to help diminish the defiant and aggressive behaviors of very disturbed children—children who typically need at least a year of weekly therapy sessions to make progress (Mordock, 2001). In this example, I present an abbreviated case, actually a vignette, of a less disturbed child who was referred for outpatient treatment in an effort to avoid his placement in special education classes for children with behavior disorders. This presentation also presents the stages of psychodynamic play therapy, as well as some interview goals and general aims.

Hector was a fifth grader referred by the staff of his elementary school because he started fights with younger children on the playground. Hector's teachers and his mother also reported that he was friendless, appeared sad and unhappy, and devoted little energy to school tasks. Because 10-year-olds have been described by some play therapists as "too old to play, yet too young to talk," these therapists often use table games, such as checkers, to engage latency-age children while they try and talk with them. In an earlier work (Mordock, 2001) I discussed a child with presenting problems identical to Hector's with whom I used checkers productively, as the game had a special meaning for the child. However, typically I do not use structured table games, as I have found that they often contribute to the child's resistance to reveal feelings and fantasies—the steppingstones to uncovering the roots of problems.

The First Stage: Establishing the Working Relationship

The major tasks of the first stage of psychodynamic play therapy are forming a working relationship, allaying anxiety, and defining the nature of therapy.

THERAPIST: Your mother brought you to see me today because she and your teachers are concerned about your temper. They say you start fights with younger children, and they're afraid you will hurt some kid badly. They also say that you have no friends and seem sad and unhappy. [Interview goal of establishing that the interview has relevance to Hector's problems and that it can help him to meet his needs.]

HECTOR: I have friends!

THERAPIST: So you don't agree with your mom and teachers that you have no friends and are unhappy?

HECTOR: (*Fidgets in silence.*)

THERAPIST: You can move around if you want; we can talk without having to sit.

HECTOR: I don't want to talk.

THERAPIST: Talking about worries and troubles is hard for most children. Nevertheless, talk helps us to keep the worries inside us from bursting out in behavior toward others, especially behaviors that get us into trouble with adults and other children.

HECTOR: (*Gets up from his chair and opens a cupboard where play materials are stored.*) Do you have any checkers? I play checkers with my mom.

I could have asked Hector if he played checkers with his friends and perhaps gotten an admission that he had no friends with whom to play. Nevertheless psychodynamic play therapy is not a place to get a child to confirm his or her shortcomings, but rather a place to start a process, a place to fulfill one of the aims of psychodynamic treatment: *to strengthen relationships with caretakers*, including the therapist. Consequently, I proceeded as follows.

THERAPIST: No, but there is lots of drawing paper, crayons, and magic markers, and you can draw anything you like. [Interview goal of letting Hector tell "what's on his mind" in his own way.]

HECTOR: I don't draw!

THERAPIST: Okay! I will draw part of a drawing and you can finish it (*therapist draws a stick figure of a woman seated on a chair at a table with a checker set on it* [stick figures downplay drawing skills]).

HECTOR: (*Adds a stick figure of himself sitting at the table.*)

THERAPIST: Did your mom teach you how to play checkers?

HECTOR: Yes!

THERAPIST: And you enjoy playing with her. I'll bet you'd like to play games with her more often. Maybe after you see me for a while, she will play with you more often, but I can't promise you that! [I knew from my interview with Hector's mother that she had stopped playing table games with him because he always cheated and threw tantrums when he lost. I adhered to the second part of the first interview goal and to the aim of establishing hope for improved relationships with others.] Your mother told me that she stopped playing table games, like checkers, with you. Why do you think your mom did that?

HECTOR: (*Silence.*)

THERAPIST: Why don't we draw something else together? I'll start a drawing of your family doing something together. (*Draws a stick figure of the mother in a kitchen.*)

HECTOR: (*Takes a new piece of paper and struggles to draw a rudimentary truck.*)

Drawings that a child makes early in treatment may not be particularly revealing, but often are understood in retrospect. In Hector's case, his absent father was a truck driver, but I didn't know it at the time (I should have taken a more detailed case history) and therefore missed an opportunity to explore his feelings about his father. In the next session, I tried again to get Hector to draw his family doing something, but he didn't follow my example of a stick figure. Instead, he took another piece of paper and tried to draw a realistic image and experienced some difficulty, but no more so than other children who don't draw much. As a result, he ripped up the paper, called me stupid, and tried to leave the playroom.

THERAPIST: I know how bad some kids feel when they can't do something well. In our first session together, you said you didn't draw, and I'm sorry I asked you to do something you don't think you're good at. Perhaps we should do something together that you are good at. Can you make things with clay?

Like lots of troubled children, Hector was not an "arts-and-crafts" kid, but rather one who managed anxiety with gross motor play—and such play is limited by the small playroom setting (and should be discouraged if such efforts are made). As a result, he destroyed his imperfect productions, regardless of the modality employed, insulted the therapist, and wanted to leave the therapy room.

THERAPIST: I kind of get the feeling that while you call me *stupid*, you have been called *stupid* by others because you think that they think you're not good at anything!

HECTOR: (*Gets out the miniature people and creates a scene of boys teasing and ridiculing another boy, followed by the boy attacking the others and throwing them to the ground.*)

THERAPIST: Since they make him feel bad, the boy beats them all up, but now none of them will ever play with him again, but the ones much bigger than him may still tease him and call him *stupid*. I also suspect that your mother stopped playing with you because you hated to lose at checkers, and although you didn't try to beat her up, you blamed her for your failure and threw temper tantrums.

HECTOR: (*Takes a miniature mother figure and calls a miniature child figure "a poor loser."*)

In these initial sessions, the therapist and, more importantly, Hector obtained an initial understanding of Hector's problems. In a tactful and supporting manner, the therapist and Hector (albeit symbolically) agreed that his behavior not only was troublesome to others, but also was troublesome to him. It cost him some loving attention from his mother, as well as friendships. He also felt poorly about himself, believing himself to be stupid and incapable of normal childhood achievements. The therapist gave Hector the message that therapy will address these issues and help him to do something about them.

The Second Stage: Analysis of the Problems and Their Cause

The "cause" of Hector's problems, established in the initial sessions, was Hector's feeling stupid and resenting others whom he perceived as pointing out his weaknesses to him. The next steps were to help him to peel away more layers. Further sessions revealed that Hector held unrealistically high standards for himself that he maintained by fantasies of grandiosity and that his illusions were temporarily shattered by perceived failures. (Studies too numerous to mention have demonstrated that depressed individuals tend to judge their performances on tasks as poor regardless of their achievement level when compared to the self-judgments of nondepressed controls, a phenomenon often called "depressive pessimism" [e.g., see Norem, 2001].)

It also became apparent that his high standards were misguided efforts to win adult approval, especially from his absent father, who not only criticized him when they lived together, but also saw him as a rival for his wife's attention. In addition, Hector needs help to accept that he may never get his father's approval and, more importantly, that he can win approval more easily from others by displaying other behaviors. He also needs to learn that he misperceives intentions and that the teasing among children often characterizes their interactions with one another.

As therapy progressed, it became obvious that Hector had considerable ego strength. He rarely needed interpretations within the metaphor, as direct interpretations did not interrupt his play (a sign of increased anxiety) and his subsequent play usually became more productive, an indication that he had assimilated an interpretation rather than resisted it. He also talked

openly about some of his concerns, rare in most child treatment situations.

The Third Stage: Establish and Implement a Formula for Change

THERAPIST: We have both learned that you thought your dad left because you were not perfect and, as a result, you became overly sensitive to criticism and overreacted to teasing, as well as failed to understand that teasing often occurs among friends. I think that if we "talk" more about your feelings about your dad leaving, that some of your anger that gets you into trouble will begin to go away. [I use the word *talk* loosely, realizing that Hector typically starts out by creating play scenes that relate to his feelings.]

The Fourth Stage: Termination

Psychodynamic play therapy ends when the child's behavior suggests that he or she is mastering age-appropriate challenges. The child may still be symptomatic, but the symptoms are less pronounced, suggesting that the child is on the road to recovery. Successful termination can be a growth experience; elsewhere I presented some techniques to facilitate this process (Mordock, 2001). Unfortunately, in most outpatient situations, when the child has shown some progress, as was the case with Hector, the parent, or parents, stop bringing the child for therapy.

Conclusion

Stages in psychodynamic play therapy are similar to stages in growth. Well-known developmental psychologist Jean Piaget (1952; see Flavell, 1970) describes growth as transitions from one stage to another, resulting from a "set" or attitude that comes from within. What is learned at any given point is determined by what has taken place before, not merely by what the child has experienced, but more by the elements to which he or she has paid attention. "Every instruction from without presupposes a construction from within" (Flavell, 1970, p. 406).

NOTE

1. According to Freud (1962), psychological development in childhood is characterized by a series of stages he called *psychosexual stages* (he used the term *sexual* in a broad way to encompass all pleasurable actions and thoughts). In each stage, *libido* (roughly translated as sexual drives or instincts) becomes fixated on different erogenous zones that serve as sources of both pleasure and frustration. In each psychosexual stage, the child experiences a particular conflict that must be resolved before successful advancement to the next stage. The resolution of each conflict requires the expenditure of sexual energy, and the more energy expended at a particular stage, the more the important characteristics of that stage remain with each individual as he or she matures psychologically.

Both frustration and overindulgence (or any combination of the two) may lead to what Freud called *fixation* at a particular psychosexual stage. *Fixation* refers to the theoretical notion that a portion of the individual's libido has been permanently invested in a particular stage of development. Also assumed is that some libido is always invested in each psychosexual stage and, as a result, an adult's personality will reflect, in some way, behaviors characteristic of infancy or early childhood.

In the *oral phase* (0–2 years of age) all desires are met through the lips and mouth, which accept food, milk, and just about anything else infants can get their hands on to sooth themselves, with caretakers often using pacifiers to keep them calm, while keeping small objects out of their reach so they won't choke on them. The first object cathexis of this stage is the mother's breast, often transferred to autoerotic objects, such as thumb-sucking. The good mother becomes the first "love object," already a displacement from the earlier object desired, the mother's breast. The primary conflict at this stage is the weaning process, and children must become less dependent upon caretakers. Freud believed

that if fixation occurs at this stage, individuals would have issues with dependency or aggression. Oral fixation can result in problems with drinking, eating, smoking, or nail-biting.

In the *anal phase* (2–4 years of age) interest develops in a new autoerotic object: the rectal orifice. The major conflict at this stage is toilet training; children have to learn to control bodily needs. Developing this control leads to a sense of accomplishment and independence. The phase is split between active and passive impulses: the impulse to mastery, on the one hand, which can easily become cruelty (sadism), and the impulse to scopophilia (love of gazing), on the other hand. According to Freud, children's pleasure in defecation is connected to pleasure in creating something of their own, a pleasure which girls later transfer to childbearing.

In the *phallic phase*, the penis (or the clitoris) becomes the primary object cathexis. Children become fascinated with urination, which is experienced as pleasurable, both in its expulsion and retention, and masturbation (in both sexes) becomes a new source of pleasure. They also become aware of anatomical sex differences, setting in motion conflicts about erotic attraction, resentment, rivalry, and jealousy. At this age, normal parents become more modest after catching their children peeking at them when they are dressing or in the shower. The trauma connected with this phase is that of castration, which makes this phase especially important for the resolution of what Freud called the *Oedipus complex*, when boys begin to view their fathers as rivals for their mother's affections, with boys fearing punishment by their fathers for these feelings—a fear Freud termed *castration anxiety*. The term *Electra complex* is used to describe a similar set of feelings experienced by young girls. Freud, however, believed that girls instead experience *penis envy*, disputed by a number of other psychoanalysts, especially Karen Horney, calling it both inaccurate and demeaning to women. Instead, Horney proposed that men experience feelings of inferiority because they cannot give birth to children.

During this phase, children learn to defer bodily gratification when necessary. In other words, the ego becomes trained to follow the reality principle and to control the pleasure principle, although this ability is not fully developed until children successfully pass through the latency period. Children also begin to deal with separation anxieties (and with an all-encompassing egoism) by finding symbolic ways of representing the mother and thus controlling separations from her (not to mention the desire for her). Transitional objects, such as Linus's blanket in the *Peanuts* comic strip, are one example. In resolving the Oedipus and Electra complexes, children begin to identify with either their mothers or fathers, thus determining the future path of sexual orientation. Identification takes the form of an "ego ideal," which aids in formation of the "superego": an internalization of the parental function (which Freud usually associated with the father, but others have attributed to both parents) that eventually manifests itself in conscience (and sense of guilt).

Next follows a long *latency phase* (7–12 years of age) during which sexual development is more or less suspended and children concentrate on repressing and sublimating earlier desires and thus learn to follow the reality principle. During this phase, children are gradually freed from dependence upon parents (moving away from the mother and reconciling with the father) or actively asserting independence (if the male child responded to incestuous desires by becoming overly subservient to the father or if the female child becomes overly close to the father and jealous of the mother). Children also move beyond childhood egoism and sacrifice something of their own egos to others (give up narcissism, i.e., self-centeredness), thus learning how to love others.

From about 13 years of age onward (from puberty onward) development over the calm latency period allows children to enter the final *genital phase*. At this point, members of the opposite sex are desired, as well as the desire to fulfill the instinct to procreate and thus ensure the survival of the human species.

The ages provided are very rough approximations since Freud often changed his mind about the actual parameters of the various stages and also acknowledged that development varied among individuals. Stages can even overlap or be experienced simultaneously. In short, psychoanalytic theory holds that personality develops out of the need to fulfill the pleasure principle by attempting to negotiate reality demands without incurring superego strictures. Nowhere is this process more critically developed and honed than within the formative years between birth and the onset of the post-Oedipal, latency years.

REFERENCES

Adler, A. (1964). *Superiority and social interest: A collection of later writings* (H. L. Ansbacher & R. R. Ansbacher, Eds.). New York: Norton.

Alexander, F., & French, T. M. (1946). *Psychoanalytic therapy: Principles and application.* New York: Ronald Press.

Alpert, A. (1957). A special therapeutic technique for certain developmental disorders in latency. *American Journal of Orthopsychiatry, 27,* 256–270.

Bowlby, J. (1988). *A secure base: Parent–child attachment and healthy human development.* London: Routledge.

Bromfield, R. (1992). *Playing for real: Exploring child therapy and the inner worlds of children.* New York: Dutton.

Bromfield, R. (2007). *Doing child and adolescent psychotherapy: Adapting psychodynamic treatment to contemporary practice.* New York: Wiley-Interscience.

Chan, W. (1963). *The way of Lao Tzu.* Cambridge, UK: Pearson.

Crenshaw, D. A. (2006). *Evocative strategies in child and adolescent psychotherapy.* Lanham, MD: Aronson.

Crenshaw, D. A. (2008). *Therapeutic engagement of children and adolescents: Play, symbol, drawing, and storytelling strategies.* Lanham, MD: Aronson.

Crenshaw, D. A., & Mordock, J. B. (2005a). *Handbook of play therapy with aggressive children.* Lanham, MD: Aronson.

Crenshaw, D. A., & Mordock, J. B. (2005b). *Understanding and treating the aggression of children.* Lanham, MD: Aronson.

Ekstein, R. (1966). *Children of time and space of action and impulse.* New York: Appleton-Century-Crofts.

Erikson, E. H. (1950). *Childhood and society.* New York: Norton.

Fisher, S., & Greenberg, R. F. (1977). *The scientific credibility of Freud's theories and therapy.* New York: Basic Books.

Flavell, J. H. (1970). *The developmental psychology of Jean Piaget.* New York: Van Nostrand Reinhold.

Freud, A. (1937). *The ego and the mechanisms of defense.* London: Hogarth Press and Institute of Psycho-Analysis.

Freud, A. (1975). *Introduction to the technique of child analysis* (L. P. Clark, Trans.). New York: Arno Press. (Original work published 1938)

Freud, S. (1962). *Three essays on the theory of sexuality* (J. Strachey, Trans.). New York: Basic Books.

Ginott, H. G. (1961). *Group therapy with children: The theory and practice of play therapy.* New York: McGraw-Hill.

Hambridge, G. (1955). Structured play therapy. *American Journal of Orthopsychiatry, 25,* 601–617.

Holmes, M. (2010). Subject of focus: The lives of emigrants—the life of Edith Weigert (née Vowinckel) (1894–1982) (C. S. Noël, Trans.). *Psychiatry, 73,* 1–33.

Horney, K. (1945). *Our inner conflicts.* New York: Norton.

Klein, M. (1984). *The writings of Melanie Klein: Vol. 2. The psycho-analysis of children* (A. Strachey, Trans.; R. Money-Kyrle, Ed.). New York: Free Press. (Original work published 1932)

Kohut, H. (1971). *The analysis of the self: A systematic approach to the psychoanalytic treatment of narcissistic personality disorders.* New York: International Universities Press.

Lee, A. E. (1997). Psychoanalytic play therapy. In K. J. O'Connor & L. M. Braverman (Eds.), *Play therapy theory and practice: A comparative presentation* (pp. 46–78). New York: Wiley.

Levy, D. (1938). Release therapy in young children. *Psychiatry, 1,* 387–389.

Lewis, M. (1974). Interpretations in child analysis: Developmental considerations. *Journal of the American Academy of Child Psychiatry, 13,* 32–53.

Mahler, M. H. (1969). *On human symbiosis and the vicissitudes of individuation.* London: Hogarth Press and the Institute of Psycho-Analysis.

Maslow, A. H. (1954). *Motivation and personality.* New York: Harper.

Mordock, J. B. (1997). Ego-supportive play therapy for children who lack imaginative play: Building defenses. *International Journal of Play Therapy, 6,* 23–40.

Mordock, J. B. (2001). *Counseling the defiant child.* Northvale, NJ: Aronson.

Moustakas, C. (1953). *Children in play therapy.* New York: McGraw-Hill.

Moustakas, C. (1997). *Relationship play therapy.* Northvale, NJ: Aronson.

Norem, J. (2001). *The positive power of negative thinking.* Cambridge, MA: Basic Books.

Piaget, J. (1952). *The origins of intelligence in children.* New York: International University Press.

Rank, B., & MacNaughton, D. (1956). A clinical contribution to early ego development. *Psychoanalytic Study of the Child, 5,* 53–63.

Russell, B. (1917). Knowledge by acquaintance and knowledge by description. In B. Russell, *Mysticism and logic* (pp. 152–167). London: George Allen & Unwin.

Shedler, J. (2010). The efficacy of psychodynamic psychotherapy. *American Psychologist, 65,* 98–109.

Van Ornum, W., & Mordock, J. B. (1983). *Crisis counseling of children and adolescents.* New York: Continuum.

von Hug-Hellmuth, H. (1920). On the technique of child-analysis. *International Journal of Psycho-Analysis, 2,* 287–305.

Werner, H., & Kaplan, B. (1973). The organismic–developmental framework. In S. G. Sapir & A. C. Nitzburg (Eds.), *Children with learning problems: Readings in the developmental–interactional approach* (pp. 148–155). New York: Brunner/Mazel.

Winnicott, D. W. (1965). *Maturational processes and the facilitating environment: Studies in the theory of emotional development.* London: Hogarth Press.

Winnicott, D. W. (1971). *Playing and reality.* London: Routledge.

CHAPTER 6

Cognitive-Behavioral Play Therapy

Angela M. Cavett

Play therapy was originally utilized by psychoanalyst Hermine Hug-Hellmuth (Maclean & Ulrich, 1991) and since then play has been utilized in most therapy with children. However, even with the founders of child psychotherapy, different clinicians conceptualized play differently. For instance, Anna Freud (1964) considered play a means to develop relationship, whereas Melanie Klein (1955) analyzed play in the same manner that her colleagues analyzed the words of their adult patients. Play therapy has reflected the movements of adult models for therapy. Specifically, it has been utilized and adapted across a range of theoretical orientations similar to therapies utilized for adults but with developmentally sensitive approaches. Most contemporary play therapists utilize child-centered play therapy, which reflects the emphasis of child-centered theory in the major teaching facilities in the United States. However, the field of child psychology has moved more and more toward cognitive-behavioral theories. Cognitive-behavioral play therapy (CBPT) was developed by Susan Knell as an extension of cognitive therapy for young children. CBPT extends the model of cognitive-behavioral therapy (CBT) to young children by allow-ing for communication through play within the therapy. CBPT is a developmentally appropriate treatment that is sensitive to emotional, cognitive, and linguistic development. This chapter considers the theory of CBPT.

History of Cognitive Therapy and Behavioral Therapy

Cognitive therapy was developed by Aaron Beck (1963, 1964, 1972, 1976) and is based on the interactions between feelings, thoughts, behaviors, and the environment (Beck & Emery, 1985). Beck (1967, 1972) proposed that cognitions impact emotions. Changing cognitions is considered facilitative of changing feelings/emotions. The cognitive triangle is utilized in CBT to describe the relationships among feelings, thoughts/cognitions, and behaviors. Factors that are also interrelated to the cognitive triad include the environment and physiology. Cognitive therapy is utilized to make changes in the cognitive component in order to decrease pathology. Beck (1976) considered irrational or maladaptive thoughts to comprise beliefs that were associated with distress. Irrational or maladaptive thoughts are considered the cause of psychological dysfunction, including depression and anxiety and the behavioral responses to them. With young children, it may be more helpful (and less condescending) to consider "irrational" thoughts related to pathology as "unhelpful."

Behavioral therapy addresses the impact of environmental influences on behavior and pathology. Behavioral therapies utilize operant and classical conditioning and social learning theory. Operant conditioning recognizes the function of reinforcers and punishments and manipulates them to improve or change behaviors (Skinner, 1938). Parents, teachers, and clinicians use operant conditioning to increase and decrease behaviors through rewards and punishments. In the treatment of children the common behavioral strategies utilized are based on operant conditioning and include contingency management (i.e., positive reinforcement and time out), self-management, shaping, differential reinforcement of other behavior, stimulus fading, and extinction.

CBT is a related model describing how changes can be made to affect and behavior. CBT incorporates concepts and interventions from both cognitive therapy and behavioral therapy. The integration of both cognitive and behavioral strategies has proliferated among treatments for adults, adolescents, and more recently, with respect for developmental concerns, children.

Play

Developmental issues restrict the use of the predominantly verbal CBT. However, with the use of play, some of those limitations can be addressed. Play allows for several cognitive processes as discussed by Russ (2004), including fantasy/make-believe, symbolism, organization, and divergent thinking. Play also can engage several affective processes, such as expression of emotion; expression of affective themes; enjoyment of play; and cognitive integration, emotion regulation,

and modulation of affect (Russ, 2004). Russ found that play had several properties that can be utilized in play therapy. Her review of the research on play indicated that play can engage the following processes:

1. Problem solving that requires a capacity for insight.
2. Flexibility in problem solving.
3. Ability to think diversely. (I prefer to leave this divergent thinking as I believe Russ would prefer it that way.)
4. Ability to think of alternative strategies in coping with daily problems.
5. Experience of positive emotion.
6. Ability to think about affective themes (positive and negative).
7. Ability to understand the emotions of others and take the perspective of another.
8. Aspects of general adjustment.

CBPT utilizes each of these processes in helping children address emotional and behavioral problems.

History of CBPT

CBT was developed for adults. Play therapy has been considered the treatment of choice for young children. For children in the preoperational stage (Piaget, 1972), cognitive functioning has been considered an obstacle to utilizing traditional CBT techniques. However, adaptations have allowed for adolescents and children to be treated with developmentally sensitive variations of CBT. Roger Phillips (1985) proposed an integration of CBT with play therapy, and Susan Knell (2009) articulated a model CBPT as a modification of CBT for preschool and young school-age children. Traditional cognitive therapy would indicate that behavior is mediated through verbalizations or words. However, if cognitive therapy is based on cognitions and not exclusively verbalizations, then the manner in which thoughts are communicated can be verbal or nonverbal. Play is how children express most of their thoughts, fantasies, and experiences. In CBPT, concrete examples of concepts are often used to help children understand those concepts and express their thoughts. CBPT does not rely on the typical open-ended questions often used to engage adults in conversations about their emotional lives. Cognitive-behavioral play therapists have developed structured, directive play therapy techniques that address presenting problems across the full range of psychological concerns.

The processing of information through verbalizations is the focus of CBT for adults. Indeed, it is thought that verbalizations mediate behaviors (Beck & Emery, 1985). Verbal processing allows for insight into cognitions. In CBPT, communication between the child and therapist can be verbal, nonverbal, or play-based. Verbalizations are not necessarily the form of communication through which one sees a child's innermost processing. Play allows for deeper appreciation of children's experiences and for processing how those experiences impact them psychologically. Verbalization during and following play helps the child integrate the played experience and return to and reference the played experience at a later time. As the extension of played communication, the experiencing of the cognition allows the child to encode the experience as a verbal, not only an experienced, memory.

Play within CBPT helps the child communicate with the therapist in a manner that is developmentally sensitive and comfortable for the child. Garry Landreth says that "the natural medium of communication for children is play and activity" (1991, p. 7). As with child-centered play therapy, the CBPT therapist appreciates and respects that the child is able to communicate through play. Indeed, across theoretical orientations, play is considered the language of the child. How the language is utilized in the sessions varies across theoretical orientation while maintaining appreciation for the importance of play as the child's language.

With adults, CBT focuses on changing faulty or irrational ideas to rational ideas. The shift from irrational to rational thoughts is considered causal in decreasing psychopathology (Beck, 1970). Use of the Socratic method with adults, which engages higher cognitive abilities, may facilitate shifts from irrational to rational thoughts, with a concomitant decrease in symptoms. With young children, determining whether a thought is "rational" or "irrational" is not necessary or even always possible given cognitive development. However, children are encouraged to learn to verbalize their thoughts, and considering these cognitions, how they interact with feelings and behaviors, and making modifications is one component of therapy that is possible and adaptive. An effective strategy is to talk with a child about how two other children, for example, would deal with a problem and to guess each of those children's thought processes. By comparing the imagined children and their outcomes, the child in CBPT is able to reconsider how he or she will think about the situation. Due to children's reliance on parents, the therapist must also process this information with the parent/caregiver and others (e.g., teachers) who are influential in the child's life.

The integration of play therapy theories with cognitive-behavioral theories is discussed in two influential books by Eliana Gil (2006) and Athena Drewes (2009). Gil discusses the importance of listening to the child while also using the strengths of cognitive-behavioral strategies that apply to the individual child's needs. Her approach integrates directive and nondirective approaches, allowing the child's voice to be the primary driving force in selecting play interventions. Drewes's edited book provides support for the integration of play therapy with cognitive-behavioral theories.

Properties of the Approach

The following properties/characteristics of CBPT were articulated by Susan Knell (2009).

1. CBPT utilizes play to engage with the child. Play allows the child to be an active participant in the therapy. Play that is interesting to the child lowers the child's resistance and increases treatment compliance. Play is viewed as an expression of thought/language. By using play to communicate with the child, CBPT demonstrates respect for the voice of the child. By allowing the child to "voice" him- or herself through play, the child is encouraged to actively participate in his or her own therapy.

2. CBPT focuses on feelings, thoughts, and behaviors as well as addressing the environment. Knell (2009) also suggests that fantasies are addressed through CBPT.

3. CBPT can be utilized to introduce and teach coping strategies. Whereas verbalization may provide opportunity for adults to change maladaptive, irrational thoughts, play allows for processing of the child's cognitions, which may result in positive, more adaptive cognitions.

4. CBPT is problem/goal-oriented, time-limited, directive, and structured. Treatment goals in CBPT are related to the presenting problem.

5. CBPT has a plethora of research providing empirical support for its treatments. Not surprisingly, CBPT incorporates strategies and interventions (e.g., relaxation techniques, processing of trauma narratives) that are supported by research. However, the research base for CBPT as an independent treatment has not been adequately explored. CBPT is likely to elicit further study in the future, and given the structure of CBPT, research could easily be conducted on treatments specific to disorders.

The Use of Play, Toys, and Play Materials

Knell and Dasari (2011) have suggested the use of toys for CBPT. Her suggestions have been expanded to reflect varying presenting problems. Puppets, for example, across a range of emotions are suggested to allow for emotional expression consistent with the range of affect with which children may present. Puppets can represent human figures or animals. Art supplies (e.g., paper, crayons, markers, paints) allow for expression of thoughts and feelings. Many play therapy techniques consistent with CBPT require specific art materials. Typically these are described in detail, cookbook style, in the CBPT-consistent books. Toys that allow children to express responses consistent with their experiences are beneficial. A kitchen area and dress-up allow for expressions related to the child's family life.

Toys in CBPT typically include imaginative toys such as a dollhouse, furniture, and human figures. It is ideal to make available dolls or human figures that represent the people who may be in the lives of children presenting for therapy. This means that dolls/human figures should span a range of ages, genders, skin tones, and facial features to reflect diverse cultural backgrounds. It may be beneficial to have dolls that reflect different family members (e.g., parents, grandparents, children, babies). Dolls can also reflect ability differences and professional affiliations (teachers, doctors, veterinarians) that children may encounter.

A dollhouse is highly recommended for children using CBPT. If possible, several other toy buildings are suggested to allow for expression of a range of responses and experiences that may relate to children's presenting problems. A second or even third dollhouse allows children to represent different experiences, especially when the dollhouses are different sizes. For example, children may use two dollhouses to represent Mom's house and Dad's house or home and foster home. Other suggested play buildings include a hospital, fire station, police station, courthouse, and school. If the therapist does not have access to, or space for, each of these toys, the child can use other resources (e.g., a shoebox) to represent the buildings. Other human figures and perhaps those based in fantasy (e.g., superhero figures) facilitate children's expression of a wide range of thoughts and feelings in their play therapy.

Problem- and Goal-Oriented

CBPT is problem-oriented, meaning that the approach focuses on specific problems in a child's life for which treatment is sought. These problems may relate to relationships, emotions, behaviors, or other areas that impact the quality of life for the child and those around him or her. CBPT focuses on the uniqueness of each child in a supportive and empathic manner in order to assist the child and family in making changes to improve the problematic areas. CBPT connects with the child and establishes a positive relationship through which change may be facilitated based on a developmentally appropriate version of the CBPT model. At times, non-CBPT therapists may misunderstand the problem-oriented focus to mean that the problem is the focus of the sessions and that the therapeutic relationship is secondary. This is a misconception, as the relationship is fundamental in effecting cognitive, affective, and behavioral changes. The problem orientation allows the therapist to respect the child's pain and discomfort and use a model of change to establish goals with the child and family. CBPT is goal-oriented in that the child's functioning has been an area of concern; assessment provides information about domains of functioning that are problematic. Goals are based on reducing symptoms and increasing functioning.

The Role of the Therapist

As with all therapeutic models, the relationship is an important factor in the effectiveness of the therapy. Conceptually, however, the therapeutic relationship is not considered the central agent of change in CBPT. The positive therapeutic relationship is necessary but not sufficient for psychological change to occur related to the treatment. A supportive and empathic therapist pro-

vides the guidance for the cognitive and behavioral change factors to work. The positive therapeutic relationship is necessary in CBPT for the child to explore his or her experiences and associated feelings and thoughts. Rapport with a supportive and empathic person provides the safety that is necessary regardless of theoretical orientation. The therapist utilizing CBPT is directive in the process. Being directive is similar to many relationships between children and adults, including parents and teachers. The directive nature of the cognitive-behavioral play therapist allows the therapy to focus on the goals of treatment, including introducing the areas that have caused concern/difficulty in the child's life and possible strategies and interventions that may improve functioning.

Empathy within the Therapeutic Relationship

Empathy from the cognitive-behavioral play therapist for the child and the child's experiences lays the foundation for change. As the therapist works with the child to change thoughts/perceptions/cognitions that are hurtful to the child, respect for how the thoughts/perceptions/cognitions were developed is communicated. For example, if a child feels angry about parental divorce or illness, the therapist empathizes with the child and shows deep appreciation for the present feeling. Only after shared experiencing and empathizing with the child's experience does the therapist suggest, verbally or through play, that another alternative is possible. This approach allows for the child to be heard and respected. As the child feels the appreciation of the therapist for his or her experience, the child may open to the possibility of considering more adaptive responses and behaviors. The therapist can also show respect for the problematic behaviors, even maladaptive ones, that the child has displayed as a means of communicating emotion. An example, in the following scenario, depicts a therapist utilizing puppets (named by the child) to communicate with the child about his aggression and the feelings related to it.

Jamal is asked to use puppets to show an event from the past week that was described by his mother. The incident included Jamal and his brother Jerome arguing, with Jerome calling Jamal names, and Jamal acting out with physical aggression.

(Puppet shows aggression toward another puppet.)

THERAPIST: It seems like Jamal [puppet] is really angry with Jerome [puppet].

JAMAL: Yes, he hates him for saying he is stupid.

THERAPIST: It is very hurtful to Jamal when Jerome says things like that. He feels really angry when he is called stupid or other mean things.

JAMAL: Yes, I hate him when he is mean to me so I just punch him. (*Shows his puppet hitting and slapping the other puppet.*)

THERAPIST: You are really angry and it hurts you so much. You just feel like you need to show him how you feel, that you feel really angry. (*pause*) And hurt. You feel really angry and hurt and he should know that! You want him to know that!

JAMAL: Yes, I feel angry! He hurts my feelings when he says that!

THERAPIST: And when your feelings are hurt, it is really important for you to tell others how you feel. You want them to know how you feel. Jerome doesn't get to hurt your feelings and not know how much that hurts you.

JAMAL: He needs to know it is mean.

THERAPIST: Yes, he needs to know that you feel hurt and angry. He needs to know that when he hurts you, you don't like it. (*pause*) It really hurts to have someone say mean things about you, and you can tell them how much it hurts. How you feel matters.

JAMAL: Yeah.

THERAPIST: Let's think about a way words could help show someone how angry you are. Maybe words could tell someone how angry and hurt you are. Then you wouldn't have to hit and you would get in less trouble too.

Differences between CBPT and Other Play Therapies

Knell articulated differences between CBPT and other play therapies, especially child-centered and psychoanalytic play therapies (Knell, 2009).

1. CBPT is directive, whereas child-centered therapies are nondirective and follow the lead of the child. The directive quality of CBPT and the focus on problems are interrelated.

2. Therapists choose the toys in CBPT based on the needs and presenting problems of the child. Different toys are used to address different therapeutic issues and therefore are utilized with different children. Children also may choose toys in sessions as indicated by the therapeutic need. Rapport building and allowing the child space to communicate his or her experiences are components of CBPT that are facilitated by the child choosing toys.

3. CBPT includes psychoeducation dependent upon the needs and concerns of the child. The therapist draws upon knowledge about the child, family, and relevant literature to address the therapeutic concerns. In CBPT, the clinician uses play to teach concepts such as the connection between feelings and thoughts. Coping skills—such as mindfulness, labeling feelings, journaling, and changing thoughts—are directly explored and taught in CBPT.

4. Cognitive-behavioral play therapists observe and allow for nonverbal, especially play-based, and verbal communication of concerns related to the presenting

problem, including emotional concerns (i.e., feelings of worthlessness or depression) and behavioral issues (i.e., physical aggression toward siblings). Both psychoanalytic and CBPT therapists offer children possible meaning based on their communications. The CBPT therapist offers the child verbalizations consistent with the child's play and they collaboratively explore whether there are patterns of thinking that are associated with the problems. The psychoanalytic therapist offers interpretations that are often based on the unconscious. For CBPT this would be conceptualized as automatic thoughts that influence mood and behavior. The child-centered play therapist would not suggest or direct that exploration but allows the child to process through the play with the belief that this will provide what the child needs to make changes.

5. With nondirective play therapies, praise is not allowed and is considered detrimental to the process. CBPT allows for and encourages praise as a positive reinforcement of the child's adaptive behaviors.

Interventions

Assessment

Observing children's play is perhaps the most effective method of assessing their functioning across most domains, including affective/emotional, cognitive, behavioral, and language domains. Play therapists have historically utilized play as a window to the child's thoughts and experiences. For nondirective play therapists, observation without a standardized method has been acceptable and consistent with their theoretical models. However, more behaviorally oriented therapists have sought a quantifiable method of assessment. The Child Behavior Checklist (CBCL; Achenbach, 1991) provides promise for CBPT therapists who are trained and qualified to administer psy-

chological testing. This assessment as well as the teacher and youth versions provide a thorough picture of the child's overall functioning as well as problem areas related to internalizing (i.e., Withdrawn/Depressed) and externalizing (i.e., Rule-Breaking Behavior) problems. The CBCL provides promise for assessing outcomes of therapies and routine use when treating children using CBPT.

The Puppet Interview (Irwin, 2000) and the Puppet Sentence Completion Task (Cavett, 2010; Knell, 1992; Knell & Beck, 2000) were developed to provide a means to assess the perceptions of children. The Puppet Sentence Completion Task provides clinicians with sentence fragments that can guide the assessment of children. Clinicians can develop their own fragments to assist in the assessment of children based on their unique presenting problems and situations. In the Puppet Interview the child's responses to sentence stems allow the clinician insight into the experiences and thoughts of the child. By assessing themes of responses, the therapist can address issues in the play to promote change in thinking followed by mood and behavior.

In the early sessions, the therapist observes the child's play to assess for cognitions (beliefs, thoughts, perceptions of self and other). Children typically do not come to session with easily articulated positive or negative cognitions. Learning to hear the language of the child in CBPT is similar to the learning process in nondirective play therapy. The use of basic therapy/counseling skills such as reflective listening and tracking are necessary to understand the world of the individual child with whom the CBPT therapist is present in that session. The use of themes such as those articulated by Helen Benedict (2004) can be used to assess the child's play. As the child expresses him- or herself through play and this play is "heard" by the therapist, a mutual understanding is developed. Throughout CBPT, portions of sessions are spent with the child engaged in nondirective play to allow for observation of the child's spontaneous experiences. The "thoughts" expressed through the play are integrated into the working portions of the session.

Treatment Planning

Children are often brought to therapy by their parents and may have been referred by other adults (e.g., teachers) who are impacted by their behaviors. Unlike adults who typically seek out therapy for themselves, children are typically not the initiators of this process. Parental and teacher reports are considered important information in guiding treatment. Usually children are aware of the problematic feelings, thoughts, and behaviors that have resulted in their referral to therapy. Therefore, in addition to the referral information, the child's perspective is considered invaluable. The cognitive-behavioral play therapist allows the child to become engaged and an active partner in the process. Throughout the duration of therapy information is sought not only *about*, but also *from*, the child.

Treatment planning strategies in CBPT allow for the child to engage in the process by sharing what behaviors he or she would like to work on in therapy. The process of treatment planning co-occurs with rapport building, and both are primarily focused on developing the relationship between the child and therapist. During the early sessions, the cognitive-behavioral play therapist develops the relationship while learning about the child's view of self, others, and world. Interventions such as the wishing well (Goodyear-Brown, 2005) allow the child to explore how things could change for him or her. With the wishing well intervention, the child creates a split sandtray, with one side representing current experience and the other side reflecting what he or she wants his or her life to be like. A wishing well figure can be used in the center of the tray.

Another intervention, Stepping Up to Success (Cavett, 2010), is a simple activity

wherein the therapist and child create an art representation of steps out of colored paper and art supplies with precut footprints going up each stair. On each stair the child and therapist write or draw a problem that they would like to change. On the footprints, the child and therapist write interventions that will address each of the problems noted on the stairs. This intervention is used initially as a map or visual representation of what will be addressed and how in therapy. Throughout therapy, the stairs and footprints can be brought out as the process and progress of therapy are discussed.

Strategies and Techniques

Affective Understanding and Modulation

A focus of CBPT is an exploration that allows the child to better understand his or her emotions. The therapeutic relationship is the medium for the most important processing of emotional/affective content. The therapist is open and genuine in reflecting emotion both in the child's play and while discussing the child's perceptions. The therapist accepts the child as he or she is and reflects the child's experience to gain deeper understanding of his or her experience. The therapist and child work together, first, to appreciate the child's affective experience. The therapist and child then build an understanding of how the negative affective experience can change to allow for positive affective experience. Often children enter therapy with symptoms that reflect situations that are difficult, even traumatizing. To move too quickly from the place of respecting the child's experience to "trying to change" the child is not beneficial and could possibly be damaging. Only through understanding and appreciating the child's experience and his or her affective responses can true change occur. The therapist, after fully appreciating the depth of the child's sadness, anxiety, or anger, can begin to explore alternatives that are respectful of the child's earlier experiences and the process of healing. The parent or caregiver is also included in empathizing with, and building affective understanding in, the child and in the parent–child dyad.

Although the therapeutic relationship is the primary "tool" by which the child benefits from CBPT, interventions may be utilized to facilitate the process. CBPT techniques allow children to learn about affect in self and others. Affective understanding begins with identifying emotions. As the therapist listens to the child's experiences via the child's verbal and nonverbal communications, including those reflected in play, the therapist is able to teach the child simple affective skills such as the labeling of emotions. The identification of feelings relates to facial expressions and bodily sensations. "Feelings charades" help children understand the expression of feelings. When feelings charades are done with a parent, the child is able to see what a particular feeling looks like in people who are present in his or her life. Another intervention often used to begin to develop a feelings vocabulary is the Color Your Life (O'Conner, 1983) intervention.

The physiology of affect can be understood through play therapy interventions. The connections between physiological reactions and the child's emotions can be revealed within the therapy using reflective statements. For instance, a therapist may reflect to the child the expressions that he or she is displaying and then extend the conversation to asking and dialoguing about the child's internal state such as heart rate, muscle tension/tightening, and nausea.

The relationship is also used to begin discussing the concept of quantifying affective intensity. Many play therapy interventions allow for further exploration of the intensity of emotion. For instance, the parachute feelings bounce-o'meter (Cavett, 2010) allows the child to express the intensity of emotions using a parachute and balls with more intense, vigorous waving for more intensity of affect. Measuring affect allows the child to understand the intensity of the felt emotion and the frequent correlation between intensity of affect and behavior. A child with a "small" amount of anger is likely to behave differently than one with a "big" amount of anger. Many play-based interventions have been developed to facilitate understanding of the concept of measuring the affective intensity. A play-based intervention for understanding the intensity of a feeling is the *feelings abacus* (Cavett, 2010), whereby the child indicates varying amounts of emotional responding throughout and between sessions. A magnetic strip is adhered to the vertical side of an abacus. Different feelings are written on card stock cut into small rectangular strips. Circular magnets are placed on the backs of the card stock so that the feeling tags adhere to the abacus. The beads on the abacus are used to represent the intensity of the emotion. For instance, one bead beside the word *worried* indicates a "small" amount of anxiety whereas five beads indicate a moderate amount, and 10 beads indicate the "most ever." Within CBPT children are able to process concepts related to affective modulation in the context of their play.

Charting or Journaling of Feelings, Thoughts, and Behaviors

Parents are partners in therapy with children. Parents' journaling about their perceptions regarding their child's feelings, thoughts, and behaviors is seen as beneficial in CBPT. Charting or journaling may require the parent to make a couple of statements about the child each day and to rate his or her behavior to inform the next session. The child can be included in this task for several reasons. First, the child has a unique perspective on his or her own experience and state of being, and noting these in one form or another reinforces the child's ability to identify feelings in self and others and to practice perspective taking. For example, the strategy "What Teddy Heard and Saw This Week," often used by teachers, can be used in therapy with preschool and young school-age children (Cavett, in press). In this intervention, a stuffed animal "visits" the child between sessions and tells the child ("journals") about experiences in the home. The journaling is done with the child dictating and the parent transcribing the story. The child is encouraged to document what the teddy "heard and saw" in the home each day. Exploration between the child and parent about what each person in the family may have seen, heard, felt, and thought, and how each person behaved, allows for extension of thinking.

Relaxation

CBT approaches often emphasize relaxation and guided imagery interventions that are beneficial for children and adolescents. Deep breathing or four-square breathing is a helpful strategy for teaching affective modulation and relaxation. With deep breathing, the child learns to breathe at varying depths and speeds. By learning to control breathing, the child is able to learn a skill that has been shown to be effective in traditional CBT. However, most traditional CBT relaxation interventions rely on verbal descriptions or instructions. Age-appropriate interventions for children must rely on relationship and/or activity. Children benefit from learning about relaxation with their parents or showing their parents the strategies in conjoint sessions. Older children or adolescents can be taught to think of a word that calms them. For instance, focusing on a word related to their spiritual beliefs or a word that represents peaceful memories (e.g., *beach*) may be helpful. Cognitions can also serve as adequate cues for calming down for older children, such as "Think about how you blow out when you are blowing out your candles." However, younger children often need to have props that help them learn relaxation skills, such as bubbles to blow when learning deep breathing. A stuffed animal can be placed on the child's diaphragm to provide a visual for the expanding and contracting that occur during breathing. Children and their parents/caregivers will only be able to adequately use the skills related to relaxation if they practice them consistently. Practice must be fun and engaging because trying to teach relaxation to a resistant child is counterproductive. Play is an essential component in teaching children affective modulation and relaxation skills.

Typically, children begin to experience the concept of relaxation through the parent–child relationship. As the parent calms, so does the child. An anxious child calms down in the presence of a mother who is not afraid of the monsters under the bed. The calm but present parent teaches a tantruming child that his or her anger is tolerable and that the relationship is not damaged by it. When children have had positive relationships with parents and secure attachment has been formed, teaching relaxation skills in therapy is much easier. However, for children who have not experienced the calm and present parent, the therapist may be the first significant adult to begin to teach these skills. The therapist is able to hear and to tolerate the child's experience, whatever it may be. Cognitive-behavioral play therapists use the literature and research on attachment to inform reactions to the child and help him or her begin to acquire affect and relaxation/calming skills that have their foundation in an accepting and secure relationship. The therapist uses calming techniques to provide security and safety in sessions. It is beneficial to teach the skills of relaxation and calming to the parent first so that the child learns them from both therapist and parent. However, the therapist should assess the parent's ability to learn and engage these skills; psychoeducation may be needed initially to enhance the parent's understanding of the values of such skills.

Relaxation that is based in the parent–child relationship, such as parental touch, soothes and comforts the child in an ongoing relationship that is potentially present for a lifetime. When the parent is able to provide positive touch that evokes a calming effect, this resource can supplement the therapy. Simple stroking and rubbing of the forearm, at the pressure sought by the child (not the parent), can provide comfort and relaxation. Touch has been shown to decrease stress, increase oxytocin, and decrease cortisol in numerous studies across populations of varying developmental stages, including adolescents who exhibited self-harming behaviors (Field, 2005) and children with posttraumatic stress symptoms following a natural disaster (Field, Seligman, Scafidi, & Schanberg, 1996).

Several play-based interventions have been developed to teach relaxation skills, such as personalized pinwheels (Goodyear-Brown, 2005), progressive muscle relaxation from head to toe, game playing (Cavett, 2010), and Batman/Ragdoll dance (Cavett, 2010). Books for bibliotherapy related to relaxation are also beneficial in CBPT. One playful book that includes several relaxation techniques utilizing imagery, progressive muscle relaxation, and interactive exercises that children love is *Stress Relief for Kids: Taming Your Dragons* (Belknap, 2006). *A Boy and a Bear: The Children's Relaxation Book* (Lite, 1996) is an engaging book for children that depicts a boy and bear doing progressive muscle relaxation. The parent and child can read the book together and the relaxation can be practiced before and after the reading, using a stuffed bear. *Moody Cow Meditates* (MacLean, 2009) teaches meditation in a playful way, specifically by making a meditation jar and discussing the concept of relaxation with an angry calf. Following the reading of the book, the child (and parent) can make a relaxation jar to use in session and at home.

Modeling and Role Playing

Modeling and role playing are utilized throughout CBPT. Common presenting concerns that can be addressed with modeling and role play include, but are not limited to, problems in the areas of identification and expression of emotions, using positive coping skills, social skills (e.g., aggression vs. assertiveness), adaptive cognitive responses (e.g., to parental divorce), and problem solving. Modeling of cognitive responses may include puppet or doll characters with experiences similar to those of the child, for example, parental divorce or childhood cancer. The puppets act out scenarios and verbalize thoughts. Statements by the puppet allow the child to consider his or her own thoughts and have access to alternative thoughts that may allow for better functioning (decreased anxiety or decreased oppositional behaviors). For a child with depression, the puppets may act out scenarios similar to those in the child's life and make statements similar to those that adults know or assume the child feels. The puppet also models positive self-talk, allowing the child an opportunity to explore similar perceptions.

Modeling can be done with puppets, dolls, masks, or other toys. Puppets allow for verbalizations by both the child and therapist. Role plays can be constructed around the specific presenting problem. The range of toys can be broad, allowing the therapist to adapt the intervention for the individual child. For example, a child who is fond of toy cars or dinosaurs may attend and learn more from role plays and modeling that include toys related to his or her preferred interest.

Understanding the Cognitive Triangle

CBPT can be utilized to teach concepts related to the relationships among feelings, thoughts, and behaviors, often conceptualized using the cognitive triangle. The Socratic method is often used when working with adults and older adolescents to help these clients explore alternative ways of thinking. This method can be seen as a mutual exploration of options. Indeed, in CBPT the exploration of feelings, thoughts, and behaviors is done in a relationship-based manner with the child being guided respectfully through options. This exploration is conducted only after the child's current experience has been appreciated and understood. To simply "correct cognitive distortions" that the child presents with in therapy would likely be insufficient.

Children are often "corrected" and literally told what to think in many relationships, including at times the teacher–student and parent–child relationship. Having a therapist that understands and allows the child full expression of his or her experience, followed by a mutual exploration of possibilities for change, is likely the most beneficial. Padesky (1993) conceptualized the Socratic method as a *guided discovery*, not a simple changing of the client's mind. This is especially true with the child client. The child needs and deserves a relationship with a caring adult who hears his or her experience and then works through the experience of the relationship to change the perceptions that are made evident through the child's communications (play and verbal) during the therapy. Therapy can be seen as a mutual undertaking that allows the child to express experience and then be joined in a process of changing perceptions. These changes emerge through the verbalizations and play that occur during sessions. Although strategies are discussed below that involve interventions, the most influential change agent, as the child changes his or her perceptions of self, others, and the world, is the relationship with the therapist.

CBPT utilizes strategies that allow children to process information about feelings, thoughts, and behaviors in a developmentally sensitive manner. For example, using the magnetic cognitive triangle (Cavett, 2010), children add thoughts to the dynamic, play-based exercise. By making changes on the magnetic board, children can "play" with the interconnections among their feelings, thoughts, and behaviors.

Systematic Desensitization and In Vivo Exposure

CBPT can be utilized to assist in the processes of systematic desensitization and *in vivo* exposure for children with anxiety. These strategies are typically used to address generalized anxiety, specific phobias, or trauma-related anxieties. Children who have been abused may need to do exposure therapy related to trauma triggers that are innocuous. Gradual exposure with children who have experienced trauma decreases anxiety (Deblinger & Heflin, 1996). Play-based interventions, such as Pop Goes the Weasel: The Jack-in-the-Box as a Metaphor for Intrusive Thoughts and Demonstration of Anxiety Reduction with Exposure (Cavett, 2010), assist in psychoeducation about how exposure helps decrease arousal. With Pop Goes the Weasel, the therapist and child use a jack-in-the-box as they talk about reducing fears as the child is exposed to the feared but innocuous stimulus repeatedly. The therapist explains that just as the child initially jumped and was anxious when the character popped out of the box, they are also afraid of something (e.g., bathing for a child who was abused in the tub) that is not dangerous. The therapist explains that once the child learns to be exposed to that stimulus, it will no longer seem scary, just as the character that pops out of the jack-in-the-box no longer is scary. The therapist then works with the child and parent on how they can do gradual exposure to help the child become less anxious around triggers. Play-based interventions such as feelings abacus (Cavett, 2010) can be utilized to help children rate their "subjective units of distress" throughout exposure. Although play alone will not be sufficient for most *in vivo* exposures, play can be used to begin the process, discuss it in sessions, and metabolize the anxiety at each stage of the exposure hierarchy.

Narratives

Trauma narratives are essential components of CBPT to help children address trauma. When processing the trauma narrative, children, especially young children, may express their narrative through play.

Cohen, Mannarino, and Deblinger (2006) have described several methods for creating a trauma narrative, including the use of dolls, puppets, or drawings to express the narrative.

Play therapy techniques may be beneficial to process the feelings and thoughts associated with the trauma narrative, once it is complete. For example, for children who have difficulty understanding how an abuser "tricked" them into behaviors leading up to sexual abuse, the "abuser's bag of tricks" (Crisi, Lay, & Lowenstein, 1998) or the "trick hat" (Grotsky, Camerer, & Damiano, 2000) can be beneficial. For children who have difficulty understanding how they had a physiological response to sexual abuse, the PFFT . . . That's just what bodies do: Normalizing Sexual Responses in Children who have Been Sexually Abused (Cavett, 2010) technique can help children understand that having a physiological response does not mean that they wanted the abuse or that they were responsible for the abuse. The range of techniques developed to address common cognitive distortions related to abuse is vast (e.g., see Cavett & Drewes, 2012; Crisci, Lay, & Lowenstein, 1998).

Teaching Interpersonal Safety Skills

Play therapy interventions intended to enhance future safety include those that teach and reinforce healthy boundaries. For example, have the child draw an outline of the body and talk about interpersonal boundaries—which parts of the body are off-limits to which people (e.g., the hands are commonly touched—even strangers will shake hands when they meet in this culture; the back is touched by those closer to the child, such as a special teacher or a friend who pats or rubs the child's back to reassure him or her). Children can use worksheet-type materials to learn about boundaries, but rarely do they enjoy it and typically it is much less enjoyable than playing out the same concepts. Some worksheets that are child-friendly include those included in the technique "My Helpers" (Crisci, Lay, & Lowenstein, 1998), which includes worksheets describing "helpers" and scenarios that require a helper; the child matches the helper to the scenario. "My Safe Neighborhood" (Cavett, 2010) describes how to process safety issues with young children through play with toys. Having an assortment of toys available that relate to safety (e.g., fire station, police station, hospital) is essential, especially with younger children. Goodyear-Brown's (2005) door hangers and megaphones techniques both address issues related to safety. The essential therapeutic component is the processing that is done during the intervention.

Termination

Termination with children in CBPT focuses on facilitating a healthy closure to the therapeutic relationship, reinforcing the skills learned during therapy, and continuing to strengthen the relationship between the child and parents as well as other sources of caregiving. The process of ending therapy often brings up concerns about loss and grief, allowing for further processing of "endings and goodbyes" through the experience of ending the therapy and relationship. The relationship is foundational for change throughout the course of treatment and the process of termination reflects upon both the connection developed and the desire to hold onto the relationship. Allowing for the expression of loss and anger during termination is important. Interventions can be utilized to facilitate the goals of termination. For example, "From Start to Finish" (Kenney-Noziska, 2008) helps the child and therapist to process the changes that have occurred from the time the child entered therapy until the final sessions. Paper doll figures are cut out so that they remain connected to each other at the hands and feet. The first one represents the child when first entering therapy, and the therapist and child process how the child initially presented. What were his or her feelings and experiences at that time? What were his or her apprehensions and fears? The final doll represents the child during the termination stage. After discussing the first doll, the final doll is discussed. How has the child changed and grown? What kinds of experiences have facilitated this growth and change? The child and therapist explore what the child continues to need and how those needs will be met. The strengths and resiliency of the child are emphasized. The child also processes how the therapeutic relationship has changed his or her perceptions of self and others in the relationship. The dolls between the first and last are also discussed and influential experiences during the therapy are written on the middle dolls.

Clinical Case Example

Spencer's parents, Joseph and Kari, met initially with the therapist to discuss deployment concerns, including how Spencer would tolerate the upcoming change. While meeting, the therapist gathered as much detailed information about the deployment as possible in order to use the information later while acting out with Spencer, age 4, the probable experiences related to his dad going to Afghanistan. His parents were able to give critical information about where and when the family would engage in activities related to deployment. Joseph indicated that he would be dressed in his Army combat uniform. They would interact with other families who were involved in deployment at the same time and others who would have parents returning at various times during the upcoming year. The family would give their final goodbyes before his father would board the bus carrying his unit. Spencer's parents felt that he would have difficulty at various times during the week leading up to the deployment and specific nurturing and reassuring activities were planned to connect with him during those times.

The therapist made available toys that reflected the deployment, including toy buildings (shoeboxes with signage related to Army base buildings typically utilized by families). Soldier dolls and puppets allowed for Spencer to engage in play related to his father's deployment. He and his family brought supplies (boots, Kevlar, camel backs, etc.) that were commonly seen by Spencer when his father would pack for extended leaves. During the play, Spencer and his therapist acted out the scenario that his parents had articulated would be expected on the final days before deployment. The details of the specific events, including gatherings with extended family and other families in his father's unit, were enacted. His father and mother came in to sessions, and he showed them some of the scenarios. His parents noted his feelings and thoughts in the play scenarios and how similar they were to how he had felt during his father's previous deployment. Spencer was able to explore feelings of abandonment and loss, and his parents as well as his therapist were able to "hear" his perceptions. His anger and sadness were understood through his play, not as an expression that needed to be "changed" but rather as one that was acceptable and therefore he was acceptable.

As he was accepted in his expressions, Spencer was able to explore the beliefs related to his feelings. Was he unworthy of his dad's love and consistent involvement? Was his dad going to return to him? Was his dad's leaving related to him or his behavior? What did the changes mean to him and about him? These themes were beyond the "words" of a child; however, they were not avoidable in his play. He was able to depict through play the thoughts that needed exploration. As the therapist was able to put words to the play (or at times staying within the play if that seemed necessary), he was able to process his fears and the loss. In this way Spencer was supported in his feelings, and his parents were able to appreciate that he needed to express the loss he felt.

In addition to using the initial therapy for stress inoculation, Spencer was also able to use the therapy throughout his father's deployment to continue to process the day-to-day experience of being the child of a deployed parent. He and his father discussed ways they would communicate, including Skype, during his deployment. His family members participated in a session during which each used a puppet to represent a different family member. Each was supported in how he or she viewed the others and in how each member felt, and the strengths of each family member were discussed. Spencer's parents expressed appreciation for acting out the scenarios in play, as they indicated that this afforded them a deeper understanding and appreciation of the experience.

Conclusion

CBT must be adapted for utilization with children due to cognitive and verbal limitations as well as interests. Children communicate through play significantly more information than they do through verbalization. Play can be used to facilitate children's self-expression and to provide a developmentally appropriate means of teaching a skill that may not be understood through verbal-only communication. Play in CBPT allows the child to express feelings, thoughts, and perceptions.

REFERENCES

Achenbach, T. M. (1991). *Manual for the Child Behavior Checklist/4–18 and 1991 Profile.* Burlington: University of Vermont, Department of Psychiatry.

Beck, A. T. (1963). Thinking and depression: Idiosyncratic content and cognitive distortions. *Archives of General Psychiatry, 42,* 441–447.

Beck, A. T. (1964). Thinking and depression. *Archives of General Psychiatry, 10,* 561–571.

Beck, A. T. (1967). *Depression: Clinical, experi-*

mental, and theoretical aspects. New York: Harper & Row.

Beck, A. T. (1970). Cognitive therapy: Nature and relation to behavior therapy. *Behavior Therapy, 1,* 184–200.

Beck, A. T. (1972). *Depression: Causes and treatment.* Philadelphia: University of Pennsylvania Press.

Beck, A. T. (1976). *Cognitive therapy and the emotional disorders.* New York: International Universities Press.

Beck, A. T. & Emery, G. (1985). *Anxiety disorders and phobias: A cognitive perspective.* New York: Basic Books.

Belknap, M. (2006). *Stress relief for kids: Taming your dragons.* Duluth, MN: Whole Person Associates.

Benedict, H. E. (2004, October). *Using play themes in play assessment and for treatment workshop.* Presented at the 21st annual Association for Play Therapy International Conference, Denver, CO.

Cavett, A. M. (2010). *Structured play-based interventions for engaging children and adolescents in therapy.* West Conshohocken, PA: Infinity Press.

Cavett, A. M. (in press). *Play-based cognitive-behavioral therapy interventions for children.* West Conshohocken, PA: Infinity Press.

Cavett, A. M., & Drewes, A. (2012). Play applications and trauma-specific components for young children. In J. A. Cohen, A. P. Mannarino, & E. Deblinger (Eds.), *Trauma-focused CBT for children and adolescents: Treatment applications* (pp. 124–148). New York: Guilford Press.

Cohen, J. A., Mannarino, A. P., & Deblinger, E. (2006). *Treating trauma and traumatic grief in children and adolescents.* New York: Guilford Press.

Crisci, G., Lay, M., & Lowenstein, L., (1998). *Paper dolls and paper airplanes: Therapeutic exercises for sexually traumatized children.* Indianapolis, IN: Kidsrights.

Deblinger, E., & Heflin, A. H. (1996). *Treating sexually abused children and their nonoffending parents: A cognitive-behavioral approach.* Thousand Oaks, CA: Sage.

Drewes, A. A. (2009). *Blending play therapy with cognitive behavioral therapy: Evidence based and other effective treatments and techniques.* New York: Wiley.

Field, T. (2005). Touch deprivation and aggression against self among adolescents. In D. M. Stoff & E. J. Susman (Eds.), *Developmental psychobiology of aggression* (pp. 117–140). New York: Cambridge University Press.

Field, T., Seligman, S., Scafidi, F., & Schanberg, S. (1996). Alleviating posttraumatic stress in children following Hurricane Andrew. *Journal of Applied Developmental Psychology, 17*(1), 37–50.

Freud, A. (1928). *Introduction to the technique of child analysis* (L. P. Clark, Trans.). New York: Nervous and Mental Disease Publishing.

Freud, A. (1964). *The psychoanalytic treatment of children.* New York: Schocken Books.

Gil, E. (2006). *Helping abused and traumatized children: Integrating directive and nondirective approaches.* New York: Guilford Press.

Goodyear-Brown, P. (2005). *Digging for buried treasure 2: Another 52 prop-based play therapy interventions for treating the problems of childhood.* Nashville, TN: Author.

Grotsky, L., Camerer, C., & Damiano, L. (2000). *Group work with sexually abused children.* Thousand Oaks, CA: Sage.

Irwin, E. C. (2000). The use of a Puppet Interview to understand children. In K. J. O'Connor & C. E. Schaefer (Eds.), *Handbook of play therapy: Vol. 2. Advances and innovations* (pp. 682–703). New York: Wiley.

Kenney-Noziska, S. (2008). *Techniques, techniques, techniques: Play-based activities for children, adolescents, and families.* West Conshohocken, PA: Infinity Press.

Klein, M. (1932). *The psycho-analysis of children.* London: Hogarth Press.

Klein, M. (1955). The psychoanalytic play technique. *American Journal of Orthopsychiatry, 25,* 223–237.

Knell, S. M. (1992). *Puppet sentence completion task.* Unpublished manuscript.

Knell, S. M. (1993). *Cognitive-behavioral play therapy.* Northvale, NJ: Aronson.

Knell, S. M., & Beck, K. W. (2000). The Puppet Sentence Completion Task. In K. J. O'Connor & C. E. Schaefer (Eds.), *Handbook of play therapy: Vol. 2. Advances and innovations* (pp. 704–721). New York: Wiley.

Knell, S. M. (2009). Cognitive-behavioral play therapy. In K. J. O'Connor & L. D. Braverman (Eds.), *Play therapy theory and practice: Comparing theories and techniques* (2nd ed., pp. 203–236). Hoboken, NJ: Wiley.

Knell, S. M., & Dasari, M. (2011). Cognitive-behavioral play therapy. In S. W. Russ & L. N. Niec (Eds.), *Play in clinical practice: Evidence-based approaches* (pp. 236–262). New York: Guilford Press.

Landreth, G. (1991). *Play therapy: The art of the relationship.* Bristol, PA: Taylor & Francis.

Lite, L. (1996). *A boy and a bear.* Plantation, FL: Specialty Press.

Maclean, G., & Ulrich, R. (1991). *Hermine Hug-Hellmuth: Her life and work.* New York: Routledge.

MacLean, K. L. (2009). *Moody cow.* Boston: Wisdom.

O'Conner, K. J. (1983). The color your life technique. In C. E. Schaefer & K. J. O'Conner (Eds.), *Handbook of play therapy* (pp. 251–258). New York: Wiley.

Padesky, C. A. (1993, September). *Socratic questioning: Changing minds or guiding discovery?* Invited keynote address presented at the European Congress of Behaviour and Cognitive Therapies, London. Retrieved October 1, 2013, from *www.padesky.com/clinicalcorner.*

Phillips, R. (1985). Whistling in the dark?: A review of play therapy research. *Psychotherapy, 22*(4), 752–760.

Piaget, J. (1972). *The psychology of the child.* New York: Basic Books.

Robingson, E. A., & Eyberg, S. M. (1981). The dyadic parent–child interaction coding system: Standardization and validation. *Journal of Consulting and Clinical Psychology, 49*(2), 245–250.

Russ, S. W. (2004). *Play in child development and psychotherapy.* Mahwah, NJ: Erlbaum.

Skinner, B. F. (1938). *The behavior of organisms: An experimental analysis.* New York: Appleton-Century.

CHAPTER 7

Integrative Approach to Play Therapy

Eliana Gil
Elizabeth Konrath
Jennifer Shaw
Myriam Goldin
Heather McTaggart Bryan

I (Konrath) answered the phone one morning to hear Shannon L., mother of 10-year-old Myra, sounding frantic and asking for an immediate therapy appointment. Shannon arrived for the intake tired, irritable, and overwhelmed. Although I requested that she attend the initial appointment by herself, she could not find child care for her daughter—my potential client—and had to bring her along. As we began speaking, Shannon reported that she needed "some help" with Myra and shared that 5 years ago, she and her husband John had adopted Myra from Vietnam when Myra was 5 years old. Shannon could not be sure of the age because she believed the adoption agency changed the year on Myra's birth certificate.

Little was known about those first years in Myra's life, other than that she had resided in a number of foster homes, as well as an orphanage. Shannon noted that Myra was underweight and underdeveloped when they first welcomed her into their family. In exploring the reason that she and John had decided to adopt, Shannon nonchalantly shared that they'd adopted another girl, Susan, 6, the year before they'd adopted Myra. Shannon reported, "Well, we thought Susan should have a little friend, so we decided to adopt another little girl." Shannon then went on to identify the type of help she and her husband needed. She explained that the family had moved from Texas to Virginia a few months ago. During the time that they'd lived in Texas, the family became very close with their neighbors. The parents often left their two children in the care of their neighbor's 15-year-old son, Michael. Over a 2-year period of babysitting by Michael, the parents noticed that Myra and Susan began acting differently. Shannon explained that when they would leave the children with Michael, the girls would become "extremely upset, angry, screaming, shouting, begging us not to go," and in retrospect she felt guilty that she and her husband had viewed their behavior as an attempt to keep them from going out. They also began having behavior problems in school during this time. Susan became withdrawn, quiet, lethargic, whereas Myra was aggressive, ran away, and threw tantrums "at the drop of a hat." When the family moved to Virginia, Susan disclosed to her school counselor that Michael had been physically and sexually abusing them.

During the intake session and while Shannon attempted to describe Myra's current behaviors, Myra burst into the office five or six times and appeared anxious, dysregulated, and hyperactive. Shannon explained that Myra was expelled from her previous school after 1 week in the first grade. In fact, Myra's behaviors had become so uncontrollable, the morning of the intake appointment John said to Shannon, "We can try this for a month. But if Myra doesn't get any better, she's going to have to go to residential. We just can't deal with her any more . . . she's turning our lives upside down. This is her last chance." Shannon indicated that Myra "does not listen to anyone . . . she runs away from me and her father, hits me and everyone else, including her sister, is triggered by nothing and everything, doesn't ask for help, and acts like a 3-year-old sometimes!" Shannon also described Myra's sleeping difficulties, frequent nightmares, enuresis, and flinching with any sudden noise. She indicated that Myra is "extremely rigid" about the type of clothes and fabrics she wears and also shared that she cannot seem to get Myra to eat anything but Eggos, pizza, and chips.

Shannon described her relationship with Myra in the following terms: "Well, I think she loves me in her own way, but sometimes I don't think she would care at all if I wasn't her mom anymore." She also shared that Myra has difficulty forming relationships with peers and adults. When I asked how John would describe his relationship with his daughter, she looked away and said, "much, much worse than mine. Sometimes it looks like he doesn't like her at all!" I noted that given the behavioral problems, it is not unusual for parents to feel worn out, discouraged. I also inquired about Myra's sister, and Shannon noted, "She's a saint, patient and loving—they couldn't be more different if they tried, in spite of both being Vietnamese." Clearly, in this family system, Myra was the problem child and Susan was the easy, good child who presented few challenges to her parents.

By the time Shannon left my office, I was experiencing all the feelings that I am certain she felt—overwhelmed, confused, and not sure exactly where to focus first. The way Shannon had described her daughter's problems sounded overwhelming and challenging. I would need to integrate every skill and therapeutic technique I had ever learned to help Myra and her family. I knew the first step was to meet the child and begin to form a relationship with her. As I reflected on what I had learned from my meeting with Shannon, some dimensions emerged to guide me. I knew several clinical issues would take priority: establishing a relationship with Myra would be critical for therapy to be successful; the family context, particularly the parent–child relationships, required immediate attention; therapy would need to be trauma-focused; and both girls would benefit from help with self-regulation and sibling conflict. I also had a number of concerns about Myra's physical health, including her enuresis, diet, and possible sensory issues related to her rigidity about specific fabrics and clothes. An important part of integrative therapy with this child would need to also include collaboration with other professionals, such as her pediatrician and possibly an occupational therapist. Although my immediate therapeutic goals and treatment considerations were determined, the specific approaches remained undefined. Using an integrative framework, I knew that I would start to identify and select approaches as I began to know the child and her family better, and I would verify that the alleged abuse had been reported and addressed in Texas.

Psychotherapy Integration

Previously called *eclecticism, integration* has become the preferred term to describe the blending of theory, technique, and common factors. The utilization of psychotherapy integration as a treatment model has been the subject of open dialogue in the field of adult psychotherapy for decades. In the past 5 years, both adult and child models are gaining increased clinical attention and support as reliable and credible approaches to treatment. As stated by Norcross and Goldfried (2005), the integration of theory, technique, and common factors in psychotherapy has gained prominence since the 1990s.

Although important discussions about the use of integrative approaches with children are appearing in the literature, minimal empirical research on integrative models with children has been conducted to date (Drewes, 2011). Nevertheless, over the past 20 years, integration of theory and treatment has developed into a clearly delineated area of interest for clinicians (Norcross, 2005). In a survey of 423 mental health professionals, the majority reported using an eclectic form of therapy (Jensen, Bergin, & Greaves, 1990). In a 2002 survey, Norcross, Hedges, and Castle found that 36% of psychologists claimed to be eclectic/integrative. A review of the literature strongly suggests that there is a general shift away from a one-size-fits-all treatment approach because research has not concluded that any single approach appears to be clinically effective for all clients (Drewes, 2011). Phillips and Landreth (1995) found that among play therapists the most common approach reported was an eclectic and multitheoretical orientation (Drewes, 2011). It is interesting to note that proponents of established efficacious treatments for particular disorders, such as trauma-focused cognitive-behavioral therapy (TF-CBT) for child sexual abuse, are also encouraging a more integrative approach when working with young children and adolescents (see Cohen, Mannarino, & Deblinger, 2012).

Norcross and Goldfried (2005) review possible reasons for the shift in interest and inclusion of integrative psychotherapies: (1) a large increase in therapies, (2) the lack of a single theory or treatment that is adequate, (3) a rise in short-term and problem-focused treatment, (4) the rise in evidence-based treatments resulting from the identification of specific therapy effects on specific target problems, and (5) the recognition that therapeutic commonali-ties heavily contribute to outcome (Drewes, 2011, p. 23).

Current writers in psychotherapy integration suggest that this approach is moving into a new phase of development that will focus more on unification as a part of a larger movement aimed at the unification of the clinical sciences (Magnavita, 2008), whereas others caution that substantial differences exist in epistemology and philosophy of mind to slow the process considerably. Whatever the next conceptualization of integration will be, it will inevitably include application to a variety of special populations served by psychotherapy, including the psychotherapy of children (Seymour, 2011, p. 15).

Current Research on Play Therapy and Psychotherapy Integration

A review of the play therapy research over the past decade suggests an increased interest in, and increasing openness to, merging or integrating approaches and their therapeutic techniques. Play therapists in the field report that they prefer integrating evidence-based directive and nondirective models when dealing with the multilayered needs of their clients. Recent articles and books on integrative play therapy illustrate that clinicians favor the use of integrated evidence-informed treatments of choice when dealing with clients that present multiple symptoms—symptoms that cannot be addressed by one particular theoretical model (Cavett, 2009; Drewes, 2011; Gil, 2006, 2012; Gil & Shaw, 2013; Weir, 2008; Wynne, 2008). At the same time, the leading voices in play therapy have realized the need to provide stronger guidelines and expectations on how clinicians consider and incorporate empirically supported play therapy models when addressing individual children's and adolescents' needs (Kenney-Noziska, Schaefer, & Homeyer, 2012).

The research also provides evidence that play therapy has a beneficial treatment effect over comparison or nontreatment groups. The strength of play therapy research lies in its application to real-world settings that validate play therapy as a usable model in working with clients (Ray, 2006). In order for play therapy to be considered a well-established treatment, play therapy researchers continue to be tasked with improving specific ways of implementing and reporting research designs (Ray, 2006). As posited by Schaefer (2003), because child and adolescent psychological disorders are multilayered, complex, and multidetermined, a multifaceted treatment approach is necessary. With the expansion of integrative play therapies, which includes the blending of two or more models, play therapy researchers have a difficult task because even as clinicians are reporting the benefits of an integrative approach and a preference for use of such an approach, the push from stakeholders (insurance companies, agencies, funding sources) is for the use of an already identified evidence-based approach. Stricker and Gold (2008) point out that psychotherapy integration in some form is a part of every clinical and research process, as part of the learning process of psychotherapists working from a particular model and considering new ideas or techniques for possible incorporation into their existing model.

Each orientation offers worthwhile methods and notions (Lazarus, 2006). As Kenney-Noziska and colleagues (2012) note, the questions regarding which treatment, by whom, and when is most effective for any individual with a specific problem, and under what set of circumstances, are the pivotal clinical questions to explore. Bratton, Ray, Rhine, and Jones (2005) found that directive and nondirective theoretical approaches produced comparable levels of overall effectiveness, with effect sizes ranging from moderate to high (Kenney-Noziska et al., 2012, p. 246). Play researchers have accumulated evidence of differential effectiveness for specific childhood disorders (Drewes, Bratton, & Schaefer, 2011; Wethington et al., 2008), revealing that "nondirective interventions work best for certain disorders, directive interventions work best for other disorders, and an integration of the two works best for still other disorders" (Kenney-Noziska et al., 2012, p. 247).

The research does not suggest that one play therapy approach is better than the other. Rather, the answer is: It depends. Nondirective and directive theoretical approaches (e.g., relationship formation, skill building) vary in effectiveness depending on the specific disorder and treatment issue. Based on current research, if one wishes to treat a broad spectrum of childhood disorders, acquiring both directive and nondirective skills is encouraged (Kenney-Noziska et al., 2012).

It is clear that the field of play therapy is moving beyond the one-size-fits-all stance to a more integrated theoretical approach. Phillips and Landreth (1995), for instance, found that an eclectic orientation was, by far, the most common orientation reported by play therapists in their survey. Additionally, integration is a growing movement as play therapy has moved toward rapprochement of the directive and nondirective theoretical approaches to meet the needs of our clients. The number of articles (Rasmussen & Cunningham, 1995) and books on integrative play therapy (Cavett, 2009; Drewes, 2009; Drewes et al., 2011; Gil, 2006) attests to "the integrative play therapy theoretical approach rapidly becoming the model intervention in our field" (Kenney-Noziska et al., 2012, p. 247).

Obstacles to an Integrative Approach

The interest in integrating different models seems to be well documented (Drewes, 2011); however, moving toward this shift requires researchers and clinicians to reflect on the obstacles to the implementation of this approach (Kenney-Noziska et al., 2012). The most critical obstacle seems to come from "the territoriality of the purist" (Drewes, 2011, p. 33) that views one theoretical approach through a unilateral lens. This outlook of one theory being the best leads to limited educational and practical training for graduate students (Drewes, 2011). Graduate students are usually taught only one or two theoretical approaches for how to respond to childhood disorders, and they often lack the grounding knowledge to integrate various complementary schools of thoughts (Drewes, 2011; Norcross, Beutler, & Levant, 2005). The philosophical position of professors and clinical supervisors can influence the manner in which students and new professionals become acquainted with treatment models, limiting their exposure to flexible models of intervention (Drewes, 2011). In addition, clinicians who might otherwise integrate different approaches can find financial or time requirements as restrictions in becoming competent in broader theories and approaches.

Finally, a major obstacle to integration is the unyielding belief that only a particular method of demonstrating evidence of effectiveness is credible. The field of play therapy seems to be advocating for increased credibility through the implementation of evidence-based practices, although clear guidelines are still needed (Drewes, 2011; Kenney-Noziska et al., 2012). Although evidence-based models are useful and advisable when available and accessible, using an integrated approach allows for the incorporation of both practice- and evidence-informed models of treatment so that research findings are valued but do not neglect other methodologies. Specifically, there are other approaches (e.g., expressive therapies) that are acceptable and used broadly but may not yet have the bulk, number, and particular type of research to provide the evidence-based foundation.

These barriers to integration can best be overcome as therapists engage in a reflective professional journey on how to best meet the needs of their clients. Pure views of directive or nondirective interventions seem to be difficult to maintain in that directive and nondirective skills are used at different times during the therapeutic process. Similarly, commitment is needed to become proficient at delivering various play therapy theoretical modalities or evidence-based models. This commitment implies that therapists will need to invest time and money in learning and training to achieve a grounded level of expertise in different treatment modalities or they will need to be open to refer cases that would be best treated by evidence-informed practices. More research is still needed to identify the basic forces in play that produce therapeutic changes within each theoretical modality (Schaefer & Drewes, 2014).

Clinical Case Example

Based on Shannon's reports, as well as the brief interactions that I witnessed between Shannon and Myra, I determined that a first step would be to conduct a parent–child assessment. I chose the Marschak interaction method (MIM; Landaman, Booth, & Chambers, 2000), believing it would be the most efficient and useful assessment tool to gain information about the type and nature of the mother–daughter relationship and their attachment. The MIM is a structured observation technique that allows clinicians to observe parent–child interactions related to specific dimensions of relationships, including engagement, nurture, challenge, and structure (Booth & Jernberg, 2010). Each of the play activities provided in the MIM is specifically chosen to allow clinicians to evaluate these four dimensions (Booth & Jernberg, 2010; Hitchcock, Ammen, O'Connor, & Backman, 2008).

The area of engagement examines the manner in which parents can provide playful experiences of shared joy and prolonged attention to their children, while staying emotionally attuned to them. The tasks in the nurture domain evaluate parental ability to respond to children's needs for attachment and regulation using soothing, tender, and calm approaches, which help children feel worthy of love and care. Play activities in the domain of structure allow clinicians to assess how parents can provide safety, organization, and emotional regulation, as well as set clear expectations and limits. Finally, the area of challenge allows for observation of how parents build children's self-esteem and encourage their children to take risks, explore, feel confident, and gain mastery (Hitchcock et al., 2008).

The MIM revealed that both Shannon and Myra needed therapeutic interventions to address all four areas. Throughout the assessment, Myra was dysregulated, agitated, and aggressive toward her mother, and Shannon frequently missed opportunities to care for and nurture Myra. She was also unable to provide even small measures of structure or emotional and physical containment. For example, there were various times when Shannon was attempting to engage Myra, but Myra ran to the opposite side of the room and literally ran around in circles. Additionally, throughout the MIM, both Shannon and Myra seemed to miscue the other: Shannon laughed when Myra was upset, or Shannon ignored or smiled at Myra when Myra threw items at Shannon and hit her in the face.

The MIM also showed some rigidity in what Myra was willing or able to do, and she appeared to need to be in constant control. Myra's behaviors can be interpreted as including the following beliefs: "I need to be in control all the time so that I can predict what will happen"; "Adults cannot help me or understand me"; and "Adults do not comfort me when I am hurt." In watching the parent–child interactions in the assessment, it became clear to me that Myra's dysregulation and need for control were related to her feeling unsafe and unprotected and experiencing constant physical and internal disorganization. During times when Myra appeared to be disinhibited and acted out, Shannon was inhibited, withdrawn, or passive–aggressive. When Shannon attempted to set structure or limits, Myra adamantly refused to cooperate and often did

the opposite of what her mother requested. During one of the activities, in which Shannon built a block structure and asked Myra to create one just like hers, Myra threw the blocks at her mother's face forcefully. Shannon attempted to implement structure intermittently; for example, she gave a warning, but was unable to follow through with any reinforcement or redirection. Myra tolerated her mother's nurturing behaviors, as long as she could have control over how the nurturing activity occurred. Finally, the MIM also revealed Shannon's strengths of patience and calm, which were demonstrated throughout the assessment.

Once I completed the MIM interaction assessment, I was able to formulate specific goals for Myra's treatment. Her treatment plan included the following:

1. Build a healthy therapeutic relationship and establish a secure base for Myra.
   a. Respond to Myra's thoughts, feelings, and experiences with empathy.
   b. Emphasize safety through consistency, limit setting, and structure.
   c. Provide unconditional positive regard for Myra.
2. Build regulation skills in Myra and coregulation skills in the parent–child dyad.
   a. Provide external regulation and model optimal arousal levels.
   b. Model emotional attunement.
   c. Decrease anxiety by emphasizing safety, consistency, and structure.
3. Build healthy attachment between Myra and Shannon.
   a. Help Shannon understand Myra's needs and respond to them in an empathic, healthy manner.
   b. Facilitate opportunities for nurture and love between Myra and Shannon.
   c. Model for Shannon how to find ways to consistently set and maintain limits and boundaries.
4. Explore the impact of trauma with Myra and Shannon.
   a. Provide options for expressive therapy so that Myra can find ways to

communicate her experiences and design (and later process) a trauma narrative.

b. Facilitate opportunities for Myra to gain mastery and competency over her traumatic experiences.

c. Provide psychoeducation for Shannon about the impact of attachment disruption and trauma.

5. Improve physical health.

a. Communicate with, and refer Myra to, a pediatrician to explore medical causes for enuresis.

b. Refer Myra to occupational therapist for assessment of sensory integration.

c. Create plan with Shannon to improve Myra's diet and exercise.

Based on my evaluation using the MIM, I determined that the family's need for attachment-based work, including attunement, regulation, and positive interactions, should take priority over any other treatment goals. I further assessed that this child would be better able to process her trauma once she felt safe, both in therapy and in her home environment. Myra needed her mother to provide containment, structure, regulation, and empathy. This family needed tools—quickly—so I selected the best approach for the identified problem: a directive, structured therapeutic technique that would have the potential to improve the relationship in an experiential way at each therapy session. Shannon needed accessible skills that would provide here-and-now modeling of empathy and limit setting, as well as a treatment that would provide opportunities to encourage fun, positive interactions with her daughter. Theraplay® was selected as a good match for this family because it provides attachment-based therapy that is also an evidence- and practice-informed approach for a child and his or her caregiver (e.g., see *www.theraplay.org*). It is a play-based, attachment-focused therapy that directly meets a child's needs for nurture, structure, engagement, and challenge (Munns, 2011). Additionally, Theraplay is

particularly helpful for children who have suffered trauma, as it provides experiences for healthy, attuned care that they may not have received (Booth & Jernberg, 2010). Beginning Myra's treatment using Theraplay would allow us to actively work on three crucial goals of her treatment plan: building a therapeutic relationship, addressing contextual family issues (specifically, parent–child relationships), teaching Myra self-regulation skills, and strengthening the sibling dyad.

From the very first Theraplay session, Myra's behaviors were consistent with those observed in the MIM: She was dysregulated, impulsive, disorganized, and aggressive at times. She also had difficulty engaging with me and attempted to take control over every activity. For example, she would take my therapy bag, where I kept the items that we would be using to play with that day, and dump out the contents, throwing them around the room or hiding them from me. I decreased this stimulation by using minimal materials and by keeping only a few things in my pockets. I also made several modifications for her based on her history of trauma. At the beginning of each session, I reviewed with her all the activities that we would be doing, so that she was aware of what would come next. She also came up with a signal (sticking her fingers in her ears) to let me know if she felt uncomfortable or unsafe with a particular activity.

At the beginning of treatment, I conducted Theraplay activities while Shannon observed and stayed several feet away from where Myra and I played. Her task was to observe my interactions with Myra so that we could discuss her impressions after the session. Although Shannon complied with my requests, she sat with her arms crossed in front of her, disengaged, and appearing stern or critical. She seemed to alternate from ignoring to glaring at her daughter.

As our Theraplay sessions progressed, Myra made substantial improvement, especially in the structure dimension, and she made fewer efforts to control the activities, accepting my limits without interpreting them as my "being mean," or telling me she hated me. Furthermore, Myra was able to remain engaged for longer periods of time, and she was more regulated and relaxed throughout the session. Myra also became more tolerant and accepting of the nurturing activities facilitated by her mother and me. Although the relationship between Myra and me became increasingly trusting, consistent, and reliable, her relationship with her mother continued to be primarily conflicted and tense. Myra's disorganized attachment and Shannon's inability to provide consistent structure and nurture became an obstacle in treatment. Consequently, I determined that Shannon needed more individual support to process and understand why Myra was behaving the way she was, and how Shannon could respond to her in a structured, empathic way. Myra's generalized dysregulation, targeted aggressiveness and disrespect toward her mother, and her mother's inability to find successful, corrective interventions had made their relationship strained and lacking in empathy and mutual emotional validation. Myra's behaviors led Shannon to make assumptions about her daughter's intent, inferring that Myra was thriving in chaos and that she calculated and manipulated her interactions. Shannon's tense and frustrated responses to Myra contributed to Myra's lack of safety and foundational security.

In addition to shifting my therapy approaches to include individual treatment of Myra, I referred Shannon to a parent education program, called Circle of Security Parenting Course (COS-PC) based on the Circle of Security attachment model (Powell et al., 2014). I chose this program because of its goal of helping parents and children develop lasting, secure attachments. This model can be provided in a group or individual format; Shannon chose to participate in an individual format with one of my colleagues.

Shannon's Participation in COS-PC

The COS-PC model uses a DVD with examples from client interactions and specific guidelines on how to understand the developmental needs of children within the context of their relationship with a caregiver. COS-PC is designed to be delivered in eight individual and/or group therapy sessions by a certified COS-PC facilitator. Shannon and my colleague met through the course of the eight sessions, watched the DVD clips together, and followed the parenting curriculum (Cooper, Hoffman, & Powell, 2009).

Shannon seemed enthusiastic and eager to learn a new parenting model, apparently cognizant of her need to find a more effective way to manage Myra's behavioral and emotional needs; however, she overemphasized learning techniques and her follow-through was compromised in the face of intense emotions toward her child. Shannon did not yet realize how Myra's many disrupted attachments and history of sexual abuse as well as her failure to protect them from subsequent abuse had resulted in a disorganized neurophysiological makeup that would need ongoing attention. Shannon's perception that Myra was behaving with ill intent understandably caused significant stress, and helping the mother and father realize that Myra's responses could be explained in the context of trauma and its impact on the brain would likely provide needed relief (e.g., see Perry & Slazavitz, 2006; Siegel & Payne Bryson, 2011).

Shannon watched videotaped presentations of some of the basic assumptions of COS-PC, and a therapy dialogue and reflection were included in each viewing of the tape. One of the goals of COS-PC is to help parents experience a shift in their perceptions of their children so that they can develop empathy as well as more nonjudgmental stances (particularly relevant in Shannon's attitudes toward Myra). In fact, parents are encouraged to see their children's behaviors as nothing more than needs that must be met. Shannon was invited to reflect on the verbal and nonverbal messages that she gave Myra. In addition, I (Gil) conveyed great optimism to her about her potential to change the quality of her current interactions with her daughter and that those changes would play a significant role in the formation of Myra's overall relationships with others in years to come.

It was very evident that Shannon's interactions with Myra reflected an unresolved or disorganized style of attachment. In general, Shannon showed a consistently passive affect with abrupt changes that seemed unpredictable and frightening to her daughter. Her gaze shifted from short periods of interest in what Myra was doing, to disinterest and/or harshness when Myra misbehaved in her Theraplay sessions. The challenge was to help Shannon realize that long-lasting change would come only from Shannon's ability to develop specific relationship capacities, rather than from learning techniques to manage Myra's behaviors. The skills that could assist Shannon in developing a secure relationship included (1) observational capacities informed by a sound model of children's developmental needs; (2) reflective abilities to help her discern how her personal history currently impacts her expectations in her role as a mother; and (3) the capacity to participate in the regulation of Myra's emotions. Cooper, Hoffman, Marvin, and Powell (2014) assert that unless parents can stand back and reflect on their ongoing experiences with their children, they will not gain the insights or abilities needed to break their interrelational struggles. Cooper and colleagues have invoked the term *reflective functioning* to describe the ideal process through which parents reflect on their own actions and responses to their children and then modify their actions to best meet their children's needs.

Shannon and Myra had a shared and repeated negative relational experience that had the capacity to change only when Shannon could reflect on her maternal role and

begin to focus primarily on Myra's emotional needs. The "empathic shift" advocated by COS-PC developers and central to their parenting course (Cooper et al., 2000) is designed to grow and improve a secure attachment in the parent-child dyad.

The outcome of the COS-PC was mixed: Although Shannon seemed to comprehend and shift her perceptions during therapeutic dialogues and when in a calm, positive state of mind, she was unable to implement positive behaviors when her frustration or anger took center stage. Perhaps Shannon's guilt at not being able to implement positive interactions in the heat of the moment, coupled with her desire to apologize to Myra and make amends as soon as she could, were indications that she was on her way to making more consistent changes in her relationship with her daughter. As expected, habits die hard, and this parent–child dyad had been conflictual from the outset, so the therapist was left with cautious optimism.

A few other issues also seemed at play:

1. John had acquiesced to his wife's desire to adopt and, prioritizing his busy and demanding career, had abdicated his parenting role to his stay-at-home wife, who had initially embraced the idea of raising young children, stating firmly that "I'm fine raising them mostly by myself; our jobs are very clearly defined and we're both okay with that."

2. Shannon and John had ambivalent feelings about cross-cultural issues, sometimes claiming to want the children to learn about their heritage, but mostly, taking actions that subtly disregarded cultural differences. In their efforts to make the children more comfortable, they rarely spoke of cultural differences, which conveyed their discomfort about their daughters' birth culture to both their girls.

3. Shannon reluctantly and vaguely referenced her own childhood abuse, which

definitely seemed to impact her current parenting but seemed out of her conscious understanding.

Shannon was encouraged to obtain individual therapy to deal with her own history and how it was impacting her parenting today; Shannon and John were encouraged to attend marital therapy (Shannon scoffed at this notion immediately); and John was invited to attend therapy sessions with his daughter numerous times, but refused. Unfortunately, his unwillingness to invest in his children contributed to their perceptions of ongoing abandonment.

Myra's Individual Therapy

The most natural and instinctive form of communication for a child is play (Schaefer & Drewes, 2014). In fact, play has been shown to have several therapeutic benefits throughout children's development, including the facilitation of communication, expression, problem solving, mastery, role playing, and affective discharging (Schaefer, 1995). Play becomes a way to express, explore, and experience what children have ignored or denied. Therefore, it is used not only as a change agent, but also as a vehicle to communicate. "Children in play reconstruct, reenact, and reinvent their stressful experiences in order to understand them, assimilate their reality and achieve mastery over them" (Schaefer, 1995, p. 295).

Play has also been found to have benefits for children experiencing psychic trauma (O'Connor & Schaefer, 1994). In fact, play therapy is considered useful for children who have experienced traumatic events that they cannot process naturally. Furthermore, Schaefer (1995) discusses that one of the most important therapeutic elements at work during play is the ability to miniaturize the traumatic experience and to gain control over those events.

During Myra's parent–child assessment, she demonstrated a strong need to be in control. It is likely that this need manifested during her abuse, as she felt helpless, overwhelmed, and faced a high level of danger and anxiety. Although children experience and internalize trauma in very different ways and their ability to express those traumatic experiences differs, most clinicians find that the establishment of a safe and trusting relationship must precede trauma processing. Once children form reliable clinical relationships, posttrauma play may emerge and give children a sense of mastery and restoration to pretrauma functioning. Posttraumatic play is one of the most clinically effective ways to help traumatized children expose their trauma in a way that is at a *safe-enough distance.* It provides them with a natural way to express and understand experiences that provoked fear, anxiety, helplessness, and discomfort. "As a child-initiated activity, posttraumatic play is a sterling example of the power of play" (Gil, 2010, p. 48).

Although directed attachment work helped to achieve the goals for safety and security, I felt that it was time to move toward a more nondirective approach that would allow Myra to explore the impact of her trauma and provide options for expressive therapy so that she could find ways to communicate her experiences and gain mastery and competency. Child-centered play therapy offers unconditional acceptance of children and does not seek to change or correct problem behaviors. Child-centered play therapists (1) value children just as they are, (2) provide a permissive and safe environment so that children feel comfortable to express their emotional worlds through play, and (3) resist efforts to guide children in particular ways. In so doing, the solely child-directed play facilitates a restoration of internal control and mastery, encourages them to make their own decisions, and allows them to externalize their perceptions of their life experiences. The child-centered play therapist is genuinely interested and accepting, creates a feeling of safety, is sensitive to the child's feelings, and trusts the child's process. Landreth (1991) notes:

Only when the child begins to feel safe with the therapist will he/she begin to express and explore the emotionally meaningful and sometimes frightening experiences which have been experienced. The therapist must wait for this development. It cannot be rushed or made to happen. This is the child's time, and the child's readiness or lack of readiness to play, talk or explore must be respected. (p. 181)

In fact, the formation of a therapy relationship is viewed as central to all child-centered therapy; however, when children have experienced trauma, it is a necessary reparative experience for children, since this form of relationship is often new and essential in their healing process (Drewes et al., 2011).

Child-centered play therapists consider toys to be children's words, and as such, they carefully select toys for their symbolic and developmental potential. Toys offered to children should allow for the exploration of real-life experiences; facilitate explorations; and allow children to express their thoughts, feelings, and experiences while using symbolic language. Suggested toys can be divided into three categories: (1) real-life nurturing (e.g., dollhouse, baby dolls, puppets, medical kit, kitchen food, cash register); (2) toys reflecting themes of aggression or "acting out" (e.g., aggressive-looking puppets, foam swords, handcuffs, toy soldiers); and (3) materials related to creative expression and emotional release (e.g., sandtray, art supplies, magic wand, dress-up toys) (Landreth, 1991).

Although Myra had a fully stocked play therapy office at her disposal for her individual therapy, the transition from Theraplay—a directive, structured, and prescriptive approach—to a child-centered, nondirective modality proved to be a challenging, trial-and-error learning experience. As we wrapped up the Theraplay sessions, Shannon and I explained to Myra that each of them would start getting help by themselves, instead of together. She re-

ported that she was happy about that "because my mom just drives me crazy anyway." The first nondirective play therapy session I had with Myra unfortunately had to end early. It became clear that I had too quickly abandoned the structure that Theraplay offered, which Myra still needed. Without it, she became disorganized and dysregulated, and ultimately hit me several times in the face, prompting me to end the session prematurely. The following session, I provided a different format that integrated Theraplay techniques with nondirective, expressive therapy. I told Myra that the first 15 minutes of the session, I would be "in charge" and would provide three Theraplay activities (primarily focusing on the nurture and structure dimensions), and then for the next 30 minutes, she was invited to choose the activities that she desired. This integration within the session allowed for a much smoother transition, and it provided clarity and understanding of expectations for both Myra and myself (Gil, 2006).

For the first seven integrated sessions, Myra chose to play in the sandbox during the nondirective portion of our therapy. She demonstrated a tremendous ability to maintain emotional and physical regulation throughout these sessions. As she played, she would whisper quietly, then crescendo to a louder, more excited tone, followed by quiet, soft tones. She frequently made eye contact with me and remained engaged with me throughout her work in the sandbox. Myra was able to keep the sand in the sandbox with minimal redirection from me. Her play consistently involved hiding and finding items, as if she needed to discover and to be discovered or see and be seen. She frequently acted out scenarios of a battle between a victim and aggressor, where the aggressor almost always killed the victim. I viewed my role during these sessions as someone who was open to witnessing her reality without intruding on her or abandoning her.

One day Myra spontaneously suggested that we play a game, in which she was a "monster" and was going to "sneak in [your] room and kill [you] in [your] sleep." With her direction and prompting, she told me what to do and say, as we acted out this monster scenario over and over in the session. She engaged in this posttraumatic play for four sessions before eventually directing me to trade parts, and telling me to act like the monster while she became the sleeping victim. I was concerned about this interaction impacting and confusing our relationship, so in an effort to separate our actual selves from the monster–victim roles, I redirected her interest, asking her to choose puppets that would act as the victim and victimizer in her story. I told her she could do and show whatever she wanted with them and direct my participation as she wanted.

Myra chose a dinosaur puppet for the monster and a knight in shining armor for the sleeping victim. Throughout this process, Myra, playing the knight, was able to fight and successfully defeat the monster. It provided her with an opportunity to feel empowered, maintain control, and gain mastery. Myra engaged in this play repeatedly for four or five sessions, each time demonstrating more internal regulation and confidence. Interestingly, there were times during these sessions that she would call a "time out" and ask me to care for a hurt on her arm, which is a nurturing Theraplay activity. One day, toward the end of the session, Myra had conquered the monster yet again, and she spontaneously determined that the monster had some hurts and needed to be cared for. She stopped calling the puppet *monster* during this interaction, and instead referred to him as *Mr. Dinosaur.* When I spoke to Shannon in general terms about the trauma-related work that Myra was doing in therapy, she told me that Myra was more nurturing and affectionate at home during this time. She had completed the first grade, and the teachers also noticed her improved behavior, attention, and that she had stopped hitting her peers.

It was through this integrative approach that Myra and Shannon were able to achieve their treatment goals. COS-PC provided Shannon with the opportunity and foundation to understand and respond to Myra's needs differently, albeit inconsistently. Shannon also became better able to help Myra when she became dysregulated, and she was more emotionally attuned and empathic with her. The initial Theraplay sessions facilitated a healthy connection between me and Myra, one in which she accepted safe limits and structure, built regulation, and challenged her negative expectations of caring relationships (internal working models). Child-centered play therapy approaches provided Myra with many opportunities to restore a sense of personal power and control, to express her experiences of feeling powerless and chaotic, and to change those experiences through ones of mastery and empowerment provided by symbolic, posttraumatic play. Furthermore, the integration of Theraplay, particularly the nurturing activities, helped Myra feel cared for and worthy, and likely contributed to her ability to nurture the "monster" during our play. Integrating these different therapeutic approaches for both Shannon and Myra provided me with focus and intention so that I could help this family, despite the numerous treatment needs and challenges they faced.

It is worth stating that John was invited to participate in therapy many times and refused consistently. In addition, I discussed Myra's sister Susan's needs with Shannon, although she did not see any symptoms that she thought would warrant treatment. She did, however, agree to have her older daughter receive some trauma-specific work with a colleague at our agency. Eventually, sibling sessions were conducted to allow the children to create a joint trauma narrative (Myra used puppets and Susan created drawings to show what she remembered). Myra and Susan had successfully uncovered and expressed their trauma through symbols, art, stories, and play themes. My intention with them both had been to witness and be part of the process, not to guide or direct the process (Goodyear-Brown, 2009). In addition, during the sibling sessions, some interesting issues came out through play concerning their immigration to this country, their acculturation, and their feeling of not belonging in either the dominant culture or their culture of origin. These issues surprised Shannon immensely, although she was receptive to focusing differently on the fact that they were a cross-cultural family and the possibility of approaching these concerns more directly (Gil & Drewes, 2005).

My role with Shannon was to offer her attachment-based work and refer her to a colleague who could promote attachment-based principles to increase her ability to respond to Myra. She was always receptive to my feedback, although her follow-through was somewhat reticent and her insight compromised. She did eventually understand why her husband's role as a mostly absent father figure was relevant, given the children's history of abandonment. She was not, however, willing to "rock the boat" regarding their marital understanding and quid pro quo.

Conclusion

Integrative psychotherapy has been a salient topic of discussion for decades and appears to be gaining popularity among mental health professionals working with both adults and children. This topic has led to exploration of change agents or competencies within psychotherapeutic models that cause positive therapy outcomes, as well as to the need for clinical flexibility in conducting comprehensive assessments that can identify treatment areas that can benefit from specific interventions. The end result is that clinicians are becoming more conversant with varied treatment approaches in an effort to provide their clients with the most relevant and promising therapies. Clinicians are also becoming better informed and better able to choose

among evidence- and practice-informed treatments in order to strengthen therapeutic potential to assist clients.

The case illustration presented in this chapter demonstrates clinical flexibility in moving from one therapeutic model to another, weaving special responses based on special needs. A structured parent–child assessment (MIM) allowed the clinician to select a treatment approach, Theraplay, designed to increase relational health—an area of vulnerability for Shannon and Myra. In addition, Shannon was referred to an attachment-based parenting course (COS-PC), and Shannon and her husband were referred for couple therapy. A trauma-based focus resulted in individual child-centered play therapy for Myra, the identified patient in the family, while mother was also alerted to systemic issues that were likely contributing to the problem, including differential treatment of siblings, the absence of a meaningful father figure, and a color-blind approach to cultural differences. The clinician identified the mother's history of abuse as relevant to her current functioning and strongly suggested she seek additional treatment to process her own abuse. Finally, the sibling subsystem of Myra and Susan was provided with joint sessions that elicited their symbolic play about cross-cultural issues and also gave them an opportunity to develop a joint narrative about their immigration and acculturation as well as abuse they experienced in their orphanage and the abuse in Texas by their babysitter. This integrated model proved helpful in maximizing the clinical potential to be of help to most family members.

REFERENCES

Booth, P., & Jernberg, A. (2010). *Theraplay: Helping parents and children build better relationships through attachment-based play* (3rd ed.). San Francisco: Jossey-Bass.

Bratton, S., Ray, D., Rhine, T., & Jones, L. (2005). The efficacy of play therapy with children: A meta-analytic review of the outcome research. *Professional Psychology: Research and Practice, 36*(4), 376–390.

Cavett, A. (2009). A playful trauma-focused cognitive behavioral therapy. *Play Therapy Magazine, 4*(3), 20–22.

Cohen, J. A., Mannarino, A. P., & Deblinger, E. (Eds.). (2012). *Trauma-focused CBT for children and adolescents: Treatment applications.* New York: Guilford Press.

Cooper, G., Hoffman, K., & Powell, B. (2009). *Early intervention program for parents and children: A relationship parenting program, COS-PC facilitator manual 5.0.* Spokane, WA: Circle of Security International.

Drewes, A. A. (2009, October). *Integrating play therapy and cognitive-behavioral therapy.* Mining report presented at Association for Play Therapy, Clovis, CA.

Drewes, A. A. (2011). Integrating play therapy theories into practice. In A. A. Drewes, S. C. Bratton, & C. E. Schaefer (Eds.), *Integrative play therapy* (pp. 21–35). Hoboken, NJ: Wiley.

Drewes, A. A., Bratton, S. C., & Schaefer, C. E. (Eds.). (2011). *Integrative play therapy.* Hoboken, NJ: Wiley.

Gil, E. (2006). *Helping abused and traumatized children: Integrating directive and nondirective approaches.* New York: Guilford Press.

Gil, E. (2010). *Working with children to heal interpersonal trauma: The power of play.* New York: Guilford Press.

Gil, E. (2012). Trauma-focused integrated play therapy (TF-IPT). In P. Goodyear-Brown (Ed.), *Handbook of child sexual abuse: Identification, assessment, and treatment* (pp. 251–278). Hoboken, NJ: Wiley.

Gil, E., & Drewes, A. A. (2005). *Cultural issues in play therapy.* New York: Guilford Press.

Gil, E., & Shaw, J. A. (2013). *Working with children with sexual behavior problems.* New York: Guilford Press.

Goodyear-Brown, P. (2009). *Play therapy with traumatized children: A prescriptive approach.* Hoboken, NJ: Wiley.

Hitchcock, D. L., Ammen, S., O'Connor, K., & Backman, T. L. (2008). Validating the Marschak Interaction Method Rating System with adolescent mother–child dyads. *International Journal of Play Therapy, 17*(1), 24–38.

Jensen, J. P., Bergin, A. E., & Greaves, D. W. (1990). The meaning of eclecticism: New survey and analysis of components. *Professional Psychology: Research and Practice, 21*(2), 124–130.

Kenney-Noziska, S., Schaefer, C., & Homeyer, L. (2012). Beyond directive and nondirective: Moving the conversation forward. *International Journal of Play Therapy, 21*(4), 244–252.

Lindaman, S. L., Booth, P. B., & Chambers, C. L. (2000). Assessing parent–child interactions with the Marschak Interaction Method (MIM). In K. Giltin-Weiner, A. Sandgrund, & C. Schaefer (Eds.), *Play diagnosis and assessment* (2nd ed.) Hoboken, NJ: Wiley.

Landreth, G. (1991). *Play therapy: The art of the relationship.* Muncie, IN: Accelerated Development.

Lazarus, A. A. (2006). Multimodal therapy: A seven-point integration. In G. Stricker & J. R. Gold (Eds.), *The casebook of psychotherapy integration* (pp. 17–28). Washington, DC: American Psychological Association.

Magnavita, M. J. (2008). Toward unification of clinical science: The next wave in the evolution of psychotherapy? *Journal of Psychotherapy Integration, 24*, 22–28.

Munns, E. (2011). Theraplay: Attachment-enhancing play therapy. In C. E. Shaefer (Ed.), *Foundations of play therapy* (2nd ed., pp. 275–296). Hoboken, NJ: Wiley.

Norcross, J. C., Beutler, L. E., & Levant, R. F. (Eds.). (2005). *Evidence-based practices in mental health: Debate and dialogue on the fundamental questions.* Washington, DC: American Psychological Association.

Norcross, J. C., & Goldfried, M. R. (Eds.). (2005). *Handbook of psychotherapy integration* (2nd ed.). New York: Oxford University Press.

O'Connor, K. J., & Schaefer C. E. (Eds.). (1994). *Handbook of play therapy.* Hoboken, NJ: Wiley.

Perry, B., & Szalavitz, M. (2006). *The boy who was raised as a dog: And other stories from a child psychiatrist's notebook—what traumatized children can teach us about loss, love, and healing.* New York: Basic Books.

Phillips, R. & Landreth, G. (1995). Play therapists on play therapy: A report of methods, demographics, and professional/practice issues. *International Journal of Play Therapy, 4,* 1–26.

Powell, B., Cooper, G., Hoffman, K., & Marvin, B. (2014). *The Circle of Security intervention: Enhancing attachment in early parent–child relationships.* New York: Guilford Press.

Rasmussen, L. A., & Cunningham, C. (1995). Focused play therapy and non-directive play therapy: Can they be integrated? *Journal of Child Sexual Abuse, 4*(1), 1–20.

Ray, D. C. (2006). Evidence-based play therapy. In C. E. Schaefer & H. G. Kaduson (Eds.), *Contemporary play therapy: Theory, research, and practice* (pp. 136–157). New York: Guilford Press.

Schaefer, C. E. (1995). *The therapeutic powers of play.* New York: Aronson.

Schaefer, C. E. (2003). Prescriptive play therapy. In C. E. Schaefer (Ed.), *Foundations of play therapy* (pp. 306–320). Hoboken, NJ: Wiley.

Schaefer, C. E., & Drewes, A. A. (Eds.). (2014). *The therapeutic powers of play: 20 core agents of change.* Hoboken, NJ: Wiley.

Siegel, D. & Payne Bryson, T. (2011). *The whole-brain child: 12 revolutionary strategies to nurture your child's developing mind, survive everyday parenting struggles, and help your family thrive.* New York: Delacorte.

Seymour, J. W. (2011). History of psychotherapy integration and related research. In A. A. Drewes, S. C. Bratton, & C. E. Schaefer (Eds.), *Integrative psychotherapy* (pp. 3–19). Hoboken, NJ: Wiley.

Stricker, G., & Gold, J. R. (2008). Integrative psychotherapies. In J. L. Lebow (Ed.), *Twenty-first century psychotherapies: Contemporary approaches to theory and practice* (pp. 389–423). Hoboken, NJ: Wiley.

Weir, K. N. (2008). Using integrative play therapy with adoptive families to treat reactive attachment disorder: A case study. *Journal of Family Psychotherapy, 18*(4), 1–16.

Wethington, H. R., Hahn, R. A., Fuqua-Whitley, D. S., Sipe, T. A., Crosby, A. E., Johnson, R. L., et al. (2008). The effectiveness of interventions to reduce psychological harm from traumatic events among children and adolescents: A systematic review. *American Journal of Preventative Medicine, 35*, 287–313.

Wynne, L. S. (2008). Play therapy in school settings [Association for Play Therapy mining report]. Retrieved from *www.a4pt.org/download.cfm?ID=26654*.

CHAPTER 8

Attachment Security as a Framework in Play Therapy

William Whelan
Anne L. Stewart

John Bowlby's pioneering work in attachment theory advanced an evolutionary model of human bonding. In contrast to the psychoanalytic drive theories of the time, he proposed that human infants attach to their caregivers because they come into the world wired for relationships, and that moment-to-moment interactions within those relationships support the child's learning and adaptation to the environment, and enhance survival (Bowlby, 1969/1982). Bowlby was convinced that children's actual relationship experiences, not just their fantasies, shaped their emotions, thinking, and behavior and, bit by bit, created in them automatic patterns of thinking, feeling, and relationship behavior.

One of the most influential and useful ideas Bowlby offered in the theory of attachment development is the organizing influence that a compassionate, wiser, competent being can have on the experience and development of an immature being. He described this influence in behavioral systems terms, using ideas from ethology, general systems theory, communication

theory, and evolution to elucidate the powerful effects on child development of the behavioral interactions between child and parent (Bowlby, 1988). These interactions, even in infancy, are complex and become more elaborated across development. Everyday interactions continue to exert an organizing influence on the child's physical, emotional, social, and cognitive growth throughout childhood and into adulthood. Observing, appreciating, and engaging the healing impact of these relational processes in therapy is one of the play therapist's most delightful, fruitful, and challenging endeavors (Stewart, Whelan, & Pendleton, 2013).

Bowlby's research collaborator, Mary Ainsworth, conducted the first observational field studies of human infant bonding, initially in Uganda and later in Baltimore. The results were significant for several identifiable patterns of infant behavior that were consistent with the caregiving environment (Ainsworth, Blehar, Waters, & Wall, 1978). Hundreds of research studies over the last 40 years have demonstrated the importance of secure attachments for positive child development outcomes (Sroufe, Egeland, Carlson, & Collins, 2005; Sroufe & Siegel, 2011; van IJzendoorn & Bakermans-Kranenburg, 2009).

This chapter presents an attachment-based framework for observing and shaping children's emotional and behavioral patterns by the way we, as therapists and parents, think, feel, and behave in small interactions with children. In so doing, we present the use and application of attachment theory in play therapy. In particular, the concept of attachment security is used as an overall framework within which to consider therapist–child interactions, relationship development, and healing in the playroom. Given that all play therapy approaches acknowledge the importance of creating a strong relationship, we propose that the attachment security framework is compatible across theoretical approaches and has the potential of enhancing their use and effectiveness. A number of essential ideas, subsumed in the overall concept of attachment security, are also a focus of this chapter.

Attachment Security Concepts

Ainsworth identified caregiver attunement, or sensitivity, as the primary ingredient or variable for the development of secure attachment patterns in childhood (Ainsworth et al., 1978). In subsequent research, other investigators identified another caregiving variable, reflective functioning, as strongly associated with secure attachment and healthy child outcomes (Bick & Dozier, 2008; Fonagy, Steele, Steele, & Target, 1997; Steele & Steele, 2008). A third variable, coregulation of the child's experience, including the child's thinking, emotion, and behavior, has also been identified as important. Coregulation (or mutual regulation) consists of dyadic interactions and the behavioral sequences caregivers use to help a child stabilize in any given situation (Steele & Steele, 2008; Tronick, 2007). All

three of these ideas are integrated into the attachment security intervention approach.

The intervention framework focuses on the therapist–child relationship, including its organization and automatic dynamics. In particular, and given the research noted above, the focus is on enhancing the play therapist's sensitivity, reflective functioning, and coregulation of the child during moment-to-moment interactions in the playroom. Related objectives for the play therapist include developing abilities to facilitate accurate observation of child emotional behavior and relationship patterns so that the child's primary needs for coregulation of emotions, behavior, and thinking can be identified. A premise of this work is that children's behavioral sequences, in various circumstances, develop into automatic patterns over time and are best shaped and altered through relationship experiences (e.g., in the playroom), rather than through direct teaching. In this regard, the purpose and process of play therapy is to help children experience sensitive and coherent interactions with us, and with their primary caregivers, which will shape their automatic emotional and relationship behavior toward health.

Average, Healthy Development

Attachment refers to the process in which a child's central nervous system organizes physically, emotionally, and cognitively around interactions with a specific caregiver. As defined by Bowlby (1969/1982), an attachment is an affectional tie of the child to caregiver, and one that is represented "in the internal organization of the individual" (Ainsworth, 1989, p. 711). Most children and parents live and grow in circumstances of "average" stress. Even so, the experience of average stress in day-to-day life is no small thing. The caregiving needs of typical healthy children can easily fill the day and be draining or even exhausting at times for caregivers. Yet, through daily moment-to-moment interactions, most parents and children acquire deeply rooted, healthy attachment–caregiving patterns that function well enough to get them through problems and disruptions of the day, and in doing so their relationships become stronger and more broadly functional in the process. In the best of families, children and parents have ups and downs and, at times, even significant struggles, yet the "normal" trajectory of their development together provides them with adaptive automatic patterns of thinking, feeling, and interacting that most often lead them to adaptive resolutions.

In such close relationships a child is intimately privy to human activity and has a front-row seat to the unfolding physical, social, and emotional life of the family. In particular, the child experiences his or her emotions and sensations with caregivers throughout the day, and also perceives and experiences the caregiver's facial expressions, tone of voice, emotional expressions, and intimate physical behavior. The child experiences sights, sounds, motion, touch, and social life throughout the day and is largely unaware of how these experiences are integrated to build their unique relational world. An average child is born with a brain well equipped and wired for relationships (Brown, 2009). Infants "learn" and develop in a nonstop fashion, adding thousands of neural connections each minute for years (Siegel, 2012). This experiential learning in life is an ongoing process that most of us are hardly aware of at all, and become only partly aware of as we get older and grow into adulthood. One might say that life has a life of its own, and in many ways this appears to be true, given the way physical, emotional, and cognitive habits develop and tend to be transferred through the generations.

In the broad sense, the *development of attachment relationships* refers to physical, neurological, social, and emotional growth that takes place in the interface of our genetic potential and the environment, especially the emotional caregiving environment.

The outcome of this interplay, this genetic–experiential soup, is an unfolding set of habits in thinking, feeling, and behaving that, in adulthood, we describe as *personality*. In childhood, these developing patterns are shaped in moment-to-moment interactions with other people, especially with attachment figures. Among other developmental outcomes, the product of early experience as it interacts with biological capacity includes the child's growing patterns of resilience, adaptation, and vulnerability (e.g., a mixture of the child's growing capacity for hope, love, trust, determination, honesty, empathy, self-knowledge, self-reflection, forgiveness, and problem-solving abilities). These are the very outcomes we hope to shape through interactions with a child in the playroom, and the ones that usually develop on their own under circumstances of average stress.

We posit that most learning a child experiences in early development, and even across the lifespan, happens outside of the child's awareness and through the experiences of day-to-day interactions with the physical and social environment. This unconscious process appears to be true in the learning of complex physical, sensory–motor activities, both in early life (e.g., eating, crawling, talking, and walking), and in later childhood, adolescence, and adulthood (e.g., swimming, tennis, golf, driving, or piloting an aircraft). Relationship interactions form us in a similar way in terms of adaptations the nervous system makes in response to the context, availability, and functioning of coregulation in the caregiving environment. So, when a parent says "I want to learn more about my child's behavior patterns so that I can prevent us from getting into the same power struggles over and over," we can know that changes in relationship interactions will require experiential learning and real practice to bear fruit.

For the purpose of discussion in this chapter, we define average or "normal" developmental circumstances as those involving stress levels in the range of mild to moderate, and only occasionally include experiences of high stress (e.g., serious accidents, frightening events, injuries and loss, divorce, death of a loved one). It is useful for our discussion to keep in mind that the majority of family experiences, for most children and parents, are lived under circumstances of mild to moderate family stress, with occasional high levels (Abidin, 2012; Derogatis, 2004). Under these circumstances of average stress, most children automatically develop a very close partnership with a caregiver who provides moment-to-moment coregulation of emotions, behavior, and thinking, and a wonderful, personal introduction to life, love, and the interdependent ways of the world.

Attachment Security

In circumstances of average stress, the child–caregiver relationship unfolds in such a way that secure patterns of interaction become the rule or pattern, rather than the exception. In fact, in study after study the secure pattern is found around the world to be, by far, the most prevalent and represented in approximately 60–70% of children and caregivers (van IJzendoorn, Schuengel, & Bakermans-Kranenburg, 1999). What is a secure pattern? It is one in which the child exhibits little anxiety in relationship to the parent; he or she can move readily and smoothly away from the parent to explore the physical and social worlds, and then shift back toward the parent when tired or distressed for soothing and regulation of internal states. Children with secure patterns tend to reliably approach (physically or emotionally) their parents for help, make good use of the help that parents offer, feel better, and then are able to once again go about the business of exploration and learning (Sroufe & Siegel, 2011). Over time, they develop confidence in the availability of their parents; through experience they learn that their parents usually know how they feel, what they are thinking, and what they need. Children with secure patterns

learn to trust their parents and develop a habit of giving themselves over into their parents' caregiving. Figure 8.1 presents an illustration of these ideas, with the parent in a position at the center of the child's life to help and coregulate the child as needed. The white area inside the circle represents the child's close emotional needs for the parent for safety, soothing, refueling, and reassurance; the area outside the circle represents the child's exploratory needs for learning about people and the environment and becoming competent in the world.

Children with secure patterns tend to be easy to read in that, more often than not, they automatically send emotional signals that are accurate and unencumbered, with little noise to distract or misdirect the caregiver.

Secure development can be illustrated as we consider an infant in the first few months of life. When born, the nurses and physicians monitor the baby to make sure he or she demonstrates basic abilities for self-regulation, including breathing air, regulating temperature, getting nutrition, digesting breast milk, and passing waste. Along with these abilities, wake and sleep cycles usually become established in the first 6 months of life (absent medical problems or chronic stress in the environment). As these basic rhythms are established, the baby is free to experience the caregiver and, during times of low stress, explore the world. When the baby is distressed from being hungry, or cold, or too hot, or thirsty, or from some other discomfort, we imagine

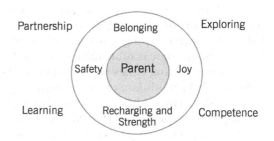

FIGURE 8.1. Attachment security.

his or her experience is like the following description.

The baby is distressed and begins crying, and then soon is crying hard. The baby can't yet think with words but is aware of strong discomfort, feeling unhappy, irritated, or in pain and continues to cry. From an evolutionary perspective, crying is an attachment behavior and usually functions to draw the parent's attention to intervene and help. If we put ourselves in the child's place, we might imagine this: I (now the baby) suddenly experience a change; my body has changed position in space (someone has picked me up). I am still distressed, but now I am held sweetly against something soft and warm and, although I don't know what it is, it feels better. Then I experience a swaying motion, back and forth. Again, I don't know what it is, but I rather like it. Then I hear something (someone is singing to me) that is sweet and comforting, and I am captivated. Then a warm, sweet liquid is in my mouth, and I am gradually, and happily, overwhelmed by the help of this beneficent other and I actually start to feel better.

Encapsulated here, in this 5-minute episode, is one of the most important relationship developments of early childhood. This infant, upset and unable to soothe him- or herself, had a transforming experience that can shape much of what is to come in the years ahead. Namely, the baby was given his or her first experience of a cycle of soothing. In the days and weeks ahead, the baby will have hundreds of similar experiences in which his or her central nervous system will get to experience and build upon these rhythms of soothing. In this way, the baby begins developing patterns of soothing (i.e., neurological subroutines) that will be activated during times of stress and will help the child modulate emotional arousal as he or she grows. Other patterns develop during these experiences as well, including rhythms of partnership behavior, synchronicity, and reciprocity. Taken together, these experiences represent the foundation for

what we will later view as the child's ability for self-control. In this regard, small episodes of reliable coregulation of experience can lead to internal integration and coherent structure in the child that, over time, will find its expression in reality-based and emotionally balanced behavior.

In the preschool and school-age years, we observe that most children no longer get upset as frequently as they used to, and typically their upsets are less intense and resolve more quickly (most of the time). Children whose internal structure contains neurological patterns of soothing and partnership behavior require less direct hands-on coregulation as they get older, and they demonstrate more abilities for self-regulation and self-control. Nonetheless, they still need help from their parents and continue to use them for close, inside needs and support for their exploration and growing competence. Bowlby wrote that attachment–caregiving bonds are important and operate from the cradle to the grave (Bowlby, 1988). Parents remain important as children reach adulthood, and children find partners and spouses that become additional attachment figures for the rest of the journey.

Caregiving Security

Caregivers with secure patterns (1) are typically accurate in their observations of their children, (2) are able to make developmentally coherent inferences about their children's internal states, (3) draw accurate conclusions about what the child needs, and (4) then generate a caregiving response that meets the need and helps the children. These caregivers appear able to provide an emotional environment that is sensitive, flexible, and can adapt to meet the needs of a particular child. Therapists with a secure approach share these same characteristics. They also tend to be genuinely curious about what is happening inside the child (i.e., reflective about the child's internal emotional and mental experiences), reflect on their own thoughts and feelings regarding the child, and reflect on the ways in which their thoughts, feelings, and behavior affect the child. They exhibit the ability to alter their own caregiving (or therapy) behavior in the moment, depending on the changing needs of the child. Another shared characteristic is an understanding of the child's sometimes difficult, oppositional, or rejecting behavior as coming from the effects of stress in the child's life. Secure caregivers (and therapists) have a developmental view of the child that helps them put difficult behaviors into perspective; therefore, they tend not to feel personally disrespected, rejected, or emotionally injured by the child's emotions and actions.

Nonsecure Patterns

Children who grow up in stressful environments may not experience the kind of sensitive and available caregiving noted above, and can miss out on the day-to-day experience of a caregiver's coregulating and shaping interactions. When caregivers are overwhelmed with environmental danger, financial crises, or when they are ill, depressed, lonely, addicted, or the subject of abuse, they may not be available for moment-to-moment partnership interactions with the child.

For some children, perhaps their primary experiences of intimacy with their caregivers have been during moments of emotional upset, loss, anger, fear, or other distress. It is not surprising then that parts of their relationship experience with caregivers can become organized and encoded internally around moments of anger, rejection, or emotional chaos. A child's patterns of overarousal, anxiety, inhibition or amplification of emotion, and dysregulated behavior can develop and recur on a predictable basis. Sometimes a specific relationship interaction or content that elicits difficult behavior may seem unconnected to current events, or "out of the blue," yet the emotional interaction pattern itself

often turns out to be recurring and predictable. In these circumstances, a simple look or tone of voice from a caregiver can elicit patterns of overarousal and difficult behavior, even when the caregiving intent was quite the opposite.

Under such relationship stress, the nonsecure pattern that develops most often is one of anxious avoidance (of intimacy) and related inhibition of emotions and needs within the attachment–caregiving relationship. This pattern occurs in about 20–25% of children in the general population, and at much higher proportions in the high-risk or clinical samples (van IJzendoorn et al., 1999; Whelan & Marvin, 2011). In contrast to children with the secure pattern, those with the anxious-avoidant pattern have trouble connecting with their parents directly for help in times of mild to moderate stress. Instead, when they are in need of help in regulating their experience and emotions (e.g., in need of protection, soothing, or assistance in exploration), they tend to stay to themselves, behave as if they don't need help, actively reject their parent's (or therapist's) help, or distract themselves. In this regard, the child's emotional and attachment signals to the parent are "noisy" and difficult to read, and tend to obscure the child's need of the parent in the moment (see Figure 8.2).

Sometimes the child inhibits, moves away, or acts out when he or she needs

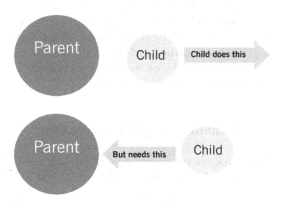

FIGURE 8.2. Noisy attachment signals.

the caregiver. As an example of this, consider a child who has had a difficult day on the playground or at school and is upset, scared, angry, or embarrassed. Upon returning home, the child goes straight to his or her room instead of connecting with the parent in some way to elicit much needed comfort and refueling. In the playroom, therapists can often tell that a child is worried, fearful, or upset about something but instead of signaling this directly, or indirectly, the anxious-avoidant child may seem to shut down, sit in a heap on the sofa, or sit on the floor just fiddling with toys and make little use of the therapist.

In contrast to this pattern, consider a child who, due to a history of family stress, loss, or trauma enters the playroom in a frantic, dysregulated way, is too rough with everything, throws toys, knocks things over, and resists the therapist's help, saying, "Leave me alone! I'm just having fun." In these instances, the child's emotional signals are noisy and obscure his or her needs, and have the unintended effect of pushing the parent (or therapist) away, or leave the caregiver feeling unwanted and ineffective. These automatic behavioral sequences are not thoughtful or intentional on the child's part but, nonetheless, are likely to have disruptive and negative relationship consequences unless the caregiver or therapist can identify them as noise in the system and formulate a response that will shape and change the child's experience and patterns. Without such sensitive intervention, the child's patterns of overarousal and anxiety will likely continue, and the development of healthier rhythms of soothing and partnership behavior will remain elusive.

Attachment Security Intervention

The process of therapy is personal, emotional, and takes place within the relationship of child and therapist. This therapeutic endeavor involves harnessing and directing the healing aspects of human interactions for the benefit and health of children. In this regard, the primary goal of play therapy is developing a relationship that, through moment-to-moment interactions, will help form more coherent internal structures and patterns of thinking, feeling, and behaving in the child. That is, the goal is to help shape and develop in the child healthy internal patterns that may not yet be present, or ones that are currently underdeveloped, due to experiences of chronic stress or trauma in the child's life. In this regard, the main therapeutic mechanisms at the play therapist's disposal are sensitivity, reflection, and coregulation of the child's experience.

The intervention begins with an observational assessment of child–parent interactions (e.g., often involving a separation–reunion procedure) to identify relationship patterns and determine which of the child's automatic emotional and behavioral responses represent accurate signals about internal experiences and needs, and which signals represent "noise" in the system that can lead us astray. With the results of such an assessment, the caregiver and therapist can look for opportunities, within this developmental framework, to shape the child's experience and scaffold behavior and emotions toward health. In play therapy, an assessment of the child's interactions with the therapist is also important for the same reasons, and can be accomplished, with parents' permission, through analysis of videotaped interactions in the playroom.

Sensitivity

Mary Ainsworth's (1967, 1978) concept of sensitivity to a child's attachment needs incorporates three components: making observations, correctly interpreting the child's signals, and providing an appropriate caregiving response. From an intervention perspective, the first order of business is observing a child's interactions to gather accurate information about internal experience and relationship needs. To become accurate observers, therapists need an observational framework and practice in observing children's attachment behavior. This involves tracking children's behavior in several ways within the attachment security framework. Therapists observe a child's behavior in the playroom (with parents and separately with therapist) in terms of proximity and contact seeking, interaction maintenance, body orientation, tone of voice, content of speech, affect, eye gaze, and body language. From the observations and in reference to a developmental framework, therapists will distinguish accurate signals from noise and make inferences about the child's feelings and thoughts in a given interaction sequence. Once this is done, therapists then draw conclusions about the child's close, inside needs, and the outside exploratory needs in a given interaction episode (i.e., a playroom episode, or an episode at home for use in consultation with the parent).

Reflective Functioning

Reflection, in this context, refers to seeing the child's behavior within family relationships and within the therapeutic relationship from a developmental point of view, and using that perspective (as it evolves) to make inferences about the child's internal states and needs, and to draw conclusions or plans about what to do next with the child in the playroom. In addition, reflection includes tracking one's own thoughts and emotions in relationship to the child in order to regulate oneself for the child's benefit. One of the primary functions of an attachment, and of a therapeutic, relationship, is to protect the child from harm, from dangers in the environment, and from the emotional reactions of other people, including the therapist. For example, as therapists our own emotional arousal, anxiety, or fear may propel us to move ahead prematurely into problem-solving mode, trying to fix things or trying to teach the child a strategy, rather than *being with* the child to share and

shape his or her experience within small moments of relationship interaction. In our training and supervision of play therapists, this is one of the most common dilemmas encountered in the playroom.

Coregulation of Experience (What to Do)

Coregulation of the child's experience occurs when we combine sensitivity and reflection to generate a caregiving (i.e., therapeutic, helpful) response that has a good chance of meeting the child's relationship need (of us) in the moment and shaping new patterns of emotion and behavior. The response we settle on necessitates taking a developmental view; setting a safe and accepting emotional tone and leading in relationship interactions with the child when needed, including soothing and protecting the child, narrating the experience, and scaffolding the child's exploration of toys, emotions, ideas, and relationship events (past and present). This dynamic and complex process of facilitating attachment security through coregulation is depicted in Figure 8.3.

Clinical Case Example

The attachment security framework helps play therapists understand and address a child's emotional needs by guiding the clinician's thinking, feeling, and behaving in the playroom. The following clinical case shows an application of the attachment security framework of observing the child's behavior (seeing), making inferences about what the child is experiencing and needing (reading), and then responding. The example is a composite case, based on the authors' collective clinical experience. The case presentation includes a discussion of how to use attachment security dimensions of sensitivity, reflective functioning, and coregulation to inform decision making and action inside (within the child–therapist relationship) and outside (within

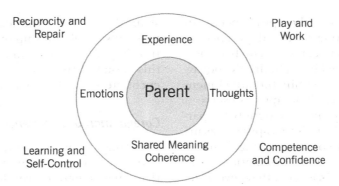

FIGURE 8.3. Attachment security: Coregulation.

the caregiver–therapist relationship) the play therapy sessions.

Creating a Nurturing Environment

Jayden, a slightly built 4-year-old boy, perched on Maria's lap. Maria was Jayden's new foster mother. He held on tightly to her sweater, sporadically and furtively risking glances at me. Ms. Cretzner, a social worker from the child protective services department, had contacted me requesting play therapy services for Jayden 5 weeks prior to this meeting. When I (Anne) first received the call, I could hear the distress in Ms. Cretzner's voice as she described Jayden's circumstances. She related that a child had been brought to the hospital emergency room by his great-aunt 6 days prior. He was severely dehydrated, had a broken leg, cracked ribs, and multiple bruises on his face and body. The physical exam showed evidence of other earlier injuries. Charges had been filed against his biological father and his girlfriend, and both were incarcerated. The department was busy setting up services. While both maternal and paternal grandparents and the child's biological mother were demanding immediate custody and vying for visitation, a well-regarded and seasoned foster family was in place to receive him upon discharge from the hospital; a primary care physician was assigned for close medical follow-up; and a guardian ad litem, an attorney with

the responsibility to provide independent recommendations to the court about the child's best interests, had been appointed. And now the child protective services department worker was interested to know how soon I could begin play therapy.

We completed and faxed the necessary permission forms and, as we resumed the conversation, I took a deep breath and considered the scenario that had been described to me: the child's serious physical injuries and pain, his fear, sadness, and anger, and his significant psychological loss and confusion; the extended family members' upheaval; and the urgency to begin services expressed by the protective services worker. Using the attachment security framework, I started by reflecting on Jayden's experience. He would leave the hospital soon, still needing a great deal of physical care, live in a different home, and be with a different family. And he was 4 years old.

I considered the inner circle of needs that were likely activated for Jayden—needs for protection, for comfort, for basic physical and psychological safety. I considered my own feelings of sorrow and worry for this young child and my desire to help him be safe and well. I thought of the research evidence regarding the positive impact of secure attachments and the negative developmental outcomes associated with adverse childhood events and toxic environments (Biglan, Flay, Embry, & Sandler, 2012; Chapman et al., 2004; Yoshikawa, Aber, &

Beardslee, 2012). As I considered the turmoil present in the extended family and tried to look at the world from Jayden's perspective, I began to wonder if adding me to the mix of new relationships would be value added at this time. I decided, yes and no: *yes*, to exploring with the social worker on how my knowledge of attachment security might be beneficial in guiding treatment planning (including the likelihood of introducing play therapy at a later time); and *no*, for initiating another new relationship, at a new place, at this time for Jayden.

As the phone call continued, I listened to the authentic concern expressed by Ms. Cretzner. I tried to respond with sensitivity to the multiple stressors and worries she was negotiating. I acknowledged how challenging it was to see a child suffering from such extreme maltreatment, how hard it was to sort through the competing and blaming stories from his extended family, and I affirmed the positive actions she had already completed to move forward in a helpful, protective manner. I then shared my perspective that Jayden's world was full of unfamiliar people and places right now and that perhaps I could be of better assistance to her and the foster parents in a consultative role, as they moved forward to create a safe and secure refuge for him. Ms. Cretzner seemed less centered on just getting a play therapy session scheduled and was curious and receptive to participating in the dialogue as Jayden's intervention plan unfolded.

When I met with Ms. Cretzner and the foster mother, Maria, 1 week later, they expressed deep concern about Jayden's behavior. Maria said that for most of the day, Jayden sat still and rarely spoke. She was concerned that he did not ask about where he was or inquire about his mother or other family members. She said that he was often crying for "no reason."

MARIA: So he sits by the window in the living room—just quiet-like. It seems like he's asleep with his eyes open. He will be sitting there and—nothing happens—but

he starts crying, big, big tears. No sound, but huge tears. We haven't said or done a thing.

THERAPIST: So this still, quiet sitting and big tears seem like a mystery to you, and it is clear, you are worried that he is so upset.

MARIA: You're right, it is a mystery and I'm worried. I expect kids to have to get used to us and to a new place. I get it that they haven't been treated well. But we have the pets, so many toys . . . we don't yell or hit. But we have had him, and only him, for almost a week and he still seems so . . .

THERAPIST: (*quietly*) So . . . ?

MARIA: So sad . . . so sad. He seems unhappy to be in our home.

THERAPIST: You are really worried about him . . . you want so much for him to feel better, to feel happy. Sounds like you are worried he is not feeling better more quickly, and maybe you're worried about how to be of help to him?

MARIA: Yes, yes for all that! Do you think he should be in a different home?

Using the attachment security framework as my guide, I was able to respond sensitively to Maria's heartfelt concern for Jayden. Furthermore, I was able to get a glimpse of how challenging it was for Maria to witness and be with such sustained sadness, so much so that she wondered if she could help or if Jayden would be better off leaving.

I commented to Maria and Ms. Cretzner about how much of what Maria was already doing was part of an approach to understanding children's needs, especially children who had experienced harsh and hurtful parenting. I complimented Maria on how much she had noticed about Jayden's behavior and how curious she was about his emotional world. I said I agreed with how important it was to understand this mystery. I told her I had some ideas, shown in a drawing that might help us map out and understand what was happening in this little boy's heart. I introduced the attachment security graphic (see Figure 8.1), and we proceeded to use it to picture what Jayden was feeling and thinking, informed by what he was doing.

As we reflected on what Maria noticed as Jayden was crying in the chair, we imagined having a video of the scene, and periodically using the "pause button" or "close-ups" to examine the situation thoroughly and compose a "Jayden Story." Collectively, we explored many areas: "What was Jayden doing?" "What did his face look like?" "Where was he looking?" "What did he say?" "How did he move?" "Who else was there?" and finally, responding with our best guess(es). "What were his needs at that moment?" As the discussion proceeded, Maria began to wonder if she was leaving Jayden alone too much.[1] In telling the story of his silent crying, she shared that she had not wanted to upset him further by "disturbing" him. Now, using an attachment security framework to imagine Jayden's inner circle needs, she realized that his stillness and tears did not mean he wanted her to stay away. Maria realized that Jayden actually needed her presence in a very specific way to begin to experience relationships with adults as loving, helpful, trustworthy, and responsive.

The information from consultation sessions helped me understand how I could support Jayden's healing by assisting Maria to stay emotionally available and attuned as he expressed intense emotional needs. I could imagine that, fueled by her genuine concern, Maria would want to move too quickly into bright, distracting activities or perhaps prematurely offer reassuring comments that did not let Jayden know his distress could be experienced as something besides overwhelming and confusing. His strong feelings, with his foster mother's help and over time, did not have to be inhibited but could be welcomed, organized, and understood.

Consultation sessions were conducted with Maria for 4 weeks. More detailed information about the attachment security framework was shared as we composed numerous "Jayden Stories" to explore and problem-solve how to best support his healing. The stories permitted Maria to practice "seeing," "reading," and "responding" to Jayden's needs, not just to his behaviors. As her observational ability increased, she began to recognize his miscues—that is, the times when he did not clearly and directly communicate his needs. Jayden's miscues were largely instances of inhibiting and not communicating his needs for comfort and protection, particularly when he was hurt physically or emotionally upset. One poignant example occurred during our second consultation visit at the foster home. Jayden was walking quickly with an armload of toys and abruptly fell, his elbow making a sharp crack as he hit the tile floor. I exclaimed, "What a tumble! Your arm hit the floor hard!" Although the fall was just a few feet in front of Maria, she did not move toward Jayden, but turned to me and said, "Oh, he is okay." Indeed, Jayden was already proceeding to collect the toys and seemed not to notice us. She continued, "I wonder if he even feels pain sometimes. He falls a lot and never cries or asks for help."

On the spot, we created a "Jayden Story" to imagine what his needs might be. Even though the fall was clearly painful, Jayden's automatic response (actually, the lack of a response) was built from a relational history of neglect and harm. His reaction was an unhappy example of a noisy signal that was leading his foster mother away from meeting his needs. Maria, in her attempt to make sense of his unusual behavior, had concluded that it was another instance of his not needing her. Using the attachment security approach, she now realized that this was a particularly compelling example of an inaccurate, noisy signal and that it was vitally important for her to respond to everyday hurts with attention and care—to create cycles of soothing with him. Using "Jayden Stories," Maria continued to make progress in her ability to read through the "noise," move in to meet his needs, and establish a relationship in which he felt her concern and the safety she could provide. After 4 weeks of consultation, Maria, Ms. Cretzner, and I agreed that Jayden's adjustment to his foster family was sufficiently established that it was an appropriate time to initiate play therapy.

I conducted play therapy in Jayden's foster home, using a suitcase playroom for 7 months. I used my knowledge of the attachment security framework to evaluate Jayden's attachment patterns during play interactions with Maria and with me. Remarkably, he demonstrated a solid mix of secure and anxious-avoidant attachment patterns and grew rapidly in his ability to use his relationships with each of us for healthy exploration and play. He clearly enjoyed interacting with us and was able to let us partner in his exploration. Following a complicated court decision, Jayden transitioned to his great-aunt's home as a foster placement with the goal of adoption. When Jayden began living with his Aunt Rose, the guardian ad litem and Ms. Cretzner were able to obtain support for a comprehensive attachment evaluation and in-home services using an attachment security model through the court and family assessment and planning team. Thus, the opportunity for Aunt Rose to learn and parent from the attachment security perspective with a designated in-home clinician was put in place (including viewing videotaped interactions with Jayden). As parenting and childrearing values are understandably shared across generations, this therapeutic support was crucial. The addition of this team member allowed the in-home provider to take responsibility for sharing the attachment security approach with Aunt Rose, and I modified my role to focus on Jayden's progress in play therapy, with periodic joint consultations with Aunt Rose and the in-home clinician.

Jayden's Journey in Play Therapy

When I had greeted Jayden in the living room at his initial foster home, I was encouraged to see that he was appropriately reticent to engage. More importantly, he was quickly able to use Maria's presence as a secure base to build a strong therapeutic relationship with me during our phase of in-home play therapy. When Jayden moved to his Aunt Rose's home, we also moved our play therapy location and began meeting in a traditionally equipped clinic playroom. I continued to use the attachment security framework to help me respond in attuned and helpful ways to his changing needs.

Play with Me: Introduction to the Playroom

Jayden stopped short a few steps into the playroom. Using a variation of the staple introduction to the playroom from child-centered play therapist Garry Landreth, I said, "Jayden, this is a room where you can talk and play with things in most of the ways you would like to." Jayden looked around the room and then turned his face up to me, with a look of amazement. With a mixture of anticipation and confidence, he pronounced, "Play with me."

I moved along with Jayden as he explored the playroom thoroughly and, at first, haphazardly. He appeared to be a bit overwhelmed, pulling out drawers and opening cabinets, unable to settle on any activity or toy for an extended period of time. I tracked his behavior and reflected possible emotions he might be experiencing. I commented about the many new things in this new room; that it was hard to figure out what to do; that he looked excited or a little worried or confused. Jayden did not verbally respond but gradually his movements slowed down, and he became more deliberate in his actions. *Coregulation*, I thought! Jayden was busily using my interest and reassuring demeanor to feel safe—safe enough to explore this new environment in a more organized and satisfying manner. He eventually stopped in front of the dollhouse, looked at me intently, and with a hint of a question, repeated, "Play with me?" He began to play by collecting all the family figures and sliding them, one by one, down the roof. He let each figure plummet to the floor.

JAYDEN: (*glancing expectantly at me*) He dead.

THERAPIST: He fell all the way down the roof and now he's dead.

Jayden continued to gaze at me, and then in a methodical and organized manner continued to slide the figures down the roof to the floor, each time stating, in a matter-of-fact manner, that they were dead. I verbally continued to reflect on the demise of each character, matching Jayden's affect.

All at once, I felt a jolt of doubt. At his foster home, Jayden's play had moved from just putting toys in jail to varied, reciprocal interactions, full of turn taking and more differentiated developmentally appropriate play. Now, in his play everyone was unsafe, sliding to their deaths, with no help in sight. I used my anxiety as a signal to apply the basics of the attachment security model, namely, I turned my attention to observing Jayden. I noticed his body was actually relaxed, not tense; he was making eye contact, he was not distressed, and he was actively engaged in the, albeit repetitive, play activity with me. I reflected to myself that Jayden knows that I am curious, supportive, and can keep him safe as he explores joyful and disturbing parts of his experience.

When I said that we had 5 minutes left in the playroom, Jayden abruptly stopped the sliding activity. He began placing the family figures on the top edge of the roof. He added two baby carriages to the rooftop. He asked me to help him put a tall cylindrical block with a police figure on top of the roof and then instructed me to get a large toy tow truck. He placed family figures in the

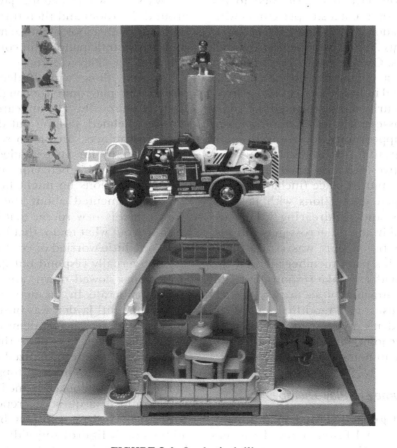

FIGURE 8.4. Jayden's dollhouse.

truck and pointed for me to put it on the front edge of the lower rooftop. (A photo of his creation is shown in Figure 8.4.) It is interesting to note the precariousness of the figures, carriages, and truck atop the roof and that Jayden's foster family's vehicle was a large blue truck. Whatever symbolic meaning the content may have, Jayden's satisfaction with what he made was evident. Jayden stepped back, smiled at me, and said he was ready to go see Aunt Rose. I witnessed with Jayden that when children are feeling safe inside the relationship, they can benefit from coregulation and have the psychological energy to explore novel, challenging, hopeful, joyful, and inexorably difficult material.

In play therapy Jayden continued to experience my responsive support and to take delight in his own explorations. In partnership, we explored themes of hurt, threat, protection, comfort, and nurturance. In the context of our relationship, he (or figures, trucks, or puppets) sometimes accepted help in troubled times and sometimes miscued the need for care with rejections, controlling play, or acting as if the hurt, worry, or fear was not real and help was not needed. Over a total of 15 months of intervention, I used the attachment security framework in play therapy and in numerous consultation meetings with the child protective services worker, the guardian ad litem, the physician, preschool teacher, and both Jayden's foster mother and kinship adoptive mother.

One month prior to termination, Jayden entered the playroom and held up his finger.

JAYDEN: It hurt!

THERAPIST: Oh, goodness! You have an *owie* on your finger? Let me see.

JAYDEN: (*moving closer*) Yes, see? (*Points to his finger, but no mark is evident.*)

THERAPIST: I am so sorry your finger is hurt and so glad you let me know! That is just the thing to do if you are hurt!

JAYDEN: I need a Band-Aid. Get me one?

THERAPIST: Yes, absolutely. Let's go get one—I know just where they are.

My heart was soaring. The child who had not acknowledged pain was pointing out a hurt to me and asking for a Band-Aid! Jayden was experiencing the outcomes of secure caregiving: He could communicate his needs more directly, and his caregivers were seeing, reading, and responding in ways that let him feel safe, protected, cared for.

Conclusion

One of John Bowlby's motivations for building an evolutionary- and ethology-based theory of attachment was to understand the troubling and mysterious behavior problems of the children he served and find ways to help them and ease their suffering (Bretherton, 1992). His work, together with the research of Ainsworth and many others since the 1960s, has provided a rich mix of child development knowledge for use in helping us make sense of mysterious child behavior problems, particularly in the context of moment-to-moment relationship interactions. The attachment security framework brings key components of healthy relationship development into focus for use in the playroom, in parent consultation, and in the larger community to shape children's attachment experiences and development toward health. With so much "noise" in the multiple systems encountered, this framework can help the play therapist stay focused on the evidence at hand (i.e., actual patterns of relationship behavior); avoid being distracted and overwhelmed by an onslaught of noisy, inaccurate signals (from multiple sources); and decipher the child's attachment needs. Being sensitive and reflective of those needs, the play therapist can then coregulate the child's experience, thoughts, and emotions to build new patterns of soothing, partnership behavior, and healing.

NOTE

1. In the conversation I was able to rule out seizure activity and dissociation as primary issues in Jayden's presentation.

REFERENCES

Abidin, R. R. (2012). *Parenting Stress Index* (4th ed.). Lutz, FL: PAR.

Ainsworth, M. D. S. (1989). Attachments beyond infancy. *American Psychologist, 44*(4), 709–716.

Ainsworth, M. D. S., Blehar, M. C., Waters, E., & Wall, S. (1978). *Patterns of attachment: Psychological study of the strange situation.* Hillsdale, NJ: Erlbaum.

Ainsworth, M. D. S. (1967). *Infancy in Uganda: Infant care and the growth of love.* Baltimore: Johns Hopkins Press.

Bick, J., & Dozier, M. (2008). Helping foster parents change: The role of parental state of mind. In H. Steele & M. Steele (Ed.), *Clinical applications of the Adult Attachment Interview* (pp. 452–470). New York: Guilford Press.

Biglan, A., Flay, B., Embry, D., & Sandler, I. (2012). The critical role of nurturing environments for promoting human well-being. *American Psychologist, 67*(4), 257–271.

Bowlby, J. (1982). *Attachment and loss: Vol. 1. Attachment.* New York: Basic Books. (Original work published 1969)

Bowlby, J. (1988). *A secure base: Parent–child attachment and healthy human development.* New York: Basic Books.

Bretherton, I. (1992). The origins of attachment theory: John Bowlby and Mary Ainsworth. *Developmental Psychology, 28*(5), 759–775.

Brown, S. (2009). *Play: How it sharpens the mind, opens the imagination, and invigorates the soul.* New York: Bantam Books.

Chapman, D. P., Whitfield, C. L., Felitti, V. J., Dube, S. R., Edwards, V. J., & Anda, R. F. (2004). Adverse childhood experiences and the risk of depressive disorders in adults. *Journal of Affective Disorders, 82*(2), 217–225.

Derogatis, L. R. (2004). *Symptom Checklist-90–Revised.* Bloomington, MN: NCS Pearson.

Fonagy, P., Steele, M., Steele, H., & Target, M. (1997). *Reflective function manual for application to Adult Attachment Interviews.* London: University College.

Siegel, D. J. (2012). *The developing mind: How relationships and the brain interact to shape who we are* (2nd ed.). New York: Guilford Press.

Sroufe, L. A., Egeland, B., Carlson, E. A., & Collins, W. A. (2005). *The development of the person: The Minnesota Study of Risk and Adaptation from Birth to Adulthood.* New York: Guilford Press.

Sroufe, L. A., & Siegel, D. J. (2011, March/April). The verdict is in. *Psychotherapy Networker,* pp. 34–39, 52–53.

Steele, H., & Steele, M. (2008). *Clinical applications of the Adult Attachment Interview.* New York: Guilford Press.

Stewart, A. L., Whelan, W. F., & Pendleton, C. (2013). Attachment theory as a road map for play therapists. In C. A. Malchiodi & D. A. Crenshaw (Eds.), *Creative arts and play therapy for attachment problems* (pp. 35–51). New York: Guilford Press.

Tronick, E. (2007). *The neurobehavioral and social–emotional development of infants and children.* New York: Norton.

van IJzendoorn, M., & Bakermans, M. (2009). Attachment security and disorganization in maltreating families and orphanages. Retrieved from *www.child-encyclopedia.com/documents/van_IJzendoorn-Bakermans-KranenburgANGxp-Attachment.pdf.*

van IJzendoorn, M., Schuengel, C., & Bakermans-Kranenburg, M. (1999). Disorganized attachment in early childhood: Meta-analysis of precursors, concomitants, and sequelae. *Development and Psychopathology, 11,* 225–249.

Whelan, W. F., & Marvin, R. S. (2011, April 2). *Caregiver patterns that moderate the effects of abuse and neglect.* Presentation of results from the Virginia foster care study (NIH Award No. GC11456) at the biennial meeting of the Society for Research in Child Development, Montreal, Quebec, Canada.

Yoshikawa, H., Aber, L., & Beardslee, W. (2012). The effects of poverty on the mental, emotional, and behavioral health of children and youth. *American Psychologist, 67*(4), 272–284.

CHAPTER 9

Child–Parent Relationship Therapy

A 10-SESSION FILIAL THERAPY MODEL

Sue C. Bratton
Kristie Opiola
Eric Dafoe

The importance of a secure parent–child relationship on children's socioemotional development has been well documented (Perry & Szalavitz, 2006; Ryan & Bratton, 2008; Siegel & Hartzell, 2003). For children who have experienced distressing life events, the caregiver–child attachment holds even greater significance. Children look to their parents to help them regulate emotions and handle adverse experiences (Schore, 2001). However, parents may lack the experience and skills to help their children cope in times of difficulty. Parental stress, including stress in the parent–child relationship, can further hinder parents' ability to respond appropriately to their children's social, emotional, and behavioral needs. Child therapy interventions that focus on strengthening the parent–child bond while also providing emotional support for caregivers and increasing parental efficacy are gaining recognition for their effectiveness in treating a wide range of childhood problems (Eyberg, Nelson, & Boggs, 2008; Guerney

& Ryan, 2013; Landreth & Bratton, 2006; Powell, Cooper, Hoffman, & Marvin, 2013; Webster-Stratton, Rinaldi, & Reid, 2011).

Child–parent relationship therapy (CPRT; Landreth & Bratton, 2006) is a play therapy-based parent training model with over 40 studies demonstrating its effectiveness for a broad range of child mental health issues. Founded on the filial therapy model of Bernard and Louise Guerney, at the heart of CPRT is the premise that a secure parent–child relationship is the essential and curative factor for children's well-being. In a supportive group environment, parents learn child-centered play therapy (CCPT) skills to respond more effectively to their children's emotional and behavioral needs. In turn, children learn that they can count on their parents to reliably and consistently meet their needs for love, acceptance, safety, and security. This chapter briefly describes the history, rationale, and theoretical tenets of the CPRT model, summarizes research to support its use with a variety of presenting issues across diverse populations and settings, provides an overview of the structure and format for implementing CPRT, and includes a brief case example to illustrate the process.

History and Development

CPRT (Landreth & Bratton, 2006) is based on the innovative parent training model developed by Bernard and Louise Guerney in the mid-1960s. The Guerneys founded their approach based on their belief in the significance of the parent–child relationship and their confidence in parents' ability to learn the necessary skills to become therapeutic agents in their children's lives (VanFleet, 2005). To reflect the importance of the familial bond, they used the term *filial therapy* to describe their pioneering approach to treating children's emotional and behavioral difficulties (L. Guerney, 2000).

In the Guerneys' original filial therapy model, a small group of parents met weekly for an unspecified period of time that sometimes extended beyond 1 year (B. Guerney, 1964). Building on the work of the Guerneys, in the 1980s Garry Landreth developed a more structured and condensed 10-session filial therapy training format with the objective to increase parent participation by reducing financial and time constraints (Landreth & Bratton, 2006). Consistent with the Guerneys' model (B. Guerney, 1964), parents in CPRT are taught CCPT principles, attitudes, and skills to use with their own children in supervised play sessions to facilitate their children's healing and to increase overall family functioning. Landreth and Bratton (2006) formalized the 10-session training model in a text, *Child Parent Relationship Therapy (CPRT): A 10-Session Filial Therapy Model*, to distinguish the model from other filial therapy approaches. The CPRT protocol was manualized by Bratton, Landreth, Kellam, and Blackard (2006) to provide practitioners and researchers with a tool for ensuring treatment integrity in implementing the intervention.

Theoretical Assumptions

CPRT is grounded on several theoretical assumptions, including those underlying attachment theory, person-centered/child-centered theory, and the significance of play in children's development. First, a secure parent–child attachment is essential for a child's well-being and holistic development (Siegel & Hartzell, 2003). A parent's ability to communicate empathy, understanding, and acceptance promotes the kind of attuned parent–child relationship that is crucial for developing secure attachments and healthy relationships in the future. The attuned caregiver is seen as emotionally responsive and consistent. Securely attached parent–child relationships help children explore the world around them, respond flexibly, organize their thoughts, and regulate emotions and behaviors.

Next, CPRT is a strength-based approach grounded in the person-centered therapeutic perspective of Carl Rogers (1951) and the nondirective play therapy principles of Virginia Axline (1947). Both Rogers and Axline believed in the innate human capacity of children and people of all ages to strive toward growth and development. As in person-centered theory, the relationship—in this case between caregiver and child—is the primary mechanism of change. In a secure relationship characterized by parental attunement, acceptance, empathy, consistency, and responsiveness, children thrive. By teaching parents basic CCPT principles, attitudes, and skills (Landreth, 2012), they learn to create an environment free from judgment, convey empathic understanding and acceptance to their child, and facilitate the child's innate tendency toward growth and wellness. Whereas most popular parenting models are problem focused and teach parents strategies to change the child's behavior, in CPRT the focus is on helping parents understand their child's needs and increasing parental efficacy. Parents are taught to nurture an internal locus of control in their child with the long-term objective of facilitating their child's self-control, self-motivation, and self-direction.

Finally, CPRT is grounded in a developmental understanding of children and focuses on weekly special parent–child playtimes. As in CCPT, play is acknowledged as the primary means that children communicate, express their worries, and make sense of their world (Landreth, 2012). In play, a child is able to regress, learn, mature, contemplate, and ultimately gain a greater understanding and acceptance of self and others. In CPRT, play is utilized as the means of enhancing the parent–child relationship and provides a lens through which caregivers can become more sensitive and attuned to their child's needs and better understand their child's view of the world.

Objectives

CPRT is unique in that it targets improvement in the child, the caregiver, and the caregiver–child relationship. Because the relationship is viewed as the medium for change, the primary objective is to enhance the caregiver–child relationship to increase trust, security, and closeness within the dyad of focus and ultimately between other family members (Landreth & Bratton, 2006). With increased trust, warmth, and affection, family members can improve communications, problem-solving strategies, and expressions of affection and familial enjoyment.

CPRT aims to help parents increase parental acceptance and empathy, understand and respond sensitively to their children's emotional needs, establish more realistic developmental expectations and limits on their children's behavior, and ultimately gain greater confidence as parents. Parents are taught CCPT principles and skills to use in the weekly special playtimes to accomplish these objectives, with an overarching aim to help parents find delight in being with their child and rediscover the joys of parenting (Landreth & Bratton, 2006).

Additionally, the support group format encourages parents' self-acceptance and insight into their own experiences and needs and the reciprocal effect on their relationship with their children.

The objectives for children in CPRT are similar to those for children receiving individual play therapy services (Landreth & Bratton, 2006). Through play and within the safety of a secure relationship, children can express their needs and feelings, including repressed feelings and tension, and ultimately learn more appropriate and satisfying ways to express, regulate, and meet their needs. CPRT offers the additional advantage of providing children with the opportunity to directly work through negative perceptions of their parents by experiencing a more positive, trusting, and secure relationship.

Role of the Therapist

CPRT requires that the treatment provider is a licensed mental health professional with specialized training in the CPRT protocol (Landreth & Bratton, 2006). CPRT is not a family therapy model in which the therapist is the agent of change responsible for directing therapy sessions. The role of the therapist is to train and closely supervise parents to become therapeutic change agents for their children. Toward this end, the therapist must be a highly skilled group facilitator, play therapy trainer, supervisor, and fallible mentor. Initially, the primary role of the therapist is to create a safe and supportive environment in which parents feel comfortable sharing and discussing their parenting struggles (Bratton, 1998). Over time, the therapist trains the parents in the skills and principles of CCPT, demonstrates for parents how to conduct special play sessions with their children, and then provides direct supervision of parent–child play sessions. Balancing the parents' needs for emotional support with the required didactic training and information within 10 two-hour sessions is an ongoing challenge even for the most experienced CPRT facilitator. Landreth and Bratton (2006) recommend the use of coleaders to balance the multiple roles.

CPRT in Practice

Central to the success of CPRT is the requirement that treatment providers are first trained and supervised in CCPT principles and skills (Landreth, 2012; Ray, 2011), and then trained and supervised in the 10-session CPRT manualized treatment protocol (Bratton et al., 2006) to ensure treatment fidelity. The treatment manual includes the 10-session training protocol, therapist's guide, parent notebook, supplemental resources, and a CD-ROM containing all parent training materials to print for each CPRT group. We caution against rigid adherence to the protocol; rather, they emphasize that the protocol is intended to be applied with clinical judgment regarding the therapeutic needs of parents and children. Additional training resources include the CPRT text (Landreth & Bratton, 2006), which contains comprehensive transcriptions of a 10-session CPRT group with six parents and the CPRT demonstration videos illustrating the process and procedures of a CPRT group with four couples (Bratton & Landreth, 2013). Readers are directed to these resources for a full description of the 10-session protocol, the CPRT training format and process, and strategies for successful implementation. But, again, we emphasize that the materials are not intended for use without formal training and supervision.

Overview of Structure and Format

CPRT uses a small, supportive group format weaving together didactic and supervision experiences. This dynamic and interactive process distinguishes CPRT and other group filial therapy models (Guerney & Ryan, 2013) from other parent training programs, which tend to be primarily educational in focus. In CPRT, a group of six to eight parents typically meet once per week for 2 hours, although CPRT has been successfully used in more intensive formats, and in some cases, the treatment time has been extended to meet families' needs (Landreth & Bratton, 2006). The CPRT group format requires a careful balance of didactic and support group components aimed at maximizing parents' success in learning and applying the CPRT skills. Initial treatment objectives include creating an environment of safety, acceptance, and encouragement, while helping parents normalize their experiences through sharing with other group members. Parents are given information about child development and CCPT philosophies, techniques, and skills that positively influence the parent–child relationship. Equipped with developmentally responsive ways of communicating, parents are able to strengthen their relationship with their children.

Arguably the most critical element of the CPRT model is the supervision component in which parents video-record required 30-minute play sessions with their children and receive feedback from the therapist and the group members. During these special playtimes, parents set up a specific group of toys in a designated area of their home and conduct weekly, child-led play sessions (B. Guerney, 1964; Landreth & Bratton, 2006) in which they apply CCPT attitudes and skills aimed at fostering a more attuned and empathic parent–child relationship. A parent's ability to communicate empathy within the parent–child relationship assists in the child's development of self-regulation and age-appropriate social behaviors (Carnes-Holt & Bratton, in press). Promoting secure attachment relationships between parents and children through the weekly play sessions is central to the success of CPRT. Ryan and Bratton (2008) emphasized the importance of both sides of the attachment relationship, arguing that effective filial therapy addresses the emotional needs of caregivers and children. Thus, sensitive support of parents' emotional needs is essential to the supervision process.

During the group process component of CPRT, the therapist facilitates connections between parents and creates an environment of safety and acceptance. As parents receive emotional support and directly experience the interpersonal relationship skills (e.g., empathy, encouragement, reflective responding) that they are learning to apply with their own children (Landreth & Bratton, 2006), they are more willing to explore their often difficult feelings and experiences. The case illustration provided below offers a glimpse into the CPRT training content and process over the course of treatment.

Clinical Case Example

This case demonstrates the flexibility of the CPRT model and illustrates how the basic principles and process of CPRT were utilized with a challenging parent in the group process. Change within the parent is often the most significant factor in children's growth and healing. Therefore, in this case example we focus primarily on how change was facilitated within the parent through the group process, the parent–child play sessions, and the supervision process to effect a stronger bond between the parent and the child. The parent of focus participated in a 10-session CPRT group that I (Bratton) facilitated. Identifying information was altered to protect confidentiality.

Ms. C., a single, 30-year-old European American graduate student, referred her 6-year-old son, Nate, to the clinic due to problems at home and school. She reported that he was a gifted child, but also angry, manipulative, oppositional, and out of control. Ms. C. reported that she was struggling financially and personally, and blamed Nate for her overwhelming distress. Ms. C. divorced Nate's father, who was Af-

rican American, when Nate was 3. She reported an adversarial relationship with her ex-husband who now lived out of state and saw his son infrequently. Ms. C. believed that Nate struggled with being biracial and that his behavior was a result of anger toward his father.

The clinical needs of the family were assessed through a detailed parent intake, information obtained from Nate's school, and a structured family play activity to assess parent–child dynamics. The assessment indicated serious problems in the mother–son relationship. Nate's behavior problems seem to stem from his emotional response to Ms. C.'s lack of acceptance and warmth toward him. I determined that CPRT was the appropriate course of treatment, although my observations indicated that Ms. C. would likely require considerable emotional support and encouragement to repair the relationship with her son and learn more effective ways of interacting with him.

Sessions 1–3: Learning CPRT Principles and Skills

Establishing an atmosphere of safety, acceptance, and encouragement is the top priority in the first three sessions, especially for this population of parents who need opportunities to share and normalize their experiences. Still, the CPRT model requires that the therapist be mindful of balancing parents' need for support with teaching the foundational CCPT attitudes and skills in preparation for parents to begin their play sessions with their child after week 3. To ensure success in skill attainment, CPRT relies heavily on demonstration and role play of skills. Beginning skills include following the child's lead, reflection of feelings, and reflection of verbal and nonverbal content of child's play. More importantly, parents are taught that during the weekly 30-minute special playtime with their child, they are to focus their full attention and convey a genuine interest in and acceptance of their child by communicating the four "be-with" attitudes: (1) "I am here," (2) "I hear you," (3) "I understand," and (4) "I care" (Landreth & Bratton, 2006). These attitudes and expressions of acceptance on the parents' part are at the core of developing a closer and more secure parent–child bond and facilitating healing within the child.

Ms. C. immediately stood out in the filial group made up of seven other single mothers. She arrived 20 minutes late to the first session, yelling at Nate from the time they entered the front door of the clinic until she left him in the child care area. Ms. C. entered the room looking defeated and helpless, and the other parents in the group were unsure of how to respond. After normalizing the experience as an embarrassing happening to which all parents could relate, Ms. C. relaxed and seemed to enjoy the support the group offered. She later told me that coming to the group was like an oasis in her week, a rare time when she didn't have to "deal with Nate." This pattern of being late and struggling to get Nate to the clinic continued for the next several weeks.

During Sessions 2 and 3, Ms. C. appeared to benefit from the supportive group experience, but she remained unconvinced of the value of the CCPT skills and resisted the idea that playing with her son to form a closer relationship would be helpful. Rather, she focused on what she could do to "improve Nate's behavior." Ms. C. listened with interest to other parents as they shared their fears and struggles, but she shared little of herself. When she did, she tended to focus on the negative in herself and her son. The Session 3 role play of CCPT skills is critical because parents typically conduct their first play session with their child during the week between Sessions 3 and 4. Ms. C. was clearly uncomfortable role-playing the CCPT skills, particularly when she played the role of the child. I believed that Ms. C. would benefit from additional support before she could successfully conduct home play sessions. Based on my observations over the past 3 weeks, I expected that she would need individual attention and closer supervision to develop a closer and

more accepting relationship with her son before she would be able to focus on skill development. I talked with Ms. C. after Session 3 and arranged for her to conduct her first play session at the clinic under my supervision, rather than at home.

Ms. C. and Nate came to the clinic a few days later. I met with Ms. C. briefly to review the basic procedure and methods for the play session while Nate played in the waiting room. Ms. C. expressed reluctance and doubt in her ability, so we determined that while Ms. C. observed behind the two-way mirror, I would conduct a brief play session demonstration with Nate, in which I would focus on the CCPT attitudes of "being with" and allowing him to direct the play. The process was explained to Nate, and I showed him where his mother would watch while he played with me.

Following the 10-minute demonstration, I met with Ms. C. to discuss what she had noticed in preparation for her play session with Nate. Next, she conducted a 10-minute playtime with Nate while I observed behind the mirror and noted positive interactions between mother and son. I chose to limit their play session from the typical 30 minutes based on my observations of mother–son interactions over the past 3 weeks. At this point, I believed she needed emotional support and encouragement from me more than she needed skill practice. I provided Ms. C. with immediate feedback after the play session. I encouraged her efforts, and we role-played a few instances in which she struggled with responses. She readily agreed to my suggestion to conduct another 10-minute playtime to gain more practice. We ended with approximately 15 minutes of video-recorded supervision in which I pointed out positive moments between Ms. C. and her son. Although Nate nonverbally and verbally expressed distrust of his mother's new behavior with him, there were moments when he was obviously enjoying his mother's full attention. Based on her view that Nate was more "difficult to handle" than other children, Ms. C. asked if she could continue her play sessions at the clinic for the next few weeks. I agreed that the one-on-one supervision would be helpful to Ms. C. and allow her to receive additional emotional support outside of the group process.

Sessions 4–10: Group Process of Supervised Play Sessions

Skill refinement through supervision and processing of parent–child play sessions is the major activity in Sessions 4 through 10. Each session begins with all parents sharing their experiences during the special play-times with their children, with the majority of time spent viewing videos and giving feedback to the two parents of focus for that week. The use of video playback holds parents accountable, facilitates greater insight as parents view themselves, provides more opportunities for vicarious learning, allows parents to see the impact of the play session on their children, and permits the therapist to reinforce skills demonstrated and suggest alternative responses and actions when needed. Perhaps more important, viewing play sessions within the group format permits the therapist to offer parents support and encouragement in a more concrete and meaningful manner, while also providing opportunities to build group cohesion as parents are able to share their struggles and receive support from other parents. In Sessions 4 through 8, foundational skills continue to be emphasized, along with the added skills of limit setting, choice giving, encouragement, and self-esteem-building responses. To ensure success during this practice phase, parents are restricted to practicing the CCPT skills only during the 30-minute play sessions, thus avoiding feelings of failure that inevitably arise when parents try to apply their new skills too quickly to daily problems that arise. In the final two sessions, parents are helped to generalize and apply their new skills to everyday interactions with their children.

In Session 4, there was a subtle change in Ms. C.'s behavior. She expressed relief to hear the other parents express their inse-curity as they described the happenings in their first play session. She chose to be last to report on her play session, and although she maintained her typical self-critical stance, she was able to share two positive comments. As planned, Ms. C. continued to bring Nate to the clinic for their weekly special playtime. Ms. C. demonstrated small gains over the next 2 weeks in her ability to allow Nate to direct the play. However, her nonverbal attitude toward Nate continued to limit her ability to fully convey acceptance, which is foundational to CPRT's success. In addition, Ms. C. was unable to effectively set limits on Nate's behavior in the playroom, generally reverting to "Don't do that" or "I told you to stop," after which Nate would respond by getting angry. Most of these incidents centered around Nate's use of a Nerf ball shooter that made a loud noise Ms. C. did not like. Of course, it was Nate's favorite toy! Nate was a master at "pushing his mom's buttons" in order to get her to respond in the way that was familiar to him.

Ms. C.'s most significant area of growth over CPRT Sessions 5 through 8 was in self-acceptance. As Ms. C. experienced acceptance from me and the other parents, she became less self-critical and began to show more acceptance of Nate's behavior *in some* situations. This acceptance did not extend to those situations in which Ms. C. perceived Nate's behavior as aggressive. For example, when Nate would shoot the Nerf ball shooter, as he did in every session, Ms. C. perceived his actions as aggressive behavior toward her and continued to respond to Nate in a critical manner. By the fifth play session (after CPRT Session 7), Ms. C. had learned to refrain from responding harshly, but she could not convey verbal or nonverbal acceptance of Nate's feelings when he engaged in what she considered aggressive play.

The most dramatic shift in Ms. C. and in Nate occurred in their sixth play session. The play session took place the day after CPRT Session 8, during which parents had spontaneously initiated a discussion about unconditional and conditional acceptance. I emphasized the importance of parents accepting both positive and *negative* feelings in their children during their weekly 30-minute playtimes and related their children's needs to their own needs to have all their feelings accepted. Ms. C. was visibly emotional as the parents discussed their experiences of rejection and the need to experience the same kind of acceptance I asked them to give to their child. Ms. C. chose not to share her feelings within the group, but the other parents' empathy was obvious as they offered her support and encouragement.

In their play session the next day, Ms. C. was able to convey acceptance of Nate's aggressive behavior by reflecting how he was feeling. The change in Nate's behavior was dramatic; he immediately became calmer and began to hum while he played with the Nerf shooter in a more creative and less aggressive manner. After several minutes he lost interest in playing with the toy and invited his mother to paint at the easel with him for the remainder of their playtime. Ms. C. was noticeably more relaxed and able to respond with greater empathy, acceptance, and enjoyment. During feedback after the play session, Ms. C. expressed amazement at the change in Nate's behavior and commented on how much she enjoyed playing with her son.

I helped her take credit for facilitating the change in their relationship and the changes she saw in Nate. I asked her to reflect on what was different about the play session. She reported that the discussion about the importance of accepting children's negative feelings had been on her mind all week. She had genuinely felt more accepting of Nate in the session, even when he was playing aggressively. As usual, we ended supervision with a video review of a portion of her session. I cued the video to the segment where she reflected to Nate that he was angry with her. Ms. C. became overwhelmed with emotion as she observed the dramatic effect on Nate. Ms. C. then shared what she had not been able

to express in the last group. "Growing up, I never had anyone who cared about my feelings. It was not okay to be angry or sad. I stuffed all my feelings inside. I was good at that and eating was a way I could feel better, but eventually I would explode." This kind of comment is common as parents begin to make a connection between their own feelings and experiences and the parenting difficulties they are having.

In the ninth CPRT session, Ms. C. chose to show her video-recorded play session during the group for the first time. After receiving positive feedback and support from the other parents, she tearfully shared some of her early experiences of "never feeling good enough," particularly in regard to her father and men, and made the connection between those experiences and her inability to accept her son at the beginning of CPRT. During the next week, before the 10th CPRT session, Ms. C. conducted her first home play session and reported that both she and Nate enjoyed their time together. Perhaps the most noticeable change in their interactions was their arrival to the clinic for the last two group sessions. Ms. C.'s yelling and Nate's refusal to comply were now replaced with laughter and obvious enjoyment of their time together.

Ms. C. came to the clinic for supervision one additional time after the group ended. The parents in the group asked for follow-up meetings to hold them accountable to continue their play sessions. Ms. C. attended both the 1-month and 3-month follow-up sessions. During that time, she chose to seek personal counseling to explore feelings that had surfaced as a result of the CPRT process. In the last follow-up meeting, Ms. C. reported continued improvement in Nate's behavior at home and school and reported a significant improvement in their relationship. I again encouraged Ms. C. to take credit for facilitating the changes she was seeing.

Ms. C. called occasionally over the next 3 years with concerns about Nate as he entered new developmental phases and struggled with life transitions. I met with her a few times to lend support and encouragement prior to their relocation out of state for Ms. C.'s new job. Ms. C. showed more improvement than any parent with whom I have conducted CPRT; yet, her skill level at the end of 10 weeks was among the weakest of any parent in her group. The greatest shift I observed was in her attitude of acceptance toward herself and toward Nate, and most importantly, the development of a closer, more affectionate mother–son relationship. Through the confidence and skills she gained as a result of CPRT and the closer relationship she enjoyed with her son, Ms. C. was now better equipped to handle the challenges she faced as a single parent.

Evidence Base for CPRT and Filial Therapy

CPRT is a well-researched child therapy treatment model with numerous studies investigating its effectiveness. Just as CPRT is grounded in the original filial therapy model developed by Bernard and Louise Guerney, the substantial body of CPRT research rests firmly on the empirical foundation they built. From their inception of filial therapy in the 1960s, the Guerneys and colleagues were committed to investigating its efficacy as a therapeutic modality (Guerney & Ryan, 2013; Guerney & Stover, 1971; Stover & Guerney, 1967). Although early filial therapy studies lacked the methodological rigor of contemporary studies, the encouraging findings from the Guerneys' groundbreaking research provided the catalyst for the significant body of research that currently exists on the 10-session CPRT model (Bratton, Landreth, & Lin, 2010).

Since the first published study almost two decades ago (Bratton & Landreth, 1995), the evidentiary base for CPRT has grown as studies' methodological rigor increased. An impressive 36 studies, involving almost 1,100 participants, employed a control group design to examine CPRT's effects. Of these 36 studies, 19 employed experimental designs regarded as the "gold standard with regards to questions of treatment efficacy" (Nezu & Nezu, 2008, p. vii). The remainder of the studies used quasi-experimental designs largely due to limitations in conducting research in real-world settings that interfered with random assignment. As an indicator of the high level of treatment fidelity in CPRT research, 32 of the 36 controlled studies were conducted by investigators who were directly trained and supervised in the CPRT protocol (Bratton et al., 2006).

Bratton and colleagues (2010) provided the most comprehensive review of CPRT research to date. Although the majority of outcome studies focused on the effects of training and supervising parents as therapeutic agents, almost one-third of CPRT research examined the benefits of the CPRT model delivered by teachers and mentors. The vast majority of studies showed statistically significant results and moderate to large treatment effects for the superiority of CPRT over control groups. Given the quantity of studies and comprehensive number of participants, several conclusions can be drawn from reviewing the findings from the body of research. Overall results indicate that CPRT is effective in reducing children's behavior problems, decreasing parental stress, and increasing parental empathy (Bratton et al., 2010). Specifically, studies show CPRT's efficacy across a variety of issues and populations, including sexually abused children; children living in domestic violence shelters; adopted/fostered children with attachment difficulties; children whose mothers or fathers were incarcerated; chronically ill children; and children diagnosed with learning differences, pervasive developmental disorders, speech problems, adjustment difficulties, or assorted internalized and externalized behavior problems. CPRT's wide applicability and transportability are further demonstrated by its successful use in a variety of real-world settings, including hospitals, churches, shelters, prisons/county jails, Head Start programs, public and private schools, and community agencies.

The level of multiculturalism addressed in CPRT research is another strength of this treatment model. Multiple studies show CPRT's efficacy across ethnic, socioeconomic, and cultural groups, including immigrant Latino, second-generation Latino, African American, Native American, immigrant Chinese, immigrant Korean, Korean, and Israeli populations. Finally, the age range of child participants (2–11 years) indicates CPRT's responsiveness to the developmental needs of very young children through preadolescence. With a participant mean age of 5 years 3 months, CPRT seems particularly sensitive to the treatment needs of young children and, as such, responds to the scarcity of evidence-based child therapy treatments for young children (Chorpita et al., 2011; *www.effectivechildtherapy.com*).

Meta-analytic research supports and strengthens the findings from individual CPRT/filial therapy studies (Bratton, Ray, Rhine, & Jones, 2005; LeBlanc & Ritchie, 2001). Researchers found stronger outcomes for studies in which caregivers were trained and supervised in filial therapy methodology to use with their children than play therapy studies in which professional play therapists provided treatment. Using the meta-analytic data from Bratton and colleagues (2005), Landreth and Bratton (2006) analyzed only those studies using the CPRT model to calculate an overall effect size. CPRT demonstrated a very large treatment effect size of 1.25 (Cohen, 1988), meaning that the average child–caregiver dyad receiving CPRT performed more than one and a quarter standard deviations better on outcome measures compared to the average child–caregiver dyad not receiving the treatment (Bratton et al., 2010).

In summary, the current evidentiary base of research supports CPRT as an intervention for training caregivers to utilize CCPT skills to address the therapeutic needs of children. According to criteria established by the American Psychological Association (Chorpita et al., 2011), the strong empirical support of CPRT positions it as a "promising treatment" for several presenting issues and populations. CPRT research has increased in rigor over its relatively short history by investigating clearly defined populations and target behaviors, by the use of a manualized protocol and treatment fidelity checks, and by the use of randomized controlled trials with larger sample sizes. However, a continued focus on these areas, along with replication of well-designed studies by independent researchers, is needed to move CPRT toward recognition as a well-established treatment for specific childhood disorders.

Conclusion

The importance of a healthy parent–child relationship on children's holistic development has been well documented. Child therapy interventions that focus on strengthening the parent–child bond are gaining recognition for their effectiveness in treating a wide range of childhood problems (Eyberg et al., 2008; Landreth & Bratton, 2006; Powell et al., 2013; Webster-Stratton et al., 2011). CPRT is a manualized, play therapy-based intervention that is responsive to the developmental needs of children through its focus on the use of play to help parents understand and communicate their child's needs and to foster a secure and predictable caregiver experience for the child. Parents whose children are experiencing social, emotional, and behavioral problems are often plagued by feelings of guilt and powerlessness to help their child. As parents begin to better understand and respond to their children's needs through successful application of CCPT skills, they are empowered and develop confidence in their ability to effectively parent and help their child in times of difficulty. Furthermore, the emotional support offered to caregivers within the group meetings can serve as a healing force that facilitates their personal well-being.

Positive, robust research outcomes for CPRT highlight its efficacy and confirm that training caregivers in CCPT is a valid treatment for addressing the mental health needs of children (Bratton et al., 2010). The strong research base for CPRT has implications for child therapists who are ethically responsible for accountability to their clients. All major mental health professional organizations in the United States have called upon their members to use interventions for which there is empirical support. CPRT's manualized protocol contributes to its ease of replication by practitioners and researchers. Research findings (1) support its efficacy with a broad range of populations, settings, and presenting concerns and (2) demonstrate CPRT's transportability across settings and its potential for successful application with a variety of clinical populations. The use of CPRT cross-culturally is strongly indicated by the overwhelmingly positive findings from research with several nondominant groups. Furthermore, meta-analytic results suggest that parents trained in CCPT techniques can be more effective with their own children than a trained professional, and that results can be achieved in as few as 10 sessions. Landreth and Bratton (2006) emphasized the importance of treatment fidelity in achieving the treatment results indicated by the research and proposed key training components that are critical to the overall success and effectiveness of CPRT:

- The requirement that treatment providers are first trained and supervised in CCPT principles and skills, and then trained and supervised in the 10-session CPRT treatment protocol (Bratton et al., 2006).
- The requirement that parents conduct weekly, video-recorded play sessions with their children and receive direct supervision by the CPRT-trained therapist.
- The structured use of the video-recorded play sessions as well as supervised role play within the group format, so that parents receive support and specific feedback on their use of the CPRT skills.

The empirical support for CPRT holds further implications for practitioners governed by the dictates of managed care to provide treatments that are proven and economical. CPRT can be provided in a time-limited and group format, thereby enabling practitioners to provide effective care. Moreover, it is plausible to suggest that training parents in CPRT serves a preventive function by equipping them with skills that can be infused into their daily interactions with their children, thereby helping them respond more effectively to difficulties in the parent–child relationship long after treatment has ended.

While these results are compelling and clearly support the need for play therapists to strongly consider using CPRT with their clientele, there are cases when presenting issues or parent or child characteristics would dictate the use of play therapy conducted by a professional over CPRT or as an adjunct to CPRT (Landreth & Bratton, 2006) and instances when parents lack the motivation or personal resources to commit to the significant investment required in this approach. Nevertheless, the robust findings for CPRT's effectiveness with a variety of problems and populations suggest that if a child and a parent are both suitable candidates, CPRT should be strongly considered as the treatment of choice.

REFERENCES

Axline, V. (1947). *Play therapy*. New York: Ballantine.

Bratton, S. C. (1998). Training parents to facilitate their child's adjustment to divorce using the filial/family play therapy approach. In J. M. Briesmeister & C. E. Schaefer (Eds.), *Handbook of parent training: Parents as co-therapists for children's behavior problems* (2nd ed., pp. 549–752). New York: Wiley.

Bratton, S. C., & Landreth, G. L. (1995). Filial therapy with single parents: Effects on parental acceptance, empathy, and stress. *International Journal of Play Therapy, 4*(1), 61–80.

Bratton, S. C., & Landreth, G. (Producers). (2013). *Child parent relationship therapy (CPRT) in action* [DVD]. Dallas, TX: Child Parent Relationship Therapy Institute.

Bratton, S. C., Landreth, G., Kellam, T., & Blackard, S. (2006). *Child parent relationship therapy (CPRT) treatment manual: A ten session filial therapy model for training parents*. New York: Routledge.

Bratton, S. C., Landreth, G., & Lin, Y. (2010). Child parent relationship therapy (CPRT): A review of controlled outcome research. In J. N. Baggerly, D. C. Ray, & S. C. Bratton (Eds.), *Child-centered play therapy research: The evidence base for effective practice* (pp. 267–294). New York: Wiley.

Bratton, S. C., Ray, D., Rhine, T., & Jones, L. (2005). The efficacy of play therapy with children: A meta-analytic review of treatment outcomes. *Professional Psychology: Research and Practice, 36*(4), 376–390.

Carnes-Holt, K., & Bratton, S. C. (in press). The efficacy of child parent relationship therapy for adopted children with attachment disruptions. *Journal of Counseling and Development, 92*(3).

Chorpita, B., Daleiden, E., Ebesutani, C., Young, J., Becker, K., Nakamura, B., et al. (2011). Evidence-based treatments for children and adolescents: An updated review of indicators of efficacy and effectiveness. *Clinical Psychology Science and Practice, 18*(2), 154–172.

Cohen, J. (1988). *Statistical power analysis for the behavioral sciences* (2nd ed.). Hillside, NJ: Erlbaum.

Eyberg, S. M., Nelson, M. M., & Boggs, S. R. (2008). Evidence-based treatments for child and adolescent disruptive behavior disorders. *Journal of Clinical Child and Adolescent Psychology, 37*, 213–235.

Guerney, B. G., Jr. (1964). Filial therapy: Description and rationale. *Journal of Consulting Psychology, 28*(4), 303–310.

Guerney, B. G., Jr., & Stover, L. (1971). *Filial therapy: Final report on MH 18264-01*. Unpublished manuscript, Pennsylvania State University, University Park.

Guerney, L. (2000). Filial therapy into the 21st century. *International Journal of Play Therapy, 92*, 1–17.

Guerney, L., & Ryan, V. (2013). *Group filial therapy: The complete guide to teaching parents to play therapeutically with their children*. London: Jessica Kingsley.

Landreth, G. (2012). *Play therapy: The art of the relationship* (3rd ed.). New York: Routledge.

Landreth, G., & Bratton, S. C. (2006). *Child parent relationship therapy (CPRT): A 10-session filial therapy model*. New York: Routledge.

LeBlanc, M., & Ritchie, M. (2001). A meta-analysis of play therapy outcomes. *Counseling Psychology Quarterly, 14*(2), 149–163.

Nezu, A. M., & Nezu, C. M. (2008). *Evidence-based outcome research*. New York: Oxford University Press.

Perry, B. D., & Szalavitz, M. (2006). *The boy who was raised as a dog and other stories from a child psychiatrist's notebook: What traumatized children can teach us about loss, love, and healing*. New York: Basic Books.

Powell, B., Cooper, G., Hoffman, K., & Marvin, B. (2013). *The Circle of Security intervention: Enhancing attachment in early parent–child relationships*. New York: Guilford Press.

Ray, D. (2011). *Advanced play therapy: Essential conditions, knowledge and skills for advanced practice*. New York: Routledge.

Rogers, C. R. (1951). *Client-centered therapy: Its current practice, implications, and theory*. Boston: Houghton Mifflin.

Ryan, V., & Bratton, S. C. (2008). Child-centered/non-directive play therapy with very young children. In C. Schaefer, P. Kelly-Zion, & J. McCormick (Eds.), *Play therapy with very young children* (pp. 25–66). New York: Rowman & Littlefield.

Schore, A. (2003). *Affect dysregulation and disorders of the self*. New York: Norton.

Siegel, D. J., & Hartzell, M. (2003). *Parenting from the inside out: How a deeper self-understanding can help you raise children who thrive*. New York: Penguin Putnam.

Stover, L., & Gurney, B. G., Jr. (1967). The efficacy of training procedures for mothers in filial therapy. *Psychotherapy: Theory, Research, and Practice, 4*(3), 110–115.

VanFleet, R. (2005). *Filial therapy: Strengthening parent–child relationships through play* (2nd ed.). Sarasota, FL: Professional Resource Press.

Webster-Stratton, C., Rinaldi, J., & Reid, J. M. (2011). Long-term outcomes of Incredible Years parenting program: Predictors of adolescent adjustment. *Child and Adolescent Mental Health, 16*(1), 38–46.

CHAPTER 10

Theraplay®

REPAIRING RELATIONSHIPS, HELPING FAMILIES HEAL

Phyllis B. Booth
Marlo L.-R. Winstead

Nine-year-old Lindsey was less than enthusiastic about coming to therapy. Her parents, Sandy and Jim, understood that the difficult behavior of their "precious little girl" was related to her early experiences of neglect and sexual abuse while in the care of her biological mother. However, this understanding did not help them know what to do when Lindsey was oppositional and defiant with them, exhibited compulsive traits rooted in anxiety, and acted out sexually with children at school. Lindsey's parents sensed that she was hurting—she chewed her nails until they bled—and tried to comfort and care for her, but she rejected each approach by drawing away. She covered her ears when they made statements of love and concern.

Because Lindsey was very rejecting toward her adoptive mother and father, I (Winstead) asked them to observe the first few Theraplay® sessions while I found the best way to help Lindsey feel safe and more accepting of our interactive play. As I expected from her parents' report, Lindsey was reluctant to respond to my efforts to engage her. She seemed to be trying to sabotage the activities I initiated. When we played a game of balloon

tennis with the goal of keeping the balloon in the air for as long as possible, Lindsey repeatedly bopped the balloon over my shoulder and onto the floor. During a hand-stacking game, in which Lindsey and I were to alternate one hand over the other till our hands were way above our heads, Lindsey quickened the pace, placed her hand on the stack out of order, and reversed the stacking direction at will.

As sessions continued, Lindsey became more trusting and her need to maintain control lessened, although it was always present. When her parents actively joined the sessions, however, Lindsey was very rejecting toward them. She made derogatory comments about her mother's weight and rude statements targeting dad's "thick glasses." In our next parent session, they expressed their fear that Lindsey wasn't making as much progress as they had hoped.

In the seventh session a sudden breakthrough calmed Sandy and Jim's fears. The four of us were playing balloon tennis using our elbows and knees to keep the balloon in the air; our announced goal was to make it to 50 hits. After six unsuccessful attempts Lindsey became discouraged, but I urged the family to keep trying. On the ninth attempt, as the count neared 45, the tension in the room was high. Lindsey bopped the balloon with her elbow and said, "Forty-nine, we're almost there." As she tried to bop it with her knee for the victory point, she stumbled. But just as a look of disappointment washed over her face, Sandy saved the day by hitting the balloon into the air with her knee. Lindsey immediately jumped up, ran over to her mom, threw her arms around her neck, and said, "You did it, we did it, we're awesome!"

Bowlby's (1969/1982) theory of attachment is the foundation of the Theraplay philosophy and model. The wealth of research spawned by his theory helped us focus our work around the qualities of parent–child interaction that lead to secure attachment, support healthy brain development, and create long-term mental health.

Many of the behavior problems that lead parents to seek help for their children have as their basis relationship issues that need to be addressed before the difficult behavior will diminish. Because of its basic and universal applicability, Theraplay has been helpful for children of all ages with many kinds of presenting problems and family constellations or living situations in many cultures around the world. Research demonstrating the efficacy of the Theraplay model has been completed in Germany (Wettig, Coleman, & Geider, 2011), Hong Kong (Siu, 2009), South Korea (Kim, 2010, 2011), and the United States (Weir et al., 2013). Through sensitively timed and highly attuned interactions, the therapist guides the parent and child through the regulatory process central to the formation of a secure attachment in order to foster an environment in which they can create or re-establish healthy patterns of relating.

In this chapter we present a picture of how Theraplay works. First, we describe the research and theory that support our approach. Then we use a case example to illustrate the typical sequence of Theraplay treatment.

Theory and Research

Theraplay is modeled on the sensitive, responsive, playful give-and-take that occurs naturally between parents and their infants and young children. The goals of treatment are to create a secure attachment, including positive internal working models for both parents and child, the capacity for self-regulation, good social skills, the ability to learn, and long-term mental health.[1]

Core Concepts

The core concepts or basic principles of Theraplay support and guide our work. Here we briefly describe each concept along with its supporting theory and research relating to attachment, brain development, and the elements that lead to therapeutic change.

Interactive and Relationship-Based

In Theraplay, the focus of treatment is the parent–child relationship itself. We bring parents and their child together and guide them so that they can create the dance of attunement and joy that is so essential to long-term mental health. Healthy parent–infant relationships are supported by two important innate drives: a drive to stay close to be safe, and a drive to share meaning and the joy of companionship. Feeling safe is essential before it is possible to share meaning and companionship.

Our understanding of what is involved in these instinctive impulses guides us as we attempt to create a new or healthier relationship. Babies signal their need for comfort and protection by crying, smiling, gazing, and clinging. Loving parents instinctively respond in ways that protect and reassure their infants. Many things can interfere with this natural response—for example, illness, stress, poverty, drug abuse, or the parents themselves did not receive adequate parenting. One of the goals of treatment is to help parents respond to their child's sometimes confusing signals and create a sense of safety and security.

The second important innate drive supports our ability to share meaning and companionship. It is made up of overlapping elements that guide our Theraplay approach: the capacity to resonate with the feelings of others (Trevarthen & Aitken, 2001) and to mirror and synchronize our behavior with others (Iacoboni, 2008). These capacities make it possible for parents to attune to their baby's needs, to coregulate his or her experience, and to reconnect when things don't go well (Tronick & Beeghly, 2011). Well-defined neural circuits support shared social engagement behaviors and the defensive strategies of fight, flight, or freeze (Porges, 2011). These capacities make it possible for babies and responsive parents to achieve what Trevarthen and Aitken (2001) call *intersubjectivity*; that is, a shared view of the world. They are present to each other, and have similar vitality levels and congruent intentions (Hughes, 2007; Siegel, 2006). A child who has experienced neglect, abuse, or ongoing trauma, however, has learned that it is not safe to get close to anyone and therefore is unable to enter into this experience of connection and companionship.

Our goal in Theraplay is to create a felt sense of safety for both parent and child so that they can be open to new experiences of connection and companionship. Our simple games create shared, synchronous interactions between parent and child and intense "moments of meeting" (Tronick et al., 1998). We give parents a direct experience of Theraplay for themselves to help them understand their child's feelings and to provide missing intersubjective experiences from their own childhoods. As therapists, we make full use of our own capacities to resonate, synchronize, regulate, and read the intentions of both child and parents.

Direct, Here-and-Now Experience

Change in a relationship can best be achieved by interacting affectively in the moment. Attachment patterns and their accompanying internal working models are stored in nonverbal and movement-oriented memory. Playful, accepting responses, not congruent with what the child has come to expect, challenge the child's negative internal working model and open up possibilities for change. We are playful, accepting, curious, and empathic (Hughes, 2007). We guide parents to provide the attuned responses that will repair the disrupted relationship and form a positive connection. These can be subtle, microscopic moments that change the neural circuits bit by bit (Hart, 2008). Or they can be moments of great excitement that suddenly shift the child into a state of joyful connection, as we saw with Lindsey. These moments of intense connection and synchrony, referred to as "now moments," lead to a major shift in internal organization and sense of self (Mäkelä, 2003; Tronick et al., 1998).

Guided by the Adult

Because regulation is at the heart of the attachment process, Theraplay therapists carefully guide and structure the child's experience so that the child feels safe and well regulated. We provide guidance and regulating structure for parents as well. The coregulation that attuned parents provide for their infants—maintaining body temperature, providing food, soothing the agitated infant—is the first step in the process of coregulation that leads to the capacity for self-regulation. The child gradually becomes less dependent on external regulation for survival, but she still needs a great deal of help to modulate her level of excitement, organize her experience, and help her make sense of the world. Rather than creating dependency, adult guidance and supportive structure are the foundation for self-reliance.

Attuned, Empathic, Responsive, and Reflective

The Theraplay model is based on the attuned, empathic, mindful responsiveness of the healthy parenting that leads to secure attachment and the development of a positive internal working model. The ongoing experience of being together allows the parent to attune to the level and tone of the child's emotion. This attunement signals to the baby that his feelings are understood and, in turn, he learns that others have feelings as well.

When a parent and baby are comfortable together, each makes gestures to connect. Often the connection is brief, followed by a turning away and then a reconnection. Responsive parents create an experience in which both parent and child gain confidence that they can interact in positive ways and maintain a healthy connection (Tronick & Beeghly, 2011). When a parent is unresponsive, the baby becomes disorganized. When this unresponsiveness persists, the child gives up hope that a connection can be made. The neglect that Lindsey experienced in her first years of life is at the root of her inability to trust.

In order to make attuned responses, parents must be able to reflect on their own as well as their child's internal states (Fonagy, Gergely, Jurist, & Target, 2002). This capacity for reflection and insight makes it possible for parents to understand the link between behaviors and underlying mental states and thus to respond sensitively to their child's signals (Slade, 2002). A major goal of our work with parents is to help them gain more insight into the meaning of their own and their child's experience. Through discussions, watching videotaped interactions, and their own interactive Theraplay experience, parents are helped to get in touch with their own feelings as well as to understand their child's feelings.

Preverbal, Social, Right-Brain Focus

Schore and Schore (2008) suggest that effective therapy must be "rooted in an awareness of the centrality of early dyadic regulation, a thorough knowledge of right hemisphere emotional development, and a deep understanding of the dynamics of implicit, procedural memory" (p. 17). This understanding supports our focus on meeting the child's younger emotional needs and on finding ways to calm the dysregulated and frightened child.

During the first 2 years of life, just at the time when attachment is forming, rapid neuronal growth takes place, especially in the right, social–emotional structures of the brain. Interactive experiences with caregivers create neural connections and organize the developing brain. The right-brain limbic system along with the developing orbitofrontal cortex attunes to the social environment and regulates the internal state of the body. "Loving connections and secure attachments build healthy and resilient brains, while neglectful and insecure attachments can result in brains vulnerable to stress, dysregulation, and illness" (Cozolino, 2010, p. 180).

Based on our understanding of brain development, we focus our Theraplay treatment on the child's current state of arousal and level of emotional development. In this way we are able to provide interactive experiences that reorganize the brain of a troubled child. As we provide these experiences, we make use of the nonverbal language of the right brain—voice, facial expression, eye contact, movement, rhythm, rocking, singing, and touch—to create the deep levels of neural integration that make it possible to communicate on the mentalizing and narrative levels later on.

Multisensory, Including Touch

The lively, nurturing care that parents give to their baby provides stimuli to all the senses. These tactile, vestibular, and proprioceptive experiences lead to a clear sense of self and of how to interact with others (Williamson & Anzalone, 1997). In Theraplay we provide a wide range of safe, appropriate, therapist–child and parent–child touch and physical play, as well as calming touch and soothing sensory experiences. We resonate with the child's autonomic nervous system through body communication and thereby contribute to the child's affective sense of self. Parents are encouraged to engage in active, physical play, and to use touch to become their child's source of comfort and safety.

Touch is fundamental to the human experience (Brazelton, 1990). From the very beginning infants require the warmth of body contact to support their immature regulatory system. Touch and warmth raise the levels of the hormone oxytocin, which is calming to both adult and child and aids in the management of stress (Tronick, Ricks, & Cohn, 1982).

Playful

Play is the essence of our Theraplay approach. We encourage the joyful, interactive play that occurs naturally between parents and their young children and helps to create a strong emotional bond and a feeling of being alive and full of energy. It is important to note that this play is quite different from the symbolic play so important to most play therapy models in which toys and expressive art materials are used to create opportunities for symbolic expression. The play of Theraplay is aimed at the developmentally younger needs of a child who has experienced distress or disruption in his early attachment relationships. This kind of play can be an important first step in creating the safety and optimism that will help a child heal.

Parents who meet their children with joy and interest generate a sympathetic arousal in children's nervous system that promotes a sense of connectedness and empathy, as well as creating spontaneity and resilience in the face of stress (Sunderland, 2006). The better the nervous system is at handling high arousal levels without disintegrating, the more flexible and resilient the child will become. Play episodes create affective synchrony, enhancing development of brain synapses (Hart, 2008).

What Made the Difference for Lindsey?

Using the Theraplay core concepts, we can understand how Lindsey's early experi-

ences (described at the beginning of this chapter) affected her current behavior as well as the components of Theraplay that made the difference. During her first 2 years, Lindsey was cared for by a neglectful, abusive mother. She had to work out her own survival strategies to feel safe, which included making sure she was in control at all times. She missed out on the regulating experience provided by an attuned responsive parent. And most importantly, she felt that she could not connect safely and interact positively with others.

Lindsey's first efforts to play the balloon game were hampered by her lack of trust ("Will I be safe if I let someone else take the lead?"), her lack of experience engaging in healthy give-and-take, and her lack of self-regulation. The balloon bops went way off base not because she was being "oppositional," but because she was excited and unsure of how to interact in a successful give-and-take manner.

During Lindsey's early sessions, her therapist focused on helping her learn a new way of interacting. The therapist organized activities so that they were calm and well regulated, and she attended to every subtle sign that Lindsey was not feeling safe and adjusted her behavior. Lindsey gained a sense of competence and self-esteem from the experience of playing together with her therapist, whose cheerful acceptance of "mistakes" convinced her that she was valued and that they could connect and have fun. Once that foundation was in place, the parents were brought in and helped to learn what they needed to do to make playing together possible. Lindsey's happy announcement, "You did it. We did it. We're awesome!" brings it all together. She has become an integral part of a loving team, which expands her sense of herself and her capacity to move forward.

Over time Lindsey was able to generalize the skills she learned in therapy to other environments so that she became successful as a student, daughter, friend, and member of a soccer team and dance troupe. Two years after graduating from therapy, Lindsey's parents unexpectedly conceived naturally and gave birth to a little boy. They were very worried about how Lindsey would respond. She did regress a bit as her security in the family was shaken by the addition of the new baby. However, the knowledge Sandy and Jim had gained from Theraplay provided them with tools to meet Lindsey's needs as they integrated another child into the family.

Clinical Case Example

To illustrate the process of treatment, we describe the strategies and techniques of Theraplay using the example of Jacob and his adoptive parents, Rebekah and Philip.

Theraplay treatment includes an assessment period followed by treatment. The assessment takes place during the first three to five sessions (depending on the number of caregivers involved) and includes the intake and the Marschak Interaction Method (MIM; Booth, Christensen, & Lindaman, 2011). Treatment includes a feedback session, a parent session, and sessions with the child. The length of treatment varies, depending on the severity of the problems and the extent of positive parental involvement, from 24 sessions to over a year. Parent sessions without the child are scheduled regularly after every third or fourth session. As termination nears, there is a gradual countdown ending with a "graduation party."

Assessment

The Theraplay assessment procedure includes an intake interview in which we talk about the parents' concerns and gather as much information as possible about the child's and the parents' history, particularly that which relates to their attachment experiences. Next we observe the interaction between the parents and child using the MIM (Booth et al., 2011). After that we meet for a feedback session with the parents without

the child, in order to share our observations and understanding of the child's difficulties, show them video clips from the interactions that highlight the strengths in the relationship, and begin to plan treatment to meet their goals for change within the family. Our overall goal for this feedback session is to create a supportive, collaborative relationship with the parents as a basis for our ongoing work together.

Intake Interview

During my (Winstead) intake interview with Jacob's adoptive parents, I learned that Rebekah and Philip met Jacob when he was almost 3 years old. Their first impressions were that he was a handsome, happy, well-adjusted little boy. Over the course of their visits in preparation for adoption placement they began to see, hidden beneath his surface charm, the effects of Jacob's early experiences. Being neglected as well as having multiple foster caregivers had left him wary of trusting adults. He had difficulty following directions and accepting or asking for help. He had very intense tantrums at times, and he was very difficult to console.

Rebekah and Philip were concerned about the challenges they would face as Jacob's parents, but they did not question moving forward with the placement and adoption. The couple had tried to conceive naturally for several years and engaged in fertility treatments for several more years. Their dream of having a child became a nightmare as each month passed. Adoption was the answer to their pain, and they expected wholeheartedly to love the child they waited for such a long time to name and claim as their own.

Jacob was 3½ when he came to live with Rebekah and Philip. It was not long before his behavior became more difficult. Jacob would unravel emotionally at what seemed to be "nothing," and it was not uncommon for his raw emotional state to last for 3–5 hours. It was exhausting, frightening, saddening, and worst of all, Rebekah and

Philip felt utterly helpless. They tried many strategies (e.g., distraction, comforting, consequences, soothing, time outs) in an attempt to help Jacob move through his day and to avoid hours of emotional turmoil.

I completed the Adult Attachment Interview (AAI; George, Kaplan, & Main, 1985) with each parent separately after the initial intake, which gave me additional information about their own childhood experiences. Rebekah and Philip were certainly committed to Jacob, and to each other, but there were elements of their own attachment histories that posed challenges as they added "Mom" and "Dad" to their titles. Rebekah's internal working model resulted in a very controlling and structured parenting style, whereas the parenting Philip had experienced led to avoidance and passivity when interacting with Jacob. The radical difference in their approach to parenting caused strife in their marriage and confusion for Jacob as he attempted to learn the family's language.

Marschak Interaction Method

To learn more about Jacob's relationship with his parents, I (Winstead) asked them to participate in the MIM. I explained:

"I want to learn more about how Jacob relates to each of you by observing him doing some simple activities with you. I'll tell you what activities to do. This usually takes between 30 and 45 minutes. I will videotape the interaction so that we can look closely at it. At our next session we can talk about what it was like for you. I will tell you what I have learned from watching each of you together with Jacob. I'll show you a few video clips so that we can try to understand more about Jacob's feelings and responses. And finally, we will talk about our treatment plan."

The MIM is a structured play-based technique for assessing the quality of the relationship between a caregiver and child. Par-

ents interact with their children in many ways that can be categorized in terms of four dimensions: structure, engagement, nurture, and challenge. In the MIM simple tasks are designed to elicit interactions within each dimension. We look for the parent's guidance and the child's responsiveness as well as their emotional availability in each dimension. We are particularly interested in the child's ways of coping with stress and the attunement of the parent in regulating that stress.

The parents each participated in an MIM assessment with Jacob: first Philip and then a week later, Rebekah. For the first MIM Philip and Jacob sat side by side at a table on which I had placed a set of nine instruction cards, along with the materials needed for the activities. I gave Philip the following instructions: "Please read each instruction aloud. There's no right or wrong way to do the activities. You can decide when to go on to the next one." Then I left the room and observed the session from behind a one-way mirror.[3] At the end of the MIM session, I reentered the room and asked Philip a few questions:

"Did I get a good picture of how things go when the two of you are together?"
"Were there any surprises?"
"What activity do you think Jacob liked best? Why?"
"What did he like least?"
"What did you like best?"
"What did you like least?"

I followed the same procedure a week later with Rebekah and Jacob.

Analyzing the MIM Using the Theraplay Dimensions

Following the completion of each MIM, the family went home and I carefully reviewed the videos in preparation for sharing my observations with Jacob's parents during the feedback session. I used the dimensions to organize my analysis of the interaction and my plans for treatment. We first describe each dimension and then describe an interaction with the child and each parent that illustrates his or her pattern of interaction in that dimension.

STRUCTURE

Secure parents structure their child's experience in many ways that create an atmosphere that is safe and well regulated. Tasks in this dimension assess the parent's ability to take charge, to set limits, and to provide a safe, orderly, understandable environment for the child. Does the parent structure the interactions or look to the child for structure? We are equally interested in the child's ways of responding to the parent's structure. Does the child accept the parents' guidance or insist on doing things his or her own way?

Structure Example. The task—"Adult and child each take paper and pencil. Adult draws a quick picture, encourages child to 'Draw a picture just like mine' "—shows a clear difference between the parents in their ways of providing structure for Jacob. While Philip was reading the task, Jacob quickly grabbed the paper and pencil out of the envelope and started drawing. Dad repeated the instructions and sheepishly attempted to have Jacob cooperate, but Jacob was already drawing a giraffe and quickly convinced his dad to copy his giraffe. Without much hesitation, Dad went along with Jacob's idea. Dad and Jacob had fun together, but did not complete the task. This is one example of many in the MIM with his father where Jacob responded to a task by doing it on his own terms.

When Rebekah read the task, she held on to the materials so that Jacob was unable to launch into the activity on his own. Mom said, "I'm going to draw a picture and then you'll copy me. Do you know what *copy* means? It means you do exactly what I do. I'm going to hold the pencils until it's your turn, but you can hold your paper."

Jacob watched closely as Mom drew several shapes, but as she got to the third of six shapes, his legs started to move in a nervous manner and a look of worry appeared on his face. Mom gave Jacob his pencil and instructed him to copy her picture. He drew several shapes, but none of them matched Mom's drawing. When Mom redirected Jacob, he started to whine and say that it was too hard, but within moments he said, "I just want to draw what I want to draw, not what you want me to draw." Recognizing Jacob's uncertainty, Mom guided him to draw one shape at a time. Although none of his marks resembled her drawings, she accepted them and moved on. Just before putting the paper back in the envelope, he scribbled something on the page and said, "And I put a mouse." Mom provided a high level of structure for Jacob throughout the task, both verbally and physically. Jacob accepted several of the directives, but when he had the opportunity, he made his own decisions.

ENGAGEMENT

Parents engage their young children in many ways that provide excitement, surprise, and stimulation, creating opportunities for connection and for sharing positive feelings. Responsive parents attune to their child's affective state in order to maintain an optimal level of arousal. Tasks in this dimension assess the parent's ability to encourage interactive engagement that is appropriate to the child's developmental level and emotional state. We are looking also at how the child responds to his parents' bids for engagement. While playfulness can be part of any interaction, it is clearly an important factor in engaging the child in joyful shared interactions.

Engagement Example. The task "Adult and child play a familiar game together" allows us to see the parent and child's capacity for creating engagement. Jacob initiated a game of hide-and-seek with Philip, which was familiar to both of them as they easily entered into the preestablished rituals of the game. However, there was not much eye contact or physical contact between Jacob and Philip. Jacob made the majority of the decisions in structuring the activity; who would hide first, who would count first, where Dad should hide, and when the game was over. When Jacob found Philip, he got so excited that he jumped on his back in a very rough way. Although Philip's face signaled discomfort, he did not comment on Jacob's action.

Without knowing that Jacob and Philip had played hide-and-seek, Rebekah quickly initiated the same game. Jacob was very excited to hide from his mom, managed to wait patiently as she counted to 10, and was also very excited to be found. He took his turn as the seeker, and the two enjoyed a comfortable, familiar game in which they showed delight in one another's company. There were several indicators of healthy engagement throughout the activity—cooperation, eye contact, physical contact, and give-and-take.

NURTURE

Within the parent–infant relationship there are many opportunities for nurturing activities that create feelings of comfort and calmness as well as a sense of being loved and cherished. Tasks in this dimension assess the parent's ability to respond to the child's developmentally appropriate needs for nurture, as well as to recognize tension and stress in the child and to use a calming, nurturing response that helps the child regulate emotionally. We assess the child's ability to accept the parent's nurturing care and to turn to the adult for comfort as well as the child's capacity for appropriate self-soothing and self-regulation.

Nurture Example. In contrast to his comfort with exciting, engaging activities, Jacob found it very difficult to accept the calming, nurturing tasks in the MIM. These tasks included "Adult and child put lotion on each other," "Adult and child feed each other," and "Adult tells child about when you came to live with us." With Dad, Jacob was very controlling in each one of these tasks: He snatched the lotion out of Dad's hands and only allowed Dad to apply lotion if he chose the spot. Jacob demanded that he feed himself, and when Dad insisted on feeding him, Jacob bit Dad's finger very hard. Whenever Jacob responded in a negative way, Philip quickly changed his approach. He would say, "Okay, okay, what do you want to do? We can do anything you want to do," and Jacob would immediately calm down and change the activity.

Jacob was just as unable to accept Rebekah's offers of nurture as he had been with Philip. However, she did not change her approach, and she seemed determined to find ways to nurture her little boy. She did this in very quiet, sensitive ways, trying to soothe and calm Jacob by rubbing his back, hugging him, speaking to him softly, and singing to him to help him stay with the activities. Jacob whined, cried, and wiggled around as his mom tried to care for him. At the end of each nurture activity, Rebekah let out a deep sigh, as if to collect herself from the hurt and confusion of being rejected by her child who, at the same time, constantly demanded her attention.

The MIM task "Adult leaves the room for one minute without child" allows us to assess attachment issues, including how the child manages stress. We look for evidence of the parent's sensitivity to the child's possible distress as shown by how the parent prepares the child for the separation, and how he or she repairs the break in the relationship upon reunification. What the child does during the separation gives us a glimpse into the child's typical coping and self-regulating strategies.

When Dad left the room he prepared Jacob by encouraging him to count to 60, "And then Daddy will be back." Initially Jacob wandered around the room, looked at the materials for the next tasks, and quickly went to the door and said: "Daddy, are you out there?" "Yes Jacob, I'm here." "Loud counting so I can hear you!" Jacob demanded. Philip counted out loud and reentered the room just as he said *60* to find Jacob standing at the door with his ear glued to the doorframe. It is clear that Jacob was very anxious when he was left alone and needed to quickly reconnect with his father.

When Mom read the task aloud, her face showed concern. She thought quickly and chose an activity that she knew would help him handle the separation: "You find a place to hide and I'll go out of the room and count and when I come back in I'll find you." Jacob's face lit up, and he promptly hid behind a large potted plant where he stayed until Mom returned. Mom scooped Jacob up when she came back into the room, asked him what he had been doing while she was gone, and gave him a kiss on the head and a rub on the back. Jacob allowed Mom to put him on her lap, and to reconnect with him, but did not reciprocate the warmth and care. Rebekah was very sensitive to Jacob's needs, and her use of a familiar game sustained Jacob for the 60 seconds that she was away.

Although Philip recognized that Jacob would need something to help him deal with the separation, his choice of counting to 60 was not enough to help Jacob handle his anxiety; it was up to Jacob to demand the support that he needed from Dad. Mom provided an ongoing connection with Jacob using the familiar hide-and-seek game that sustained him through her absence. Each parent initiated contact with Jacob when they returned to the room, letting him know that they had missed him. Although Jacob accepted their gestures, he did not initiate contact with either of them, and he did not show excitement.

CHALLENGE

Activities in the challenge dimension encourage the development of competence and confidence. Healthy parents support their child's impulse to learn, to explore, and to become more independent. They provide the scaffolding that makes it possible for the child to be successful at each new step. Appropriate challenges give the child a sense of mastery and lead to realistic self-expectations. Tasks in this dimension assess the adult's ability to stimulate the child's social, emotional, and physical development, to set developmentally appropriate expectations, and to take pleasure in the child's achievement. We look for the child's willingness to try something new, to do something where success is not certain, or to persevere in order to achieve.

Challenge Example. The task "Adult teaches child something child doesn't know" again highlighted interesting differences between the two parents' approaches. Philip chose to teach Jacob how to change a flat tire on a car. Jacob wasn't interested in this adult activity and eventually suggested that they sing "The Wheels on the Bus." Dad happily took up this suggestion without finishing his story.

Mom said, "Hmmmmm, what to teach you? Oh, do you know 'The Itsy Bitsy Spider' song?" Jacob answered, "No," and Mom said, "Great, I'll teach it to you. Watch first and then we'll practice together." Jacob watched intently as Mom sang and moved her hands, but he started to wiggle around as the song continued. When it was his turn to join in, he had difficulty singing and doing the motions at the same time. Mom offered verbal direction, but Jacob grabbed the bag of materials, saying, "Let's do another one." Mom said, "We need to practice this one first and then we'll do another one." Jacob let go of the bag, but turned around in his mother's lap so that his back was facing her and started singing a different song. Rebekah turned him around and very slowly talked through 'The Itsy Bitsy Spider' while clearly demonstrating the hand motions. Jacob followed her briefly, but as the difficulties mounted, he started crying, and said, "This is too hard, I can't do it, I never ever can do anything." Mom said, "Okay, we're going to move on now, but we'll practice it later." Rebekah was excited to teach Jacob something new; she made it fun and appealing for him, and slowed the pace when he struggled—all valuable and effective techniques. Jacob's low tolerance for frustration and his fear of failing make it necessary for Rebekah and Philip to provide help at a younger developmental level.

Treatment and Outcome

Feedback

The feedback session was scheduled the following week, and I planned to meet for 1½ hours to discuss the MIM. In preparation for this session, I reviewed each of the films carefully. I could see that Rebekah's and Philip's individual strengths as well as areas of difficulty were clearly demonstrated in the MIM. Philip engaged Jacob in creative ways, and was present and available to his son. Philip's structure was very loose, and he allowed Jacob to make the majority of the decisions, thus avoiding most conflicts during the MIM. Philip also had unrealistic expectations of Jacob (e.g., "Count to 60 while I'm gone"), which likely stemmed from a lack of interaction with small children.

Rebekah clearly had many good ways to connect with Jacob. She showed skill in structuring the activities. She was also extremely patient when Jacob did not follow her directions, and she utilized many soothing actions to help Jacob regulate his emotions and behaviors. However, her need for Jacob to complete tasks "correctly" overshadowed her ability to attune to him at times, and she placed unrealistically high expectations on him.

In spite of his early negative experiences, Jacob had many ways of connecting with his parents. However, there were several important areas where he needed help:

1. He was uncomfortable receiving nurture unless it is on his terms.
2. He found it very difficult to accept adult direction and structure.
3. He was easily overwhelmed by too much input, as shown by his wiggling around when his mother went on a long time with an activity.
4. He lacked self-confidence and avoided challenging tasks by diverting attention to other activities.

In order to prepare for the feedback session, I carefully selected segments that served multiple purposes: (1) to demonstrate the effective skills and strategies that Rebekah and Philip were already using in their parenting; (2) to show them examples where a shift or change in approach would enhance their relationship with Jacob; (3) to learn more about Rebekah's and Philip's individual and mutual understanding of their son, his needs, his struggles, and his strengths; and (4) to launch a conversation about collaborative treatment planning as we prepared to include Jacob in therapy in the coming weeks. A major goal for this meeting would be to make a good connection with them and give them hope that, together, we could create the happy relationship for which they so longed.

I chose the following MIM tasks to show Philip: "Draw a picture," "Play a familiar game," and "Feed." I emphasized Philip's creativity and willingness to be playful with Jacob; there were many moments when Jacob and Philip made eye contact and connected through laughter. Because Philip expressed a lack of confidence as a new parent in earlier meetings, I decided not to show the video of the feeding, but to discuss it with him. "I noticed that Jacob was resistant to being fed initially, but you stuck with the directions of the task. How was that for you?" Philip told me that he was very worried that Jacob would become upset. He said, "I often 'back down' and let Jacob have his way just to avoid tantrums." During the discussion I learned about Philip's fears. He was afraid that he would not live up to his own expectation of being a "perfect dad." And he feared that he might trigger or re-create Jacob's painful early experiences if he insisted on something when Jacob was upset. This information helped me understand why Dad had difficulty directing Jacob and providing structure.

For Rebekah I selected the following tasks to discuss: "Teach your child something," "Leave the room," and "Lotion." I focused on Rebekah's patience with Jacob, her ability to provide clear directions for him, and her ongoing use of gestures to promote physical connection and regulation. There were several instances when Jacob displayed a lack of self-confidence (e.g., "Draw a picture," "Teach the child something") in response to his mother's high expectations. I gently explored this with Rebekah to gain a better understanding of her desire for Jacob to succeed, and to see if she was aware of his nonverbal indicators of distress. Mom's capacity to provide structure and nurture were good, but knowing when to structure Jacob and when to nurture him was really difficult for her. Therefore, attunement was the primary issue. During the session Rebekah talked about her struggle to be flexible in several areas of her life. Learning about this area as a challenge for her, I better understood why Mom was overstructured at times and entered into power battles with Jacob that contributed to his escalating behaviors.

The overarching goal of treatment was to strengthen the bond between Jacob and his parents. We discussed the treatment objectives that would support this goal, which included (1) increasing Jacob's ability to accept nurture from his parents, (2) increasing Jacob's self-esteem and confidence through the use of challenge activities, (3) helping Jacob accept adult direction through structure activities, and (4) strengthening Rebekah's and Philip's confidence as Jacob's parents by facilitating opportunities for Dad to successfully implement structure, and honing Mom's ability for attunement

and responding to Jacob's cues. I planned to provide education regarding healthy development in order to help the parents have realistic expectations of their son. Above all, I wanted to create many experiences of shared joy for Mom, Dad, and Jacob.

Parent Session

The next session in the treatment protocol is an experiential session with the parent(s). I met with Rebekah and Philip, and together we did the activities that I planned to include in Jacob's first session:

1. "Check-Up," to help Jacob feel noticed and important.
2. "Lotion," to nurture him by caring for his special freckles and hurts.
3. "Beep-Honk," to encourage reciprocal engagement and provide structure.
4. "Popping Bubbles," to rehearse regulation and practice structure.
5. "Feather Blow," to give him a mild challenge and a way to practice give-and-take.
6. "Feeding," to help him feel well cared for.
7. "The Twinkle Song," to give Mom and Dad a way to express their love for Jacob in a tender manner.

The purpose of this session was to provide Rebekah and Philip with the same personal, attuned experience that their son would be having soon, to explore their thoughts about how Jacob would respond, to answer their questions about the treatment modality, and to identify areas of comfort and discomfort that would likely impact their participation in the sessions with Jacob.

Mom and Dad were both very playful and enjoyed the engaging physical activities. They each said that during the nurture activities, they felt "vulnerable" and "cared for" at the same time. An example was the feeding activity. I fed Mom one cracker, then Dad one cracker, and then had Mom and Dad feed each other several crackers. Rebekah said, "It was kind of weird at first, but then I just told myself, 'It's okay, let someone else take care of you,' and that helped me to relax and enjoy." This was a good opportunity for me to say, "How do you think Jacob will feel when we feed him; how do you think he will respond?" At the end of the session, I told them what I would expect from Jacob during a session and how I would respond to behaviors that he might use to avoid being in relationship with me and/or them.

Jacob's Treatment

As planned, both Mom and Dad participated in each Theraplay session. I had Jacob sit in his mother's lap during the early sessions to provide him with a sense of safety and security as well as containment and structure. Dad sat next to Mom and Jacob. In the beginning I did the activities with Jacob while they watched so that they could learn through modeling. I signaled playfulness from the very beginning when I knelt down in the waiting room and said, "Okay, Jacob, we're going to play in the room at the end of the hall. Let's hold hands and count how many big, big steps it takes us to get down there. Mom and Dad are coming too. Here we go." Jacob accepted, and we walked down the hall, hand in hand, counting each big step: "One, two, three. . . . We made it in 12 big steps—hurray!"

As expected, during the initial sessions Jacob was resistant to many of my attempts to connect with him. He pulled his hands away from me when I tried to count his fingers, but they would reappear like an invitation to reconnect when I turned to counting Mom's or Dad's fingers. This reinforced my assumption based on the MIMs that Jacob had a longing for intimacy. When I said, "I'm going to blow this feather into your hands and then you blow it back to me," Jacob said, "Actually, how 'bout you throw it and I'll whop it." I responded by saying, "You have some great ideas, but

we're going to blow the feather. Here we go, get your hands ready." He often had suggestions for activities that he would rather do, or that would be "more better than the stupid things" that I wanted to do.

Because of his fear of failure and lack of self-confidence, Jacob was reluctant to try new things and strongly avoided challenging activities. For example, in the fourth session when I asked him to mimic my short clapping rhythm, he started telling me all about his birthday party; when I attempted to reengage him in another clapping rhythm, he wiggled nervously in his mom's lap as he told me about a rock he'd found on the sidewalk and an egg that he'd cracked on the counter. To help him get beyond his ambivalence, I had Rebekah hold Jacob's hands and I said, "Now I'm going to do three claps, and you and Mom will copy me together." With his mom's help, he was successful.

As we saw in the MIM, nurture was very difficult for Jacob to accept. In the first three sessions he put a pillow over his head when I sang to him. I had prepared Mom and Dad for this type of response beforehand, so they understood that although he was not looking at me he was still able to hear the song, and that the provision of nurture was not contingent on his behavior. During the feeding activity, Jacob chewed loudly with his mouth open and full of food and then asked, "Doesn't this gross you out? It grosses Mom and Dad out." Instead of reacting negatively, I said: "Wow, you have some great chompers in there. I can see all of your teeth and your tongue and your food in your mouth. When I give you this next one, let's see if you chew it with your mouth open or closed."

In spite of Jacob's many attempts to reject his parents and me, we continued to try to connect with him in sensitively timed and attuned ways. When I wanted to put lotion on his hands, Jacob hid them behind his back. In response I sang the children's song "Where Is Thumbkin?" Not only did the song help Jacob join me in a playful, hide-and-seek thumb game, but more importantly he experienced a response that was patient and respectful, in contrast to the criticism and rejection he had come to expect from his birth mother. The combination of a controlled environment, a therapeutic atmosphere of repair, and my empathic responses created a safe place for him to process the feelings that created his need to reject all his parents' and my earlier attempts to connect.

As treatment continued, I gradually increased Mom's and Dad's involvement in the sessions. This participation significantly contributed to Dad's growing feelings of competence and confidence as a parent. I assigned the family homework between sessions, and Rebekah and Philip adopted a Theraplay attitude toward parenting. Jacob's ability to trust adults slowly improved both in and out of session, and he used fewer strategies to resist getting close. He laughed more and cried less, his tantrums decreased in frequency and duration. He became much more accepting of care and loving attention from his parents. During Session 17 he fell asleep in Philip's arms as his parents sang a special song to him at the end of the session. As Philip and Rebekah gazed at their sleeping boy, Dad looked up with tears in his eyes and said, "I'm his Daddy, I'm really and truly his Daddy. I haven't really felt that until this very moment."

Rebekah, Philip, and Jacob participated in Theraplay for approximately 1 year.[4] Gradually their relationships strengthened and they began to achieve their treatment goals. Although Jacob's early experiences were not erased, the positive, healing interactions with his parents led to a shift in his internal working model from mistrust and anxious self-reliance to trust and joyful acceptance of his parents' loving care.

Conclusion

Many life circumstances cause disruptions in families. No family is immune to the pain that comes along with daily life—physical, emotional, psychological, spiritual, relational. The litmus test is how well members come together to support, connect, and care for each other. If, for any reason, parents are unable to do this for their child, the wound grows deeper instead of getting better. As the healing agent, Theraplay helps family members, like those you have read about in this chapter, repair their damaged relationships and experience joy, connection, and love again.

NOTES

1. For full descriptions and supporting research, see Chapter 2 of Booth and Jernberg's *Theraplay* (2010).

2. Both case examples have been carefully disguised to protect the privacy of the clients.

3. A one-way mirror is ideal, though not necessary, to complete the assessment.

4. A child with a history of significant trauma will need to process his or her early experiences using a model designed specifically to process trauma (Booth, Lindaman, & Winstead, 2014). When Jacob was ready, we integrated other treatment modalities into our therapy.

REFERENCES

Booth, P., Christensen, G., & Lindaman, S. (2011). *Marschak Interaction Method (MIM): Manual and cards* (3rd ed.). Chicago: Theraplay Institute.

Booth, P., & Jernberg, A. (2010). *Theraplay: Helping parents and children build better relationships through attachment-based play* (3rd ed.). San Francisco: Jossey-Bass.

Booth, P. B., Lindaman, S., & Winstead, M. L.-R. (2014). Theraplay in reunification following relational trauma. In C. A. Malchiodi & D. A. Crenshaw (Eds.), *Creative arts and play therapy for attachment problems* (pp. 130–157). New York: Guilford Press.

Bowlby, J. (1982). *Attachment and loss: Vol. 1, Attachment.* New York: Basic Books. (Original work published 1969)

Brazelton, T. B. (1990). Touch as a touchstone:

Summary of the round table. In K. E. Barnard & T. B. Brazelton (Eds.), *Touch: The foundation of experience.* Madison, WI: International Universities Press.

Cozolino, L. (2010). *The neuroscience of psychotherapy: Healing the social brain* (2nd ed.). New York: Norton.

Fonagy, P., Gergely, G., Jurist, E. L., & Target, M. (2002). *Affect regulation, mentalization, and the development of the self.* New York: Other Press.

George, C., Kaplan, N., & Main, M. (1985). *An Adult Attachment Interview: Interview protocol.* Unpublished manuscript, University of California, Berkeley.

Hart, S. (2008). *Brain, attachment, personality: An introduction to neuroaffective development.* London: Karnac Books.

Hughes, D. A. (2007). *Attachment-focused family therapy.* New York: Norton.

Iacoboni, M. (2008). *Mirroring people: The science of empathy and how we connect with others.* New York: Farrar, Straus & Giroux.

Kim, Y. K. (2010). The effect of group Theraplay on elderly women living alone. *Korean Journal of Play Therapy, 13*(4), 153–169.

Kim, Y. K. (2011). The effect of group Theraplay on self-esteem and depression of the elderly in day care center. *Korean Journal of Counseling, 12*(5), 1413–1430.

Mäkelä, J. (2003, Fall/Winter). What makes Theraplay effective?: Insights from developmental sciences. *Theraplay Institute Newsletter,* pp. 9–11.

Porges, S. W. (2011). *The polyvagal theory: Neuropsychological foundations of emotions, attachment, communication, and self-regulation.* New York: Norton.

Schore, J. R., & Schore, A. N. (2008). Modern attachment theory: The central role of affect regulation in development and treatment. *Clinical Social Work Journal, 36*, 9–20.

Siegel, D. J. (2006). An interpersonal neurobiology approach to psychotherapy. *Psychiatric Annals, 36*(4), 248–256.

Siu, A. F. Y. (2009). Theraplay in the Chinese world: An intervention program for Hong Kong children with internalizing problems. *International Journal of Play Therapy, 18*(1), 1–12.

Slade, A. (2002, June/July). Keeping the baby in mind: A critical factor in perinatal mental health. *Zero to Three,* pp. 10–16.

Sunderland, M. (2006). *The science of parenting: Practical guidance on sleep, crying, play, and building emotional well-being for life.* New York: DK Publishing.

Trevarthen, C., & Aitken, K. J. (2001). Infant intersubjectivity: Research, theory, and clinical applications. *Journal of Child Psychology and Psychiatry, 42*(1), 3–48.

Tronick, E. Z., & Beeghly, M. (2011). Infants' meaning-making and the development of mental health problems. *American Psychologist, 66*(2), 107–119.

Tronick, E. Z., Bruschweiler-Stern, N., Harrison, A. M., Lyons-Ruth, K., Morgan, A. C., Nahum, J. P., et al. (1998). Dyadically expanded states of consciousness and the process of therapeutic change. *Infant Mental Health Journal, 19*(3), 290–299.

Tronick, E. Z., Ricks, M., & Cohn, J. F. (1982). Maternal and infant affective exchange: Patterns of adaptation. In T. Field & A. Fogel (Eds.), *Emotion and early interaction* (pp. 83–100). Hillside, NJ: Erlbaum.

Weir, K., Song, L., Canosa, P., Rodrigues, N., McWilliams, M., & Parker, L. (2013). Whole family Theraplay: Integrating family systems theory and Theraplay to treat adoptive families. *Adoption Quarterly, 16*(3–4), 175–200.

Wettig, H. G., Coleman, A. R., & Geider, F. J. (2011). Evaluating the effectiveness of Theraplay in treating shy, socially withdrawn children. *International Journal of Play Therapy, 20*(1), 26–37.

Williamson, G. G., & Anzalone, M. (1997). Sensory integration: A key component of the evaluation and treatment of young children with severe difficulties in relating and communicating. *Zero to Three, 17*(5), 29–36.

CHAPTER 11

Sandtray and Storytelling in Play Therapy

Theresa Kestly

Discovering the sandtray was a joyous experience for me, and I knew immediately that it would be an important modality in my play therapy practice. Eight-year-old George[1] validated my intuitive feeling about the sandtray when I first added it to my play therapy room. He asked, "What's that?" I replied, "Oh, this is a place where you can build a world and tell a story, if you like." With clear skepticism in his voice, he said, "What can live in the sand?" Simultaneously he saw my first-time small miniature collection, and he reached out for several figures, saying, "Oh, trees! Now the animals can live here." He placed four trees firmly in the sand. Without any explanation from me, his storytelling brain knew exactly what to do to bring the sandtray to life for the animals, and as it turned out, after a number of sessions playing in the sand, he also knew how to bring healing and "new life" to himself.

I was hooked! Clearly something had shifted in George's therapy. As a new clinician in my first play therapy job, I was relieved to find a modality that promised to be effective with children who, like George, found talking quite difficult. Enthusiastically, I began researching and looking for further training opportunities. I read everything I could find

on sandtray and sandplay therapy. I consulted and found a mentor and supervisor who'd had extensive training, including an intensive hands-on seminar with Dora Kalff, founder of sandplay (a Jungian version of the sandtray method). In the tradition of Margaret Lowenfeld, founder of the sandtray method (along with the children who showed her how it worked), I studied, and I observed, and I learned from George and my other child clients just how well the sandtray worked when children were given the freedom and support to tell their life stories. Over and over again, I witnessed the power and healing of the storytelling that emerged from the sandtray worlds.

Now, 27 years after first using sandtray therapy in my playroom, and then teaching the method to many other therapists, I still feel enthusiastic, and I still experience deep joy when I sit as a witness to children or adults using the sand and miniatures to tell the stories of their lives, a process that brings integration to their hearts and minds. One of the things I love about teaching this method is witnessing the joy and enthusiasm that often comes when others discover how easy it is to access the deep layers of life stories through playing with wordless images in the sand. The enthusiasm that clinicians often feel when they first encounter the sandtray modality is also the part that sobers me because I know of numerous cases where inadequate preparation and misunderstanding about the depth of this kind of play on the part of the practitioner has produced hurtful results. A school counselor once told me that she offered the sandtray to a 7-year-old and was quite surprised by his quick reply, "I don't want to make a sandtray. I did that with my counselor at my old school, and all she did was preach, preach, preach." Fortunately, this young one had good boundaries and knew how to protect himself. Unfortunately, he may have lost an opportunity for personal storytelling that could have been healing.

A Powerful and Invaluable Modality

Doing No Harm

On the positive side, all mental health specialists (counselors, psychologists, psychiatrists, and social workers) are bound by ethical principles of *doing no harm*, and that helps to mitigate the problems of inadequate training that we saw in the example above. Dora Kalff (1980) clearly understood the potential for this kind of harm with the sandtray, and she addressed it in her book *Sandplay: A Psychotherapeutic Approach to the Psyche*. Following are her words, standing alone on the first page of her book, right before the Prologue. The passage begins with the word *Caution*, an apt heading for those of us who love using the sandtray modality.

Caution

In the hands of a properly prepared therapist, sandplay is a powerful, invaluable modality. The operative word is "powerful." To the extent that any method can heal, so can it do harm.

Therefore, I urgently advise that even a psychotherapist highly experienced in other methodologies, who contemplates practicing sandplay, should have had a deep personal experience doing a sandplay process as a patient with a qualified sandplay therapist and an extended period of careful supervision— anything less would be irresponsible. (Kalff, 1980, p. 8)[2]

Although Kalff's words of caution were intended for practitioners of *sandplay* (a term coined by Kalff pointing to a Jungian-based use of the modality), in my opinion her words are equally important to any clinician who offers sand and miniatures for healing purposes. In this chapter I want to talk about Kalff's deep respect for the sandtray and how we might think about her words of caution. I seriously doubt that she wanted to scare anyone away from using this powerful modality. I believe she simply understood its potential for harm and wanted to guide us toward responsible and ethical uses of the tray. I also want to draw from the work of Margaret Lowenfeld, one of Kalff's teachers, to deepen our understanding of how the mind works in the context of the sandtray modality. Although neither of these founding women had the benefit of current neuroscience findings, both of them pointed us toward guiding principles that are consistent with what we are now discovering in scientific studies of brain and mind. Intuitively, like Lowenfeld and Kalff, many of us recognize the power of the nonverbal sandtray as a core method of accessing inner intelligence and, curiously enough, bringing this intelligence into verbal form through the brain's love of storytelling. We can now more easily articulate the power of this nonverbal process in scientific terms.

What was difficult for me at the beginning of my work with the sandtray was my inability to explain why this modality was so effective. I could see how it healed, but I struggled to find the words to explain it. I once had a mother contact me about her

11-year-old daughter, Sheila, who was being seen by a psychiatrist for medication. The psychiatrist told the mother that she needed to find another sandtray therapist for her daughter because she said she had noted progress as long as Sheila was doing her sandtray therapy, and now that the mother had pulled her daughter out of the therapy, she felt that Sheila was no longer progressing. When the mother first described the situation to me, she was somewhat annoyed with the psychiatrist because, she explained, the reason she had stopped her daughter's previous sandtray therapy was because the therapist could not explain to her how the sandtray worked. In response to the mother's questions about the sandtray, the therapist had told the mother, "You just have to trust me." The mother complained to me that *trust* was not enough. She needed to *know*.

I had just finished writing a dissertation about brain laterality, and so as best I could, I explained to her that the sandtray allowed us to use both halves of our brain in therapy, and that that would be a decided advantage in making the therapy go faster. I told her that the right hemisphere was able to use nonverbal and sensory images to solve problems. I said, "For instance, it would be easier for your daughter to resolve some of her conflicts with her peers if she could play them out with the sandtray figures in a safe and nonthreatening environment where I can support her attempts to create positive relationships. And then we can help her articulate that in her left hemisphere. We won't be relying on just half of her brain." The mother said, "Oh, okay, I just needed to know. That makes perfect sense." My explanation was quite simple, but it did help reassure the mother that there was science-informed knowledge behind this modality, and even though there was much more for me to learn, I knew we were headed in the right direction. Fortunately for me, we were at the dawn of a new era in brain science, and as the decade of the brain unfolded, it

became clear to me that we were going to find many ways to articulate how sandtray therapy helps with the integration of brain and mind. Our new understanding of interpersonal neurobiology also points the way toward ethical and effective use of the tray supporting Kalff's words of caution.

In this chapter I touch on a few discoveries from neuroscience that will help us use the sandtray modality, with caution, knowing that we are on solid ground about following our ethical principle of *doing no harm*. Drawing from a number of neuroscientists, I consider some of the components and aspects of the process that make the sandtray powerful: (1) the "fit" between the sandtray, the miniatures, and the storytelling capacity of the brain; (2) the presence of a free and protected space; (3) the metaphorical thinking that is evoked; and (4) the hand–mind connection. I also discuss the importance of mindfulness in sitting as a witness to the sandtray process and the *spiral of play* that emerges naturally and authentically when we pay attention to how brain laterality works. I also address the concept of becoming *science-informed* as the basis for developing an *evidence-based* practice. Rather than talking about these points as separate topics, I interweave them, providing headers only to alert the reader that I am introducing a new idea to be woven into our discussion. I also consider this material in the context of our 8-year-old, George, to see how current neuroscience concepts may help to provide guidance in the ethical and effective use of this wonderful modality.

What Is Sandtray Therapy?

Before we talk about what makes the sandtray modality powerful, let's begin with a simple description (Kestly, 2004) that I have found useful in my training program:

> Sandtray therapy is a dynamic process in which clients use miniature figurines, trays

of sand, and sometimes water to create miniaturized versions of their worldviews. The therapist witnesses this process and provides a safe container in which the client is free to explore and create what needs expression. Because the sandtray process is a nonverbal medium, it can access experience that lies beyond the reach of language. By giving thoughts and feelings concrete form through expressive play in the sandtray, clients can represent their life experiences in a context where they can control, organize, and eventually integrate them. Drawing from the unique perspectives of both the right and left hemispheres in the brain, clients are often able to interweave the embodied experiences of the right and the narrative knowledge of the left to tell their life stories in a coherent way. This integration often results in healthier perceptions, behaviors, and relationships.

Many clients benefit from this nonverbal, playful, and nonthreatening way to explore and express inner fears, conflicts, questions, and unresolved experiences. By telling these stories to a caring and mindfully attentive therapist, clients can often develop a deeper understanding of the issues at hand. When clients create and re-create their own worlds in miniature form, in the presence of a skilled therapist, they often can integrate and master what has previously been disjointed and chaotic. In short, clients are able to work with their worldviews on a comfortable scale until the pieces fit and an inner shift occurs. It is this inner shift that clears the way for new experiencing and interacting with the world.

Witnessing the Sandtray Mindfully

Interdisciplinary studies across a number of scientific perspectives over the last two decades have drawn our attention to the practice of mindfulness in mental health (Baer, 2006; Siegel, 2007). We are beginning to understand that mindful awareness, or becoming aware of all that's happening around and within us without judgment, is a function of our prefrontal cortex, the part of our brains that helps us to integrate the whole. Daniel Siegel (2007) writes, "Being aware of the fullness of our experience awakens us to the inner world of our mind and immerses us completely in our lives" (p. 3). He describes the benefits:

> Research on some dimensions of mindful awareness practices reveals that they greatly enhance the body's functioning: Healing, immune response, stress reactivity, and a general sense of physical well-being are improved with mindfulness. Our relationships with others are also improved perhaps because the ability to perceive the nonverbal emotional signals from others may be enhanced and our ability to sense the internal worlds of others may be augmented. In these ways we come to compassionately experience others' feelings and empathize with them as we understand another person's point of view.
>
> We can see the power of mindful awareness to achieve these many and diverse beneficial changes in our lives when we consider that this form of awareness may directly shape the activity and growth of the parts of the brain responsible for our relationships, our emotional life, and our physiological response to stress. (p. 6)[3]

Mindfulness with George: Turning Inward and Listening Deeply

I was grateful when I first read *The Mindful Brain* (2007) (including the words in the above quote) by Daniel Siegel because it helped me to explain an experience with 8-year-old George that I'd had many years ago when I was new to play therapy. When George's mother first brought him to me for play therapy, I did not have a sandtray, but I had a lot of other play therapy resources in my playroom. Despite what I thought was a welcoming and inviting playroom, George was always reluctant to come with me. He seemed to prefer his mother's lap in the waiting room, and I must confess, I found that a little unnerving. Although I was quite uncertain about how to engage George in the play therapy, I will never forget what I learned about being a play therapist during George's fifth session.

At this turning point session, I had convinced him to come to the playroom by himself. He walked in, and without saying a word to me, or even looking at me, he took a large piece of paper and with a black magic marker, he drew the outline of a large house that filled about half of the page. He then chose a red marker and, for the rest of the session, proceeded to fill in the outline quite laboriously. He looked miserable. I tried to reflect without being intrusive. No response! I tried again, and when I still got no response, I became a little more vigorous (and yes, a little intrusive). I was now anxious. Still nothing. I persisted, and he refused all my efforts to connect. I finally got it! He was not going to talk to me, or even look at me.

At this point my misery began. Mindlessly, my brain began struggling with my failure as a play therapist. I got very quiet—quiet enough to acknowledge the feelings that were arising in me. I really did not like being with this child. And immediately I felt ashamed as soon as I heard that inner thought because here I was, professing to be a child therapist, and I was having trouble liking this child. It frightened me, and I sank further into my misery thinking that perhaps I had chosen the wrong profession. "What had made me think that I could ever be a child therapist anyhow?"

As I descended into my misery, I felt myself being drawn into paying careful attention to the misery I was feeling, and I realized that these feelings might well be what George was feeling every day in his life, living in a world of adults who really did not like being with him. As I imagined what that must be like for him, my heart filled with compassion for George. I did not say anything. I just felt very deeply. We were almost at the end of our session time, and so I just sat with the feelings of deep compassion. I now know that these feelings of compassion arising in me when I did not know what else to do except to turn inward and listen deeply were the beginnings of a mindfulness practice for me.

At our next session, George brought some play dough—the homemade kind comprised of flour and salt. He had made the dough at school, and when he came into the playroom, he showed it to me. He began molding a small dog, and when he handed me a chunk of the dough, I began molding a small cat. When he saw what I was making, he pretended to have his dog chase my cat. I could see that we were both ready (now that we could play together) to build a relationship. Perhaps, as Siegel said (in the above quote), as I was drawn into a state of paying attention to George with mindful awareness and compassion, our relationship could begin because my ability to perceive his emotional nonverbal signals and his internal state had been enhanced. Without any words between us, it was clear to me that George understood and received my internal shift.

Therapeutic Relationship, First, Modality and Technique, Second

About 10 sessions later, when I introduced the sandtray modality into my playroom for the first time, George began to tell his nonverbal story more vigorously. Repeatedly he created sandtray worlds where vulnerable little animals had to protect themselves from dangerous predators. He dug holes in the sand where the rabbits could live safely, and he fenced many small areas for the piglets, the chickens, and the goats. He especially liked the little rabbits, and he used them consistently in almost every world as he showed how they learned to deal with a dangerous environment where rattlesnakes and hungry coyotes lived.

Looking back, I am deeply grateful for George. He taught me that words were not necessary for healing to occur. George was mostly nonverbal during his sessions, but through playing with images in the presence of my emerging mindfulness practice and compassion, he could find his way to human relationships and healing. Most important, he helped me to see that the therapeutic relationship precedes modality or technique. I knew then that a good therapeutic relationship would always be at the heart of healing. I also had a hunch that the sandtray, grounded in interpersonal relationship, had had an important part in George's healing because of its capacity to allow him to tell the story of his life experiences without words.

Often I would invite George to tell me about his worlds. Most of the time, he would shrug his shoulders with an "I don't know" look on his face. I never pressured him for words because, with the introduction of the sandtray modality into my playroom, I had learned about the importance of nonverbal communication in healing. Linda Hunter's (1998) description of sandplay is poignant in this regard:

> Sandplay provides an opportunity to process life experience through a tangible, visible procedure which is both fun and intensely meaningful, both intimately revealing and symbolically concealing. The process of healing takes place while playing with the sand and figures, without the need for interpretation, verbalization, or conscious awareness. The tray provides the reflection used in play therapy. The tray absorbs the fear and anger and hurt as these feelings are revealed in the scenes, rather than being painfully voiced as in verbal therapies. (p. 4)

Numerous times I have reread this paragraph to myself because it helps me to stay steady when I am tempted to use the language thoughts that arise in my left hemisphere too quickly. Once again, there is now an abundance of scientific evidence supporting the ideas that Hunter conveyed in her description of sandplay. In this next section, we turn to the neuroscience of storytelling to explore what this might mean for us in our use of the sandtray in our play therapy practices.

The Storytelling Brain

Antonio Damasio (1999), seminal neuroscientist, talks about the naturalness of wordless storytelling and how it is a nonlinguistic process that is inherent in the brain's tendency to select, sort, assemble, and integrate the objects that it encounters in its environment. He says, "Telling stories precedes language, since it is in fact, a condition for language, and it is based not just in the cerebral cortex but elsewhere in the brain and in the right hemisphere as well as the left" (p. 189). Damasio believes that storytelling begins nonverbally (for all of us, throughout our lifespans) as we try to assemble a coherent picture of our "lived" moments each time we encounter (or experience) the objects of our environments. As we "live" these encounters with objects (including other people), we experience a "feeling of what happens" and our brains map these bodily feelings in the right hemisphere (Damasio, 1999), creating embodied implicit memories.

Damasio's ideas fit with Margaret Lowenfeld's (1979) intuitive understanding that we think first in images, and then, and only then, can these "image thoughts" come to the level of language where we can share common words with one another to tell our life stories. Damasio points out that this concept may be hard to grasp because once we are skilled in language production, words follow so closely after our "image thoughts" that it appears we are thinking with words, but in fact, we are thinking in images.

Daniel Siegel (2012; Siegel & Bryson, 2011; Siegel & Hartzell, 2003) suggests that storytelling may be one of the primary ways the brain integrates itself. I often ask parents to read Chapter 2 in *Parenting from the Inside Out* (Siegel & Hartzell, 2003) because it describes how we perceive reality by constructing the stories of our lives. It helps to explain the storytelling function of the brain. From that perspective, I can talk about the naturalness of storytelling in the sandtray and how the tray may be helpful in play therapy as we work on various ways to help their children integrate their brains and minds in healthy ways. It is also a good introduction for talking about integration of the differentiated parts of the brain as a core concept of mental health and resilience. Siegel (2012) says that good storytelling requires mental integration in a number of ways: left and right hemisphere collaboration (horizontal); bottom-up and top-down processing (vertical); weaving together the past, present, and future of the self across time (temporal); social context requiring a storyteller and an audience (interpersonal); and linking implicit and explicit ways of remembering (memory).

Over the course of therapy, I also recommend to parents *The Whole-Brain Child* (Siegel & Bryson, 2011) because it helps to explain Siegel's proposal that we can understand mental health and resilience in terms of the differentiation and linkage of the subsystems of the brain/mind (application of complexity theory). For example, Siegel and Bryson (2011) say:

> What kids often need, especially when they experience strong emotions, is to have someone help them use their left brain to make sense of what's going on—to put things in order and to name these big and scary right-brain feelings so they can deal with them effectively. This is what storytelling does: it allows us to understand ourselves and our world by using both our left and right hemispheres together. To tell a story that makes sense, the left brain must put things in order, using words and logic. The right brain contributes the bodily sensations, raw emotions, and personal memories, so we can see the whole picture and communicate our experience. This is the scientific explanation behind why journaling and talking about the difficult event can be so powerful in helping us heal. In fact, research shows that merely assigning a name or label to what we feel literally calms down the activity of the emotional circuitry in the right hemisphere. (p. 29)

This description fits with Lowenfeld's idea of the multidimensional nature of the sandtray (Lowenfeld, 1979). She was interested in helping children heal from trauma, and she believed that language alone was inadequate for this task. The sandtray can help with this because it allows patients to play simultaneously with the tactile and visual images, the bodily sensations, the implicit memories, the raw emotions, the personal memories, and the relational aspects impacting their well-being. Language, produced by the left hemisphere alone, is linear, and it falls short of what is necessary for healing to occur. Healing requires a number of dimensions to be open simultaneously, including the nonverbal aspects of the whole experience.

Bonnie Badenoch (2011) draws from numerous research studies to describe the neurobiological nature of storytelling:

> We are storytelling beings; the propensity for meaning is written into our genes. Our brains drive us to make meaning of our experiences, resolve conflicts, and prepare for the future. It has also become clear that this activity does not begin when we consciously shape experience into language. The internal process of knitting together neural networks related to our history and its impact on what we will do next goes on all the time, below the level of conscious awareness. (p. 83)

Like Damasio, Badenoch is pointing clearly to the origins of storytelling that precede language. Damasio (1999) says that from the moment we awaken, our brains are telling stories each time we encounter any object, beginning before a word is even formed. As Badenoch (2011) says, it is going on all the time without our conscious awareness. For a long time I have watched this storytelling process as it takes place in sandtray play, and I have come to trust this deep biological nature of the storytelling process. Even when children appear to be distracted from what they are doing in the sandtray (telling me something that seems unrelated to the images they are placing in the sand), I can have confidence in the scientific studies that point toward this consistent storytelling nature of the brain. Instead of trying to direct the language of what children or adults are telling me about their sandtrays, I try to make room for this deeper, nonverbal, nonconscious storytelling that goes on all the time.

George's 10-Second Sandtray—the One I Almost Missed

I almost missed an important turning point in George's therapy. That is how swiftly and efficiently the nonverbal integration of the right hemisphere works below the level of conscious awareness. It happened in an unusual session when George came into the playroom and pointed to Candyland on the shelf where I kept a few board games. At this point, he was pretty invested in the sandtray, and usually preferred it to all the other play possibilities. For some reason (a therapeutic error on my part, no doubt), I picked up the Candyland box and read out loud, "For ages 3 to 6" (I had an old version of the game). Placing both hands at his waist in a playful and defiant gesture, he shot back, "Then I'll be 6!" George was almost 9 years old at this point, but he let me know that he could accept my challenge of whether or not he was picking the right, age-appropriate game. From that moment on, he taunted me every time my piece got stuck or got sent backward instead of forward on the path that led to the candy castle. The victory of winning was his only goal—at any cost. Playfully (looking at me with a smile on his face) he picked up the deck of cards and shuffled through it until he found the "Plumpy" card—the one that sends you back to the very beginning. He placed it on top and said, "Your turn." I played along. Usually, depending on therapeutic goals, I would call children on cheating (in a therapeutic way, of course) during structured games, but this time I sensed a different energy in the room, and I simply took my turn. I groaned and complained

about having to go all the way back. He gloated, raising both arms in a gesture of victory. The entire session went this way. He was going to win, and he was determined that I was going to lose. When I told him that our time was up, he walked over to the door and just before I opened it, he put both hands into the middle of the sandtray at the bottom, and with an upward sweep made two opposing circles, then swiftly raised his hands out of the tray. He said emphatically, "Cobra." I could clearly see the head of a cobra looking right at me. I responded, "So, you are going to leave a cobra in my office?" He said (now really gloating), "Yep!"

At first I thought it was just his way of ending our session in the spirit of the playful competition that we had both engaged in throughout the session. I did not see his cobra shape in the sand as an actual sandtray, and so I decided not to take a picture of the tray even though I had been carefully recording all of his trays. This was before digital cameras, so photographing trays was more expensive than it is now. As an afterthought, however, I decided that maybe I should take a photo—just in case.

I was glad that I had changed my mind about the picture taking because months later as I was preparing a sandtray case for a group of colleagues, I realized just what had happened in that 10-second tray. I had decided George's experiences would be a good way of talking about the benefits of having a tool for working with the nonverbal part of the brain in play therapy. As I was assembling the photos and my case notes for my presentation, I saw that George's *Cobra Tray* was a critical turning point in his therapy. Up to that point, he had been working very hard in every sandtray to make the worlds safe for the vulnerable animals—digging tunnels and rabbit holes, fencing off areas and using shrubbery to shelter the animals. In the *Cobra Tray*, in a split second, he had filled the tray with danger, and he left it for me to hold. He seemed to have confidence that I could hold it—that I could hold the lethality of living in a dangerous world. Indeed, the bitter divorce of his parents, who had frequently shouted at one another when he was only 2 years old, had been deadly for him. George needed to know if I could hold this death-dealing energy with him and for him. To me this was a test of the strength of the sandtray container, held within the being of the therapist, whose task, according to Dora Kalff, is to hold a free and protected space.

A Free and Protected Space

Metaphorically, the physical dimensions of the miniature sandtray serve as a container for this free and protected space. Dora Kalff (1980, 2003) described her sandtray apparatus and how she put it together in her playroom in the same way that Margaret Lowenfeld had done for her *World Technique*. Kalff credited Lowenfeld with this setup, saying that Dr. Lowenfeld "understood how to place herself in the world of the child. With ingenious intuition she created a game that enables the child to build a world, his world, in a sandbox" (2003, p. 16). She goes on to describe in more detail her understanding of the free and protected space in terms of the physical dimensions of the sandbox and the child's freedom to choose objects. She wrote:

> The size of the box corresponds exactly to what the eye can encompass. From among the numerous objects, the child chooses those that particularly appeal to him and are meaningful. He forms hills, tunnels, planes, lakes and rivers in the sand in the same way he views the world from his own situation. He allows the figures to act as he experiences them in his fantasy. The child has absolute freedom in determining what to construct, which figures to choose and how to use them. The same limitations that are prerequisite for genuine freedom in the real world are present in the measurements of the sandbox. They are scaled down to one-person size, thereby forming limits to what can be represented and providing a frame wherein transforma-

tion can take place. Quite unconsciously, the child experiences what I call a free, and at the same time, protected space. (2003, pp. 16–17)

This free and protected space of the sandtray resides both in the physical container and in the strength of the therapeutic relationship. Kalff (1980, 2003) pointed this out when she said, "This free space occurs in the therapeutic setting when the therapist is fully able to accept the child so that the therapist, as a person, is as much a part of everything going on in the room as is the child himself. When a child feels that he is not alone, not only in his distress but also in his happiness, he then feels free and protected in all his expressions" (p. 7).

The Day the Humans Arrived in George's World

I believe that this free and protected space was a necessary part of George's play therapy. Metaphorically, he needed the physical limitations of the small tray[4] (typically 28.5″ × 19.5″ × 3) to give him the emotional and psychological protection he needed to express the dangerous and lethal part of his inner world. One of the primary reasons his parents brought him to therapy was his physical violence in his school classroom. He had shoved a desk toward his teacher in defiance of her authority. In addition to the physical limitations of the sandtray, he needed me to be a relational, emotional, and psychological container capable of holding this lethal energy without being destroyed by it. This would play out metaphorically at his next session when he returned to find me intact despite the fact that he had left a cobra in my office. Neither of us mentioned the cobra that he had created in the sandtray the week before. This turning point in his therapy happened below the level of conscious awareness. It was not until I consciously engaged my left hemisphere (preparing my photos and notes for a collegial presentation) that I saw what had happened.

Prior to the *Cobra Tray* there were never any humans in any of his sandtrays. Not long after this tray, a farmer came into the world with some food in his hands. As soon as the man's feet touched the sand, George made all the rabbits dart into their holes that he had so carefully prepared for them before he incorporated the man. Each rabbit was standing close to its hole. Taking cues from George, I rarely talked while he was building his trays because he rarely talked (and I wanted to join his emotional energy), but this time, I said, "They feel much safer in their holes." He paused for a moment, and then looked at me and said, "They're not really that afraid." One by one, he brought each rabbit out of its hole. Slowly George began bringing other humans into his worlds. He brought a young girl with a pail of water, and then grandparents, or "old fogies" as he called them, followed by a young boy with a fishing pole. There were still themes of danger in George's worlds, but at this point he could experience what it meant to have caring and nurturing others in his world.

Metaphor and the Divided Brain

We have been talking about the storytelling brain and how the sandtray serves as a metaphorical container for both freedom and protection. To explore this concept of metaphor in the divided brain more fully, we turn now to the work of Iain McGilchrist (2009), psychiatrist and philosopher, who draws from a large body of scientific research to explain the wisdom of our skull brains being divided into two asymmetrical halves (left and right hemispheres), and why metaphor is a crucial aspect of language. In his book *The Master and His Emissary: The Divided Brain and the Making of the Western World*, McGilchrist describes in great detail the unique differences between the perspectives of the right and left hemispheres of the brain, but he also points out their similarities and shows us how they

collaborate with one another and also how they sometimes inhibit one another. Acknowledging that both hemispheres are activated in everything we think, feel, and do, he focuses on *how* each hemisphere attends to the world. He uses the example of a bird to show us why we need a divided brain. The bird, he says, needs the focusing ability of its left hemisphere to pick out a single grain of corn in a gravel field, and it needs its right hemisphere to simultaneously look out over the whole environment for predators. The bird needs this more global right-hemisphere function to avoid becoming someone else's lunch. The two viewpoints, taken together, support the survival and thriving of the organism. In the human brain, the right mode of attending opens us to the world of immediate experience and the relational perspective, whereas the left mode focuses us on organizing that experience for manifestation in the world of precision and systems.

McGilchrist's way of describing the relationship between the two hemispheres can help us understand the storytelling brain. We can begin to sense how important it is to have the full participation of, and the collaboration between, both modes of attending. We also can sense the unique contribution of each perspective, and that we cannot tell coherent stories with either one in isolation. In addition, McGilchrist (2009) says that storytelling requires a special kind of journey through our right and left hemispheres. He explains how language evolved primarily, but not totally, in the left hemisphere. The right continues to be the domain of words expressing fresh experience, poetry, and, significantly, metaphor. Like Damasio (1999), who said that storytelling begins with the mapping in the right hemisphere of "the feeling of what happens" when we encounter objects in our environments, McGilchrist also says that language has its origins in the bodily experience of being in the world. As language evolved in the left hemisphere into its current form, however, it became more abstracted from its origins in the body. This abstraction enables us, says McGilchrist, "to refer to whatever is *not present* in experience: language helped its re-*presentation*" (p. 125).

Our divided brains allowed the denotative elements of language (enabling precision of reference and planning) to develop in the left hemisphere while the connotative and emotive functions remained in the right hemisphere. As we journey from our right-centric experiences (origins of wordless stories) into our left mode of attention, the bits and pieces of our experiences can be processed and named with precise words in a linear fashion, making sense of time and planning (re-*presentation* of our experiences using words).

However, it is important to remember that if we are to experience language at its highest level, we must return once again to the right to make sense of the words in a narrative where words and embodiment come together, helping us to retain our connection to the world of lived experiences. This blending of word and lived experience is potentially what can happen as the embodied storytelling that is unfolding in the sand finds its way into words. McGilchrist's (2009) main point is that each hemisphere, taking its unique perspective of the same experience, can ultimately inform the other. He shows us that "metaphor is the crucial aspect of language whereby it retains its connectedness to the world" (p. 125)—the way we experience ourselves through our right-hemisphere processing. He contrasts this with language processing that potentially goes on in the left hemisphere, where words move us away from contact with the reality of experience that is unfolding from the perspective of the right. If we disconnect from our embodied experience and go more completely into the perspective of the disembodied left, then language dies. He goes on to describe the special journey we can take through the hemispheres via metaphorical processing, which allows our hemispheres to collaborate at a higher level. He says, "There is an important shape here which we will keep encountering: something that arises out of the world of the right hemisphere, is processed at the middle level by the left hemisphere and returns finally to the right hemisphere at the highest level" (p. 126).

The Spiral of Play

Staying with McGilchrist's (2009) idea of this potential relationship between the ways the two hemispheres attend, we can see a movement from right-mode experience to left-mode processing that must then return to the right hemisphere if language is to be understood in its highest, most living form. This right–left–right progression, one of McGilchrist's main themes, can be useful as we search for ways to collaborate with the way our patients' brains and minds work. If we first support the nonverbal origins of their thought processes, grounded as they are in bodily experiences, we can then invite them into the world of the left-based attention through reflecting their bodily experiences as they present them in gesture, sound, or word, moving gradually toward re-*presentation* without losing the felt sense of the experience. As their bodily experiences flow toward language, we can mentor them through this process within our therapeutic relational context. This continued focus on relationship can help the right-mode of experience stay connected with the left-mode of words.

For example, I believe that George used the word *cobra* (perhaps arising simultaneously from both hemispheres or just from the right[5]) to describe his 10-second sandtray in an attempt to show me how lethal and dangerous it felt in his inner world (the map of his bodily experience in his right hemisphere). In response, I could say to him playfully, "So you are going to leave a *cobra* in my office," to support him in his naming of the right-hemisphere experience of danger in a way that allowed him to return to his right hemisphere metaphorically, where he could process his experience at a higher (more integrated) level. My response to him metaphorically communicated that I could hold his lethal feelings without being destroyed because we were "just playing." In the broader context, we were "safe" in our play. To me, this right–left–right progression is a *spiral of play* that, with mindful awareness, I can watch, helping me to know when and how to join in this natural interweaving of the brain when it is operating at its highest level. This flowing interconnection between the perspectives of the hemispheres helps us to make sense of our experiences in the body and in the narrative. It keeps us from getting stuck in one hemisphere or the other, and it allows us to tell our life stories in an embodied and coherent way. When we have this coherence, we often feel a deep sense of settling, supporting better interpersonal connections and greater capacity for attention. This spiral progression allows us to make meaning of our lives in the context of the whole in an ever-expanding and irreversible flow.

The Hand–Mind Connection

Something else comes to mind when I think about George's cobra tray: "thinking with your hands." I first came across this phrase when I was reading about Lego® Serious Play® (LSP), a specific way of using Lego play in corporate, business, and government settings to help adults come up with creative solutions to serious problems. Typically, a trained facilitator invites these "serious" adults to play "seriously" with a set of Lego bricks so that they can build something with their hands in an effort to access potential solutions that may already lie deep within. "If you don't know what to make, just start building," says the facilitator. This instruction is given with confidence, based on scientific knowledge that neurons are distributed throughout the body, and that each hand is connected to the opposite side

of the brain; the right hand connects to the left hemisphere, the left hand to the right. Neurologist Frank Wilson (1998) wrote an entire book about how the use of the hand shapes the brain, language, and human culture. He says:

> This book has been an inquiry into the premise that the hand is as much at the core of human life as the brain itself. . . . The hand is involved in human learning. . . . For a great number of people, the hand is the focus of years of specialized training and becomes the critical instrument of thought, skill, feeling, and intention for a lifetime of professional work. (pp. 277–278)

So perhaps it is not such a stretch to say, "We think with our hands," or as some would say, "with our bodies." At least, this is how LSP is used to help business people, architects, engineers, and government officials rethink serious problems. They use a hands-on environment to play with the bricks. There is never a point in an LSP session where the trained facilitator asks participants to merely sit back, write down, or chat about the issues at hand without building their response first. *Build, then talk* would be a good, simple description of what happens in LSP.

I think this is what happened when George suddenly and swiftly swept his hands up and over in opposite directions making a sand image of a lethal cobra in the sandtray. Both hands, both sides of his brain, participated. And it began in the right hemisphere where, as McGilchrist, Damasio, and Badenoch point out, meaningful stories begin. We can imagine that this swift movement was a *felt experience* for George, and as it quickly moved over into the left hemisphere, he was able to name it. McGilchrist (2009) says that we "unpack" things in the left hemisphere as we analyze, sort, categorize, organize, and name our experiences. This left-hemisphere process helps us make sense out of our experiences, and if we can keep from getting stuck in the left-hemisphere naming, we can return to the right hemisphere where we can reconnect to our bodily experiences at a higher and more integrated level. Perhaps that well-used quote by Carl Jung (1969) says it best, "Often the hands know how to solve a riddle with which the intellect has wrestled in vain" (p. 180).

The Power of the Sandtray to Heal

We have been talking about some of the reasons that the sandtray is (in Kalff's words) "a powerful, invaluable modality." The question many ask is, "How do you know?" What scientific evidence is there for the effectiveness of the tray? Although we are beginning to see a few studies that try to meet the rigorous criteria of *evidence-based* practices (experimental studies using randomized experimental and control groups), there is still a need for more in-depth research on the sandtray and sandplay modalities. At the same time, it is important not to devalue a modality purely on the grounds that there have not been enough experimental studies to demonstrate its effectiveness. We do now have a lot of *science-informed* data that help us to articulate not only the legitimacy of this modality but also the core need to utilize these kinds of practices that align themselves with how the brain/mind works.

In this chapter and elsewhere (Kestly, 2014), I have drawn from a wide variety of neuroscientific studies supporting our use of the sandtray modality. In our eagerness to be accepted in the mainstream of the behavioral sciences, we may grasp prematurely for "evidence." This effort can inadvertently create an imbalance in how we conduct our research, sometimes leaving out crucial aspects of the brain/mind that are not easy to measure, such as recognizing the power of relationship to heal, accessing life experiences that language cannot reach, and creating safety for the nervous system through providing opti-

mal zones of social engagement where the brain/mind can function most effectively. If we could change our language a little to use the term *science-informed* as well as *evidence-based* practices, I think we could advance our scientific understanding without undermining our need to know and to provide the most effective modes of healing. If we skip over the *science-informed* to reach the predictive power of the *evidence-based*, we may err on the side of the limited left mode of attending when it operates in isolation, as if the right mode did not exist. In the introduction to his book, McGilchrist (2009) tells a story from Nietzsche of a master and his emissary to help us understand this point. He writes:

> There was once a wise spiritual master, who was the ruler of a small but prosperous domain, and who was known for his selfless devotion to his people. As his people flourished and grew in number, the bounds of this small domain spread; and with it the need to trust implicitly the emissaries he sent to ensure the safety of its ever more distant parts. It was not just that it was impossible for him personally to order all that needed to be dealt with: as he wisely saw, he needed to keep his distance from, and remain ignorant of, such concerns. And so he nurtured and trained carefully his emissaries, in order that they could be trusted. Eventually, however, his cleverest and most ambitious vizier, the one he most trusted to do his work, began to see himself as the master, and used his position to advance his own wealth and influence. He saw his master's temperance and forbearance as weakness, not wisdom, and on his missions on the master's behalf, adopted his mantle as his own—the emissary became contemptuous of his master. And so it came about that the master was usurped, the people were duped, the domain became a tyranny; and eventually it collapsed in ruins. (p. 14)

Applying McGilchrist's idea that metaphor takes us to the highest level of language processing in our right hemispheres, we can use this metaphor of the master and his emissary to see that we may need to choose wisely, choosing consciously, how we go about accessing this amazing potential for collaboration and wholeness of our divided brains. Of the relationship between our hemispheres, McGilchrist (2009) says: "If the relationship holds, they are invincible; but if it is abused, it is not just the Master that suffers, but both of them, since the emissary owes his existence to the Master" (p. 428). We can make conscious decisions to respect and nurture this potential for collaboration between our two hemispheres in our personal lives, in our professional practices, and in the way we approach our scientific research. As McGilchrist says, the relationship is *invincible*. In the absence of this collaboration, we suffer.

The Healing of George's Suffering

Over time and very gradually George found more words to describe his trays, but his preference was to play primarily with the sandtray without words. I could see clearly, however, that his wordless stories were being conveyed through the miniatures he chose and through his actions upon them. Lowenfeld (Urwin & Hood-Williams, 1988) described this mode of expression in children: "Action, not language, is the natural mode of expression of children and the use of objects for expression and feeling is much more natural to them than the use of words" (p. 357). George often set up his sandtray as if setting a stage set for action. For example, he dug the holes for the rabbits before he brought the farmer in, and then he made them dart into their holes with well-timed precision.

Danger in George's worlds was always present, even to the very last tray, but how he had come to manage the danger in the environment was very different. In his last tray, he made a beautiful scene in a densely wooded area with a tranquil pond of water in the middle. Wild animals abounded, including a bear, a skunk, a fox, many little rabbits, and a rattlesnake. There were fish in the pond. Beside the pond there was a large log, and on top of the log, George placed one of the little rabbits. He faced the rabbit toward the upper right corner of the tray where the rattlesnake was coiled. George said, "Now the rabbit can see where the danger is." The rabbit no longer had to stay right beside his hole because he had developed a different perspective where he could keep track of the danger without inhibiting his movement in the woods.

It was clear to me that George had found a way out of his suffering by gaining access to a part of his brain/mind that had been cut off from his ability to express himself. Where he had been isolated within the anxiety and fear, he could now be confident through awareness because he had found a vehicle for expressing himself within the free and protected space of his trays and our relationship. Though he still spoke few words, with the few words he did choose, he could tell his whole story in a new and coherent way, where suffering yielded to playfulness and joy.

NOTES

1. The clinical examples in this chapter are based on composite material drawn from a number of individual cases. I have done it this way to protect confidentiality of patients while preserving authenticity of case examples.

2. This quote appeared on a page by itself right before the Prologue written by Harold Stone, PhD. When Temenos Press republished Kalff's book in 2003, the passage was preceded by the words, "Advice from Dora Kalff." Several other sentences were added, perhaps to clarify the certification process of sandplay therapy by the International Society for Sandplay Therapy.

3. Siegel (2007) includes the following reference in this quote to provide the source of his research information: Davidson, R., Kabat-Zinn, J., Schumacher, J., Rosenkranz, M., Muller, D., Santorelli, S. F., et al. (2003). Alterations in brain and immune function produced by mindfulness meditation. *Psychomatic Medicine, 65*(4), 564–570.

4. Kalff (1980, 2003) explained that the prescribed small size of the sandtray (28.5″ × 19.5″ × 3) would confine the patient's imagination, thus acting as a regulating, protecting factor (p. 8).

5. Language is often thought of as a left-hemisphere mode of processing, but it does not always arise from the left. Both hemispheres are activated in everything we think, feel, and do, and the right mode continues to be the domain of words expressing fresh experience, poetry, and, significantly, metaphor.

REFERENCES

Badenoch, B. (2011). *The brain-savvy therapist's workbook*. New York: Norton.

Baer, R. A. (Ed.). (2006). *Mindfulness-based treatment approaches: Clinician's guide to evidence base and applications*. Burlington, MA: Academic Press.

Damasio, A. (1999). *The feeling of what happens: The body and emotion in the making of consciousness*. San Diego, CA: Harcourt.

Hunter, L. (1998). *Images of resiliency*. Palm Beach, FL: Behavioral Communications Institute.

Jung, C. (1969). *The collected works of C. G. Jung: Vol. 8. Structure and dynamics of the psyche* (2nd ed.). Princeton, NJ: Princeton University Press.

Kalff, D. (1980). *Sandplay: A psychotherapeutic approach to the psyche*. Boston: Sigo Press.

Kalff, D. (2003). *Sandplay: A psychotherapeutic approach to the psyche*. Cloverdale, CA: Temenos Press. (Original work published 1980)

Kestly, T. (2004). *What is sandtray therapy?* Unpublished handout.

Kestly, T. (2014). *The interpersonal neurobiology of play: Brain-building interventions for emotional well-being*. New York: Norton.

Lowenfeld, M. (1979). *The world technique*. London: George Allen & Unwin.

McGilchrist, I. (2009). *The master and his emissary: The divided brain and the making of the Western world*. New Haven, CT: Yale University Press.

Siegel, D. J. (2007). *The mindful brain: Reflection and attunement in the cultivation of well-being*. New York: Norton.

Siegel, D. J. (2010). *Mindsight: The new science of personal transformation*. New York: Bantam Books.

Siegel, D. J. (2012). *The developing mind: How relationships and the brain interact to shape who we are* (2nd ed.). New York: Guilford Press.

Siegel, D. J., & Bryson, T. P. (2011). *The whole-brain child: 12 revolutionary strategies to nurture your child's developing mind*. New York: Delacorte Press.

Siegel, D. J., & Hartzell, M. (2003). *Parenting from the inside out: How a deeper self-understanding can help you raise children who thrive*. New York: Tacher/Penguin.

Urwin, C., & Hood-Williams, J. (Eds.). (1988). *Child psychotherapy, war and the normal child: Selected papers of Margaret Lowenfeld*. London: Free Association Books.

Wilson, F. (1998). *The hand: How its use shapes the brain, language, and human culture*. New York: Vintage Books.

CHAPTER 12

StoryPlay®

A NARRATIVE PLAY THERAPY APPROACH

Joyce C. Mills

Storytelling is recognized as the oldest and most respectful means of communication transculturally (Campbell, 1991; Mills & Crowley, 2014). Whether through art, music, dance, or play, it is the story, the *narrative*, which captures attention, evokes emotion, and transforms consciousness.

The symbolism embedded within a story allows the listener to enter his or her own world and discover meanings that are personally relevant to him or her. It is the ultimate client-centered approach, inviting children to enter the garden of their imaginations and discover solutions as one would a blossoming bud after a winter's frost.

There is no doubt that narratives and storytelling are vital for healthy brain development (McGilchrist, 2009; Mills & Crowley, 2014; Ramachandran, 2011; Siegel & Bryson, 2012). Brown professes that "storytelling has been identified as the unit of human understanding" (2009, p. 91). With the neuroimportance of metaphors, cre-

ativity, and play at its center, this chapter highlights the six roots of StoryPlay®, an Ericksonian, resiliency-based, indirective[1] model of play therapy that focuses on how to identify, access, and utilize inner resources, skills, and gifts as invaluable "gems." The goal of StoryPlay is both to move beyond diagnosis and to effect *transformational change* for children and adolescents who have experienced trauma and adversity (Mills & Crowley, 2014).

Differing from narrative therapy (White, 2007; White & Epston, 1990), wherein the narrative therapist *asks questions* in order to generate "experientially vivid descriptions of life events" (*http://en.wikipedia.org/wiki/Narrative_therapy*), the StoryPlay therapist *utilizes* the symptom and all forms of the client's story to evoke behavioral and emotional transformational change. (*Utilization* is a major cornerstone of Erickson's body of work.)

Also included in this chapter are two metaphorical activities, called "StoryCrafts," which provide patients with a *resiliency pathway* for healing (Carey, 2006, pp. 207–213; Geary & Zeig, 2001, pp. 507–519; Mills, 1999, 2011; Mills & Crowley, 2014).

The Six Roots of StoryPlay

Just like a tree's roots anchor and store resources for healthy growth, each of the six roots of StoryPlay carries valuable principles, resources, and teachings that provide substance and information to ensure the solidity of this model (see Figure 12.1):

1. The taproot—principles of Milton H. Erickson.
2. Transcultural wisdom and healing philosophies.
3. Real life, myth stories, and metaphors.
4. Play therapy.
5. The natural world.
6. Creativity.

The branches of StoryPlay extend beyond play therapy and can be applied to the fields of education and coaching.

Root 1: The Taproot— Principles of Milton H. Erickson

Just as most trees begin life with a *taproot* to anchor and ensure the healthy growth of new roots, the StoryPlay model stems from

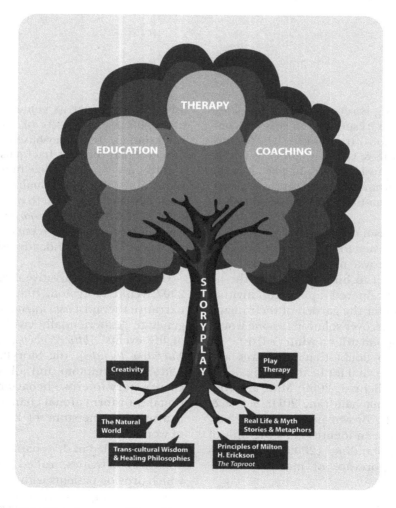

FIGURE 12.1. The six roots of StoryPlay. From Mills (2011). Reprinted by permission.

the resiliency-focused principles of Milton H. Erickson as its metaphorical taproot—the main anchoring root from which all other roots sprout (Mills, 2011; Mills & Crowley, 2014; O'Hanlon, 1987).

Ericksonian therapeutic principles are founded on a belief in the inherent healing potential of recognizing, activating, and utilizing a patient's skills, inner resources, and gifts to achieve "small successes that reach into the future" (Short, Erickson, & Erickson-Klein, 2005, p. xx). Ericksonian approaches are not focused on analyzing the past or the pathology, but instead they are attentive to the present and to the utilization of hidden potentials and inner resources to facilitate positive change. In Erickson's words, "Children have a driving need to learn and to discover, and every stimulus constitutes, for them, a possible opportunity to respond in some new way" (1958/1980a, p. 174). Taking a closer look at Erickson's statement, it becomes evident that his views coincide with the new brain-based discoveries related to *neuroplasticity* (Siegel, 2012; see also Doidge, 2007; Ramachandran, 2011).

Clinical Case Example: Surfing the Waves

While living on the Hawaiian island of Kaua'i, I had the opportunity of working with Peter, a 13-year-old boy, who had been severely abused both physically and emotionally. Peter was failing school and breaking the law to an extent that could prospectively land him in the juvenile justice system. In order to give him the opportunity to turn his life around, he was sent to a residential program, where I was working, to learn how to make positive choices.

During our first session, I noted that Peter was wearing the usual tank shirt, surfer shorts, and slippers that most of the kids wore. After introducing myself, I placed my hand on top of a thick file folder in front of us and told him that I hadn't read the file, which contained his reason

for admittance to our residential program. I told him that what I really wanted to know was what he liked to do. Peter looked at me with a wrinkled brow as well as an inquisitive and disbelieving expression. After a few quiet moments, he responded by saying, "Surfing." I then became curious about a number of things related to surfing and asked him, "What kind of board do you use?" . . . "Where's your favorite surfing spot?" . . . "How do you know how to read the waves?" . . . "What do you do when faced with a powerful undertow?"

Peter perked up almost immediately and told me the kind of board he uses, where he likes to surf, and how he learned to read the waves. Our conversation continued to focus on surfing for the whole session. At one particular point, I leaned in a bit closer and asked, "What do you do when you get 'wiped out' by a huge wave?" Peter laughed and said that he gets back on his board and paddles out again to catch the next wave.

At that moment, I took the opportunity to utilize surfing as a metaphorical narrative theme, saying: "Peter, sounds to me like you know a lot more about surfing than I ever will. You know how to read those waves and paddle out just at the right time to catch a good one to ride. And when you see those big 30-footers coming, instead of fear, you see them as a challenge and take 'em on with respect and courage. You also said that when you wipe out, you get back on your board and paddle out to meet the next one. Well, Peter, I ask you this. . . . How would it be for you to *surf life*?" Peter smiled and said in pidgin,[2] "Aunty, how you do that?"

"Peter, sometimes waves come in different forms. Some can take you down, and some can carry you a long way where you'll enjoy the ride. Seems to me, it's important to know when it's time to recognize the difference." I continued, "Maybe the next time you grab your board and stand before the ocean, something important that can help you will come to mind. Enjoy discovering what that might be."

As we ended the session, Peter gave me the "shaka" sign with his right hand, and shook his head as if to communicate he understood. We worked together, creating a plan for Peter to "surf life" successfully. Over the many weeks, he had his ups and downs while confronting the waves of emotions that manifested when realizing what he had endured as a young child. Through it all, Peter remained connected to the metaphor of surfing, which kept him balanced, steady, and ready to meet the waves.

Root 2: Transcultural Wisdom and Healing Philosophies

For close to three decades, I've been intimately involved with Native American, Hawaiian, African American, and other transcultural wisdom teachings related to life, spirituality, and healing (see Mills, 1999). The depth of what I've learned came through participating in rituals, ceremonies, many life events, and by living and working on Kaua'i for 9 years (Hammerschlag, 2012; Mills, 1999). The foundations of the teachings and principles that follow may look simple, but they each carry profound cultural healing principles and wisdom.

Historical Trauma

Before each of the three transcultural wisdom and healing principles are presented, I respectfully note that the effects of historical and intergenerational trauma are often minimized, and, worse, overlooked when speaking about cultural issues in therapy (Brave Heart, 1998; Duran, 2006; Duran & Duran, 1995; Glover, 2005, pp. 168–179; Hammerschlag, 2012). The answer is not simply to have multicultural toys in the playroom; more importantly, it is to develop an understanding about the impact that historical and intergenerational trauma has had, and continues to have, on children, adolescents, families, and communities.

Working toward restoring a sense of "soul healing" (Duran, 2006) is at the core of the StoryPlay principles.

WHEEL OF BALANCE[3]

Hozjo is Diné (Navajo) for *balance and beauty*. In a comprehensive article written by Robert S. Drake (2004), he writes, "It is about health, long life, happiness, wisdom, knowledge, harmony, the mundane and the divine." Therefore, the first philosophy being addressed is, as I have previously said, "woven within the Native American Medicine Wheel, wherein there must be balance between mental, emotional, physical, and spiritual aspects of the self in order to achieve harmony. If one aspect is neglected, it is believed that the person is out of harmony with his or her well-being."[4]

In the StoryPlay model, it is essential to create a plan that will address all four of these aspects when working with children, adolescents, and families. I developed Figure 12.2 in order to assess areas of strengths and areas that are in need of attention. I often give a copy of this graphic to children, teens, and families so that they can self-assess how well they are taking care of themselves.

Additionally, the Wheel of Balance can be used with sandtray play therapy. Using a round sandtray, I ask clients to choose various miniatures representing how they are taking care of themselves in each of the four areas. Once completed, a story emerges related to the miniatures they have chosen. They become aware of how they are taking care of themselves, as well as what area(s) need attention.

HAWAIIAN CULTURAL VALUES[5]

The next set of teachings is inherent to Native Hawaiian people.[6] These values are the foundation of Na Pua No'eau (The Blossoming Flowers), a center for gifted and talented Native Hawaiian children. Parents,

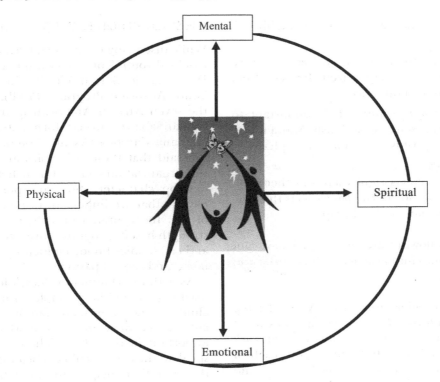

FIGURE 12.2. The "Wheel of Balance" handout.

children, teachers, and related staff are encouraged to memorize these principles as well as to *live* them.

When I first learned of the following ideals, I realized that not only do they address significant aspects of the Hawaiian culture, but they are also strong elements for strengthening all child and family relationships. Since then, these cultural values have become important components in the StoryPlay model.

• *Aloha—the "Breath of Life."* The word *aloha* means many things, including "love" and "spirit." It represents the connectedness (life stems) between people. Parents are encouraged to say *aloha* when waking their children up to go to school, rather than using an alarm clock to jolt them into wakefulness. This sets a positive tone from the very beginning of the day.

While working with Kalani Flores, a respected Hawaiian *Kumu* (source teacher), I learned that *alo* means "I greet you face to face." The syllable *ha* means "the breath of all of life." Joining those two syllables together, the word has a deepened meaning, which is "I greet you face to face with the breath of all of life."

• *Ho'omana–spirituality* (daily *pule*, prayer). Children and parents are encouraged to reflect on blessings they have received. In addition, each person should express his or her own spirit, which connects him or her with a greater good and flows through to others.

• *Laulima–cooperation and support.* Listening to the words and feelings of others is encouraged as well as the sharing of our own feelings.

• *Pa'ahana–devotion and diligence.* Commitment to family and goals is highly valued.

- *Kokua–positivity, helpfulness.* Positive behaviors are emphasized for children, family, and community.

- *Le'ale'a–playfulness.* It is important to not take ourselves so seriously. Maintaining a playful spirit is an important emphasis.

- *Ho'oponopono–to cleanse and make right.* Deal with issues right then and there. Do not hurt the spirit. *Ho'oponopono* is the original Hawaiian family therapy.

The following are two ways I have put these values into practice with children and families.

1. *Family value assessment.* After sharing the cultural story, I give this assessment (Figure 12.3) to family members and ask them to evaluate themselves in each of the areas. Zero indicates no value and five, the highest value. Family members are then able to see where their strengths are and where they are in need of help.
2. *Creating a collage.* Family members can create a collage by using pictures that represent each of the values. This exercise is intended to expand words into symbolic representation, which can deepen the connection to each value.

THE SEVEN PRINCIPLES OF NGUZO SABA

While discussing the importance of helping troubled youth from a cultural perspective, Dr. Alexander Sutton, Vice President of the Youth Advocate Programs (YAP),[7] shared the seven African American principles of Nguzo Saba (Kwanzaa), formulated by Dr. Maulana Karenga (Asante, 2009). Dr. Sutton said that these principles are part of the organization's program to help youth develop character and learn positive behaviors that are important to honoring all of life. Incorporated into their numerous strength-based programs are storytelling and ceremonies honoring identity, achievement, and rites of passage.

As with the Hawaiian values, I feel these teachings should be a template for helping children, adolescents, and families from all cultures reconnect to a sense of what is truly important in their lives. These principles speak to the core of cultural healing and, at the same time, help us to understand that the parts are no greater than the whole.

1. *Umoja (oo-mow-jah)–unity.* To strive for and maintain unity in the family, community, nation, and race.
2. *Kujichagulia (koo-gee-cha-goo-lee-ah)–self-determination.* To define ourselves, name ourselves, create for ourselves, and speak for ourselves instead of being de-

Family Value Assessment	0	1	2	3	4	5
Aloha—giving and receiving love						
Ho'omana—spirituality						
Laulima—cooperation and support						
Pa'ahana—devotion and diligence						
Kokua—positivity, helpfulness						
Le'ale'a—playfulness						
Ho'oponopono—deal with issues right away						

FIGURE 12.3. Assessment for family value strengths and weaknesses.

fined, named, created for, and spoken for by others.

3. *Ujima (oo-gee-mah)–collective work and responsibility.* To build and maintain our community together, make our sisters' and brothers' problems our problems, and to solve them together.

4. *Ujamaa (oo-jah-mah)–cooperative economics.* To build and maintain our own stores, shops, and other businesses and to profit from them together.

5. *Nia (nee-ah)–purpose.* To make our collective vocation the building and developing of our community in order to restore our people to their traditional greatness.

6. *Kuumba (koo-oom-bahj)–creativity.* To do always as much as we can, in the way we can, in order to leave our community more beautiful and beneficial than we inherited it.

7. *Imani (ee-mah-nee)–faith.* To believe with all our heart in our people, our parents, our teachers, our leaders, and the righteousness and victory of our struggle.

Each of these sacred African American principles is integral if we are to offer paradigm shifts in our therapy. At the core of StoryPlay is the respect for cultural diversity and, conversely, our human connectedness with one another.

Root 3: Real Life, Myth Stories, and Metaphors

"Once upon a time, a long time ago. . . . " Our attention is immediately captured. With these words, we are transported through time and space into symbolic worlds of adventure, discovery, and mastery. Ramachandran (2011), a neuroscientist, tells us that " . . . the use of metaphor and our ability to uncover hidden analogies is the basis of all creative thought" (p. 105). Daniel Siegel, noted expert on neurobiology, explains that "we are storytelling creatures, and stories are the social glue that binds us to one another" (2012, pp. 31–32).

Stories and metaphors convey a message or idea in an indirect yet paradoxically more meaningful way, bypassing resistance and opening the doorway to receptive communication (Erickson & Rossi, 1979; Mills, 2011; Mills & Crowley, 2014). Erickson's innovative use of metaphor over the span of his 50-year career is regarded as nothing short of masterful. Additionally, Erickson is recognized as the first clinician to assign the heading of *metaphor* to represent a special class of interventions (Erickson & Rossi, 1979; Short et al., 2005).

The sharing of personal life experiences, metaphors, favorite myths, and fantasy stories help a child explore new ways of seeing obstacles, overcoming problems, awakening inner resources, and developing creative solutions. Using the StoryPlay model, the child is not asked to relive the story or trauma in any way. Instead, a metaphor is offered to reframe the problem and provide a pathway for resolution. In much the same way as a chrysalis protects the transformation of a butterfly, so too does the metaphor protect the *process* of change. Nothing is analyzed, interpreted, or explained cognitively; rather, the actions, miniatures, and play themes are *utilized* as symbolic *Imaginal Discs*[8] to support a child's quest to reach his or her full potential (Mills, 1999, 2007).

Suggestions for Releasing the Storyteller within[9]

The following are four ideas that can support the process of becoming more proficient as a storyteller.

1. Gather pieces of jewelry, photographs, or a special object that were given to you.
2. Find a quiet time and see what stories connect with these items.
3. As the stories begin to emerge, write them down.
4. Share the stories with a colleague or someone special in your life.

I tell the participants in my trainings, "Enjoy discovering the story seeds that give substance and meaning to your lives."

Root 4: Play Therapy

Another root of StoryPlay comes from the theories and principles of play therapy, wherein children are encouraged to express their experiences, thoughts, desires, and emotions through the medium of play to resolve problems (Allan, 1997; Axline, 1947; Brody, 1997; Crenshaw, 2008; Freud, 1946; Gil, 1991, 1994; Guerney, 1997; Jernberg, 1979; Kestly, 2001, in press; Landreth, 1991; Lowenfield, 1979; Moustakas, 1959/1992; Norton & Norton, 1997; Oaklander, 1998, 2007; O'Connor & Schaefer, 1994; Schubach De Domenico, 1988; VanFleet, 1994). In his groundbreaking book *Play*, Stuart Brown writes, "When we play dilemmas and challenges will naturally filter through the unconscious mind and work themselves out" (2009, p. 128).

Traditionally, play therapy has been divided into two approaches: directive and nondirective (child-centered). A more recent addition to this list is *integrative play therapy* (Drewes, Bratton, & Schaefer, 2011), wherein, as the term suggests, a more eclectic and blended approach is practiced.

As stated previously, StoryPlay introduces a new resiliency-focused, Ericksonian, and *indirective* model of play therapy. Rather than having traumatized or abused children create their *trauma narratives*, StoryPlay focuses on the creation of *strength-based narratives* in various forms that include storytelling, play, artistic metaphors, StoryCrafts, and therapeutic rituals and ceremonies (Carey, 2006; Mills & Crowley, 2014). The trauma event isn't ignored, by any means. Instead, it is utilized and reframed so that unconscious association patterns can be activated to create new pathways of response.

The StoryPlay is always patient-centered and can be directive when needed. StoryPlay is also an integrative process because, as it is in Ericksonian principles, it accepts other models as well as provides important new elements that are not included in other modalities—namely, *interspersed suggestions* (Erickson, 1966/1980b; Lankton & Lankton, 1989; Lankton & Matthews, 2008; Mills & Crowley, 1986/2014; Short et al., 2005). Rossi termed Erickson's extraordinary communication skills as "two-level communication" (Erickson & Rossi, 1976/1980). Rossi was referring to Erickson's ability to provide the conscious mind with one message, while simultaneously providing the unconscious mind with "therapeutic messages" *interspersed* within a larger context (e.g., a story, metaphor, play). These "therapeutic messages" are gleaned from what the client wants to have in his or her life (Erickson, 1966/1980b, p. 271). For example, in our book *Sammy the Elephant and Mr. Camel*, suggestions such as "can easily hold everything within," "trust you can do it," and "learn that now" were *interspersed* throughout the story in order to help children with bedwetting problems (Mills & Crowley, 1988, 2005).

In the StoryPlay model, the therapist's response to a child's playful action does not direct the child to do anything, nor does it only reflect back what the child says or is doing. Instead, the therapist's response is meant to expand the healing process and tap into the *resilient inner core* of the child by delivering the message in a clear, understandable manner to his or her unconscious mind. Similar to a vitamin that releases essential elements for well-being, the intention of this *indirect message* is woven within the broader response and is absorbed in the child's unconscious mind, thereby facilitating healing and fostering resilience (Geary & Zeig, 2001, pp. 507–519).

Root 5: The Natural World

Beyond the Internet, books, and even toys lies our *Natural World Library*, which proves to be another valuable source of information for learning life lessons and achieving comfort for healing. StoryPlay uses the seasons, the weather, leaves, feathers, shells, butterflies, animals, flowers, and even annoying insects such as flies as educational and healing instruments to facilitate transformational change.

Clinical Case Example: Ant Medicine

"Dr. Joyce, I can't handle one more thing! My life sucks big time!" Those were the words exclaimed by 15-year-old Olivia as she stormed into my office and flopped herself down on the couch. Wrapping her arms around Barstow, my soft stuffed bear puppet, she crumbled into tears.

Olivia's life had been fraught with learning challenges, which left her feeling overwhelmed and fearful every time she had to face a test in one of her subjects. She had a competent 504 plan in place, but the 6 years prior to her being diagnosed with dyslexia had left Olivia with residual feelings of failure.

With strong interest in nature and photography, Olivia loved hiking and camping. During our sessions, we swapped stories about Native American philosophies related to ecology and the natural world. Olivia spent many years listening to her Diné (Navajo) grandmother's stories until she moved from New Mexico to Phoenix.

It was now time for finals. Squeezing Barstow even tighter, Olivia told me she didn't know how she was going to pass. It didn't matter how hard she studied, it was all "too f'ing heavy."

At that point, a story popped to my mind like a corn kernel pops when heated. "You know, Olivia, as I'm listening to you, I'm reminded of a story. Remember I told you I used to live in Hawai'i?" Olivia nodded, and I continued.

"Well, it was the night before a huge exam I had to pass in order to be relicensed as a therapist. The last time I took a test such as this one was in 1979. Olivia, I was a wreck because I'm dyslexic too, and I've been out of school for years. Sure, I studied all of the material, but I was really scared. If I didn't pass, I wouldn't be able to work.

"Finally, I knew I had to get some sleep. With all of my study materials spread out on the floor, couch, and table, I said a prayer asking for a sign to let me know I'd be okay. Then I closed my eyes and went to sleep.

"I jumped up as the alarm sounded at 6:15 A.M. and went to gather the scattered papers. Olivia, to my surprise, everything was covered with what looked like zillions of small black ants." Olivia grimaced and said, "Yuck!"

"That's what I thought at first. Well, Olivia, you know I'm a little weird and believe that all aspects of nature are teachers and talk to us in many ways. So I said to myself, 'Okay, little ants, what have you come to teach me?' And then it came to me; ants can carry 100 times their weight. They can travel over all kinds of terrain through all kinds of weather to get to their destination. Nothing stops them. They are determined.

"Olivia, somehow these ants were the sign I had asked for. They told me, 'Don't worry, you can handle it. You know all that you need to know in order to pass this exam. Let go of your doubt and keep going forward.'"

I paused for a few moments and then said, "I don't know what this story may say to you, but to this day, every time I see these little ant relatives, I smile and remember how they came to me just when I needed reassurance. And, by the way, I passed the exam."

Olivia looked noticeably more relaxed and asked if we could look at the Medicine Cards (Sams & Carson, 1998) and see what they say about ants. She often asked to use the cards and stories during previous sessions. Sure enough, there on page 165, we found the teaching, "Patience. . . . What is yours will come to you."

At the end of the session, I gave her a small, plastic ant I had in my miniature bug collection. I told her to find a special place for it and let it teach her something that would be helpful before she took her exam.

Two weeks later, Olivia came in for her next session, this time with a smile on her face. She handed me a collage of all kinds of ants she'd found on the Internet and in nature magazines. She had written *Ant Medicine* across the top. Smiling, she said, "Dr. Joyce, I passed my exam." We both laughed and wondered if Walgreens would be selling *Ant Medicine* any time soon.

Root 6: Creativity

At the core of all new ideas and problem solving is the ability to use our creative, imaginative minds to generate transformational change for those with whom we work. StoryPlay encourages the activation and utilization of the creative imagination to explore, innovate, and discover new pathways of healing, thinking, and being. The noted neuroscientist V. S. Ramachandran notes that "indeed, far from being mere decoration, the use of metaphor and our ability to uncover hidden analogies is the basis of all creative thought" (2011, p. 105).

The intention of StoryCrafts is to build a healing bridge between both worlds; namely, between *metaphor* and *creativity*. They were originally designed to inspire a reconnection to an inner core of resilience that may have been shrouded by the dark clouds of life's storms (Mills, 1999, 2011; Mills & Crowley, 2014).

The following are two examples of the numerous StoryCrafts[10] that were created and implemented in response to catastrophic events—in these cases, Hurricane Iniki (September 11, 1992, the worst natural disaster to hit the Hawaiian island in the last century), and the World Trade Center bombing (September 11, 2001). Since then, these StoryCrafts have been included in all StoryPlay Foundations trainings, Camp PlayMore Retreats,[11] and the Turtle Island Women's Healing Journey retreats.[12]

StoryCraft 1: Life-Story Puzzle[13]

The greatest legacies we have to give to our children are our stories. Stories help us become whole in a fragmented world. Some contain elements of tragedy, whereas others contain experiences of joy. As it is with all puzzles, every story is made up of the sum total of its parts. One piece is not more important than the next, as they all must interlock in order to reveal the total picture (Mills, 1999, 2011).

The Life Story Puzzle practice can be used with individual clients, in groups, and in family play therapy practices. It helps children create a new form of narrative that is uniquely theirs.

SUGGESTED MATERIALS

These include poster paper or foam board of various sizes, depending on if you're working with individuals or groups; markers, paint, or crayons. *Optional:* glue, glitter, glue-on colorful (flat-back) rhinestones, and feathers.

INSTRUCTIONS

Initially, I suggest drawing five to seven interlocking lines to represent pieces to a puzzle. Next, I ask the client to cut out each piece so that they are all separated. For younger children, or to maximize creative time for the craft, pieces can be cut out prior to session.

I ask the child to draw symbols representing aspects of his or her life on each piece. The symbols do not need to be in any sequential order. Splashes of colors, shapes, stick figures, and line drawings are fine. The symbols only need to make sense to the client(s).

Finally, I ask the client to take his or her time fitting the pieces back together. I suggest taking a few reflective moments to look at the whole picture and then I ask the client to notice what he or she experiences while looking at this picture.

For Groups or Families. I ask participants to choose a piece from the already drawn and cut out puzzle frame. Next, I ask them to draw a symbol on that piece. When they are finished, they are asked to come back to the circle and share it with the group. At the end of the group or family session, the pieces can be rejoined to indicate the connection to the whole. The Life Story Puzzle can be made in various shapes (e.g., turtles, butterflies, hearts).

Figure 12.4 is a photograph taken in a classroom of third graders who created their Life Story Puzzle with the guidance of StoryPlay practitioner and teacher Joy Rigberg.[14]

StoryCraft 2: Dreaming Pots[15]

Many years ago, while I was visiting one of my favorite spots in Arizona (the Heard Museum), I came upon an exhibit from the Mimbres tribe displaying beautiful painted pots with holes in the bottom. Although little was known about the specifics of the bowls, it was hypothesized that they were placed in burial sites to bring good spirits to those who had died and that the holes allowed the departed spirits to travel freely (Mills, 1999; Mills & Crowley, 2014).

After meditating for a while, the idea of creating what I called *Dreaming Pots* with the children and families with whom I worked came to mind. The children would

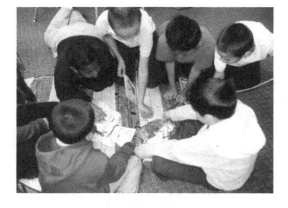

FIGURE 12.4. Creating a Life Story Puzzle.

be given small clay pots and asked to decorate them with symbols from their good dreams. The holes were created to allow an exit for their bad dreams. Families were given larger pots, and each member decorated the pot with his or her own symbols. Stories then emerged about the symbols, evoking positive conversation. Little did I realize at the time in private practice that Dreaming Pots would become an integral StoryCraft for children and communities who experienced catastrophic disaster.

After Hurricane Iniki ferociously ripped through Kaua'i, children and families slept on floors in the homes of others or in tents. They were afraid to go to sleep and experienced many nightmares. As part of the Kaua'i Westside O'hana Activities Project,[16] Dreaming Pots became one of the *natural healing activities* offered to the community. The intention was for those who made their Dreaming Pots to put them by their sleeping places, so that they could be reminded of their good dreams. The Dreaming Pots gave them something tangible on which to focus that brought comfort and a sense of inner control.

In response to the aftermath from the bombing of the World Trade Center, I was invited to be part of a team that was involved with engaging Healing and Recovery after Trauma (HART)—a special project specifically designed to provide free-of-charge, community-based programs and services to the youths and youth-serving professionals in counties directly adjacent to New York, and/or which had a significant number of residents who worked in New York. We designed nine modules, one of which was Dreaming Pots. Participants created their pots and then shared whatever they wished. Everyone expressed gratitude for our program's focus on strengths.

Dreaming Pots continue to be used in a variety of settings, including classrooms, domestic violence groups, and grief groups, as well as in treatment settings following other natural disasters.

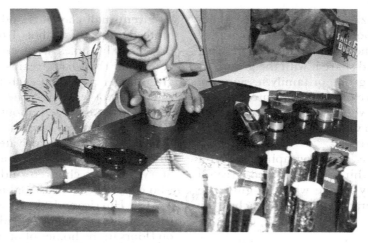

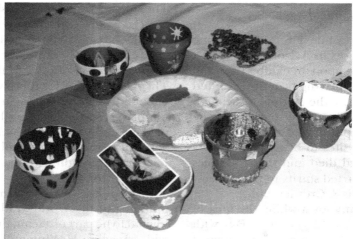

FIGURE 12.5. Creating Dreaming Pots.

Conclusion

My hope and vision is to create a resiliency-focused community where we all learn to look beyond that which we see with everyday eyes and see with the vision of our hearts; to stimulate discussions and develop programs that connect children to their strengths and inner gifts, so they can move beyond the traumas that they have endured and embrace the brilliant possibilities that lie before them.

NOTES

1. Indirect suggestion is well documented in Erickson & Rossi (1981); Gilligan (1997); Lankton & Lankton (1993); and Lankton & Matthews (2008).

2. *Pidgin* is defined as a mixture of two or more languages for cultural communication. Pidgin is commonly spoken in Hawai'i.

3. Healing and Recovery after Trauma was the first module in a resiliency-focused project specifically designed to provide free-of-charge community-based programs and services to the

children and adolescents who were exposed to and affected by the 9/11 tragedy (Hines, Mills, Bonner, Sutton, & Castellano, 2007). Because the acronym was HART, a heart replaced the StoryPlay logo.

4. For more information about the use of the Medicine Wheel, see *The Sacred Tree* (Bopp, Bopp, Brown, & Lane, 1984/1985).

5. Edited and excerpted with permission from Mills (2011).

6. These Hawaiian values were shared as part of a conference on Hawaiian Healing, February 5, 1994, in Waimea, Kaua'i, HI.

7. YAP (Youth Advocacy Program) is an organization dedicated to helping troubled youth from the inner cities.

8. *Imaginal Discs* are special cells that lie dormant in the body of the caterpillar. Within the chrysalis the caterpillar breaks down in structure and at that point the *seeds of change* are released. These cells transform the caterpillar into the butterfly.

9. Adapted with permission from Mills (1999, p. 207).

10. StoryCrafts were originally designed for the children, youth, and families on the west side of Kaua'i, Hawai'i, in the aftermath of Hurricane Iniki, funded by the Office of Youth Services, Child and Family Services—Kaua'i. Since then, they have been globally used to treat children, adolescents, families, and communities who have experienced abuse, trauma, and grief (Hines et al., 2007; Mills, 1999; Mills & Crowley, 2014).

11. Co-led with Teri Krull, award-winning psychotherapist, author, and registered play therapy supervisor.

12. The Turtle Island Project is a nonprofit organization dedicated to research, education, and healing (see *www.turtleislandproject.com*).

13. Adapted with permission from Mills (1999, pp. 136–138).

14. Joy Rigberg is a bilingual teacher, counselor, and addiction life coach. She and I coauthored a grant proposal to bring The StoryPlay® Life Skills Enrichment Program into the school setting.

15. Excerpted and adapted with permission from Mills (1999, pp. 17–21).

16. A three-part program offering direct services and culturally respectful opportunities to youth and families needing to move past the prevailing posttraumatic stress disorder (PTSD) focus into a model more centered on posttraumatic stress healing (PTSH).

REFERENCES

Allan, J. (1997). Jungian play psychotherapy. In K. J. O'Connor & L. Braverman (Eds.), *Play therapy theory and practice: A comparative presentation*, (pp. 100–130). New York: Wiley.

Asante, M. K. (2009). *Maulana Karenga: An intellectual portrait*. New York: Wiley.

Axline, V. (1947). *Play therapy: The inner dynamics of childhood*. Boston: Houghton Mifflin.

Bopp, J., Bopp, M., Brown, L., & Lane, P., Jr. (1984/1985). *The sacred tree: Reflections on Native American spirituality*. Lethbridge, Alberta, Canada: Four Worlds International Institute.

Brave Heart, M. (1998). The return to the sacred path: Healing the historical trauma and historical unresolved grief response among the Lakota through a psycho-educational group intervention. *Smith College Studies in Social Work, 68*, 287–308.

Brody, V. (1997). *The dialogue of touch: Developmental play therapy*. Lanham, MD: Roman and Littlefield.

Brown, S. (2009). *Play*. New York: Avery Press.

Campbell, J. (1991). *The power of myth*. New York: Anchor Books.

Carey, L. (2006). *Expressive and creative arts methods for trauma survivors*. Philadelphia: Jessica Kingsley.

Crenshaw, D. A. (2008). *Therapeutic engagement of children and adolescents: Play, symbol, drawing and storytelling strategies*. Lanham, MD: Aronson.

Doidge, N. (2007). *The brain that changes itself*. New York: Penguin Books.

Drake, R. S. (2004). Hozho: Diné concept of balance and beauty. Retrieved from *www.roberts-drake.com/files/Hozho.htm*.

Drewes, A. A., Bratton, S. C., & Schaefer, C. E. (2011). *Integrative play therapy*. Hoboken, NJ: Wiley.

Duran, E. (2006). *Healing the soul wound*. New York: Teachers College Press.

Duran, E., & Duran, B. (1995). *Native American*

postcolonial psychology. Albany: State University of New York Press.

Erickson, M., & Rossi, E. (1981). *Experiencing hypnosis: Indirect approaches to altered states*. New York: Irvington.

Erickson, M. H. (1980a). Pediatric hypnotherapy. In E. Rossi (Ed.), *The collected papers of Milton H. Erickson on hypnosis: Vol. 4. Innovative hypnotherapy* (pp. 174–180). New York: Irvington. (Original work published 1958)

Erickson, M. H. (1980b). The interspersal hypnotic technique for symptom correction and pain control. In E. Rossi (Ed.), *The collected papers of Milton H. Erickson on hypnosis: Vol. 4. Innovative hypnotherapy* (pp. 262–278,). New York: Irvington. (Original work published 1966)

Erickson, M. H., & Rossi, E. (1979). *An exploratory casebook*. New York: Irvington.

Erickson, M. H., & Rossi, E. (1980). Two-level communication and the microdynamics of trance and suggestion. In E. Rossi (Ed.), *The collected papers of Milton H. Erickson on hypnosis: Vol. 1. The nature of hypnosis and suggestion* (pp. 430–451). New York: Irvington. (Original work published 1976)

Freud, A. (1946). *The psychoanalytic treatment of children*. London: Imago.

Geary, B. B., & Zeig, J. K. (2001). Ericksonian play therapy. In B. B. Geary & J. K. Zeig (Eds.), *Handbook of Ericksonian psychotherapy* (pp. 576–521). Phoenix, AZ: Milton H. Erickson Foundation Press.

Gil, E. (1991). *The healing power of play: Working with abused children*. New York: Guilford Press.

Gil, E. (1994). *Play in family therapy*. New York: Guilford Press.

Gilligan, S. (1997). *The courage to love*. New York: Norton.

Glover, J. (2005). *Commentary: Socrates, Freud and family therapy*. New York: Wiley.

Guerney, L. F. (1997). *Filial therapy: Strengthening parent–child relationships through play*. Sarasota, FL: Professional Resources Press.

Hammerschlag, C. A. (2012). *Kindling spirit: Healing from within*. Phoenix, AZ: Turtle Island Press.

Hines, P., Mills, J. C., Bonner, R., Sutton, C. E., & Castellano, C. (2007). Healing and recovery after trauma: A disaster response program for first responders. In *Systemic responses to disaster: Stories of the aftermath of Hurricane Katrina* (Winter AFTA Monograph Series, pp. 61–68). Available at *www.afta.org/files/2007_Monograph.pdf*.

Jernberg, A. M. (1979). *Theraplay: A new treatment using structured play for problem children and their families*. San Francisco: Jossey-Bass.

Kestly, T. (2001, September). *Articulating the value of play*. Paper presented at the New Mexico Association for Play Therapy, Albuquerque, NM.

Kestley, T. (in press). *The interpersonal neurobiology of play: Brain-building interventions for emotional well-being*. New York: Norton.

Landreth, G. L. (1991). *Play therapy: The art of the relationship*. Muncie, IN: Accelerated Development.

Lankton, S., & Lankton, C. (1989). *Tales of enchantment: Goal-oriented metaphors for adults and children in therapy*. New York: Brunner/Mazel.

Lankton, S., & Matthews, W. (2008). An Ericksonian model of clinical hypnosis. In S. Lynn, J. Rhue, & I. Kirsch (Eds.), *Handbook of clinical hypnosis* (2nd ed., pp. 209–238). Washington, DC: American Psychological Association Press.

Lowenfield, M. (1979). *The world technique*. London: Allen & Unwin.

McGilchrist, I. (2009). *The master and his emissary*. New Haven, CT: Yale University Press.

Mills, J. C. (1999). *Reconnecting to the magic of life*. Phoenix, AZ: Imaginal Press.

Mills, J. C. (2007). *Butterfly wisdom®*. Phoenix, AZ: Imaginal Press.

Mills, J. C. (2011). *StoryPlay foundations*. Phoenix, AZ: Imaginal Press.

Mills, J. C., & Crowley, R. J. (1988). A multidimensional approach to the utilization of therapeutic metaphors for children and adolescents. In J. K. Zeig & S. R. Lankton (Eds.), *Developing Ericksonian therapy: State of the art* (pp. 302–323). New York: Brunner/Mazel.

Mills, J. C., & Crowley, R. J. (2005). *Sammy the elephant and Mr. Camel* (2nd ed.). Washington, DC: Magination Press.

Mills, J. C., & Crowley, R. J. (2014). *Therapeutic metaphors and for children and the child within* (2nd ed.). Philadelphia: Brunner-Routledge.

Moustakas, C. (1992). *Psychotherapy with children*. Greeley, CO: Carron. (Original work published 1959)

Norton, C. C., & Norton, B. E. (1997). *Reaching children through play therapy*. Denver, CO: Publishing Cooperative.

Oaklander, V. (1998). *Windows to our children.* Moab, UT: Real People Press.

Oaklander, V. (2007). *Hidden treasure.* London: Karnac Books.

O'Connor, K. J., & Schaefer, C. E. (Eds.). (1994). *Handbook of play therapy: Vol. 2. Advances and innovations.* New York: Wiley.

O'Hanlon, W. H. (1987). *Taproots.* New York: Norton.

Ramachandran, V. S. (2011). *The tell-tale brain.* New York: Norton.

Schubach De Domenico, G. (1988). *Sand tray world play: A comprehensive guide to the use of the sand tray in psychotherapeutic and transformational settings.* Unknown binding.

Short, D., Erickson, B. A., & Erickson-Klein, R. (2005). *Hope and resiliency.* New York: Crown.

Siegel, D. J. (2012). *The developing mind: How relationships and the brain interact to shape who we are* (2nd ed). New York: Guilford Press.

Siegel, D. J., & Bryson, T. P. (2012). *The whole-brain child: 12 revolutionary steps to nurture your child's developing mind.* New York: Bantam Books.

VanFleet, R. (1994). *Filial therapy: Strengthening parent–child relationships through play.* Sarasota, FL: Professional Resource Press.

White, M. (2007). *Maps of narrative practice.* New York: Norton.

White, M., & Epston, D. (1990). *Narrative means to therapeutic ends.* New York: Norton.

ADDITIONAL READINGS

Benard, B. (1991). *Fostering resiliency in kids: Protective factors in the family, school, and community.* Portland, OR: Western Center for Drug-Free Schools and Communities.

Blum, R. W., Beuhring, T., Shew, M. L., Bearinger, L. H., Sieving, R. E., & Resnick, M. D. (2000). The effects of race/ethnicity, income, and family structure on adolescent risk behaviors. *American Journal of Public Health, 90,* 1879–1884.

Brown, J. H., D'Emidio-Caston, M., & Benard, B. (2001). *Resilience education.* Thousand Oaks, CA: Corwin Press.

Butler, K. (1997, March/April). The anatomy of resilience. *Family Networker,* pp. 22–31.

Cameron-Bandler, L. (1978). *They lived happily ever after.* Cupertino, CA: Meta.

Duran, E., Duran, B., Brave Heart, M. Y. H., & Yellow Horse-Davis, S. (1998). Healing the American Indian soul wound. In D. Yael (Ed.), *International handbook of multigenerational legacies of trauma* (pp. 341–354). New York: Plenum Press.

Gil, E., & Drewes, A. A. (2005). *Cultural issues in play therapy.* New York: Guilford Press.

Haggerty, R. J., Sherrod, L. R., Garmezy, N., & Rutter, M. (1996). *Stress, risk, and resilience in children and adolescents: Processes, mechanisms, and interventions.* New York: Cambridge University Press.

Hammerschlag, C. A. (1988). *Dancing healers.* San Francisco: Harper & Row.

Hammerschlag, C. A. (1993). *Theft of the spirit.* New York: Simon & Schuster.

Heller, S., & Steele, T. (1986). *There's no such thing as hypnosis.* Phoenix, AZ: Falcon Press.

James, B. (1989). *Treating traumatized children:* Lexington, MA: Lexington Books.

James, B. (1994). *Handbook for treatment of attachment-trauma problems in children.* Lexington, MA: Lexington Books.

Kopp, R. R. (1995). *Metaphor therapy: Using client-generated metaphors in psychotherapy.* Bristol, PA: Brunner/Mazel.

Krovetz, M. L. (1999). *Fostering resiliency: Expecting all students to use their minds and hearts well.* Thousand Oaks, CA: Corwin Press.

Leffert, N., Benson, P. L., Scales, P. C., Sharma, A. R., Drake, D. R., & Blyth, D. A. (1998). Developmental assets: Measurement and prediction of risk behaviors among adolescents. *Applied Developmental Science, 2,* 209–230.

Mills, J. C. (1989). No more monsters and meanies. In M. Yapko (Ed.), *Brief therapy approaches to treating anxiety and depression* (pp. 150–170). New York: Brunner/Mazel.

Mills, J. C. (2006). The bowl of light: A storycraft for healing. In L. Carey (Ed.), *Expressive and creative arts methods for trauma survivors* (pp. 207–213). Philadelphia: Jessica Kingsley.

Mills, J. C. (2009). *StoryPlay® therapy* [DVD]. Pheoniz, AZ: Imaginal Press.

Werner, E. E. (1995). Resilience in development. *Current Directions in Psychological Science, 4,* 81–82.

Werner, E. E., & Smith, R. S. (1992). *Overcoming the odds: High risk children from birth to adulthood.* Ithaca, NY: Cornell University Press.

Werner, E. E., & Smith, R. S. (2001). *Journeys from childhood to midlife: Risk, resilience, and recovery.* Ithaca, NY: Cornell University Press.

CHAPTER 13

Family Play Therapy

PRACTICAL TECHNIQUES

Greg Czyszczon
Scott Riviere
Dianne Koontz Lowman
Anne L. Stewart

George Bernard Shaw once said, "A happy family is but an earlier heaven," and certainly for many families the memories created growing up are some of the happiest memories of all. Other families experience great difficulty generating positive memories and experience significant challenges when attempting to move beyond the confines of their earliest family-of-origin patterns of thinking, feeling, and behaving. Most families bequeath to their children a varied and complex set of memories, full of helpful and less helpful patterned ways of responding to people, everyday events, and stressors. As a relatively new intervention weaving play into family therapy modalities, family play therapy (FPT) invites family members to engage with one another in ways that are mutually satisfying and relationally edifying.

Scott Eberle of the Strong National Museum of Play describes the functions of play that can also be applied to desired qualities of satisfying family dynamics: anticipation, surprise, pleasure, understanding, strength, and poise (as cited in Brown, 2009). As desirable elements of family life, these qualities are evoked in the simple process of play—a process that families in distress may find difficult to access owing to trauma or stress. The practice of FPT aids families in moving beyond obstacles in order to experience joy while providing a context for a deeper vision of what family can be.

Theoretical Foundations and Current Context

FPT takes its place in a long history of therapeutic methods designed to address both the well-being of family members and the family as a whole. According to Nichols (2012), most sources point to the period after World War II as the period that set the stage for the development of family therapy. Four different clinical and scientific developments contributed to the emergence of family therapy. Researchers such as Bateson, Schism, and Bowen, concerned about the family's role in the development of schizophrenia, proposed a new and controversial conceptualization: namely, that disturbances in the family relationships caused mental disorders (Nichols, 2012). Marriage and premarital counseling that focused on treating couples' relationship difficulties and the child guidance movement also considered the prominent role the family played in determining behavior in adulthood. Lastly, Bion and Klein's work on group process and dynamics stressed the need for dealing with current problems in the "here and now" and emphasized that the group is a unit within itself and a carrier of change (Goldenberg & Goldenberg, 2007, p. 112).

In the 1990s, distinct schools of thought faded in a move toward integration and eclecticism, with overlap and borrowing between the different perspectives. At the same time, managed care fueled the search for brief techniques. Constructionists encouraged family therapists to help families examine their belief systems rather than attempting to change underlying structural or behavioral patterns (Goldenberg & Goldenberg, 2007). Today's family therapists pay close attention to class, ethnicity, gender roles, cultural, and spiritual influences in the family members' lives. Evidence-based interventions are emphasized by researchers, consumers, and insurance companies to provide effective (and cost effective) clinical services (Nichols, 2012; Stanton & Welsh, 2012).

It is in this contemporary context that FPT emerged as a way to bring the power of play to families. In keeping with her role as a leader in the field in the United States, Eliana Gil first wrote of FPT in her book *Play in Family Therapy* (Gil, 1994). Gil outlined in great detail the historical threads knitting the modality together and provided specific interventions for practitioners. Other works followed, including contributions by Lowenstein (2010), Mullen and Rickli (2011), and Munns (2009).

Related to FPT are other play-based family and filial therapy approaches that incorporate parents in the therapeutic process (see Ariel, 1992; Booth & Jernberg, 2009; Landreth & Bratton, 2006; Schaefer & Carey, 1994; VanFleet, 2005). Higgins-Klein (2013) outlines nine characteristics of what she calls *mindfulness-based play–family therapy* (MBPFT): conducting an evaluation phase, having parents present with the child when significant issues are being discussed, keeping the child's play imaginary, maintaining versatility, holding a multicultural perspective, using contextual family therapy, using mindful parent meetings, including multiple family members, and maintaining ongoing cooperation and collaboration with other professionals (pp. 23–27).

In our conceptualization, FPT contributes anew to the field of family therapy in that it operates as a systemically informed modality at the level of *family vision* by inviting families to imagine and participate in creating an alternative vision of what *family* can be (Waters & Lawrence, 1993). Families often come to therapy in some manner of crisis, a reactive space in which they are responding primarily to events that emerge from day to day, "putting out fires" without being able to enter into more satisfying modes of action. Family therapy approaches support families differently, potentially allowing family members to engage with deeper action modes. For example, structural family therapy is well known for inviting families to create a more satisfying organization of family roles as members experience how to relate to one another differently. FPT offers an intergenerational rootedness that may require parents to challenge their own patterned ways of relating, as members often do not see play as vital to family functioning. In this manner, FPT interventions invite caregivers to examine family values, and in so doing, they provide substantial leverage for change. Affecting a shift in the family's vision is a sure way to shift the mental models, structures, patterns, and events that define daily life. We might imagine a family's vision as similar to a seed from which all other attitudes and behaviors spring. If a seed does not include playfulness, love, acceptance, caring, and empathy, the fruits will not contain those qualities.

Parents who bring their children for play therapy are often struggling with challenging behaviors and turn to a therapist to help "fix" the child. Although individual play therapy is a profoundly important and useful modality, often a systemic view of a child's behavioral and emotional difficulties is helpful and allows for work with the family as a whole (Stanton & Welsh, 2012). When parents are exceedingly frustrated, angry, "at their wit's end," and looking for relief, they may be stuck in unsatisfying patterns that ignore the family's strengths, unique moments of joy and connection, and resilience. FPT addresses each of those areas, appealing to parents to take the lead in shaping a playful present and future.

Clinical Application

It is said that the family that plays together stays together. Clinically, a therapist must consider when and where FPT might be a useful modality for a family so that play can be used most effectively to support more satisfying relationships within the family.

Foundational Skills

Foundational skills for the therapist include the following:

• *A genuine interest in working with families.* Feeling confident and being competent with the population served will have a positive impact on the therapeutic alliance.

• *Enjoyment of family therapy.* Family therapy can sometimes be a challenging modality because of the different dynamics and the amount of relational information present in the room to make sense of at any given time.

• *Being comfortable with ambiguity.* Particularly when working with families that have young children, a level of uncertainty will likely emerge that can aid the therapist in maintaining an attitude of openness and curiosity.

• *The ability to focus and attend in a particular way.* Noticing small moments that illustrate larger relational patterns requires that we practice staying mindful and immediate for the entirety of a session.

• *The ability to convey respect.* Understandably, it is often difficult for families to enter into the therapeutic process or to make that decision to go to therapy. Some members may be more engaged in treatment than others (especially if family members were "forced" to attend). As a clinician, it is important to respect and honor the different levels of engagement of family members from the moment they come through the door until termination.

• *Emotional stamina.* Working with families can require much more emotional energy than individual work.

• *A genuine sense of humor.* A lighthearted approach to some of the heavier issues that family members bring can help them change their perspectives and look at their situations in a way that makes healing seem possible.

• *A playful style.* Part of this work is learning how to be comfortable with who you are and recognize that your unique style may be the agent of change that the family needs (Hughes, 2013).

Considerations for the Family

Therapists should consider the use of FPT to meet specific objectives in the course of treatment and be mindful of scenarios for which its use might be overwhelming for a family. It is crucial for the therapist to assess the level of physical and psychological safety in the family. Some questions to ask of families for whom a therapist is considering this modality are the following:

- Can the members tolerate the level of openness necessary in FPT, or is the family so rigidly bounded that such ambiguity represents too much of a psychological threat?
- Do family members have sufficient capacity for emotional reciprocity that FPT can build more of this ability?
- Have any members been traumatized or abused by others in the family so that trust cannot be safely established yet?
- Are there any members who are so hostile and angry that they are unable to interact without verbal violence and threats toward others?

Finally, the primary focus of FPT is the "process" and not the "product." The activities we present later in this chapter are a means to an end, not an end in themselves. *How* a family completes an activity is the essential component in coming to understand, support, and develop the family's capacity to grow into healthier, more satisfying and playful functioning. In FPT, the focus is on each person's contribution, as well as the "tenor" of the family as a whole. Challenging family members can sometimes help them see that they can do things that previously seemed impossible. The therapist is in the role of noticing moments in which a gentle suggestion, a nod of support, or an empathic phrase can hold a family member's tender attempt to step out of an old role and into a new way of being within the family. Such moments typically emerge during later stages of FPT; it is to the stages of the work that we now turn.

Stages of FPT

We have worked with hundreds of families in our collective experience, all different. However, the process that families go through when entering therapy is relatively consistent. An awareness of the consistent stages of this process is helpful as the therapist tracks a family's overall progress through therapy. We provide a general outline of the process, with the recognition that each therapist will approach this modality somewhat differently. Our hope is that therapists will integrate their own theoretical orientation, clinical skill, and awareness of their own family-of-origin legacy into a unique, meaningful, and effective FPT approach.

Initial Stage

In the initial stage of therapy, family members are entering into an experience that may be quite new for them. Whether new or familiar, it is likely that participation will vary, and family members may exhibit confusion about what is expected. Additionally, family members may express doubt regarding the effectiveness of the therapy and may demonstrate a low level of commitment and trust in the process. Parents may have a strong sense that the child is the problem and may feign play as though role playing. At this point in the therapy, it is crucial for the therapist to hold all of this anxiety while simultaneously establishing that FPT is emotionally safe for the family. It is helpful for the therapist to role-model what is expected and to provide clear structure during this stage.

CLINICAL CASE EXAMPLE

Mr. and Mrs. Dean referred their 8-year-old son Jeffery for counseling due to his difficulties in dealing with his anxiety, anger, disrespect for authority, and low self-worth. During the assessment, it was noted that Jeffery had failed to develop peer relationships appropriate to his developmental levels. He didn't play well with the boys in the neighborhood or his younger brother at home. He was bossy and resistant to authority at home. Observations indicated that he had difficulty correctly reading or imitating nonverbal behaviors, including facial expressions. These difficulties made it hard for him to navigate basic social interactions. He was intensely preoccupied with trucks and ambulances beyond what would be expected for his age; he demonstrated repetitive motoric activity, including walking on his tiptoes and picking at sores. There was no evidence of a delay in his language development or in cognitive development or skills. The parents reported he had recently been identified by the school system for special education services as a child with autism spectrum disorder.

During the initial session, Mrs. Dean indicated that her husband felt Jeffery was misbehaving and should be able to control his behavior; in addition, she said that Mr. Dean felt she was too "soft" on Jeffery. Mrs. Dean said that "Jeffery behaves better for his father," and it was clear that his father was extremely stern and somewhat authoritarian at times. According to the parents, at home Mrs. Dean did activities with the children, whereas Mr. Dean had relatively little interaction with them.

Case Analysis. In the initial stage of this case, we first did a comprehensive assessment of the family that included meeting first with the parents for a clinical interview and developmental history. In the next two sessions we administered the Marschak Interaction Method Behavior Rating Scale (Booth & Jernberg, 2009; McKay, Pickens, & Stewart, 1996) to each parent and the child, and we met with the entire family to begin the process of introducing the modality of play. Initial impressions of these interactions included our observation of many satisfying, attuned interactions between Jeffery and each of his parents. Additionally, we noticed that Jeffery's younger brother appeared to struggle with his own developmental issues. Both parents appeared overly focused on task completion and demonstrated little spontaneity in various play activities. Of significance at this stage was Mrs. Dean's sense of herself as not being a good play partner with her child and Mr. Dean's level of frustration with Jeffery, in particular.

Our goal was to use play with the family as well as with Jeffery and each of his parents in order to support the parents in recognizing their children's delight in the process of play. We also wanted to build on the parents' underutilized capacities to provide leadership with their children in an environment of safety and enjoyment, with the recognition that doing so would provide crucial experiences of emotional coregulation. For the parents, the experience would involve recognizing their children's signals more clearly and providing leadership as a soothing presence; for the children, the experience would be one of feeling safe enough to allow themselves to be soothed. We would then help the parents gradually learn to apply those same coregulatory experiences in situations where their children needed them to help regulate feelings of fear, sadness, or anger.

Transition Stage

As families gain a degree of comfort with the process, they move through a transition stage that has its own unique set of observable behaviors. In this stage, family members, particularly children, may push against the rules, boundaries, and limitations set by the therapist. Family members may struggle with how much to engage in the process of play as they discern how (and whether or not) to enter into new ways of experiencing themselves in the family. Parents, in particular, may struggle to trust the emotional safety and effectiveness of the play atmosphere as they find ways to move into genuine and playful engagement with each other.

In this stage the therapist's mindful attention affords the sensitivity to notice the delicate moments when new attitudes and behaviors are possible. Here the therapist can invite such risks by family members while maintaining a "whole-family" stance as the nature of play may challenge long-held and possibly distorted ideas about power and authority. The therapist follows the child's natural inclination to play while inviting the parents to join more deeply and authentically with the process. The issue of trust with the therapist may become overt for parents as the therapist creates the safety necessary for genuine play.

Conflict may emerge in a particular way at this stage and manifest as "stuckness." Whereas a simple acknowledgment is sometimes sufficient to get the family moving forward (e.g., "It seems like we are stuck?" or "What is not being said right now?"), other families may require individual, dyadic, or subsystem (parental, couple, or sibling) check-ins if addressing the conflict directly in the room is too difficult. During this time, the therapist can help the family member clarify what needs to be said and some appropriate ways to communicate the message. The therapist can rehearse with the various family members and help them communicate their individual wants, needs, and desires more effectively.

CLINICAL CASE EXAMPLE

We now find the Dean family in the transition stage of FPT. Theraplay activities, which are part of an attachment-based approach, were initiated with each parent and Jeffery to increase the parents' sensitivity, foster security of attachment, and foster spontaneous delight in playing. After 5 weeks of Theraplay activities with Jeffery and his mother and one week with Jeffery and his father, the parents came in to talk to the counselor. They said that, although they thought that Jeffery enjoyed playing with them in the sessions, they felt that nothing had changed in Jeffery's behavior at home. As a team, Jeffery's parents and the counselor discussed a recent incident that took place at a local activities center. The counselor wondered how Jeffery might approach this highly stimulating and unstructured environment. Mr. Dean said that it was helpful to think about how Jeffery might be thinking and viewing the world. He wondered if it would be helpful for him to spend more time with Jeffrey playing and giving him attention.

Case Analysis. Since we observed that many of the challenges at this point involved Jeffery specifically, we sought to focus our work on his relationships with his parents in the context of the family. We still viewed the family as a system that would benefit from strengthening the bonds between each parent and Jeffery. Unfortunately, the father's work schedule made it difficult to meet with him as frequently as all would have liked; however, we were able to maintain a whole-family stance while working with different subsystems of family members (parent–child, siblings, parents). We maintained a connection with the father by jointly composing messages to deliver to him after any family play session he could not attend.

Consistent with this stage in the process, Jeffery's parents wondered how much their work in play therapy was helping. For them, relief from the struggles they had been experiencing with Jeffery's behavior in the home was paramount. We responded to their concerns by maintaining our FPT sessions and providing some specific suggestions regarding how they might approach Jeffery during his more difficult moments. We also consulted with Jeffery's teacher and linked them with a well-respected child development clinic to conduct a comprehensive psychological evaluation with individualized recommendations for the school and home. We thoughtfully supported their efforts in beginning to wonder about how each of their children was thinking and feeling at any given moment. In supporting their capacities to notice joy and contentment, we gradually helped build their capacities to notice moments in which each of their children began to show subtle signs of anger and hurt. We coupled this with considerations of each child as being on the autism spectrum, recognizing that each child had unique needs.

Working Stage

During the working stage of FPT, trust and connection with the family members increases, and communication tends to be more open and accurate. Power and authority begin to be shared, and members are more likely to take risks and receive acceptance. Conflict is recognized and dealt with openly, and feedback can be given freely and without judgment. More and more, family members feel supported in their attempts to change.

Although the family is typically making progress toward its goals, it is important to stay vigilant during this stage and be mindful of regression of any family member. Therapists should continue to model appropriate behavior while they provide support to members to confront any remaining obstacles. Commitment to the therapeutic process is an important part of the working stage with families. Initially, the concept of commitment can be addressed through an overt discussion of what the family can expect to do during FPT, the importance of attending the sessions consistently, being fully present (mindful) during the sessions, and inviting oneself to be as open and honest as possible. It is not uncommon for one or more members of the family to have difficulty maintaining their commitment, so the therapist should monitor this area throughout the therapeutic process and explore when appropriate. It is the therapist's job to support the family in questioning the effectiveness of the work and being sufficiently invested for change to take place. Another way of thinking about commitment to the therapeutic process is to imagine it as instilling hope. One way of helping members commit to FPT is to continue to give each one a voice on setting up how the time will proceed.

Toward the end of this stage, the therapist may step back and challenge the family to create activities that will increase family cohesion (e.g., "What do you want to do today?"). Additionally, the therapist should help the family transfer insights learned during the sessions into action. We now return to the Dean family to see how this stage has played out in their process.

CLINICAL CASE EXAMPLE

With the Dean family, the next series of counseling sessions involved a combination of one or both parents (when the father wasn't working), Jeffery, and his little brother. During this time, Mrs. Dean asked for some assistance with Jeffery's little brother, who appeared also to demonstrate characteristics of a child with autism spectrum disorder (ASD). Specific strategies (e.g., a visual schedule, choice board, wait card) were suggested and added to the individualized education program (IEP) at school. The family developed a family vision collage that illustrated a family that was both unconventional and happy. The family brainstormed ways to give both parents time with each child and with each other. Looking to the future, Mr. and Mrs. Dean were able to see both children finding something each was passionate about and following that as a career.

Case Analysis. Having moved through the transition stage, the family was now ready to work more specifically on dyadic and triadic relationships as well as on their family life with everyone in the room. It was here that the parents became more open to and engaged in exploring the relational challenges confronting both of their children. The parents held different opinions regarding the diagnoses of ASD. Mrs. Dean was much more open to the idea of the children having a diagnosis of autism, possibly because she did most of the caregiving and had more contact with them. Mr. Dean was reluctant to consider such diagnoses and tended to attribute behaviors and compromised affect regulation strategies to his older boy's (in particular) just being bad and needing more direct control. Here the reader is reminded of the initial few sessions in which Mr. Dean indicated that he thought Mrs. Dean was "too soft" on the kids; part of the working stage was to evoke from the Deans a more balanced approach when addressing what they considered to be problematic behaviors in the home.

In this stage we were able to support the family in articulating a clear and satisfying vision, using the exercise we describe below. In describing their family as "unconventional but happy," the Dean's vision captured a resilient quality, something that we consistently nurtured with a strengths-based approach to the family's interactions. Mr. and Mrs. Dean were also able to develop a vision for their children's future, something that had been difficult to imagine in the midst of the many crises they were attending to when therapy began.

Additionally, the parents' narrative regarding behavioral difficulties in the home began to shift from one in which they saw their children as misbehaving to one that put a primacy on each child's unique developmental needs. Mr. and Mrs. Dean deepened in their ability to consider empathically what each child was thinking and feeling and to respond with a greater sense of understanding for each child's tendencies. In addition to ameliorating some of the tantrums, this new parenting approach also provided the Deans with a frame that helped them understand, support, and engage with their children in more satisfying ways.

Termination Stage

The final stage in FPT is termination, a time full of mixed emotions. The therapist's guidance in the termination stage is critical in preserving the changes that have been made while allowing for a successful goodbye. Family members may feel excitement as well as anxiety and sadness regarding termination; after all, family members at this point in therapy have learned how to have fun together. Some family members may withdraw, others may worry about being able to continue the skills that they have learned, and some may even disagree that termination should occur.

During this stage of the process, the therapist should continue to assist family members in identifying and expressing their emotions, especially those in response to the upcoming termination. In addition, the therapist and family should co-create a maintenance plan to support family members' efforts when they are on their own. Activities can be very helpful during this time to aid family members in developing a sense of confidence in their ability to continue the changes they have made.

CLINICAL CASE EXAMPLE

The Dean family experienced positive changes in their therapy and was eager to continue with those. The children had become close to the counselor and did not want to leave therapy. In the closing sessions, the counselor was able to bring discussions into the room about accepting oneself as unique and growing up "on the spectrum." The counselor shared contact information for a national movement in which individuals with autism are increasingly describing themselves as "neuroatypical" and resist attempts of "neurotypicals" to put limitations on them. In this way, the counselor helped the Deans to see that their children have a unique and important view of the world that embraces the idea that "I like who I am." The counselor and the Deans co-created a plan to involve the Deans in a local support group for parents with children with ASD. The counselor was able to involve all family members in creating a closing ritual (discussed in the Strategies and Techniques section) that highlighted the important work that had been done, the contributions of each family member, and their hopes for the future. The Dean family said goodbye after many thank-yous and wishes for continued growth.

Case Analysis. Termination with the Dean family went very well, and the counselor was able to help each of them consolidate the changes they had made and integrate their emerging understanding of autism. Play was a consistent vehicle for the changes the Deans made in their view of themselves and their view of their family. At this last stage, the counselor was mindful of the power of co-creating a strength-based healing narrative for the family and did so thoughtfully; this process had the effect of supporting the Deans' new experience of authority as a collaborative and effective experience. The counselor's relationship with the parents was isomorphic to the parent's relationship with their children: as parents, they were now able to be in charge without needing to be in control.

Considerations for the Therapist Regarding Special Populations

Therapists are likely to work with families who are experiencing stressors that result from adoption, medical issues, or developmental delays of children in the family. Because consideration of such challenges is important in the practice of FPT, we provide general recommendations for therapists to consider. First, therapists should have a good understanding of the nature of the difficulty, how long it has been occurring, and the manner in which the family has come to adapt to the needs of the child in question. A thorough intake assessment will achieve these objectives. A therapist should have some notions about how the parents view the difficulty and the degree to which the parents accept their child's challenges. It can sometimes be the case that a child has not yet been diagnosed, and part of the family's struggle is in managing behaviors and emotions for which they have no context. As shown in the case example above, part of the utility of FPT is in supporting parents to meet the child's unique needs more consistently and effectively. Part of the work involves educating parents about the particular challenges or disorder (in this case, of ASD) and in helping them to manage the emotions that invariably arise when confronted with unexpected or previously unknown information about one's children. The manner in which a therapist welcomes parents' emotional experience is a powerful model for the manner in which parents can learn to attend to a child's need for emotional co-regulation.

Strategies and Techniques

We offer several activities a therapist can consider using to address the therapeutic goals of families in FPT. These activities can be used to meet specific goals at a given stage in the process. Remembering that the purpose of each activity is the relational process, the therapist should provide attuned support, guidance, and encouragement as families interact and play together.

"The Rules Rule" Activity

Rules are important for many reasons, but the main benefit of this activity is to help family members understand that they have a say in the process of how the time in therapy is going to be used. The structure inherent in having rules also gives permission to assert needs; rules can create a sense of safety and security within the session and help families see the value of knowing what to expect.

To complete this activity, provide every family member with a different color of marker, and tape a large piece of paper to the wall. The therapist starts a conversation about the importance of rules that goes as follows: "We are ready to begin our family playtime, so that means we are ready to figure out what rules we want to start with. Everyone will have turns. Dad and Mom, each of you please tell us a rule you would like to be considered and write it on the paper." Continue around the room until everyone has had opportunity to name potential rules. If needed, the therapist should encourage parents to assist younger children in writing their rules. Lead the family in a conversation to select and modify the rules they wish to adopt for their FPT time. It is important to share that families often learn rules through interacting and unknowingly break a rule that is important to another family member.

After the rules are determined, you can ask, "Who do you think should have to follow the rules in here?" Most kids will say that they do; the ideal answer is "all of us." Affirm their response by acknowledging that everyone will follow the rules and that they all will get to discuss the proposed rules and suggest changes.

As an alternative, you may wish to conduct the Rules Rule activity by introducing a number of rules for the family to consider and edit. You can start the activity by noting that some rules are important in making family members feel comfortable. The rules can be put in a basket and pulled out by family members or just presented by the therapist and discussed together. We have found it helpful to write the rules on pieces of tagboard or paper plates to create some kind of tangible and visual reminders. The therapist and family members can "look over" the rules and consider them together. The first rule might be *Nobody gets hurt*. This rule helps to establish that physical safety will characterize this time spent together. Talk briefly about physical boundaries and the limit of the time so that everyone can feel safe. Another rule could be *No laughing or making fun of serious stuff*. This rule helps to establish the emotional safety of the therapy experience. The therapist can briefly discuss situations that may have come up with friends or family in which an emotional topic was brought up and they either laughed about it or minimized the seriousness of it. The *We can talk about anything* rule can be used to establish a level of permissiveness in family sessions that the family may not have at home. Obtaining verbal permission from all the members when this rule is suggested can be beneficial. For example, ask the parents, "Mom and Dad, is it okay if we talk about things that make you happy? Is it okay if everyone talks about things that make them sad? Makes them mad? Makes them scared or worried? Can we talk about the past? Talk about the present? Talk about the future?" Most parents respond with a yes, and after several questions and affirmative replies, a lighthearted laugh emerges from the children to hear their parents says yes over and over.

The next rule, *Tell the truth*, emphasizes the importance of being honest with each other. If a family member knows that another person has done something, have the courage to tell the person rather than ask. In the same way, it is important that the therapist speak openly and honestly with the family as well. Another potential rule is *We can have fun*. The therapist will spend some time talking about how some issues experienced by families are often not funny, but that doesn't mean families can't have fun learning how to cope and deal with difficult things. After everyone has completed the rules and identified the things that they need to make the time feel safe and secure, each person (including the therapist) signs the document to acknowledge agreement with the rules.

Although rules help family members feel safe, security is another important concept of family health that needs to be addressed. Security comes from consistency and predictability, from having rules and from acknowledging when a rule is broken. Initially, the therapist may play an important role in modeling how to respectfully confront a lapse. Of course, this must be done in a culturally congruent manner. Members of the family may test to see if the rules are going to be enforced. Examples of rule breaking include making fun of another family member, threatening to cross a physical boundary, or talking about things that other people said outside of sessions. When a rule is broken, it is important that someone immediately acknowledge that the rule was broken. Initially this responsibility will likely fall on the therapist, but eventually the members of the family should be encouraged to confront rule breakers in a timely manner. The simple technique of acknowledging the breaking of a rule can have a tremendous therapeutic benefit toward establishing security. The acknowledgment that a rule was broken helps create an opportunity for the offending person to take responsibility and make amends. Ideally, family members will begin to stand up for the rules that they established for themselves.

Spider Web Activity

One of the challenges family members sometimes face is in recognizing their particular role in an unsatisfying family dynamic. The Spider Web activity can help illustrate the concept of family systems theory (Bowen, 1978) and assist family members in seeing that everyone in the family has a role in the current situation.

For this activity, the therapist needs a ball made of approximately 100–150 feet of yarn. This size ball should be sufficiently large to accommodate the several unravelings involved in the activity. The family sits in a circle in the room and the therapist's instructions are as follows: "This activity is called Spider Web. I'm going to start off by wrapping this end piece of yarn around my hand and ask a question. I will gently toss the ball of yarn to someone who will then answer the question. That person will wrap the yarn loosely around his or her hand and toss the ball to another family member, who will do the same. We will keep playing until everybody has answered the question at least one time. After that, I will ask another question [or introduce another topic]." This activity takes anywhere from 30 minutes to an hour depending on how many questions you ask, the ages of the children, and how much each member of the family discloses. The therapist is encouraged to participate in this activity to increase the solidarity and connection/commitment to the family. The first round question is typically something that is easy to answer and focuses on the positive. For example: "What is something that you do that makes your family life better?"; or "What is one thing that you would like to do in your family?"; or "What is your favorite memory in your family?"

After each person answers that initial question, introduce a second question that may be a little more intimate. For example: "What is something you do that causes stress in your family?"; "What is something you do that creates conflict in the family?"; "What is something you do that makes the family angry?"; or "What is something you do that scares other members of the family?"

The third round of questions might consist of even more difficult topics to talk about. For example: "What is something that you have a hard time letting go of?"; "What does your family need to do or stop doing in order to be happy?"; "What are the things you do for which you tend to blame others?"; or "What are things you have a hard time changing?" Each person answers the question and wraps the string around his or her hand each time. The question for the final round tends to be one that calls upon family members to change. For example: "What is something you are willing to do this week that will make your family life better?"; or "What are you willing to stop doing this week so that your family gets along better?"

After several rounds of answering these questions, the entire family and therapist are connected together with this yarn in what looks like a big spider web. The spider web is used to illustrate the concept of a family as a system in which the actions of one affect all in some manner. The activity proceeds with the therapist asking each family member to pretend that he or she is having a good day or a bad day (each member can pick). The therapist then asks each member of the family to pull his or her string (one at a time), and if another member of the family feels that pull, he or she simply raises his or her hand. Play several rounds of the game, so that each member can see that his or her actions have an effect on the other members. Next, open a discussion on how we can influence what effect we have on others. That effect can be a positive one or an unpleasant one. This activity can help increase parents' insight into how the current situation may be more of a family problem than just labeling a particular member of the family as the primary obstacle.

"What I Like about You" Activity

This activity invites each family member to list the things he or she likes about the others. Each person will need something to write on and something to write with; paper plates work well. Instructions for this activity are as follows: "I want each of you to take a paper plate and on one side of that plate, write your name and decorate it any way you wish. Once everyone is finished with decorating one side of their plate, we are going to start an activity called 'What I Like about You.'" Once everyone is done decorating their plate, give the following instructions: "Please pass your plate to the person on your left. That person is going to flip the plate over and write one thing that he or she likes about that person. For example, you may recall something that a family member does or does not do that has helped you. After everybody completes the first round, pass the plate to the next person, and the game will continue until each person's plate has been signed by every member of the family." After the plates have rotated around the circle several times, each person should get his or her original plate back. The back side is typically filled with affirmations from each member of the family. Family members are encouraged to take their plates home and hang them up in a place where they can be reminded of what their family enjoys about them.

Mirror Blocks Activity

This activity requires two identical sets of 7–10 wooden blocks (in a variety of shapes). The instructions for this game are simple, and most families can complete this activity within a 30-minute period. Instructions go somewhat like this: "I will need somebody in the family who thinks he or she is good at communicating to volunteer for one role, and I will need somebody in the family who thinks he or she is good at listening to volunteer for another role. Finally, I will need

somebody to volunteer to help. The goal of this activity is for the good communicator to create a design with the blocks and for the good listener to be able to re-create the exact design without being able to see what the first person did." Once the members of the family have volunteered for each of those three positions, the therapist asks the person who volunteered to be the good communicator to sit on one side of the table and the person who volunteered as a good listener to sit on the other side of the table. The therapist sets up a simple barrier between the two people so that they cannot see what the other person is doing (I typically use the lid to a board game turned on its side). Once the people are across from each other with the barrier between them, the therapist distributes the blocks to each person so that each has an identical set of blocks that are different shapes.

The therapist explains to the person in the good communicator role to place one block on his or her side of the barricade, and then write on a small index card what he or she just did. The good communicator volunteer then hands the written note to the helper, who in turn gives it to the person who volunteered to be the good listener. The good listener then reads the note and follows the instructions that the good communicator wrote. After the good communicator has placed the second block of the design, he or she then writes what was done on another index card, hands it to the helper, who then gives it to the good listener—who will follow the instructions that were written and place the second block. This activity continues until the good communicator has placed all of his or her blocks, passed written instructions for each step, and the good listener has completed the design.

After this activity is finished, if it has been done correctly, the design on each side of the barrier should be the same. However, it is often the case that the design does not match. The therapist's role in this activity is simply to watch how this family is completing this task. Do they follow the rules? Does one person try to sneak a peak? Are subtle, nonverbal cues given that a block was placed correctly or not? Once the activity is completed, the therapist takes the instructions that have been written on the index card and reads them out loud in the order that they were received just so the good listener (and everybody else in the family) can check or cross-check to see if the blocks were placed correctly. Once the instructions have been reread out loud, the barrier is removed so that each person can see his or her creation. It is always rewarding to see the joy that is on the faces of family members when the design is similar or exact.

The therapist then uses this opportunity to talk a little bit about the three types of communication and what each part of the game symbolizes. The design that was created by the person who thought he or she was a good communicator is labeled *What I wanted to say*. What was written on the card goes under the category *What I did say*, and the design that is on the other side of the barrier is called *What I heard*. The therapist then asks each family member to self-assess what each one thinks are his or her particular strengths or weaknesses: "Are you good at communicating what you really want or need?"; "Are you good at perceiving what was said, or do you sometimes misinterpret what the person was trying to say?"; and "Are you good at identifying the things you actually want to say versus having difficulty communicating your needs or wants?"

After all members of the family have identified their strengths and weaknesses, the therapist then spends some time talking about techniques that they can use to improve their particular weaknesses. For example, if a person realizes that it is difficult for him or her to identify what he or she is thinking or feeling, the person might be able to use a feeling word list to help recognize what emotions he or she is experiencing. If a member has difficulty communicating accurately what he or she is thinking or feeling, the person might benefit from letter writing or finding a song that accurately expresses what he or she thinks or feels. If a person misinterprets what other people say, he or she could practice the skill of reflective listening and repeating back what the other person says.

Before-and-After Sandtray

Supplies needed for this intervention are a sandtray, an assortment of miniatures, two index cards (one with the word *Before* on it and the other with the word *After* on it), and then some type of fencing down the center of the tray. The therapist sets up the sandtray by placing the fencing down the middle of the tray vertically and placing the *Before* card on the back side of the left-hand side of the tray and the *After* card on the back of the right side of the tray. The instructions for this activity go something like this: "We are going to do what is called a *Before-and-After Sandtray*, and I will need somebody to volunteer to go first. Using the miniatures, make a scene in the sandtray to express what your life was like before the event happened. (The event is a significant happening for the family, such as divorce, loss of a family member or friend, move to a new home or new city, etc.) Then on the right side of the tray, I want you to create a scene that shows what your life has been like afterward."

After the person is finished, the family will go into the playroom and the volunteer is given the opportunity to explain each side of the tray. After the person has finished explaining the tray, the therapist can ask if he or she is comfortable answering questions that people may have about the story. If the person agrees, then the family members as well as the therapist can ask questions. The therapist can ask questions that clarify the emotional content on each side. For example, "How did you feel over here versus over there?"; "What did you have to let go of to get here?"; "What was the hardest of the *after* section?"; "What was the best part of the *before*?"; "What was the worst part of the *before/after*?"; "How is your life better now versus how is your life worse?" Process questions such as these can help the person gain insight about the story that he or she may not have been aware of, and/or it can help the person communicate things verbally that might have been difficult to do otherwise.

After the person is finished, the therapist can ask if the individual wants a photograph, and a cellphone camera can be used to commemorate the process. The sandtray is then disassembled and made ready for the next family volunteer to create a Before-and-After Sandtray. The next person is given the opportunity to share the story of his or her sandtray and questions are asked if consent is given. This activity continues until all family members have had the opportunity to participate.

The Family Vision Collage

The supplies needed for this activity include several magazines, scissors, glue, and poster or tagboard. Encourage the family members to have fun with this activity and to create a collage that they would be willing to hang up somewhere in the house. The instructions to this activity are as follows: "What I would like for you all to do is to create a collage of the hopes and vision you have for your family for the next year to 5 years." Family members then decide on the time frame that they want the collage to encompass. Ask members to go through the magazines and cut out words or pictures that best describe how they would like for their family to be within the time frame that they chose. This activity can take anywhere from 60 minutes to two or three sessions. Encourage conversation throughout the process of cutting out their pictures or words. Sample statements and questions might include: "Say a little bit about why you picked that picture"; "How does that word represent how you want your family to be?"; "What are you going to need to do different in order to achieve that?" Ques-

tions like these can prompt each family member to open up about his or her hopes and dreams and wishes for the family.

After the collage is complete, family members are asked where they want to display it. Encourage them to select a place where they can see it daily to be reminded of what they want to achieve. Examples include using their collage as a covering for their coffee table; framing their collage and hanging it up in the home or taping it to the refrigerator. The value of the family vision collage is that it helps the family focus on aspirations for the future and encourages members to dream about the possibilities for their family. In addition to generally engaging the family in a fun, positive activity, the collage making can also help each person identify what things he or she needs to change or work on. The Family Vision Collage is also a very good closure or termination activity for a family. It helps all the parties involved to create a transitional object from the scheduled therapeutic time in the therapy office back to the real life in their home.

The Goodbye Game

Termination is a very important part of the therapeutic process, and having a way of assisting the family through this phase can be beneficial. The Goodbye Game instructions are as follows: "Sometimes in life we don't get an opportunity to have a good goodbye. When this happens, we are often left wishing that we could have said something or told that person how we really felt. So in this activity we are going to take an opportunity to tell each other what we like about him or her or what changes we have seen the person make. One of you will go first, and you will pick a family member and share what you like about him or her, what changes you have seen the person make, or perhaps what hopes you have for him or her. After you tell the person your comment, all he or she can say is "Thank you." You will then go to the next family member and do the same thing, until you have told everybody what you think or how you feel. Somebody will then volunteer to go second and third and so on, until everybody has had an opportunity to share." The therapist is encouraged to participate in this activity with the family as a way to role-model acknowledging feelings about termination and to give family members an opportunity to express their thoughts and feelings about the time together.

Conclusion

FPT is an exciting and useful therapeutic modality that can be implemented with a variety of families. This format challenges therapists and families alike to reinvent their vision as one that includes play as an ongoing, constructive, and important aspect of what it means to be a family. Although FPT is a relatively new way of working with children and families, in some ways it is as old as humanity in its emphasis on play as relationally edifying.

REFERENCES

Ariel, S. (1992). *Strategic family play therapy*. Somerset, NJ: Wiley.

Booth, P. B., & Jernberg, A. M. (2009). *Theraplay: Helping parents and children build better relationships through attachment-based play* (3rd ed.). Somerset, NJ: Wiley.

Bowen, M. (1978). *Family therapy in clinical practice*. New York: Aronson.

Brown, S. (2009). *Play: How it shapes the brain, opens the imagination, and invigorates the soul*. New York: Penguin.

Goldenberg, H., & Goldenberg, I. (2007). *Family therapy: An overview*. Boston: Brooks Cole.

Gil, E. (1994). *Play in family therapy*. New York: Guilford Press.

Higgins-Klein, D. (2013). *Mindfulness-based play–family therapy: Theory and practice*. New York: Norton.

Hughes, D. A. (2013). *Eight keys to building your best relationships*. New York: Norton.

Landreth, G. L., & Bratton, S. C. (2006). *Child parent relationship therapy (CPRT): A 10-session filial therapy model*. New York: Routledge.

Lowenstein, L. (2010). *Creative family therapy techniques: Play, art, and expressive activities*. Toronto, Ontario, Canada: Champion Press.

McKay, J., Pickens, J., & Stewart, A. L. (1996). Inventoried and observed stress in parent–child interactions. *Current Psychology, 15*(3), 223–234.

Mullen, J. A., & Rickli, J. A. (2011). *How play therapists can engage parents and professionals*. Oswego, NY: Integrative Counseling Services.

Munns, E. (2009). *Applications of family and group Theraplay*. Lanham, MD: Rowman & Littlefield.

Nichols, M. (2012). *Family therapy: Concepts and methods* (10th ed.). Boston: Allyn & Bacon.

Schaefer, C. E., & Carey, L. J. (1994). *Family play therapy*. Northvale, NJ: Aronson.

Stanton, M., & Welsh, R. (2012). Systemic thinking in couple and family psychology. *Couple and Family Psychology: Research and Practice, 1*(1), 14–30.

VanFleet, R. (2005). *Filial therapy: Strengthening parent–child relationships through play* (2nd ed.). Sarasota, FL: Professional Resource Press.

Waters, D. B., & Lawrence, E. C. (1993). *Competence, courage, and change: An approach to family therapy*. New York: Norton.

CHAPTER 14

Animal-Assisted Play Therapy

Risë VanFleet
Tracie Faa-Thompson

Robbie had spoken little and played tentatively during his prior 10 play sessions. He seemed to trust no one after years of maltreatment at the hands of his mother's boyfriends. He appeared to be unsure of himself and the situation, and he entered the playroom tentatively each time, manipulating some of the toys but not really playing as one might expect of a 6-year-old boy. Although I (VanFleet), his therapist, had considerable play therapy experience, I had been unable to connect well with him because of his ever-present suspiciousness. He seemed to like me well enough, but he was not about to let himself go, even though the playroom seemed safe enough. He had been brutally punished too many times to let his guard down with any human adults.

On this particular day, I met Robbie accompanied by my play therapy partner, Kirrie, whom Robbie had met the session prior. Kirrie is a highly trained play therapy dog, a rescued border collie–hound mix with an ever-present desire to play. Remembering what he had learned last time, Robbie told Kirrie to sit, and she did. He then held out his left hand, palm open toward the dog, and told Kirrie, "Kiss me!", and she touched her nose to his hand. Robbie giggled, "Kirrie remembers me!" During the play session that ensued, Robbie talked excitedly to Kirrie, offer-

ing her some small treats in exchange for her doing some "tricks," such as jumping through a hoop, picking up a toy and dropping it in a basket, and spinning around, first one way and then the other. There was little trace of Robbie's earlier reticence as he showed me the things he could get Kirrie to do, with a broad smile and an air of confidence. I reflected, "You're really pleased that Kirrie remembers you! . . . It's funny to you the way that Kirrie spins around. . . . You like it when she listens to you and does what you ask." Later, Robbie and I taught Kirrie a new trick, hopping into a big box and lying down.

When the session was over, Robbie asked if he could show the box trick to his foster mother, and he did so, narrating what he was doing and explaining how he had taught her this new trick. His foster mother marveled, "He's like a different kid!" Indeed, Robbie's behavior had changed rather dramatically, thanks to Kirrie's presence and responsiveness to him, and his ability to teach her something new. In just two sessions with the dog, Robbie was showing the impact of the social lubrication effects of a therapy dog. It was clear that animal-assisted play therapy (AAPT) was likely to be an excellent modality through which Robbie could learn to trust and grow.

Background

AAPT represents the full integration of two empirically supported approaches: play therapy and animal-assisted therapy (AAT) (see VanFleet, 2008). AAPT has been defined as "the involvement of animals in the context of play therapy, in which appropriately trained therapists and animals engage with children and families primarily through systematic play interventions, with the goal of improving children's developmental and psychosocial health as well as the animal's well-being. Play and playfulness are essential ingredients of the interactions and the relationship" (VanFleet, 2008, p. 19). AAPT is applicable to children, adolescents, and adults, and in individual, group, or family sessions. Play, playfulness, and humor help create the emotional safety necessary for clients to tackle their difficult emotions and problems in therapy. Although the types of play used might shift with the age of the client, a lighter atmosphere is invaluable in encouraging therapeutic progress in any-age client.

AAPT can be used as a nondirective, or child-centered, approach, or it can be used to teach skills or address specific problem areas through directive and cognitive-behavioral play therapy. Families can be involved in a variety of ways, as well. Because AAPT is grounded in play therapy, it has the same versatility as play-based interventions do.

The practice of AAPT has become more widespread in the past decade, although some play therapists have systematically incorporated dogs in their work for over 25 years (Marie-José Dhaese, 2012, personal communication), and others have written about their work and research with this modality (Crenshaw, 2012; Parish-Plass, 2008, 2013; Thompson, 2009; Trotter, Chandler, Goodwin-Bond, & Casey, 2008; VanFleet, 2008; VanFleet & Colţea, 2012; VanFleet & Faa-Thompson, 2010, 2012, 2014; Weiss, 2009). Dogs and horses are the species involved most frequently, but cats, rabbits, donkeys, turtles, and other species have been included as well (VanFleet, 2007).

In AAPT, the therapist includes a properly trained dog in play therapy sessions with clients or arranges for clients to visit a farm or stables for interventions involving equines. The animals function as partners in the therapeutic process, serving in a number of different roles designed to facilitate progress. AAPT practitioners typically are play therapists or family therapists who have learned to work with an animal partner in playful ways to address a wide range of possible therapeutic goals.

There are considerable benefits to clients in the use of AAPT, but there are also significant risks. It is critical that therapists obtain the appropriate training for themselves and their animals to ensure the safe and ethical practice of AAPT. The next section outlines the principles underpinning the practice of AAPT, and the rest of the chapter outlines some of the competencies, methods, ethical considerations, resources, and certification in AAPT. Illustrative case examples are included.

Principles

It is vital that AAPT is conducted in ways that support the high quality of play therapy and other psychotherapy intervention while simultaneously recognizing and protecting the animals' needs and welfare. Not only is it critical to consider animals' welfare for their own well-being, but to ensure that appropriate models of interaction are provided for children. The therapist–animal relationship serves as a metaphor for the therapeutic relationship as well as for relationships in general. Steps to create and demonstrate a positive relationship based on mutual respect and consideration with therapy animals must be taken. For example, if a therapy dog shows stress signals when children intrude in the dog's space, the therapist needs to address that behavior so the dog's comfort is restored. This intervention, in itself, is therapeutic for clients, and the therapist can process the need for such boundaries with clients in a variety of ways. Therapists who continue to work with tired, anxious, or bored animal partners are providing a very poor model of humane treatment and empathy for their clients. Principles that guide the therapeutic practice and decision making in AAPT can be found in VanFleet and Faa-Thompson (2010). (Space limitations do not permit their inclusion here, despite their importance for effective and ethical practice.)

Competencies Needed for AAPT

It is part of the ethical code of most mental health professions that therapists must practice within the scope of their competencies. This means that for any new treatment modality, they must obtain the appropriate training and supervised practice. In the case of AAPT, not only must the therapist develop new skills, the animals must be appropriately selected and fully prepared for the work as well. Although it might be tempting to take one's very sweet dog into play sessions to see how children respond, this can lead to serious problems for the dog, the clients, the therapist, and the entire field of AAT and AAPT. (Most of us would not want to be a surgeon's first patient for a new procedure if that surgeon had not been properly trained and supervised in the method!) Most practitioners of AAPT realize that it is one of the most complex forms of therapy they have learned and conducted. The following sections describe some of the key competencies that therapists must acquire to conduct AAPT effectively and ethically.

Competence in Play Therapy

Therapists must be skilled and experienced in all the major forms of play therapy, and they need to be able to use spontaneity, creativity, and playfulness during sessions.

They must also know how to select appropriate play interventions to meet child and family goals.

Competence in Knowledge of Animals

Therapists must develop considerable knowledge about the animals with whom they work. This includes understanding and respecting the unique species and individuals that they are and what drives their behavior. Therapists must also learn to read the animal's body language and communication signals in real time, and to interpret what those mean about the animal based on the whole body and the context. Despite living with animals their entire lives, most therapists who enter the field of AAPT learn that there is a whole other world of learning to take place. It is a critical skill to read body language in real time to ensure the well-being of the animal and to prevent potential injuries from occurring.

Competence in Animal Selection, Husbandry, Training, and Handling

In the case of dogs, therapists must learn what it means to select appropriate dogs for the work; socialize them; train them using dog-friendly, nonaversive methods; and then to work with clients to help them train or interact with the dogs. Therapists who work with horses must understand many of the same things about equines, as well as how to interact safely and positively with them, or a herd of them. Competence in these areas provides the foundation from which therapists can also help children develop humane attitudes and behaviors.

Competence in Facilitating Client–Animal Interactions and Relationships

This area represents some of the most complex features of conducting AAPT. Therapists must develop the ability to split their attention between client and animal, ensuring the well-being of both. They must also learn the most effective responses at any given moment and within different types of play therapy, all with an eye toward facilitating therapeutic goals. Therapists need to be versatile, sometimes teaching children about animals and their emotions, sometimes recognizing the metaphors and play themes through their empathic responses, sometimes reinforcing appropriate child behaviors with the animals, and using a wide range of counseling strategies to foster self-understanding, self-regulation, and behavior change. AAPT practitioners must keep track of a great deal, all the while keeping the goals of the clients in mind. The therapist needs to be able to use real-time moments to strengthen the process.

Competence in the Unique Challenges in AAPT

Inviting a nonhuman animal into the playroom adds new relationships into the therapeutic mix. The therapist has a relationship with the animal, most often because the animal lives with the therapist and is a companion. The child not only creates a relationship with the therapist, but also with the animals who are introduced. Sometimes, in the case of children who cannot trust humans, the relationship with the therapist is created through the social lubrication effects of the animal. Related to these effects is the issue of countertransference, which is far more likely in sessions in which the therapist is involving one of his or her own animals in the process. It is important for therapists to be aware of these critical dynamics and how the presence of the animal partner affects them and their work.

Developing these competencies takes time, training, experience, and supervision. On top of this, each animal involved in sessions needs to be assessed for appropriateness, trained, and prepared for the work. Much of the extensive preparation required to practice AAPT safely and effectively is fascinating, and it is likely that practitioners will find it rewarding. A certi-

fication program specifically in AAPT has been developed, and more information is available at *www.playfulpooch.org*.

Goal Areas of AAPT

There are five major goal areas that can be addressed through the use of AAPT (VanFleet & Faa-Thompson, 2010). In many cases, more than one area can be addressed simultaneously. Goal areas include (1) self-efficacy, (2) attachment/relationship, (3) empathy, (4) self-regulation, and (5) problem resolution. These areas are discussed in greater detail in VanFleet and Faa-Thompson (2010, 2014).

Child-Centered (Nondirective) AAPT

The principles and skills used in child-centered play therapy (CCPT) (Landreth, 2012; VanFleet, Sywulak, & Sniscak, 2010) are essential to the practice of all forms of AAPT, including more directive approaches. The use of empathy, attunement, imaginary play, and limits is valuable even when the therapist operates from a more directive stance or is working with groups. This section, however, focuses specifically on CCPT sessions used in a nondirective format, where the child selects the toys and how to play with them, and the therapist creates a safe and accepting environment in which the child can feel free to explore, play, and work through life's challenges in the playroom as he or she feels the need to do. Dogs are the primary species used in the types of CCPT sessions as described by Landreth (2012) and VanFleet and colleagues (2010).

Dogs for Nondirective AAPT

It takes a special type of dog to work in CCPT sessions. Nondirective play therapy dogs must have the right temperament to be interested and engaged in a range of playroom activities as selected by the child as well as to lie quietly in the corner of the room should the child decide not to include the dog in his or her play. The dog must also be trained to a significant degree, learning many skills and cues that can be used creatively by children. The dog, with minimal cueing from the therapist, must be able to take part in a wide range of play themes and choices, remaining relatively unperturbed by moving or noisy toys, swashbuckling children, and rapidly changing play scenarios. This is not to say that dogs must tolerate things that they truly dislike. At no time is a dog expected to put up with frightening or threatening gestures, uncomfortable costumes, or intrusive touching. Structuring and limit setting are used to help children treat the dog humanely and respectfully at all times. Even so, in CCPT, the dog needs to be comfortable with motion, noise, involvement, or no involvement, as the case may be. Anxious dogs need not apply. This is a job for a stable, people-oriented dog who is very adaptable.

Nondirective AAPT Play Sessions

During the play sessions, as with CCPT without animals, the child chooses which toys to play with and how to play with them; the child also determines the play sequences and themes. In AAPT, the therapist not only tracks and empathically listens to the child's primary play themes and feelings, engages in imaginary play when asked, and sets limits when necessary, but helps the dog do what the child wishes as well. This requires close attention to the child and his or her play, but also to the dog to ensure that the dog can play along as needed while remaining safe and comfortable. Sometimes the therapist "gives voice" to the dog, empathically listening through the dog or "speaking" for the dog when a role calls for this intervention. For example, the therapist might reflect through the dog, "Kirrie, Martin is putting on his policeman's hat. It looks like he's getting ready to go to

work. . . . Uh-oh! Kirrie, did you see that? Martin's chasing those bad guys! Things look pretty dicey there. . . . Martin caught them! Oh, Kirrie, Martin's very proud that he got those bad guys."

During imaginary play, the therapist helps the dog play the role as envisioned by the child. For example, when Sally says she is the teacher and Kirrie is her pupil, the therapist asks Kirrie to sit and stay in her "seat" in the classroom, and if Teacher Sally asks Kirrie if she knows the answer to a question, the therapist might cue Kirrie to give a "wave"—which approximates raising her hand in class. At the same time, the therapist might continue empathically listening (unless playing another role in the drama, in which case that role would take precedence): "Teacher Sally is asking tough questions. Looks like Kirrie has put up her hand!" Things can be even more complicated if the child has asked both the dog and the therapist to play different roles, and the therapist plays out his or her own role while helping the dog to do the same.

Limits during CCPT with a therapy dog are expanded to ensure the safety of the dog, but they are set in the same way as they are with other types of limits. The therapist states the limit specifically and then provides a general redirecting statement in order to permit the child an opportunity to solve whatever problem has come up. The therapist might say, "June, you're curious about Kirrie's ears, but one of the things you may not do is pinch Kirrie. You can do just about anything else." This gives June the chance to redirect her feelings and behavior away from an action that might hurt the dog. If the child attempts to break the same limit a second time, a warning is given, such as, "June, remember I said you may not pinch Kirrie's ear. If you try to do that again, we will have to leave the special playroom for today. But you can do just about anything else." Here, the limit is restated, followed by a warning of what the consequence will be, giving the child another chance for self-direction. The general redirection statement is included as before. Finally, if the child attempts to breach the same limit a third time, the therapist enacts the consequence as stated during the warning stage: "June, remember I said that we would have to leave if you tried to pinch Kirrie's ear? You chose to pinch again, so we must leave the special playroom for today." Once outside the playroom, the therapist can reassure the child that the dog and the therapist will see the child at their next session.

One additional consideration with play therapy dogs is to consider teaching the dog a cue to come immediately and move behind the therapist to safety—an "emergency cue" given when things are moving swiftly and the dog is in imminent danger of being hurt. This gives therapists the option to get the dog out of harm's way quickly while then establishing the limit with the child.

At all times during CCPT with a play therapy dog, the therapist attempts to stay within the principles and skills used in CCPT when no therapy dog is present. It can be rewarding for the child to forge his or her own unique relationship with the dog while working through various issues, but nondirective AAPT is not for the faint of heart. It requires superb CCPT skills and the ability to shift one's attention quickly back and forth from child to dog and back to the child. It is perhaps the most challenging form of AAPT to conduct properly.

Clinical Case Example (Therapist: VanFleet)

Jackie was 9 years old and in the fourth grade. She had missed several months of school the prior year due to injuries from a car accident. When she had returned to school, she had been whiny and demanding with her peers, perhaps due to residual pain and the stress of enduring intrusive medical treatments. Her classmates had at first been compassionate, but her demands for help and to do things her way eroded that over time, and by the end of the school year, she was largely left alone. Although her classmates had not been cruel to her, no one wanted to play or eat lunch with her anymore. Her parents brought her to play therapy, hoping that she would make a better adjustment to the accident experience that might in turn improve her peer relationships. When her parents learned that a therapy dog was available, they eagerly gave permission for Jackie to have sessions with Kirrie.

I first held a couple of play sessions with Jackie to get acquainted and for her to experience the nondirective atmosphere. Because of the loss of control she had experienced during the accident and treatment, as well as her pain and subsequent poor social adjustment at school, I thought that CCPT would offer her a number of benefits to make choices in her play that would be helpful to her. The family planned to participate in filial therapy (Guerney & Ryan, 2013; VanFleet, 2014a) with me later in the summer when their work schedules would be better.

During her first two play sessions, Jackie explored the playroom without settling on any one thing for long, as is typical of early play sessions. Jackie knew about Kirrie and asked when she would meet her. After finishing her CCPT session in the first 30 minutes of the second session, we used the remaining time to talk about how things might work with Kirrie. I taught Jackie how to meet and greet dogs safely, and gave her a letter that Kirrie had "written" featuring her picture and information about how she liked to play with children a great deal. I also taught Jackie some of Kirrie's primary cues, and we practiced using them with a life-sized stuffed toy dog, all done in a playful manner.

Kirrie joined us for the next several play sessions. Jackie was delighted and spent the first several minutes petting Kirrie and giving her treats when Kirrie performed the behaviors that Jackie cued. Jackie then told Kirrie that she was a "doggie doctor" and Kirrie was her patient. When Jackie moved to Kirrie with the stethoscope and doctor's kit, I provided empathic listening responses: "Kirrie, Jackie needs to check you out. You seem to need a doctor! . . . Here comes Dr. Jackie, the Doggie Doctor. She has her equipment all ready." I did not tell Kirrie to sit or stay because Jackie knew how to do that herself if she wanted to. Jackie did not give those cues, though, and kept following Kirrie around the playroom. I could see frustration growing in her nonverbal communication, so I reflected, "Kirrie isn't staying still for you. It's frustrating!" Jackie nodded and kept following Kirrie around. Eventually she turned to me and said, "Can you tell Kirrie to quit walking?" Again I reflected, "You want Kirrie to stay still so you can examine her." She nodded and looked at me expectantly. "And you'd like me to help with that." She nodded again. Because she had asked me directly, both verbally and nonverbally, to help, I then followed her lead and did so. I called Kirrie over nearer to the table where Jackie had the doctor's kit and told her to sit and stay. Jackie then examined Kirrie very carefully. Jackie looked at me and said, "Your dog is sick! Very, very, very, very sick." Since she had implicitly put me into an imaginary role, I played it as I believed she wished me to: "Oh, Dr. Jackie, I'm so sorry that she is sick, and I'm very, very, very worried." Jackie looked at me and said, "It's okay, lady, I know what I'm doing." This occurred near the end of the session, and Jackie left without incident. She went to the waiting room and told her mother that she was now Dr. Jackie, the Doggie Doctor. Later, her mother told me privately that she was amazed that Jackie had begun doctor play so quickly, as she had resisted attempts at the hospital to get her to play with the medical equipment and toys.

During her next session, Jackie resumed her Doggie Doctor play, very much as before. This time she said she had to give medicine and then "make Kirrie take it" because it was so yucky. She commented that she might have to "burp" Kirrie to get her

to take it. I reflected, "It's going to be very hard for Kirrie to take that awful medicine. She is not going to like it one bit." Jackie pretended to give Kirrie some medicine from a little plastic bottle, then moved behind Kirrie and stood at her side: "Kirrie, I'm going to have to burp you to make you swallow!" Jackie raised her hand high above Kirrie's back, and I could see her imminent plan was to strike Kirrie's back. I immediately set a limit in a calm, but firm voice: "Jackie, I see you want to burp Kirrie, but one of the rules in the special playroom is that you may not hit Kirrie at all. You can do just about anything else." Jackie looked disappointed but then began looking around the room. I empathically responded, "You're disappointed you couldn't burp Kirrie to get that medicine down; now you're looking around." Jackie then spied the small bottle of dog treats sitting on a table by the door. She picked that up and asked me if she could give some to Kirrie. I responded, "You'd like to give some to Kirrie and want to know if it's okay. Yes, you may give her some of those." Jackie smiled and said, "It's *medicine!*" She gave Kirrie several treats and declared Kirrie all better.

This play was repeated during the next two sessions, although the treatment changed from giving medicine to taking X-rays (Kirrie had to lie down while Jackie passed a horizontally held piece of drawing paper over her about a foot in the air above her) and bandaging her leg (Jackie found and used a self-sticking purple bandage). Jackie engaged in much more touch with Kirrie, stroking her gently and telling her she was "okay." She ended both of these sessions sitting on the floor with Kirrie lying beside her, stroking and massaging Kirrie's neck. Near the end of her fourth session with Kirrie, Jackie declared that Kirrie really was all better and did not have to see the doctor anymore. Kirrie and I, playing the roles Jackie had given us, thanked the Doggie Doctor, and I reflected what I saw on Jackie's face, "You're pretty happy when you make your patients all better!" Jackie smiled and said, "Yeah, sometimes they get better and they don't have to see the doctor anymore." I replied using empathic listening, "It's such a relief when they are all better and no more doctors."

Jackie's mother reported that after the second play session with Kirrie, and Jackie's fourth overall, she had been quite different at home, seeming happier and more relaxed. By the end of the fourth session with Kirrie, her mother said she was "like her old self again," with far less whining and demanding and much more playing and dancing around the house.

Kirrie continued to be part of Jackie's play sessions, but Jackie never again asked her to visit the doctor. Their roles became those of friends, and Jackie pretended that Kirrie was her best friend. It was not long after this that we began filial therapy sessions, and we gradually phased out Kirrie's and my individual work with Jackie as we phased in the filial therapy play sessions. By the time Jackie had to face some final medical procedures, her parents were well prepared to help her with her fears and discomfort through their parent–child play sessions and empathizing with her feelings. I later heard from Jackie's mother that she had made a good adjustment back at school and that things were going well in all regards.

It is entirely possible that Jackie would have found other ways of playing through her fears and regaining a sense of control over her life had AAPT not been available to her. I have worked with many children with medical problems using play therapy and filial therapy, and it is common for them to cope better with their problems and resolve issues surrounding pain, treatment, loss of control, feeling "different," and many other difficulties related to their illnesses or injuries through the use of play interventions. What made this case notable was how quickly Jackie was able to engage in the sessions with Kirrie, how focused her play was, and how thoroughly she was able to express her feelings about physical

injury and treatment. Her problems, which had lasted for months, abated in six play sessions, four of which included the dog. Although more sessions were held, the presenting problem was noticeably better according to her parents, and it remained so.

It seems likely that Jackie responded rapidly and thoroughly both because of the safety inherent in the play therapy process and because of a living therapy dog willing to play out the patient role with her. Kirrie responded to Jackie's ministrations with an occasional lick to Jackie's arm, or leaning against Jackie as they sat together on the floor. Kirrie not only could allow Jackie to play out her feelings about her medical experience, but she also provided the important medium of touch. For Jackie, whose injured body, out of necessity, had been treated with intrusive and sometimes frightening procedures, the ability to touch and be touched by the dog was important. Perhaps Kirrie also represented for her a more vulnerable being than herself— someone she could take care of in ways that she wished she would be taken care of. She was empowered by the doctor role in which she could dole out the treatments rather than be subjected to them. Many dynamics were at play, and it seemed that Kirrie was able to enhance them during this nondirective AAPT course of treatment.

Directive AAPT

Directive play therapy generally refers to a wide range of interventions in which the therapist plays a larger role in selecting the toys and/or the activities in which the child, adolescent, family, or group engages. Within the many directive play therapy options, there is a continuum of directedness. At one end, the therapist provides some light structure and gentle suggestions at the start of the session, and then plays a relatively nondirective role thereafter, reflecting feelings and supporting the clients through the process. On the other hand, the therapist might suggest a very specific activity designed to build psychosocial skills, or help clients work on designated need areas. The therapist might facilitate the interactions heavily in some cases, such as when a child learns to clicker-train a dog or a horse, where instruction in the method is important to prevent confusion to the animal and to help the child have a successful experience. AAPT can be applied all along this continuum.

Animals for Directive AAPT

Some dogs are more suited to directive AAPT, sometimes due to their higher energy levels, their tendency to "suggest" games to play, or their need for greater attention from the people involved. The wide array of interventions along the directive continuum means that there is a broad range of canine personality types who might be suitable for this work. There are some who are not appropriate at all, of course. An online course is available that provides guidance to play therapists in selecting puppies or rescued dogs who are likely to be more successful in this type of work (VanFleet, 2014b).

Horses, by virtue of their size, require outdoor space or a barn or arena, and this configuration typically produces greater structure than one might need to implement in a playroom. There are safety considerations as well, just as there are with dogs and any other species. Some structure in presenting activities adds to the physical and emotional safety of the program, although undue emphasis on safety can backfire by creating greater anxiety for clients. Some horses are well suited to working with children or family groups. In general, they are stable individuals who do not spook easily, who remain calm despite noise or movement, and who approach people readily and with interest. As with dogs, therapists must know a great deal about the nature of their animal partners, and at all levels: species, breed, and individual, with individual being the most important. In all cases, animal partners need to enjoy a trusting, reciprocal relationship with the therapist. A certification program in AAPT includes a thorough assessment of each animal on an Animal Appropriateness Scale, trained behaviors, and the therapist's plan for involving the animal, showing full awareness of the fit between the animal's unique strengths and needs and the therapeutic work planned (International Institute for Animal Assisted Play Therapy Studies, 2013; see also *www.playfulpooch.org*).

Directive AAPT Play Sessions

Directive AAPT sessions can be individual, group, or family in nature, and they run the full spectrum of relatively unstructured activities with a minimal amount of directedness to heavily structured interventions with much greater directedness, such as teaching the child or group a specific skill to use with a dog or horse or other animal. The therapist selects an activity involving the animal that can facilitate the clients' work toward particular therapeutic goals. Children might teach a new trick to the play therapy dog as a way to build their sense of competence and confidence; lead a horse through an obstacle course using only a ribbon to develop communication and problem-solving skills; pay attention and respond to animals' body language to work on emotional awareness and sensitivity; play an arousing game with a dog, interspersed with calm periods to improve impulse control; groom or massage a horse for empathy and relationship building; or work with a family or group to accomplish a fun challenge with a therapy animal that might seem impossible without teamwork and helping behaviors.

Play therapists blend their skill in conducting various play therapy interventions with the creative inclusion of the animal in the process. This integration of play therapy with AAT occurs throughout the process: when planning the activities; facilitating them in a lighthearted, playful manner as they occur; and debriefing them for very short periods at the end, mostly to learn clients' impressions, struggles, lessons learned, and sense of accomplishment or happiness. Sometimes the interventions are as simple as standing or sitting with the animal. As I (Faa-Thompson) have commented during workshops, "Standing close to horses may not be a cure-all, but it's as good a place as any to start." Other interventions create rather challenging tasks that show faith in the children's ability to solve them. The sense of accomplishment and mastery that follows hard work, persisting through frustration, facing one's fears, creative problem solving, and working together can provide tremendous therapeutic benefit. Other resources provide further examples of the breadth and depth of this approach (e.g., see Faa-Thompson, 2012a, 2012b; Trotter, 2012; VanFleet, 2008; VanFleet & Faa-Thompson, 2010, 2012, 2014).

Some play therapists might be interested in equine-facilitated play therapy but have no access to horses to do so. One model of practice that fits well with play therapy is that of the Equine Assisted Growth and Learning Association (see *www.eagala.org*). In this, certified mental health specialists team up with certified equine specialists to facilitate interventions as co-therapists. Often, the equine specialist has horses available.

Clinical Case Example (Therapist: Faa-Thompson)

Sometimes during AAPT, the animals lead the session in ways that the human therapists never could. When the therapist and the animal partner have a strong, mutual relationship, there is a give-and-take and trust that occur, sometimes resulting in changing roles within a session. Therapists who listen to what their animals are offering are sometimes rewarded with outcomes they might never have brought about using only their own ideas. Two case studies,

based on the same AAPT intervention involving horses, illustrate two very different ways of working. One might ask if one way is better than the other, and the answer lies in whether the approach used worked for the children involved. In each case, it did. The intervention is described first, followed by each of the cases.

Feelings Balls

Feelings Balls is a directive AAPT activity that could work as easily with dogs as with horses. It is excellent for children and family groups that struggle with recognizing, identifying, describing, sharing, and letting go of feelings.

The equipment consists of colored, plastic-coated, soft foam balls in the shape of small baseballs, soccer balls, and footballs that are scattered around the arena. On each individual ball is written a feeling, such as *Happy, Scared, Excited, Lonely,* and so on. Also spaced across the arena are three large plastic containers in bright colors, and about 6 feet away from each container is a Hula Hoop. One word is painted on each of the containers: *Sometimes, Often,* or *Never.* For children who cannot read there is also one with a happy face and upturned mouth, one with a downturned mouth, and one with a straight-line mouth.

During the activity, the therapist asks the children to choose a horse and then choose a ball with a feeling on it. They are then to tell the horse about a time when they might have felt like that. Once they have done this, they must walk to the Hula Hoop, stand in it, and throw the feeling ball into the tub that is appropriate for them. This permits them to get rid of the feeling if it is not a good one.

Case 1

Sandra, age 15, a twin, lived with her specialist foster parent and was one of three siblings all separated from one another. She had contact with her twin sister and her mother, but the contact often was contentious and did not meet her needs. Sandra was referred a year prior because of self-harming behaviors (cutting her arms with razors), struggling with school, and poor peer and adult relationships. There was an ongoing court case of sexual abuse in which her older brother had victimized her, and she was providing evidence against him.

Sandra very quickly made a strong connection with one of the horses, a large Gypsy Vanner gelding named *Sailor* to whom many people were drawn. As early as the second session, Sandra's self-harming behaviors had been drastically reduced, and she voluntarily handed over her razors to her foster parent. She had been funded for six hourly sessions held every other week, and she continued to do well. Sandra began doing very well at school during this time, too.

There was a gap in Sandra's service due to funding issues, and resumed funding coincided with the collapse of the court case against her brother due to the lack of physical evidence. The Feelings Balls activity was conducted during Sandra's 11th session.

It was a cold day, so the activity was set up inside a small indoor arena. Sandra immediately chose to work with Sailor and set off to catch him. Sailor kept walking away, something he rarely does, and Charlie, an Arab gelding, kept blocking Sandra's path to Sailor. Charlie kept putting his head toward the head collar that Sandra was carrying. After about 8 minutes, I asked Sandra what was going on for her. She replied that she thought Charlie wanted to work with her instead. She then decided to work with Charlie, and she began picking up balls and telling Charlie about times she felt like each of them. All was going fine until she picked up the ball marked *Bad*. Sandra was silent and started to walk toward the *Often* container. Charlie lagged behind. Seeing where she was headed, I asked her to tell Charlie what she often felt bad about. Sandra shook her head and said, "No, I *am* the bad one!" I asked her what was so bad about herself,

and she said that since the court case had collapsed and her brother was found not guilty, it must have been all her fault.

As she approached the bucket with *Often* on it, Charlie walked in front of her and blocked her from putting the *Bad* ball into the bucket. He did this four times. I asked her what was happening. Sandra said that Charlie wouldn't let her put the ball into the bucket. I wondered aloud whether Charlie disagreed that she was bad, and so was preventing her from putting the ball into the bucket. Sandra shrugged and then hugged Charlie.

After two more attempts, Sandra finally got the ball into the bucket, but Charlie refused to leave the bucket with her. After a 5-minute struggle, Sandra persuaded Charlie to leave the bucket. As they were walking away to look for another ball, my other Arab gelding, Buster, who had appeared to be dozing at the other end of the arena, purposefully strode up the full length of the arena past Sandra and Charlie, put his head in the bucket, picked up the *Bad* ball with his teeth, and dropped it on the ground. I commented that Buster also disagreed that she was bad and that it was two against one. Sandra smiled, sighed, and half-heartedly put the ball back in the bucket again. Buster again picked out the same ball despite other balls being in there, and again dropped it onto the floor. He then walked away and stood by Sailor. Sandra smiled and left the *Bad* ball there and didn't use it again in the session. At the end of the session as we were grooming the horses, I asked her if perhaps the horses knew she wasn't a bad person and that they could see through her pretense. Sandra smiled, hugged Charlie, and replied, "I guess."

Sometimes in a session as profound and astonishing as this one, the therapist may be tempted to draw the client out further with verbal processing. As seen in this example, however, the horses sensed what was needed in a way that I never could have conveyed as well. Buster had not been trained to pick out certain balls, nor had he ever picked up one of these balls before. How or why this happened as it did remains a mystery, but my role was simply one of trusting the process as much as my horses did, and then reflecting what Sandra seemed to be feeling and what the horses seemed to be conveying. Sandra did not need to say very much because the hug she gave Charlie said it all.

Case 2

Eight-year-old George was one of five siblings who were all in separate foster placements. There was an ongoing court case to decide the long-term future for George. The local authority (child services) plan for him was long-term fostering separate from his siblings, some of whom had been slated for adoption. George was involved in an excellent program for child victims of domestic violence. George's social worker had worked with him for 18 months and eventually secured funding for George and six other children to receive equine-assisted play therapy for three sessions, to be held on alternate days of the designated week.

The seven boys and girls were between the ages of 7 and 9. None of the children had met before, so they had to get to know each other quickly since only three sessions had been authorized. George, like most children who are victims of domestic violence and trauma, had learned not to trust adults easily and to keep his thoughts and feelings to himself.

The Feelings Balls activity was set up on the morning of the second day outside in the much larger arena, and it was used as a group activity. Some children chose to work in pairs with a horse, but George chose to work on his own with Charlie. After doing the activity for a few minutes, George picked up a ball labeled *Scared* and stood looking at Charlie. I suggested that Charlie would like to hear about a time when George had felt scared. George nodded and began to tell Charlie that he was scared when he heard screams coming from down-

stairs, and he went downstairs and saw his father with his hands around his mother's neck, strangling her. I said that must have been so, so scary. George nodded and said it was really scary because he thought his mother was going to die. I asked if George was often scared when things like that happened between his mommy and daddy. He nodded and said he was, then he went off to put the ball in the *Sometimes* tub.

Later, George picked up the *Sad* ball, and I again asked him to tell Charlie when he might feel like that. George said, "Same as before, Charlie." He was referring to the domestic violence incidents he had alluded to previously. After the activity ended, all the children hugged the horses and thanked them for helping them with their feelings. No further verbal processing was needed.

While the activity was taking place, I was standing with George's domestic violence counselor who had been working with him for 18 months. Up until this session with the Feeling Balls, George had never disclosed anything about what he had witnessed in his family home to his domestic violence counselor or his social worker. The counselor was amazed at how quickly the barriers to communication had come down and how quickly George was able to put his trust in the equine play therapy team.

Play therapists are used to children working through their pain and concerns in astonishing ways when the circumstances and the therapeutic facilitation are right. As these cases illustrate, adding an animal offers the potential for quicker, more intense, and more joyful healing. These case examples show how simple activities can bring about significant outcomes when a suitable and well-prepared therapist–animal team work together. Animals and therapists are skilled in the observation of others, and they are well attuned to changes in energy of the children and families. Animals do it naturally, whereas we therapists have to work a bit harder to accomplish that attunement. The longer that we work with animal partners, the more we learn about attunement, humility, keen observation, perfect timing, and most of all, how to trust the process.

Resources and Certification

There are growing resources in the field of AAPT. The reference list at the end of this chapter includes many of them, along with classic resources in AAT that are important for all practitioners to read (e.g., Arkow, 2012; Chandler, 2012; Fine, 2010; Jalongo, 2014; McCardle, McCune, Griffin, Esposito, & Freund, 2011). At the time of this writing, there are approximately 225 play therapists in the United States, 25 in the United Kingdom, and several from other countries who have attended intensive AAPT training courses, and interest is growing rapidly. In 2013, a stringent certification program specifically intended for professional AAPT practitioners and support professionals was developed, tested, and implemented. More information about this program can be found at *www.playfulpooch.org*. Although preliminary research studies show promise, more research is needed, and with growing numbers of well-trained practitioners and animals, this research becomes increasingly possible.

We have websites with considerable information (*www.risevanfleet.com*, *www.playfulpooch.org*, and *www.turnaboutpegasus.co.uk*), and we regularly conduct training seminars together in the United States and the United Kingdom. Online courses are also available that cover some of the key skills therapists need for conducting AAPT (*www.risevanfleet.com/aapt*).

Conclusion

Involving nonhuman animals in play therapy is a huge undertaking that requires complex knowledge, skills, and supervised experience even for highly qualified play therapists. However, the learning process is fun and fascinating, and the ability to facilitate play sessions with dogs, horses, and other animals offers powerful benefits to mental health practitioners. Jalongo (2004) commented, "Animals should matter to educators if for no other reason than they mean so much to children" (p. 17). The same could be said about therapists!

We know that children relate readily to animals (Jalongo, 2014; Melson, 2001; Melson & Fine, 2010; VanFleet, 2008), and in the process of developing healthy, mutually satisfying relationships with therapy animals, children can gain confidence, feel cared for, develop empathy, resolve serious problems, open up, and be touched in unique and profound ways. Sometimes suitable and properly trained animals can reach children and clients of all ages when human therapists simply cannot. At other times, children can learn from the relationship model provided by the therapist–animal partnership. Ultimately, animals help us feel part of the larger, natural world, and they bring their finely tuned sense of survival, social interaction, play, and living in the here and now with them into therapy sessions. Not only can they help our clients, but they can teach us how to be better therapists if we approach our partnerships with them with humility and respect.

REFERENCES

Arkow, P. (2012). *Latham and the link: A legacy of cruelty prevention and personal responsibility* (Vol. 1). CreateSpace Independent Publishing.

Chandler, C. K. (2012). *Animal assisted therapy in counseling* (2nd ed.). New York: Routledge.

Crenshaw, D. A. (2012). Secrets told to Ivy: Animal-assisted play therapy in a residential treatment facility. *Play Therapy, 7*(2), 6–9.

Faa-Thompson, T. (2012a). Safe touch using horses to teach sexually abused clients to value their bodies and themselves. In K. S. Trotter (Ed.), *Harnessing the power of equine assisted counseling* (pp. 53–58). New York: Routledge.

Faa-Thompson, T. (2012b). You gotta crack a few eggs. In K. S. Trotter (Ed.), *Harnessing the power of equine assisted counseling* (pp. 129–132). New York: Routledge.

Fine, A. H. (Ed.). (2010). *Handbook on animal-assisted therapy: Theoretical foundations and guidelines for practice* (3rd. ed.). New York: Elsevier.

Guerney, L., & Ryan, V. (2013). *Group filial therapy: The complete guide to teaching parents to play therapeutically with their children.* Philadelphia: Jessica Kingsley.

International Institute for Animal Assisted Play Therapy Studies Play Therapy. (2013). *Certification in animal assisted play therapy.* Boiling Springs, PA: Play Therapy Press.

Jalongo, M. R. (Ed.). (2004). *The world's children and their companion animals: Developmental and educational significance of the child/pet bond.* Olney, MD: Association for Childhood Education International.

Jalongo, M. R. (Ed.). (2014). *Teaching compassion: Humane education in early childhood.* New York: Springer.

Landreth, G. L. (2012). *Play therapy: The art of the relationship* (3rd ed.). New York: Routledge.

McCardle, P., McCune, S., Griffin, J. A., Esposito, L., & Freund, L. S. (Eds.). (2011). *Animals in our lives: Human–animal interaction in family, community, and therapeutic settings.* Baltimore: Brookes.

Melson, G. F. (2001). *Why the wild things are: Animals in the lives of children.* Cambridge, MA: Harvard University Press.

Melson, G. F., & Fine, A. H. (2010). Animals in the lives of children. In A. H. Fine (Ed.), *Handbook on animal-assisted therapy: Theoretical foundations and guidelines for practice* (pp. 223–245). New York: Elsevier.

Parish-Plass, N. (2008). Animal-assisted therapy with children suffering from insecure attachment due to abuse and neglect: A method to lower the risk of intergenerational transmission of abuse? *Clinical Child Psychology and Psychiatry, 13*(1), 7–30.

Parish-Plass, N. (Ed.). (2013). *Animal-assisted psychotherapy: Theory, issues, and practice.* West Lafayette, IN: Purdue University Press.

Thompson, M. J. (2009). Animal-assisted play therapy: Canines as co-therapists. In G. R. Walz, J. C. Bleuer, & R. K. Yep (Eds.), *Compelling counseling interventions: VISTAS 2009* (pp. 199–209). Alexandria, VA: American Counseling Association.

Trotter, K. S. (Ed.). (2012). *Harnessing the power of equine assisted counseling.* New York: Routledge.

Trotter, K. S., Chandler, C. K., Goodwin-Bond, D., & Casey, J. (2008). A comparative study of group equine assisted counseling with at-risk children and adolescents. *Journal of Creativity in Mental Health, 3*(3), 254–284.

VanFleet, R. (2007). *Preliminary results from the ongoing pet play therapy study.* Boiling Springs, PA: Play Therapy Press. Full report available at *http://play-therapy.com/playfulpooch/pets_ study.html.*

VanFleet, R. (2008). *Play therapy with kids & canines: Benefits for children's developmental and psychosocial health.* Sarasota, FL: Professional Resource Press.

VanFleet, R. (2014a). *Filial therapy: Strengthening parent–child relationships through play* (3rd ed.). Sarasota, FL: Professional Resource Press.

VanFleet, R. (2014b). *Selection of dogs for family life and therapy work, with special attention to animal assisted play therapy* [Online course]. Boiling Springs, PA: Play Therapy Press.

VanFleet, R., & Colţea, C. G. (2012). Helping children with ASD through canine-assisted play therapy. In L. Gallo-Lopez & L. C. Rubin (Eds.), *Play-based interventions for children and adolescents with autism spectrum disorders* (pp. 39–72). New York: Routledge.

VanFleet, R., & Faa-Thompson, T. (2010). The case for using animal assisted play therapy. *British Journal of Play Therapy, 6,* 4–18.

VanFleet, R., & Faa-Thompson, T. (2012). The power of play, multiplied. *Play Therapy Magazine of the British Association of Play Therapists, 70,* 7–10.

VanFleet, R., & Faa-Thompson, T. (2014). Including animals in play therapy with young children and families. In M. R. Jalongo (Ed.), *Teaching compassion: Humane education in early childhood* (pp. 89–107). New York: Springer.

VanFleet, R., Sywulak, A. E., & Sniscak, C. C. (2010). *Child-centered play therapy.* New York: Guilford Press.

Weiss, D. (2009). Equine assisted therapy and Theraplay. In E. Munns (Ed.), *Applications of family and group Theraplay* (pp. 225–233). Lanham, MD: Aronson.

PART II

Clinical Applications of Play Therapy

INTRODUCTION

Play therapists practice in a wide array of clinical and educational settings, yet they all agree that developing a clear theoretical framework and approach to guide their work is essential, that science informs interventions, and that practitioners acquire a strong foundational knowledge in child development. But since play therapists are largely practitioners in the diverse settings in which they work and practice, "the rubber really hits the road" when it comes to clinical applications.

This book is abundantly enriched by a wide range of clinical application chapters from leading practitioners in the field—a total of 17. The section begins with David A. Crenshaw, in Chapter 15, on play therapy with "children of fury." Next comes Steven Baron in Chapter 16 with an important focus on the spectrum of bullying, including the internalized bully. Many play therapists work in the schools, and Chapter 17, by Angela I. Sheely-Moore and Peggy L. Ceballos, is devoted to play therapy with school-related problems. In Chapter 18 David A. Crenshaw and Kathleen S. Tillman focus on facilitating trauma narratives in foster care in play therapy and group play therapy. Chapter 19, by Debbie C. Sturm and Christopher Hill, focuses on the compelling issue of play therapy with children of homeless families.

Perhaps no clinical problems are more frequently seen in the play therapist's office than those related to divorce, and in Chapter 20 Sueann Kenney-Noziska and Liana Lowenstein capably handle this topic. Chapter 21, by William Steele, features play therapy for children dealing with grief and traumatic loss. In Chapter 22 J. P. Lilly addresses the difficult topic of conducting Jungian analytical play therapy with a sexually abused child. Janine Shelby and Lauren E. Maltby delineate key issues in child maltreatment in Chapter 23, particularly safety-based clinical strategies for play therapists. The highly acclaimed Eliana Gil, in Chapter 24, tackles a topic often neglected in the play therapy literature: the role of play therapists in reunification.

Of great interest is Chapter 25, on play-based disaster interventions, by Anne L. Stewart, Lennie G. Echterling, and Claudio Mochi. A chapter of great relevance and timing, Chapter 26, by Jessica Anne Umhoefer, Mary Anne Peabody, and Anne L. Stewart, discusses play therapy with children of military families. Kevin Boyd Hull explores the practice of play therapy with children on the autism spectrum in Chapter 27. Another population frequently seen in schools, clinics, and private practice is that of children diagnosed with ADHD; Heidi Gerard Kaduson addresses this topic in Chapter 28. One of the most revered practitioners in the field, Louise F. Guerney, discusses filial therapy with anxiety disorders in Chapter 29, another presenting problem frequently brought to the play therapist for intervention. Next is a creative and exciting chapter on play therapy with adolescents by Brijin Johnson Gardner (Chapter 30). Finally, in Chapter 31, Diana Frey describes the application of play therapy with adults.

We are pleased that our chapter authors in this section include three recipients of the Association for Play Therapy (APT) Lifetime Achievement Award: Louise F. Guerney, Diana Frey, and Eliana Gil. Garry Landreth, who coauthored Chapter 1 on child-centered play therapy, was the first recipient of the APT Lifetime Achievement Award. These outstanding movers and shakers in the play therapy field are joined by other leading practitioners in writing the chapters in this section, and in doing groundbreaking work that is taking the play therapy field forward.

CHAPTER 15

Play Therapy with "Children of Fury"

TREATING THE TRAUMA OF BETRAYAL

David A. Crenshaw

Child of Fury

Oh, child of fury how long has it been since someone touched your heart?
Words may fail, but perhaps you can express your pain through play or art.
So many tears locked away inside, untold burdens too heavy to bear;
  How long has it been since you shed a tear?
  Too long. Too long I say! Let those tears flow.
How long since a hug, a tender touch, or kind words set your heart aglow?
Oh, child of fury play and paint with all your heart, your heart so torn apart.
—DAVID A. CRENSHAW

Children of fury are not always able to express in words the rage stemming from the many and varied forms of betrayal they have experienced. The rage may exceed words. However, these children may be able to draw, paint, create pictures in a sandtray, or use clay or puppets to express their fury when words fail. The term *children of fury* is not intended to indicate that these children invariably act out their rage. Rather, the term is meant to describe children who, due to invisible emotional wounds, harbor rage and fury. Under specific conditions, when triggered by certain internal or external events, they act out their fury.

Of all the presenting problems that play therapists are called on to treat, physical aggression tends to cause the most anxiety and stress, with the possible exception of sexualized behavior in the playroom. In addition to the anxiety related to keeping the child and therapist safe in the playroom, typically there are increased pressures from parents, schools, and other referral sources to resolve the problem quickly. The aggressive behavior unnerves parents and school officials, and may threaten the safety of other children. In discussing aggression in childhood, I am mindful of Jerome Kagan's (1998) admonitions to be careful in the language we choose. Although it may create awkwardness at times in wording, I follow, as carefully as possible, his strong recommendation that we as clinicians should never use the phrase *aggressive children*. Kagan explained that no child is aggressive all the time, even the most violent child. Some children may be aggressive at home but not at school, or vice versa. The child who is aggressive at home will not be aggressive at all times, but is quite likely to become aggressive when his older brothers tease him. The context must be supplied when talking about aggressive behavior in children.

Aggression in children is the result of multiple contributing factors. In his 1998 lecture "How We Become Who We Are" to the Psychotherapy Networker Symposium, Kagan used the analogy of a tapestry woven together in a complex way by many threads. The threads include biological factors (genetics and neurobiology); social influences, including our family and the values we are taught by our families; and our culture and its values; and even the historical moment in time in which we grow up. Children growing up today encounter a markedly different world than the one I experienced in my formative years. In addition to risk factors such as poverty, psychiatric disturbance in the parent(s), substance abuse by parents, child abuse (physical or sexual or both), criminal incarceration of a parent, and neglect (ACES Study; Anda et al., 2006), the other side of the equation also needs to be considered. Children can be remarkably resilient and hardy (Crenshaw, 2013), as illustrated by studies of Ugandan former child soldiers who were exposed and subjected to unimaginable atrocities. Viewing all of these contributing risks and assets, and their interaction with each other, makes for the weaving of a complex tapestry indeed!

Description of the Clinical Application

An Integrative Approach

An integrative approach to working with children of fury has guided my play therapy with children in residential treatment settings who display extreme aggression under specific conditions, and with children in an outpatient private practice for 36 years who

exhibited a wide range of aggressive behaviors, again within a specific context.

Child-Centered Play Therapy

Child-centered play therapy (CCPT) is the treatment of choice while working to build a strong therapeutic relationship. The attunement, curious attentiveness, empathy, genuineness, and warmth that CCPT emphasizes leads to trust, growth, and healing in children who present a wide array of problems. CCPT is especially effective when aggression is the presenting problem because many of these children will not easily trust the therapist. CCPT demonstrated positive results with a group of elementary school children (Ray, Chapter 32, this volume; Ray, Blanco, Sullivan, & Holliman, 2009). Children who participated in a 14-session CCPT group demonstrated a significant decrease in aggression, whereas children in a control group showed no significant change in aggression. In an exploratory study of disruptive behavior in a Head Start program, CCPT demonstrated statistically significant decreases in aggression as well as for problems of attention (Bratton et al., 2013).

Disrupted attachment in early life can be a contributor to aggression. CCPT has been shown to increase the child's attachment security with the therapist even when the child remains insecurely attached to the parent (Anderson & Gedo, 2013). In the Anderson and Gedo (2013) case study the child's mother was not able to participate in the therapy due to language barriers; however, the child's level of aggression still decreased as the result of CCPT. A modified CCPT approach used with highly aggressive adolescents has shown promising results as well (Cochran, Fauth, Cochran, Spurgeon, & Pierce, 2010). Cochran and colleagues (2010) viewed the person-centered approach, with its emphasis on warmth, genuineness, and empathy, as particularly well suited for adolescents who are reluctant to engage in a verbal expressive therapy approach.

Sensory–Motor Therapy

Sensory–motor therapy, based on findings from neuroscience, offers exciting new opportunities for working with young children presenting with aggressive behavior. Traditional therapy approaches may fail with children exposed to early trauma unless attention is paid to hyperarousal and the need to soothe the brainstem (Gaskill & Perry, 2014). In an exploratory study with at-risk preschoolers in a therapeutic program, use of the neurosequential model of therapeutics (NMT; Gaskill & Perry, 2014) to determine the timing, nature, and "dose" of therapeutic activities provided in the context of filial play therapy (Barfield, Dobson, Gaskill, & Perry, 2012) resulted in significant improvement in emotional regulation and impulse modulation. The NMT emphasizes that what we do may not be as important as when we do it. NMT is a promising framework to integrate into play therapy to guide play therapists in the timing and sequencing of their interventions based on brain research.

Gestalt Play Therapy

Using a Gestalt play therapy approach, Oaklander (2006) described three phases of dealing with anger in play therapy. The first phase she referred to as "talking about" the angry feelings. This initial work involved not only developing a lexicon for the feelings but also drawing or painting pictures depicting a wide range of angry feelings. She also utilized music, such as the beat of the drum, to help children express various intensities of anger. In the second phase of the anger work, Oaklander focused on new and more satisfying ways of expressing anger. She found that it was important to enlist the family in this phase of the work because the way the family expresses anger can profoundly affect the way the child deals with his or her experiences of anger, ranging from slight annoyance to out-of-control rage. In the third phase, in

the safety of the therapeutic relationships Oaklander sought to determine whether there was blocked or buried anger related to unresolved trauma or grief. The anger may be so buried as to be completely out of the child's awareness. This type of anger needs to be released in small increments so it doesn't frighten or overwhelm the child. The Gestalt approach, as best elucidated by Oaklander, has much to offer to play therapists working with problems of aggression and can be integrated with other approaches.

Psychodynamic Play Therapy

With its emphasis on dynamic forces such as unconscious motives, feelings, and impulses, psychodynamic play therapy offers a deep understanding of the child's symbolic play and creative productions whether in sandplay, art and drawing activities, or use of clay or other materials (see Crenshaw & Mordock, 2005a, 2005c; Mordock, Chapter 5, this volume). Psychodynamic theory can also guide different levels of empathic statements and interpretations in response to the symbolized play or creative expressions (Crenshaw & Mordock, 2005a, 2005c).

Key Concepts and Strategies

Identification with the Aggressor

Children brought to play therapy for problems of aggression frequently identify with the aggressor in their aggressive play action, at least in the early stages of the work. This identification is easily understood from a psychodynamic framework. Children who have either witnessed or been subjected to violence invariably feel powerless, terrified, and voiceless. In fantasy play they can assume the role of the powerful one, the victimizer instead of the victimized, which is understandably gratifying for the child. The problem arises when children get stuck in the role of aggressor; if this behavior continues indefinitely, it can lead to crystallization of their self-identity around the aggressor. This dynamic is seen in many cases of bullying (see Baron, Chapter 16, in this volume). In the event that the child gets fixated on the role of the aggressor, a directive stance is adopted by the play therapist to help the child shift to other more constructive ways of experiencing power. In some cases, they can be the police chief in the play drama, or the mayor, the judge, or any character through which power can be exercised in constructive, helpful ways. The play therapist may need to be quite active and directive to keep the child from reverting back to identifying with the aggressor. Brief sequences of playing one of the constructive, empowering roles can be useful, followed by praise to help the child to make this shift (credit goes to Kevin O'Connor for his suggestion of this intervention at a workshop I attended in 1995).

Empathy-Based Interventions

Regardless of specific theoretical approaches, it is crucial to include empathy-based interventions. Research has shown repeatedly that the lack of empathy is a hallmark of serious aggression and violence (Andershed, Kerr, Stattin, & Levander, 2002; Kolla et al., 2013). Social skills training and anger management strategies are likely to miss the mark if they don't include empathy-based interventions. Examples of specific empathy-based strategies in both individual and group work are available in previous writing along with descriptions of specific programs developed to increase empathy (see Crenshaw & Mordock, 2005a, 2005c).

Theory and Research

The contributing factors in childhood aggression are many and varied. Profound losses and rage can result from being born into and raised in poverty, growing up in dangerous and crime-filled neighborhoods,

and/or being bullied in school. When grief is buried, remaining unexpressed and unresolved, it can turn into anger and ultimately to rage. Some children never develop an adequate sense of empathy due to assaults on their dignity and humanity. To be judged harshly and narrowly because of gender, race, class, ethnic, regional, or national group membership is a dehumanizing experience. Although social toxins (Garbarino, 1999) impact many children, an extremely small percentage become violent offenders as adults (Kolla et al., 2013). Children with limited educational and vocational opportunities, faced with daily threats of violence, may turn to gangs for affiliation and protection needs. Key factors among the small number who becomes violent offenders in adulthood are the callous/unemotional traits associated with the syndrome of psychopathy (Kolla et al., 2013).

Psychopathic individuals tend not to accurately read signs of pain or sadness in others. The personality pattern of psychopathy in adult criminals is associated with an earlier onset of criminal acts compared to other criminals, commission of more violent crimes, and engaging in more violence while incarcerated (Andershed et al., 2002; Decety, Chen, Harenski, & Kiehl, 2013). It is important to hold this perspective in mind because most children seen in clinical practice for aggression or conduct problems are not headed for a life of violent crime, the parents' and sometimes the clinician's fears notwithstanding. What we most frequently encounter in clinical practice is reactive instead of proactive aggression.

Reactive aggression is defined as hostile, impulsive behavior in response to a perceived threat or frustration, in contrast to *proactive aggression*, which entails the commission of aggressive acts that are often unprovoked and directed toward possessing or controlling others (sometimes referred to as *instrumental aggression*; Dodge & Coie, 1987). Reactive aggression—but not proactive aggression—was found to be linked to childhood maltreatment (Kolla et al., 2013). Although further research is indicated, it appears that psychopathy is a critical contributing factor to the emergence of proactive aggression (Kolla et al., 2013). Again, these findings are important for the play therapist as well as the parents of the children seen in treatment who may be unduly worried that their child of fury is headed for a life of violent crime.

Aggression and destructive behavior before the age of 3 predicts later problems in preadolescence and calls for early recognition and intervention (Pihlakoski et al., 2006). Aggression in childhood can occur in 12-month-olds but was observed more commonly in 24- and 36-month-olds in a nonclinical sample (Alink et al., 2006). The rates of physically aggressive behaviors increased in the second year of life and declined beginning after the third birthday on (Alink et al., 2006).

Conventional wisdom has suggested that the greater aggression seen in young boys, as compared to girls, is the result of the difference in the ways that boys and girls are socialized in our culture. Studies by researchers in Canada (Zoccolillo et al., 2007) found that at just 17 months of age, there was a substantial gender difference in the prevalence of physical aggression, with 5% of the boys but only 1% of the girls exhibiting physically aggressive behavior on a frequent basis. There was no change in this difference at 29 months. Zoccolillo and colleagues (2007) asserted that it is unlikely that differential gender socialization could account for such marked differences at such an early age. This view could be challenged, however, by attachment researchers who have found that there are early differential ways that children present as well as ways we interact with them based on gender (Weinberg, Tronick, Cohn, & Olson, 1999).

Attachment security also plays a role in childhood aggression. Boys with disorganized attachment and children with ambivalent attachment reported a higher level (more frequent and severe) of exter-nalizing problems than did secure children (Moss et al., 2006). Pervasive hyperactivity in preschool boys combined with poor quality of mother–child interactions were predictive of higher rates of aggression and noncompliant or nonsocial behaviors as well as lower rates of peer acceptance than occurred for boys in a comparison group (Keown & Woodward, 2006). Preschool children exposed to cumulative family risk factors (e.g., parental alcoholism, parental depression, antisocial behavior, marital conflict) along with difficult child temperament showed higher levels of aggression at 18 months than children in low-risk families (Edwards, Eiden, Colder, & Leonard, 2006). Boys with high- or low-risk status had higher levels of aggressive behavior at all ages than girls. Media exposure is still another factor. A 2-year longitudinal study found that the extent of media exposure predicted relational aggression for girls and physical aggression for boys at school (Ostrov, Gentile, & Crick, 2006).

Still another factor associated with early childhood aggression is prenatal exposure to cocaine combined with gender and environmental risk factors (Bendersky, Bennett, & Lewis, 2006). Cocaine exposure *in utero* combined with being male and a high-risk environment were all predictive of aggression at the age of 5.

Metaphors to Inform the Rationale for Intervention

Play therapists can't begin to adequately treat children of fury without a cohesive rationale based on theory and research to guide the treatment plan and the choice of interventions. Helpful ways of conceptualizing the problem of aggression in children are described below.

"Fawns in Gorilla Suits"

The metaphorical phrase *fawns in gorilla suits* applies particularly to children in foster care and especially in residential treatment programs. These children often experience relational trauma at the beginning of life (Schore, 2012) and then are exposed to various social toxins (Hardy & Crenshaw, 2008; Hardy & Laszloffy, 2005) such as poverty, abuse, and neglect, along with discrimination and devaluation due to gender, class, nationality, racial, or heterosexual bias. I've used this metaphor to describe many of the children in child welfare placements (Crenshaw & Garbarino, 2007; Crenshaw & Hardy, 2005; Crenshaw & Mordock, 2005a, 2005b, 2005c) because I think it captures the essential dynamics of children suffering from complex or developmental trauma (van der Kolk, 2005). In addition to the sociocultural trauma (Hardy & Laszloffy, 2005), the children who populate residential treatment centers have experienced a high proportion of adverse childhood experiences (ACES), including physical and/or sexual abuse and/or neglect, family and/or community violence, major psychiatric disorder in one or both parents, incarceration of one or both parents, substance abuse by one or both parents, and separation or divorce of parents (Anda et al., 2006). In an unpublished study (Crenshaw & Alstadt, 2011) in one residential treatment center, 87% of the last 100 children admitted had at least four of these ACES (Anda et al., 2006). In previous studies of ACES, four or more such experiences placed a person at high risk for a range of deleterious behavioral and physical health outcomes (Anda et al., 2006).

Defensive Strategy: The Gorilla Suit

Fawns in gorilla suits typically suffer complex or developmental trauma due to three sources of trauma exposure: (1) relational trauma, (2) sociocultural trauma, and (3) ongoing exposure to ACES. A common shared and repeated experience of our fawns in gorilla suits is the assault on their dignity (Crenshaw & Hardy, 2005; Hardy &

Crenshaw, 2008; Hardy & Laszloffy, 2005). The metaphor of the gorilla suit delineates the defensive operations: the gorilla suit represents the identification with the aggressor. The aggression keeps people at a distance and is designed to protect the vulnerable, often traumatized core self that is represented by the fawn. The anger, rage, and aggression are in response to the cumulative trauma rooted in multiple origins and myriad contributing factors identified earlier.

Defensive Strategy: Brick Wall of Detachment

It should be noted that not all youngsters use aggression as a defensive function to protect the traumatized, vulnerable self (fawn). It is also common to encounter children who barricade themselves behind a *brick wall of detachment*. The children using this strategy are nearly impossible to make contact with emotionally. They are remote, unmoved, and impervious to the efforts that therapists make to establish meaningful connections with them. Children who barricade themselves behind the brick wall of detachment tend to respond only to those therapists and adults who refuse to give up on them and persevere in the face of constant obstacles and discouragement.

"Children of Fury"

I have come to realize that although fawns in gorilla suits frequent the populations of children in the foster care system and particularly those placed in residential treatment and inpatient programs, they don't account for all the enraged children that the play therapist might encounter. Play therapists work in a wide range of settings, including inpatient programs, partial hospitals, day treatment centers, outpatient clinics, schools, Head Start centers, prevention programs, and private practice. The children to whom I refer as *children of fury* can be encountered in any of these settings, and the core psychodynamic issue for these children is intimate betrayal. Of all the experiences encountered in human life, betrayal, perceived or actual, tends to provoke the most intense rage. This experience is sometimes referred to as *betrayal trauma* (Gobin & Freyd, 2013). According to betrayal trauma theory, children who have early experiences of violation and betrayal by close others may not develop certain social capabilities, including the ability to make healthy decisions about whom to trust. As a result, these children become vulnerable to repeated betrayal and the consequent cumulative rage.

The Myriad Forms of Betrayal

The descriptions of intimate forms of betrayal that follow are not comprehensive because such wounds and the accompanying fury can be provoked by both subtle as well as overt actions. The betrayal can be intended or unintended. It is always the subjective experience of betrayal that matters in understanding the fury of the betrayed, not the unassailable facts. For instance, children whose parent abuses alcohol or drugs may have a gratifying connection with the sober/clean parent and feel betrayed and enraged when the intoxicated parent shows up. In contrast, in *betrayal trauma theory* (Freyd, 2008; Freyd & Birrell, 2013)—which focuses on caretakers, upon whom the betrayed person is dependent for survival, who then abuse, neglect, or in some way significantly violate that person's sense of trust—the betrayed person is posited to be numb to reacting to the betrayal. The dependence on the caretakers for survival can "blind" the person to the betrayal (Freyd & Birrell, 2013) and can pose a formidable force in silencing the betrayed victim. Although I have treated clients who would fit the criteria of betrayal trauma, as outlined by Freyd (2008), especially in instances of sexual abuse by a caretaker and when the child is silenced by threats, more often my

clinical experience has shown that betrayal is not a silent wound, at least not over time.

I've worked with many families that suffer the extreme stress and hardship of a chronically ill family member. Clinical experience has revealed that no matter how much love is shared in the family, the devastation of chronic illness may be enraging to the other members of the family. The resources of the family are disproportionally allocated to the ill family member, leaving fewer resources in the form of time, energy, money, and activities for the rest of the family. This dramatic change in family life can feel like a betrayal and can provoke wrath in family members who experience this sense of betrayal. Children may experience guilt and shame for having such feelings, thus making it hard to talk about and resolve. The same dynamics apply to the death of a family member. Emotionally, it can feel like desertion and betrayal, even though such feelings cause great distress because of guilt and shame. Rage is often relegated to a secret chamber of the heart that gets unleashed at the most unexpected times.

Children who have been abused or neglected by the very adults who would be expected to love and protect them will almost certainly experience a sense of betrayal. An elementary school student may experience enduring fury as a result of the betrayal of a former best friend who now has joined with other peers to taunt and bully him or her. In middle school and high school it is not unusual for students to feel betrayed by a former boyfriend or girlfriend who has a new romantic interest. Sometimes the fury is directed primarily at the ex-boyfriend or girlfriend and sometimes at the person who is the new romantic partner, the one who has replaced him or her.

Betrayal can take the form of promises broken, especially if this is a pattern. I've often observed the fury of children in foster care whose parent(s) doesn't show for a visit that was promised to the child. The same applies to children of divorce when promises of regular phone calls or visits by the noncustodial parent are repeatedly broken. Secrets not kept by friends who were previously considered trustworthy can trigger rage that can be the equal to that of a scorned lover. A teacher who humiliates a child in front of the entire class is often perceived by the child as betraying his or her implicit trust.

Abuse, neglect, and betrayal permeate all levels of society and socioeconomic groups. I've encountered children of fury from affluent families. Their parents may occupy positions of occupational prestige or esteemed social status in the community, and they may be extremely generous with their time and talents to local charities and community causes. But the children of fury may feel betrayed. In their rage they sometimes portray their parents as "frauds." They explain that although their parents relentlessly pursue success in ways that are recognized by the larger community, the children feel abandoned, robbed of their parents' time and interest. The rage of these youth is sometimes striking and when introduced into family sessions, it is often shocking to the parents, who have long been oblivious to the needs and feelings of their children.

Of all the betrayals so devastating to children, the worst and the hardest to heal is, in my experience, the ultimate betrayal of a child by a parent. An example that is even hard for most people to imagine is when a parent would choose their romantic partner over the child after that partner had abused the child. Children suffering this ultimate betrayal are often placed out of the home in foster care after intervention by child protective services (Webb, 2007). The fury in these cases is understandably beyond description. The rage can reach homicidal proportions, at least in fantasies about revenge. Sadly, some of these children redirect the rage inward in the form of suicidal attempts or nonsuicidal forms of self-injury. They turn on themselves with the same contempt that the parent has shown to them, and they feel unworthy of love from anyone.

Betrayal by the Play Therapist

Play therapists can make mistakes that trigger the fury of children and leave them feeling betrayed. Children in play therapy often test therapists in a wide range of ways to see if they are trustworthy, dependable, and genuine. Keeping a secure, reliable structure and frame around the play therapy is essential with children and even more important with children of fury who have experienced prior devastating betrayals. For instance, the child will pay close attention to details, such as the therapist's (1) being on time for appointments; (2) sensitively handling and preparing the child for breaks in the treatment due to illness, vacation, or conference attendance; and (3) following up in a concerned way when a child misses an appointment. The child will be watching to see if details of the sessions are indeed kept confidential. He or she will be acutely sensitive to what is shared with parents, the school, teachers, or other referring sources.

Since therapists—like other humans—are imperfect, they will inevitably make mistakes. The point is that, when mistakes are made, it is imperative to honestly admit the failure to the child and work toward repairing the rupture in the therapeutic relationship. Play therapists must realize that with children who have prior histories of repeated betrayal, repair may take considerable time—or may not be possible.

Therapeutic Focus with "Children of Fury": Repair of the Injured Sense of Trust

Since an injured sense of trust is endemic to betrayal, the gradual development of trust in the therapeutic relationship can serve as a powerfully reparative emotional experience (Gobin & Freyd, 2009). Although therapists in the play therapy field come from different theoretical schools and approaches, a common factor in the work is providing a secure attachment relationship in the form of the therapist–child alliance. In the push to utilize evidence-based treatment, nothing is more empirically supported than the quality of the therapeutic relationship (Stewart & Echterling, 2014). In the search for "breakthrough techniques," it can be lost that one of the most potent factors in therapeutic change is the quality of the treatment relationship. If children feel secure and safe in their relationship with the play therapist and experience the therapist as trustworthy, it will be a major step toward healing the damaged sense of trust, an important emotionally corrective experience (Alexander, 1961). When a child of fury reaches a point of sufficient trust and safety with the play therapist, he or she will begin to play out, and perhaps later tell in words, to the extent possible, the story of his or her prior betrayal(s) that has underpinned the rage. When youth begin to disclose and unburden the sources of their rage, it represents "an active declaration of trust" (Bonime, 1989) that is a vital ingredient of healing for those who have suffered the intimate wound of betrayal.

"Surviving the Rage"

A valued colleague of mine, Heather Butt, introduced me to this concept of "surviving the rage," inspired by the work of Winnicott. In order to help children and adolescents of fury, as play therapists we must be able to survive their rage. We must be able to be in the presence of rage that can reach proportions that can be frightening for both the child and the therapist and somehow remain in relationship through the process. Surviving the rage is an enormous challenge. Typically the child is in treatment because a number of key people have not been able to survive the rage. If the child is unable to express the fury and process it in therapy, where is he or she to turn? It may be extremely uncomfortable for the child if, in a fit of rage, he or she breaks one of the toys in the therapy room. In fury the child may try to break

windows or smash lights in the room by throwing blocks. Obviously, this behavior calls for effective limit setting and preventive measures to keep both child and therapist safe. But the essential ingredient of surviving the rage is that the therapeutic relationship remains intact. The child learns that his or her fury does not destroy the therapist or totally consume or sweep away the child.

Even if the child doesn't deliberately break toys or furnishings in the playroom, it can be extremely distressing to witness him or her slam dolls on the edge of a table with such force that their heads come flying off. Witnessing rage of sadistic proportions can be disturbing; however, if the rage is contained in the realm of symbolic reenactment, it is far superior to behavioral reenactments in daily life that may lead to harm of self or others. It is important for the therapist to remember that this kind of rage does not arise in a vacuum and that there simply is no rage like the fury that results from betrayal and especially repeated betrayals. To have a once-trusted person be the source of pain adds aggravated insult to the injury.

Surviving the rage is another example of an emotionally corrective experience stemming from the quality and trustworthiness of the therapeutic relationship. Safety is established in play therapy not only by consistently setting limits on unsafe behaviors but also by teaching calming and soothing techniques. These techniques, which include mindfulness training and breathing practices, can be employed when the child is about to spin out of control and is unable to regulate the rage; they also help the child develop an awareness of these emotional states. Perhaps most importantly, safety is established in play therapy by building a strong and trusting relationship with the child. Psychological safety in the therapeutic relationship calms the anxiety of the child and makes it possible for him or her to undertake the arduous process of confronting their invisible wounds.

Honor the "Fighting Spirit"

Play therapists should not overlook the resilience and irrepressible spirit of a child of fury. This is a child who has not given up. She is fighting for her dignity. He feels there is something worth fighting for and defending. She is seeking redress of an intimate, searing wound. This impressive show of strength in the form of fury and outrage can be harnessed and redirected in the form of determination to take effective action to restore dignity in ways that are constructive and helpful. Redirecting the fury will only happen when the invisible wounds and the corresponding rage have been validated and the youth feels understood. Strictly cognitive interventions will fall short because the corresponding affect of the child will need to be expressed and met with empathy.

Respect and Dignity

The essential corrective emotional experience mediated by the therapeutic relationship with children of fury is predicated on treating those children with respect and dignity throughout the treatment process. Children of fury are inordinately sensitive to any offense—perceived or real—to their sense of dignity. Answering the phone during a session with such a youngster, keeping him or her waiting without a sincere apology, or failing to be fully present and attuned will stymie the therapeutic process because in the eyes of the child of fury, these are examples of significant ruptures in the attachment with the therapist.

Clinical Case Example

Background

Manny (fictitious name), a child of fury, was 8 years old when I met him for the first time. A Hispanic child, Manny was adopted by spouses who were both elementary school teachers. In Manny's view, the first betrayal occurred when his birth mother made him available for adoption because she was young and poor. She didn't feel she could give him a decent life and the father, who was also young, was not able and/or willing to help. The father was no longer in a relationship with his mother.

Manny's adoptive parents were well-intended people who had raised three children of their own and wanted to raise another child when their youngest son was a junior in high school. All three of the biological children finished college and were independent at the time Manny began treatment with me. Their oldest son is a coach in high school, their daughter works as a paralegal in a law office, and their youngest son is an engineer. All three of the biological children were supportive of Manny and their parents, although the older two expressed concern when the parents, who were well into their 40s, shared their plans for adopting a child. They worried that the parents would not have the energy to deal with the new child, especially if the child had special needs or behavior problems. In spite of the support from the family's grown children, Manny was convinced that the older children didn't accept him into the family (perceived betrayal #2), but he also believed that they would not admit to it. Manny retaliated by being aggressive toward the young children of the oldest son and the daughter when they visited their parents, which made the parents and grandparents wary and frustrated, and further reinforced Manny's belief that he was unwelcome and unwanted in their eyes. In Manny's perception, the grandchildren of his adoptive parents were preferred not only by their parents but by the grandparents (his adoptive parents) over him (subjective betrayal #3).

Manny embarrassed his adoptive parents by acting out in the school where both parents were teachers. He was frequently in the principal's office for aggressive and rough play on the playground and in the lunchroom. If he wanted to sit at a particular table next to a friend, he would push a child out of the seat in order to sit there. Manny was a hazard to other children on the playground because he would, at times, run recklessly at full speed across the play area and crash into other children, knocking them to the ground, in some cases causing minor injuries. Parents of the other children in his class became alarmed, complained to the principal, and demanded that something be done about Manny.

At other times, Manny could be quite charming. He had a nice smile and could be polite and engaging when he was in a positive mood. But Manny was predominantly a brooding, sulking, and quick-to-anger child. What was most concerning to both the school and the parents were his rages, which frightened other children at school and alarmed the adults. The rages occurred only twice a month or so, but when the fury was unleashed, it was disturbing in both intensity and duration. On some occasions it was necessary for the teacher, the principal, the behavior specialist, and sometimes the school psychologist to restrain Manny by using physical holds (they had received training for this method) to keep Manny and the other children, as well as the school staff, safe. The restraints invariably intensified Manny's fury and undoubtedly extended the duration of the episode, sometimes lasting over an hour. These physical restraints were upsetting to Manny, the school staff, and the other children, resulting in a sense of great urgency when Manny began treatment with me. In Manny's perception, teachers liked the other children in his class far better than him. In accordance with this belief, he acted in such a way to alienate both his teachers and the other students (perceived betrayal #4).

An Integrated Play Therapy Approach

An integrated play therapy approach is illustrated in the work with Manny, beginning with the use of CCPT to build a strong relationship. In addition to needed limits

and boundaries to maintain safety, I used the early sessions to follow Manny's lead as he played out numerous battles in puppet play, sandtherapy creations and enactments, and in the family playhouse.

Gestalt play therapy and specifically the work of Violet Oaklander (2006) informed the use of directive interventions, as described below. Psychodynamic play therapy informed the therapist's understanding of the emotional processes underlying Manny's play (Crenshaw & Mordock, 2005a). Sensory-based play activities (Gaskill & Perry, 2014) were utilized throughout the therapy to calm the brainstem and enable Manny to process the therapeutic experience utilizing higher cortical regions of the brain and to maintain appropriate emotional regulation to assist with safety.

My work with fury and rage in play therapy has led me to propose a developmental progression in the expression of aggression through play in the course of therapy in the form of three stages: (1) enactment of the rage, (2) displacement of the aggressive action play into symbolization, and (3) mastery of the rage through symbolic play. The three stages of working through the fury and rage with Manny are described below.

Stage 1: Enactment of the Rage

Manny's sandtray pictures of the world often expressed a degree of fury that was extreme and at times reached sadistic proportions. In a directive intervention with puppets, I took the alligator puppet and asked him to view it as a symbol of what makes him angry and to talk to the alligator about what infuriates him. He immediately grabbed a plastic whiffle ball bat and started pounding the alligator puppet with such force that I had to remove it from my hand to avoid injury. After placing the puppet on the floor, I asked him to try to use words, and in response he started screaming, "You bastard, I hate your guts!" as he continued to pound the alligator puppet with the bat, using all the force he could muster. I asked Manny if the alligator puppet represented a specific person or situation that caused him such fury. He did not answer but continued to swing the bat at the alligator puppet and screamed loudly, "I hope you rot in hell, you bastard!" The identification with the aggressor was infused with palpable affect.

In the sandtray, Manny's pictures of the world consisted of violent scenes designed to show how overpowering force always wins: Tanks and jet fighters completely decimated villages and towns in a reign of destruction and terror. Manny referred to this obliterating force as "shock and awe" (the battle cry of the U.S. invasion of Iraq in 2003). The bombardments and tank fire continued long after all the buildings were destroyed and all the people had been killed.

This extreme intensity of rage is frequently seen with fawns in gorilla suits and sometimes children of fury. The difference I observe between the two is the directly expressed affect versus the symbolized affect. Fawns in gorilla suits at times manifest minimal overt affect even though it is vividly symbolized. Children of fury almost always express intense, overt affect in keeping with the aggressive and sometimes violent action of the play. They tend to be extremely animated and loud, and I've often had my sessions with a child of fury interrupted by a knock on the door from a concerned colleague just checking to make sure everyone was okay. In Manny's case, there were multiple knocks on the door, sometimes in the same session, to make sure the occupants had survived the fierce battles. The emotional intensity of these sessions continued over a 3-month period. The symbol of betrayal Manny used in his puppet play was the alligator, whereas in the sandtray he used either the snake or the dragon. These symbols of betrayal were viciously attacked when they appeared in Stage 1 of the work.

Although fawns in gorilla suits are inclined toward aggressive actions in play, they do not consistently register overtly the degree of outrage displayed by children of fury. Partly this difference relates to the central dynamic of betrayal and its accompanying rage in children of fury, whereas fawns in gorilla suits have experienced a whole range of trauma conditions characteristic of complex trauma. The outrage and indignation are no longer as spirited as they once were in the "fawns."

Stage 2: Displacement of Aggressive Action Play into Symbolization

As the intensity of the rage diminished in Stage 2, Manny's symbols of betrayal appeared less frequently and when they did, they typically were attacked but not with the same viciousness observed earlier. It should be noted that these stages aren't linear. The child can show decreasing intensity accompanied by increased symbolization and then be triggered by a memory or an event that forcefully reminds him or her of the betrayal and abruptly moves the child back to Stage 1: enactment of the rage.

Also in this stage, Manny was less invested in his identification with the aggressor role. In addition, increasing use of symbolization was indicated by his elaborate preparation for battles that took the form of "staging the war" in artistic and creative ways. If the battle occurred at all, it tended to be toward the end of the session and enacted with much less intensity than in Stage 1. Another shift common to Stage 2 in my clinical experience was Manny's greater flexibility in response to my participation and input. For example, at one point I suggested the possibility of a peace negotiation. Such a suggestion would have been rejected vigorously in Stage 1, but Manny was open to trying it in this phase of the work (even though the peace talks failed).

Stage 3: Mastery of the Rage through Symbolic Play

In Stage 3 of Manny's therapy the symbols of betrayal in puppet dramas and in the sandtray gradually disappeared altogether. Aggression faded and gave way to still greater interest in the creative and symbolic containment of his aggression through battlefield design and strategic planning of the battles. His arrangements of the armies were so creative and impressive that he requested that I take pictures of his various colorful battlefield scenes and print them out. Also there was a corresponding decrease of aggressive behavior both at home and school.

Manny never came out of metaphor to talk directly about the injuries to his sense of trust by his perceived multiple betrayals. Like numerous other children his age, Manny needed the safe haven and face-saving cover provided by the symbolic play and the depiction through symbols and pictures to work through and resolve his invisible intimate injuries. When he reached the stage of *mastery through symbolic play*, he gradually became less and less interested in the play that previously had drawn him like a magnet each session to the puppet theatre, the family playhouse, or the sandtray. Manny knew his work was done and so did his family because instead of looking forward to his play sessions, Manny had to be encouraged to go. In addition to mastery of his invisible wounds and a contained symbolic expression of his aggression, the relationship primarily with his adoptive family but also with his therapist had increased his attachment security. This enhanced sense of relational security enabled him to develop a new social map in which there were at least some people in his relational world who could be trusted and who he no longer automatically assumed would betray him. A major part of the corrective emotional experience via the therapeutic relationship was the "survival of the rage."

Conclusion

In this chapter, the metaphor of *children of fury* is introduced to characterize a subpopulation of enraged children and is contrasted with my previous metaphorical description of *fawns in gorilla suits* as another subcategory. Children of fury can be encountered in virtually all the settings in which the play therapist works and are characterized not only by the intensity of their rage but by the core dynamic of perceived betrayal. In contrast, fawns in gorilla suits are primarily encountered in residential treatment centers and inpatient settings and most often have suffered repeated trauma that is now often called *complex trauma*. Also in this chapter, three stages of play therapy with children of fury were described: (1) enactment of the rage, (2) displacement of the action play into symbolization, and (3) mastery of the rage through symbolized play. An integrated play therapy approach was illustrated in a case study with a "child of fury."

REFERENCES

Alexander, F. (1961). *The scope of psychoanalysis*. New York: Basic Books.

Alink, L. R., Messman, J., van Zeijl, J., Stolk, M. N., Juffer, F., Koot, H. M., et al. (2006). The early childhood aggression curve: Development of physical aggression in 10- to 50-month-old children. *Child Development, 77*(4), 954–966.

Anda, R. F., Felitti, V. J., Walker J., Whitfield, C. L., Bremner, J. D., Perry, B. D., et al. (2006). The enduring effects of abuse and related adverse experiences in childhood: A convergence of evidence from neurobiology and epidemiology. *European Archives of Psychiatry and Clinical Neurosciences, 56*(3), 174–186.

Andershed, H., Kerr, M., Stattin, H., & Levander, S. (2002). Psychopathic traits in non-referred youths: A new assessment tool. In E. Blaauw & L. Sheridan (Eds.), *Psychopaths: Current international perspectives* (pp. 131–158). The Hague: Elsevier.

Anderson, S. M., & Gedo, P. M. (2013). Relational trauma: Using play therapy to treat a disrupted attachment. *Bulletin of the Menniger Clinic, 77*(3), 250–268.

Barfield, S., Dobson, C., Gaskill, R., & Perry, B. D. (2012). Neurosequential model of therapeutics in a therapeutic preschool: Implications for work with children with complex neuropsychiatric problems. *International Journal of Play Therapy, 21*(1), 30–40.

Bendersky, M., Bennett, D., & Lewis, M. (2006). Aggression at age five as a function of prenatal exposure to cocaine, gender and environmental risk. *Journal of Pediatric Psychology, 31*(1), 71–84.

Bonime, W. (1989). *Collaborative psychoanalysis: Anxiety, depression, dreams, and personality change.* Cranbury, NJ: Associated University Presses.

Bratton, S. C., Pronchenko, Y., Ceballos, P. L., Sheely-Moore, A. I., Meany-Whalen, K., & Jones, L. D. (2013). Head Start early mental health intervention: Effects of child-centered play therapy on disruptive behaviors. *International Journal of Play Therapy, 22*(1), 28–42.

Cochran, J. L., Fauth, D. J., Cochran, N. H., Spurgeon, S. L., & Pierce, L. M. (2010). Growing play therapy up: Extending child-centered play therapy to highly aggressive teenage boys. *Person-Centered and Experiential Psychotherapies, 9*(4), 290–301.

Crenshaw, D. A. (2013). A resilience framework for treating severe child trauma. In S. Goldstein & R. B. Brooks (Eds.), *Handbook of resilience in children* (pp. 309–327). New York: Springer.

Crenshaw, D. A., & Alstadt, C. (2011). *A study of adverse childhood experiences in admissions to a residential treatment center.* Unpublished study, Children's Home of Poughkeepsie, Poughkeepsie, NY.

Crenshaw, D. A., & Garbarino, J. (2007). The hidden dimensions: Profound sorrow and buried human potential in violent youth. *Journal of Humanistic Psychology, 47*, 160–174.

Crenshaw, D. A., & Hardy, K. V. (2005). Understanding and treating the aggression of children in out-of-home care. In N. Boyd-Webb (Ed.), *Working with traumatized youth in child welfare* (pp. 171–195). New York: Guilford Press.

Crenshaw, D. A., & Mordock, J. (2005a). *Handbook of play therapy with aggressive children.* New York: Aronson.

Crenshaw, D. A. & Mordock, J. B. (2005b). Lessons learned from "fawns in gorilla suits." *Residential Treatment for Children and Youth, 22*, 33–48.

Crenshaw, D. A., & Mordock, J. (2005c). *Understanding and treating the aggression and violence of children: Fawns in gorilla suits.* New York: Aronson.

Decety, J., Chen, C., Harenski, C., & Kiehl, K. A. (2013). An fMRI study of affective perspective taking in individuals with psychopathy: Imagining another in pain does not evoke empathy. *Frontiers of Human Neurosciences, 7*(1), 489.

Dodge, K. A., & Coie, J. D. (1987). Social-information processing factors in reactive and proactive aggression in children's peer groups. *Journal of Personality and Social Psychology, 53*(6), 1146–1158.

Edwards, E. P., Eiden, R. D., Colder, C., & Leonard, K. E. (2006). The development of aggression in 18- to 48-month-old children of alcoholic parents. *Journal of Abnormal Child Psychology, 34*(3), 409–423.

Freyd, J. J. (2008). Betrayal trauma. In G. Reyes, J. D. Elhai, & J. D. Ford (Eds.), *Encyclopedia of psychological trauma* (p. 76). New York: Wiley.

Freyd, J. J., & Birrell, P. (2013). *Blind to betrayal.* New York: Wiley.

Garbarino, J. (1999). *Lost boys: Why our sons turn violent and how we can save them.* New York: Anchor Books.

Gaskill, R. L., & Perry, B. D. (2014). The neurobiological power of play: Using the neurosequential model of therapeutics to guide play in the healing process. In C. A. Malchiodi & D. A. Crenshaw (Eds.), *Creative arts and play therapy for attachment problems* (pp. 178–194). New York: Guilford Press.

Gobin, R. L., & Freyd, J. J. (2009). Betrayal and revictimization: Preliminary findings. *Psychological Trauma: Theory, Research, Practice, and Policy, 1*(3), 242–257.

Hardy, K. V., & Crenshaw, D. A. (2008). Healing the wounds to the soul camouflaged by rage. In D. A. Crenshaw (Ed.), *Child and adolescent psychotherapy* (pp. 15–30). Lanham, MD: Aronson/Rowman & Littlefield.

Hardy, K. V., & Laszloffy, T. A. (2005). *Teens who hurt: Clinical interventions to break the cycle of adolescent violence.* New York: Guilford Press.

Kagan, J. (1998, March). *How we become who we are.* Paper presented at the Psychotherapy Networker symposium, Washington, DC.

Keown, L. J., & Woodward, L. J. (2006). Preschool boys with pervasive hyperactivity: Early peer functioning and mother–child relationship influences. *Social Development,* *15*(1), 23–45.

Kolla, N. J., Malcolm, C., Attard, S., Arenovich, T., Blackwood, N., & Hodgins, S. (2013). Childhood maltreatment and aggressive behavior in violent offenders with psychopathy. *Canadian Journal of Psychiatry, 58*(8), 487–494.

Moss, E., Smolla, N., Guerra, I., Mazzarello, T., Chayer, D., & Berthiaume, C. (2006). Attachment and self-reported internalizing and externalizing behavior problems in a school period. *Canadian Journal of Behavioural Science, 38*(2), 142–157.

Oaklander, V. (2006). *Hidden treasure: A map to the child's inner self.* London: Karnac Books.

Ostrov, J. M., Gentile, D. A., & Crick, N. R. (2006). Media exposure, aggression, and prosocial behavior during early childhood: A longitudinal study. *Social Development, 15*(4), 612–627.

Pihlakoski, L., Sourander, A., Aromaa, M., Rautava, P., Helenius, H., & Silllanpaa, M. (2006). The continuity of psychopathology from early childhood to preadolescence: A predictive cohort study of 3- to 12-year-old children. *European Child and Adolescent Psychiatry, 15*(7), 409–417.

Ray, D. C., Blanco, P. J., Sullivan, J. M., & Holliman, R. (2009). An exploratory study of child-centered play therapy with aggressive children. *International Journal of Play Therapy, 18*(3), 162–175.

Schore, A. N. (2012). *The science of the art of psychotherapy.* New York: Norton.

Stewart, A. L., & Echterling, L. G. (2014). Play and the therapeutic relationship. In C. Schaefer & A. Drewes (Eds.), *The therapeutic powers of play* (2nd ed., pp. 157–170). New York: Wiley.

van der Kolk, B. A. (2005). Developmental trauma disorder. *Psychiatric Annals, 35*, 401–408.

Webb, N. B. (Ed.). (2007). *Play therapy with children in crisis: A casebook for practitioners* (3rd ed.). New York: Guilford Press.

Weinberg, K. M., Tronick, E. Z., Cohn, J. F., & Olson, K. L. (1999). Gender differences in emotional expressivity and self-regulation during infancy. *Developmental Psychology, 35*(1), 175–188.

Zoccolillo, M., Keenan, K., Cote, S., Peruse, D., Wu, H.-X., Boivin, M., et al. (2007). Gender differences in physical aggression: A prospective population-based survey of children before and after 2 years of age. *Developmental Psychology, 43*(1), 13–26.

CHAPTER 16

Play Therapy with the Spectrum of Bullying Behavior

Steven Baron

Bullying is defined as the use of one's strength or status to injure, threaten, or humiliate another person without provocation. Bullying can be physical, verbal, or indirect/relational aggression (Carlson & Cornell, 2008) and occurs repeatedly over time. The relationship between bully and victim implies that there is an imbalance of power, with the bully attempting to control the victim on a repeated basis. Bullying can include direct actions such as threatening, hitting, stealing, or verbal abuse as well as indirect methods such as spreading rumors and intentionally isolating a peer socially. The most recent statistics indicate that approximately 160,000 children miss school on a daily basis due to a fear of being bullied (Bullying Statistics, 2010). One in seven students in kindergarten through 12th grade either is a bully or has been a victim of a bully. Seventy-one percent of students report that bullying is an ongoing problem; 10% of students change schools or drop out because of repeated victimization (Bullying Statistics, 2010). On average 1 in 20 students has seen a student with a gun at school. Further investigation reveals that 90% of fourth through eighth

graders report being victims of bullying and that approximately 282,000 students are reportedly attacked in high schools on a monthly basis in the United States (Bullying Statistics, 2010). Fifty-six percent of all students have witnessed a bullying crime take place while at school.

These statistics reflect bullying that occurs specifically within the school setting. With the advent of social media, the phenomenon of cyberbullying is also a reality. The latest statistics reveal that 2.7 million students are victims of cyberbullying (Bullying Statistics, 2010). Only 1 in 10 adolescents tells a parent if he or she is being, or has been, cyberbullied. One in 10 adolescents has had embarrassing or damaging pictures taken without their permission, often using cellphone cameras (Bullying Statistics, 2010). A review of the literature indicates that bullying is a phenomenon that occurs around the world regardless of culture (Beaty & Alexeyev, 2008; Forero, McClellan, Rissel, & Bauman, 1999; Harris & Petrie, 2002; Wolke, Woods, Stanford, & Schulz, 2001).

Given the preponderance of this phenomenon, it is very likely that mental health professionals will continue to be called upon not only to support victims but also to treat bullies as well. What follows is a consideration of the psychological and sociocultural factors that contribute to the occurrence of this trend.

Social-Psychological Factors

From a social learning perspective, Bandura proposed that exposure to a combative environment contributes to the acquisition of aggressive behaviors (as cited in Espelage, Bosworth, & Simon, 2000). Parenting styles have been associated with the development of aggression in children (Espelage et al., 2000; Stelios, 2008). Boys who bully have families described as lacking in warmth, more likely to use physical violence, characterized by a harsh authoritative style, and unreliable in monitoring their children's activities outside of school. In addition, these parents may teach techniques of retaliation and punish their children in a harsh, inconsistent manner. Children with parents who emphasized nonviolent solutions to conflict were less likely to engage in bullying behavior (Centers for Disease Control and Prevention, 2011; Espelage et al., 2000).

Children who experience their parents as respecting their need for independence were less likely to engage in bullying behavior (Stelios, 2008). Families whose members share warm and accepting relationships and are able to discuss and help children with difficulties, produce offspring less likely to engage in bullying behavior. Children who reported negative peer influences, had access to guns, and had concerns about their safety in their neighborhoods were more likely to engage in bullying behavior (Van Hoof, Raajmakers, Van Beck, Hale, & Aleva, 2008).

In a survey of bullies, a correlation between low levels of maternal support and engaging in bullying behavior was evident (Holt & Espelage, 2007; Stelios, 2008). Although close supervision of children by

parents helps to reduce the likelihood of a child becoming a bully, the inverse is also true: that is, increases in bullying behavior by children lead to a reduction of parental involvement and monitoring over time. The parent–child relationship can thus reciprocally influence the development of continued bullying behavior (Georgiou & Fanti, 2010). Perhaps this decrease in monitoring in response to an increase in troubling behavior is reflective of a parent's feeling increasingly powerless and therefore withdrawing from the child. Research also suggests that single parenting increases the risk that a child may engage in bullying behavior (Yang, Stewart, Kim, Kim, & Shin, 2013). In addition, the psychological or physical absence of a father figure as well as the presence of a depressive component in their mothers has been associated with aggressive behavior in boys (Stelios, 2008). Bullies reported that they experienced their families as less cohesive, more conflicted, and less organized than did their nonbullying counterparts (Stelios, 2008). Parents of bullies were more likely to feel that their child did things to bother them, was difficult to care for, and evoked angrier responses from them than parents of nonbullying children (Shetgiri, Lin, Avila, & Flores, 2012).

Data strongly suggest that the best predictor for the absence of bullying was having positive role models. This finding is consistent with the idea of a charismatic adult, introduced by Dr. Jules Segal as someone from whom a child can gather strength (Brooks & Goldstein, 2001). A child's relationship with adults is independent of peer influences in promoting the development of bullying behavior (Espelage et al., 2000). However, the degree to which children do participate in negative behaviors (e.g., destroying property, participating in illegal activities, fighting) was predictive of bullying behavior. School alienation was associated with bullying, whereas increasing support from teachers was associated with a decrease in such behavior (Natvig, Albrektsen, & Qvarnstrom, 2001). A key predictor of bullying behavior was teachers' low expectations of their students' academic performances (Barboza et al., 2009).

Research supports the notion that bullies tend to be male, aggressive, tough, impulsive, and lack empathy (Christie-Mizell, 2003; Flescher Peskin, Tortolero, & Markham, 2006; Wolke et al., 2001). Data confirm the relationship between the degree to which a boy rates himself as having traditional masculine traits and the extent of bullying behavior in which he engages (Gini & Pozzoli, 2006; Klein, 2012). Boys are more likely than girls to retain retaliatory attitudes and to utilize physical violence to resolve conflict (Bradshaw, Sawyer, & O'Brennan, 2009).

Low self-concept is a predictor of higher levels of bullying behavior in children (Christie-Mizell, 2003). The presence of aggressive friends was positively associated with increased bullying behavior (Mouttapa, Valente, Gallaher, Rohrbach, & Unger, 2004). Bullies may have larger peer groups and have earlier dating experiences (Mouttapa et al., 2004). It has been reported that bullies who date at a younger age rated their relationships as less supportive and equitable than those peers who did not engage in bullying behavior. In addition, these youngsters were more likely to engage in acts of physical or social aggression toward their partners compared to a nonbully sample (Dake, Price, & Telljohann, 2003).

Research linking bullying behavior to a child's status in school found that the risk for engaging in bullying increases through the elementary school years and peaks during middle school years, declining thereafter (Bradshaw et al., 2009; Flescher Peskin et al., 2006). Furthermore, transitional periods in a student's life appear to be related to engaging in bullying behavior as a student moves from elementary school to middle school and again from middle school to high school. Bullies tend to victimize those who are of the same age and grade as themselves as well as those peers with whom they spend time and know well (Beaty & Alex-

eyev, 2008). Bullies have greater academic difficulties and are less motivated to do well academically (Carlson & Cornell, 2008; Dake et al., 2003; Shetgiri et al., 2012).

Significant relationships between bullying and mental health conditions, such as bipolar disorder, substance abuse, conduct disorder, paranoid, and histrionic personality disorders, are evident (Vaughn et al., 2010). Being a bully can have long-term social consequences, including antisocial behaviors, criminality, and higher conviction rates (Menesini, Modena, & Tani, 2009). In fact, 70% of middle school bullies were convicted of a crime by age 24 (Vaughn et al., 2010). A relationship between depression and engaging in bullying behavior has been noted for both males and females (Beaty & Alexeyev, 2008; Holt & Espelage, 2007; Yang et al., 2013). Bullies tend to have a positive attitude toward violence as well as significant empathic limitations (Pontzer, 2010). Although bullies tend to exhibit symptoms of externalizing disorders, evidence suggests that they also experience internalizing symptoms, particularly during adolescence, such as depression, anxiety, and eating disorders as well as psychosomatic disorders (Forero et al., 1999; Menesini et al., 2009). Children who bully are at greater risk for abusing alcohol and smoking (Bazelon, 2013; Nansel et al., 2001).

Many bullies report that they are able to make friends easily, which suggests that they are not necessarily socially isolated, although many of their friends may endorse aggressive tactics to resolve interpersonal difficulties (Holt & Espelage, 2007; Nansel et al., 2001). Social identity theory (Holt & Espelage, 2007) posits that individuals derive their social identity from the group with which they affiliate. Group members favor behaviors that are consistent with group norms and attempt to preserve the group's identity by emphasizing differences between their group and other groups. Engaging in bullying behavior can be a means to preserve the group identity. Regardless of region, certain universal characteristics have been identified in bullies. These include mistakenly perceiving hostile intent in others, overreacting in an angry manner and using force quickly, obsessively holding onto rigid beliefs, viewing image as the way to gain power, and using aggressive behavior to protect their image (Hazler, Carney, & Granger, 2006). When asked directly why they bully others, the reasons most often identified were a desire for power followed by a desire for attention (Beaty & Alexeyev, 2008).

Among demographic factors a child's race/ethnicity was associated with being a bully (Shetgiri et al., 2012), with African American and Hispanic adolescents having the highest rate of bullying behavior (Carlyle & Steinman, 2007; Fitzpatrick, Dulin, & Piko, 2007; Flescher Peskin et al., 2006). European American children and Asian/Pacific Islander children have significantly lower odds of being bullies (Shetgiri et al., 2012).

Bully-Victims

Bully-victims are children who have bullied others and have been bullied themselves. In a recent study approximately a third of bullies were identified as bully-victims (Schwartz, Proctor, & Chein, 2001). These children may overreact to teasing, threats, or physical actions, predisposing them to being bullied repeatedly. In addition, they may have difficulty controlling their anger, and their inability to tolerate frustration may lead them to retaliate against others. Thus the bully-victim cycle repeats itself. Evidence suggests that bully-victims, unlike pure bullies or victims, demonstrate a broader range of emotional distress (Espelage & Holt, 2007; Forero et al., 1999; Isolan, Salum, Osowksi, Hartmann, & Manfro, 2013; Menesini et al., 2009; Mouttapa et al., 2004; Schwartz et al., 2001). Greater levels of anxiety, depression, peer rejection, and a lack of close relationships, as seen in victims, as well as greater acceptance of rule-

breaking behavior, hyperactivity, and a tendency toward the reactive aggression that characterizes bullies are present. This cluster of characteristics places bully-victims at greater risk for emotional disturbance, substance abuse, or antisocial personality disturbance. Bully-victims are often loners, and this isolation contributes to their sense of powerlessness, anger, and expression of hostility (Gordon, 2013; Holt & Espelage, 2007). Bully-victims are often less cooperative and sociable than a pure bully or victim, and they have greater difficulty reading social signals. Bully-victims have greater difficulty following classroom rules and are less engaged in their studies, reflecting the emotional distress they experience. Furthermore, bully-victims are the least likely group of bystanders to intervene in a bullying episode to help a victim.

Exposure to, as well as being a victim of, domestic abuse is more common among bully-victims than among bullies or victims alone (Centers for Disease Control and Prevention, 2011; Espelage & Holt, 1997). In addition, this group is at greater risk for considering suicide as well as for intentionally hurting themselves. Overall the broader range of symptoms for this subgroup yields a greater degree of suffering for them than for bullies or victims.

The Bully Within

For many children the need to humiliate and control others, as well as being overly harsh and excessively critical of themselves, comes from internalizing aggressive elements in their lives, such as damaging interactions with parents or peers. This internalized product, which can be called the *bully within*, serves as a persistent message to these children to demonstrate their capacity for power and mastery over others as well as limiting their capacity to accept themselves for who they are. The oppressed becomes the oppressor both of their environment and of themselves. They become the bully and bullied simultaneously. Needless to say, this dynamic can have profound effects on a child's capacity for empathy, for accurately interpreting social cues, as well as for developing a positive self-concept. These children are not happy with their world or themselves. They are ready to strike out at an environment they perceive as unrelenting in its harsh treatment of them. They repeat this pattern not only with peers but with themselves, demonstrating a very harsh level of self-criticism. They are rarely satisfied with their world or themselves, as the oppressor they have internalized operates behind the scenes exerting a profound effect.

The bully within can influence not only children but teenagers and adults as well. Although not all such individuals who struggle with this dynamic are physically aggressive, the bully within can have a more subtle yet just as powerful impact. For instance, both adults and children can be highly perfectionistic and blame themselves profusely when they experience failure. Although not physically aggressive in their behavior, these individuals, whether young or old, can be more forceful than necessary in their interactions with others. The bully within can limit how receptive individuals are to accepting praise from themselves or others for a job well done, instead focusing on a minor imperfection. In children this mindset will limit their desire to take appropriate risks because they believe they cannot achieve success. The bully within promotes a negative self-concept that is internalized and will subsequently shape and motivate behavior. From this perspective, the outer bully is expressing in behavior what is happening within. The harshness these individuals direct against themselves is projected onto the world.

Bystanders

Whereas bullying is a phenomenon that directly impacts the bully and victim, consideration has also been given to how witnessing bullying episodes influences those who observe them as well as how the presence of observers influences the bullying. The fact that the number of bystanders is potentially much larger than the number of either bullies or victims in an episode makes it important to examine the role and impact of this group. Statistics reveal that 85% of bullying occurs in the context of a group (Oh, 2007). Research indicates that only 11% of bystanders intervened in a bullying episode, 33% of bystanders reported that they should have helped the victim, and another 24% of bystanders felt that the bullying was not their business (Banks, 1997).

Four potentially different roles for bystanders have been identified (Salmivalli, 1999):

1. *The assistant.* This group of students acts as helpers or sidekicks. These students engage in behavior similar to the bullies, such as catching the victim, holding the victim down, and joining in the fighting. However, the assistants have less power than the bullies. Approximately 8% of bystanders fall within this category.

2. *The reinforcer.* This group can enhance bullying by engaging in behaviors such as giggling, laughing, and inciting the bully by shouting. The individuals in this group do not lead or initiate the bullying behavior but reinforce it by providing positive feedback to the audience. They seem to enjoy the thrill and excitement of indirect participation with the bully. Approximately 15–19% of bystanders fall within this category

3. *The outsider.* These children do not intervene at all during a bullying episode. Their inaction, apathy, and secrecy help to maintain the bullying culture. This group is actually the majority of all participants in a bullying situation (23–32%).

4. *The defender.* These students intervene in a bullying situation by taking a variety of actions. They may offer to support

or comfort the victim, staying with the victim or seeking an adult. They might even challenge the bully and take revenge; 17–19% of bystanders are defenders. These statistics indicate that the largest amount of bystanders adopt a passive approach to a bullying situation.

Although it may appear that intervening to help a victim during a bullying episode should be an automatic response, it is in fact a rather complex behavior. Whereas children may feel sympathetic to the plight of the victim and/or have positive perceptions of him or her, they must also experience a moral responsibility to intervene. Engaging in a bullying episode in front of witnesses who don't intervene sends a message to the bully that he or she can continue to humiliate the victim. There are several possibilities as to why bystanders remain in that passive role:

1. They may feel that the bullying episode is none of their business.
2. They may fear becoming the target of the bully if they intervene.
3. They may fear being labeled a *tattletale* if they seek out help.
4. Negative attitudes toward the victim may inhibit a response to intervene to stop the bullying episode.
5. They may feel that they do not know what to do and fear they will make the situation worse.

Other factors may influence a bystander's reaction to the bullying situation. For instance, girls are more likely to intervene than boys, suggesting that gender is a factor (Oh, 2007). Bystanders are more likely to intervene and help victims when witnessing relational or indirect verbal bullying than witnessing direct physical or direct verbal aggression (Oh, 2007). Age has also been identified as an important variable; children showed a tendency to decrease helping behaviors in a bystander situation from second to sixth grade, although their bully-ing behaviors increased from kindergarten to second grade. Students tended to lose their desire to help victims as they moved from elementary school to middle school (Oh, 2007). Bystanders who were bullies or bullies-victims were less likely to help victims than those who just witnessed bullying without having any past experience of bullying and victimization (Oh, 2007).

Being a bystander does not necessarily mean that the impact of the episode ends at its conclusion. Bystanders report increased use of drugs, possibly greater incidences of depression and anxiety, and their attendance at school may be impacted by their heightened fears of being bullied. In fact, research strongly suggests that witnessing repeated bullying can produce both psychological as well as physiological distress that, over time, may equal that of victims (Mouttapa et al., 2004).

Children who become active bystanders and directly intervene in the bullying situation to stop it are regarded as more empathic than those who do not (Oh, 2007). Bystanders who experienced greater levels of state anxiety (as opposed to the more permanent trait anxiety) in the bullying episode were more likely to demonstrate helping behavior toward the victim. Also, bystanders who had a prior history of being traumatized were less likely to show a positive reaction to bullying (Oh, 2007).

Research has focused on identifying differing variables as they relate to bystander status. For instance, social status has been identified as impacting a bystander's response in a bullying situation. Students who enjoyed high social status within a group or a dominant role reported that they would be more likely to intervene to help a victim (Oh, 2007). Perhaps children who are highly regarded in their peer group may be less affected by the peer pressures that maintain the bully's dominance. This possibility has implications for interventions, as empowerment of bystanders within their social standing could be a plausible strategy to reduce the incidence of bullying. Also the nature of the bullying to which students are exposed to may influence their response. Bystanders' helping behaviors decreased when others were present in situations of low potential danger but did not decrease in situations of high potential danger regardless of the presence of others (Fisher, Grietmeyer, Pollezek, & Frey, 2006).

Clinical Case Example

The following is an actual case of a child whom I treated. All potentially identifying details have been disguised to protect confidentiality.

Mr. and Mrs. Green contacted me concerning their son, James, an 8-year-old boy who was attending the second grade. James's parents were currently in marital therapy to address their very conflicted relationship. Over the course of their therapy, they had voiced increasing concern regarding their son. Their initial complaint was his difficulty keeping up with school assignments. Focusing difficulties were present, for which James was receiving medication. However, it was within the social–emotional realm that the greatest worry was evident. Of particular concern were his increasingly frequent aggressive behaviors directed toward family members and peers in school. In addition, James displayed rage reactions when denied his way as well physically lashing out at peers when they did not agree with him. James also refused to attend school consistently. He had been bedwetting for several years, with no neurological basis determined by his physicians. The parents reported that James was riddled with fears. He would often report that he was afraid of getting into a fatal accident, was afraid to sleep alone in his room, and insisted on sleeping in the room with his younger sibling. In addition, on many occasions James feared that he would lose control and harm others. James was particularly afraid of being alone, often following his parents around their home.

James was a "happy baby" who slept through the night by 2 months. Mrs. Green did not work and according to her, developmental milestones were within age expectations and his health history was negative. James was enrolled in a variety of toddler and preschool programs and showed no difficulty adapting. He would easily separate and related well to other children. He had very successful school years in kindergarten and first grade, with no behavioral difficulties noted during this period. James complied with school demands and got along well with peers. During second grade, he became increasingly defiant at home and school, refusing to complete school assignments. James also experienced academic difficulties for the first time. His parents believed that James's behavior deteriorated at this point due to an overly strict teacher.

James's parents had been in marital therapy to address their extremely volatile relationship. James's father worked long hours and abdicated responsibility for childrearing to his wife. He became increasingly withdrawn, preferring to sleep and watch television. This behavior led to a great deal of tension between the spouses, which James was privy to as they fought in a volatile manner. Both parents took medication for depression and anxiety. The couple's family therapist reported that were it not for economic reasons, the couple would have split up many years ago. A major source of disagreement was their respective parenting styles. James's father was quick to verbally berate his son and punish him by taking away videogames, which was one of James's favorite pastimes. In contrast, James's mother reported that despite being initially patient with him, she ultimately became exasperated by her son and lost her temper. When asked about James's strengths, both had to do a considerable amount of thinking before responding that James enjoyed writing and drawing as well as playing athletics.

Prior to beginning play therapy, the parents' marital therapist had suggested that

James receive a psychoeducational evaluation. The results of the assessment indicated that James was functioning within the average range of intelligence, with his nonverbal reasoning abilities more fully developed than his verbal reasoning skills. Academically, all areas assessed were either at or above age expectations. James did not meet the criteria for an attention-deficit/hyperactivity disorder (ADHD) diagnosis, nor was a learning disability detected. At the time of the assessment, the classroom teacher rated James as having elevated levels of aggressive behavior toward peers, although not to the extent cited by Mr. and Mrs. Green, whereas the parents noted aggressive, impulsive behaviors and social skills deficits. The evaluation did recommend therapy for James to address concerns noted by his parents.

Initial Assessment

In the initial parent intake session with Mr. and Mrs. Green, the level of parental discord was very apparent. The parents openly criticized each other over their respective parenting styles and their son's difficulties. Their anger toward their son was quite blatant. They both saw him as disrespectful and intentionally contrary, admitting they had little patience for him.

James was a stocky, light-haired youngster who looked his stated age and barely acknowledged me in our first meeting. Upon entering my office to begin play therapy, James fell into his seat, offering brief, unelaborated responses to queries. James did not display interest in exploring any play materials. Instead, he sat quietly in his seat and rarely spoke. The only notable exception was when I asked James to identify the things he enjoys and is talented at doing. James confirmed his parents report that he enjoys drawing and writing. In addition, he added that he "loves" to build with Legos. I told James that there was a basket of Legos in the office for him to use if he wanted, but he declined. I replied, "When you feel more like doing it, they are here

for you." James did not respond. During the first session, he did not leave his seat, said little, and made little eye contact.

For the next session, James continued to display no interest in utilizing any play materials, nor did he speak. Because I administer a projective battery to new youngsters with whom I work, I asked James if he would like to participate in some drawing and storytelling games, and he readily agreed. Although James offered mostly brief, unelaborated responses, in some instances he was more productive. He was particularly responsive on the Thematic Apperception Test and produced stories in response to the stimulus cards that highlighted pertinent family themes. These included stories in which parents fought over the father's lack of involvement in family life. In all stories, James depicted family life as aggressive and chaotic, with the child escaping from it. There was no evidence of experiencing his world as a supportive, nurturing place. Most revealing was James's Kinetic Family Drawing. When asked to draw his family doing something, he drew four small stick figures placed apart from each other with the father throwing darts. When he drew himself in the corner, he put a box around this figure, walling him off from the rest of the family. The placement of his figure as well as the metaphor of his father throwing darts was especially striking. When this perception was reflected back to James, he said, "In the picture we are celebrating my father winning the championship. He is the best at throwing darts."

James was cooperative in completing the projective assessment, and his responses provided a glimpse into his perceptions and fears. It appeared that the aggressive associations articulated were partly a defensive reaction to cope with a view of a very volatile and frightening family life. James appeared to be incorporating the provocative, threatening manner he experienced in his parents. The impact of this dynamic on the therapeutic relationship was something that I kept in mind.

Course of Treatment

The early phase of treatment was challenging, as James was reluctant to engage with me, and his behavioral difficulties were escalating in school and at home. In sessions, James was nonverbal and refused to engage in any play activities. Long periods of silence would ensue. I never put any pressure on James; instead, I would reiterate that when he was ready, he could involve himself with any of the play materials, draw, or engage in other activities. In several sessions, James sat silently and appeared drowsy, and in a few instances he actually dozed off briefly. After several sessions of this behavior, James's parents reported that he was refusing to attend sessions. Mr. Green rearranged his work schedule so that he could bring James to his appointments. Although the father's intervention helped to ensure James's attendance, it did not reduce his reluctance.

Two months into treatment I went to the waiting room to greet James and only his mother (who accompanied him to this appointment, as the father was unavailable) was present, as James had locked himself in the car, refusing to come inside. I went out to the car, and James refused to either roll down the window or look at me. In fact, he turned on the car radio loudly to drown out whatever I was saying. After several minutes, I decided to discontinue my efforts, as James was hiding on the floor of the car. A phone call later that evening from Mrs. Green revealed that her husband had taken away privileges from James, and they'd had a screaming match. Mrs. Green also reported that James was increasingly aggressive with peers and accused of stealing their belongings. In addition, his grades were plummeting.

At this point, I suggested a family session, and the parents agreed. In the session, James sat in his seat curled up in a ball as if anticipating the worst. The family sat in silence for a few moments until Mrs. Green reported that James had been saying that he

wanted to kill himself and that his life was worthless. Mr. Green viewed these statements as a manipulation. I reflected that the entire family was hurting. James interrupted, saying that he was not happy, that his father punished him for anything, and that he (James) no longer cared. The parents stated that their punishments seemed to have no impact on James. I stated that the parents could now begin to do things differently by relating to James without relying solely on punishment. This issue had been raised previously but was not accepted by the parents. At this time, however, the family seemed more receptive to implementing a positive approach. I also recommended that James's treating psychiatrist reevaluate his medication, given the escalation of his behavioral difficulties. As for therapy, James admitted that he had mixed feelings about attending. I responded that it is a common feeling and it sometimes takes time to feel very comfortable in sessions. When asked about having ongoing family sessions, Mr. Green said that he could not commit; interestingly, James said that he would be willing to attend family sessions but would prefer to meet individually.

In the sessions that followed, James attended willingly. He brought props from home to help him transition to his sessions. A favorite item of his was Pokémon cards. James took great pride in laying out his collection of cards and providing detailed explanations of the characters. This was a first attempt of positive communication. James was very knowledgeable about this topic, becoming quite animated in describing how these characters got their powers and defeated their enemies. The theme of defeating one's enemies resonated with James. He then invited me to join him and play with the Pokémon cards. As he taught me how to play, it was apparent that a shift was happening in James. He began to let his guard down while finding a forum in which to express his aggressive strivings and desire for mastery as well as attempting to connect with the therapist. For several sessions, James and I played with the Pokémon cards. After a few weeks of this, I attempted to utilize an additional strength of his. I suggested that since James knew so much about these characters, perhaps he could draw them. James liked this idea very much and for a few weeks, would do so.

I was encouraged by the positive changes during sessions. However, this positive outlook was punctured by a phone call from Mrs. Green, stating that James's behavior continued to be challenging. He was now openly lying to his parents and teachers about completing assignments, and peers were accusing him of hitting them as well as continuing to steal their possessions. In addition, Mr. Green was not utilizing the positive approach outlined earlier. My attempts to reach out to Mr. Green were rebuffed for several weeks. Mrs. Green reported that James had intentionally clogged up a school toilet and created a flood, which he initially denied but eventually admitted to. Mrs. Green ended her phone call by questioning if therapy would help her son. Apparently, Mr. Green had already written it off.

In the session following the phone call, James did not bring his Pokémon cards with him, nor was he interested in continuing to draw Pokémon characters. He entered the session and sat quietly. I silently wondered if Mrs. Green had lectured James about the phone call she'd made to me. James was quiet for a few minutes. Finally, he pulled out paper and markers and began to draw. He drew a picture of a heavyset man yelling at a child. He then put words in bubbles above each character. The man was saying, "Screw you. You suck at everything." The child was replying, "I hate you." He sat quietly and just stared at what he had drawn. I strongly suspected that this drawing reflected an argument he'd had with his father (who was indeed very overweight). After a few minutes of silence I asked James about the characters he'd drawn. He responded, "The picture says it all." Keeping in the metaphor of the picture, I asked James what had happened to the people in

the drawing. James did not respond, then took another sheet of paper and drew two figures, one taller than the other. The bigger figure held a gun aimed at the other person, with a bullet flying out of the gun. The bigger figure was saying "Die" with the other figure saying "Why?" I was trying to get a sense of what these pictures meant to James. Was he the aggressor? The victim? Both? Was he communicating his perceptions of a recent argument between himself and his father? I had more questions than answers at this point. What was noteworthy was that James was using his sessions constructively. He was expressing his emotions via a safe modality, although the feelings stirred up were clearly unsettling for him.

For the next few sessions, James would doodle or draw various characters but would not discuss them. Mrs. Green reported that her husband and James had been increasingly fighting. Mr. Green continued to refuse the therapist's requests to meet. During this time, James brought a backpack to one of his sessions and pulled out a sheet of paper from his teacher. It had imprinted on it "Certificate of Excellence" along with James's name. It said he was getting the certificate "for excellence in everything." He showed it to me and I congratulated him. As I was about to ask James about the circumstances that won him the certificate, he retrieved a marker, crossed out the phrase "for excellence in," and wrote over it "for being an idiot." He then wrote the words *idiot* and *stupid* across the sheet. All I could think about was the anger and despair James held inside of him and how it was fueling his aggressive behavior. His scrawled words also conveyed a sense of vulnerability and helplessness. I conveyed to James that it was sad he had a hard time accepting the award and wondered if something had happened. James did not say anything. Instead, he took a sheet of paper and drew a colorful montage. James was sharing his anger, depression, and hopelessness—a major shift from how he formerly used his sessions.

For the next few visits, James drew logos of hockey teams, a sport he enjoyed, but would not communicate much else. His mother reported that James had some good days interspersed with more difficult ones. One day James came into his session and asked to play the game Mad Libs (in which players are given sentences with portions missing and asked to fill in the blanks). I agreed, and James actually smiled—which he had never done in a session. He then dictated a story to me and indicated when he should leave blanks to be filled in later on by him. The story he created was about a king who had no power. He then met a queen and an emperor, explaining how he did not feel like a king and felt very sad and wanted help. He was unable to get help from them. The king thought about his situation and decided to make a speech to the country. After he did so (James did not specify what the speech was about), "the people began to listen to me more."

This statement was one of the first examples of a positive outcome in an imaginative scenario for James. It raised a sense of hope and optimism and may also be interpreted as a positive sign for therapy. Perhaps James is expressing his hope that once he is able to get some things said, he would be taken seriously. This type of play seemed to capture James's imagination. He was able to talk metaphorically about the characters and emphasize how happy the king was in the end. In the subsequent session, James created a story in which a child was worried about getting a test back from his teacher, and he went into some detail describing the anxiety the character felt. At the end of the story, he goes home and his mother tells him he received a nearly perfect score and congratulates him. This may indeed reveal a wish for such an interaction with his parents. It was the second positive story he had created and in sharp contrast to his earlier productions. It may have also been a commentary about therapy, as he experienced an accepting relationship that could offer him positive feedback.

In the third and final use of this format, which happened in the same session, James created a story in which he comes face-to-face with a famous singer. Although his reaction was to "scream," he instead "closed my mouth." I was struck by the decision of the character to exercise self-control and refrain from opening his mouth. This was indeed a marked departure in how James managed his impulses. Interestingly, the appearance of this story corresponded with Mrs. Green's reporting that James was experiencing less severe behavioral outbursts.

James became increasingly productive in his sessions. He began to introduce events that had happened at school as well as with peers and at home. This seemed to usher in a new phase for James in therapy. He had indeed come a long way from the beginning stages of treatment in which he fell asleep or did and said nothing. James was intrigued by a portable typewriter in my office (I purchased this machine to offer children another way to utilize their self-expressive skills). James began working on a story that extended over several sessions. He would either do the typing himself or dictate to me. James created a story about a number of fruits and their adventures in school. The story highlighted various conflicts the fruits had among each other and their teachers and parents. James went into detail about the characters and their motivations. James displayed a clear talent for writing. His story was lively, used puns, and was well thought out. I shared some of these impressions with James, who continued to create more stories.

Over the course of treatment, James continued to use his sessions to express his thoughts and feelings. Not only did his aggressive behavior lessen (although not completely so), he became less fearful and his depressive ideation lessened. Despite these gains, James had a very limited circle of friends and displayed empathy on an inconsistent basis. In addition, the volatile situation at home continued. Mr. and Mrs. Green abruptly ended their marital sessions and were further estranged from each other. Unfortunately, just as James was showing growth outside of his sessions, his parents abruptly terminated treatment. Efforts to get Mr. and Mrs. Green to reconsider this decision met with adamant refusal. Mrs. Green stated that her husband and James recently had a "major blowout," with Mr. Green concluding that therapy was not helpful and forbidding the continuation of sessions. In this instance, Mrs. Green felt she could not go against her husband and refused to have a parent meeting with me. My attempts to have a termination session with James were refused. I was quite disappointed by the sudden manner in which James's sessions ended. One can only speculate about how James must have experienced it.

Despite how treatment ended, James was able to demonstrate a major shift in how he used his sessions. He gradually became less defensive and frightened as he tentatively reached out to the therapist. The progress James demonstrated shows how utilizing play therapy as a treatment for children who bully is an effective tool. Letting James acclimate at his own pace allowed him to experience the therapeutic relationship as a significant and, at times, a moving collaboration.

Treating Bullies: Some Reflections

Twenty-five years of treating bullies in a school as well as a private practice setting has yielded several important but difficult lessons learned. One of the hardest is how to help the child trust me. This is the single most difficult obstacle to overcome, but the most critical. So many bullies and aggressive children struggle with achieving this trust. Establishing this trust remains an ongoing struggle for me as well as the child. Children know they are in trouble by the time they come to see me. They often feel there is no point in reaching out, as their fate is already sealed. How do I try to convey

to them that my job is not to dispense discipline? Rather I want them to feel in their hearts that I am genuinely interested in how they experience not only the immediate situation but also how they deal with life in general. I have come to see that so many of these children wear their aggression as a coat of arms to protect them from displaying the tremendous sense of vulnerability they experience underneath. During the treatment of James I was reminded of this protective mechanism on several occasions. His drawings and free play vividly communicated his trepidation in connecting with someone yet at the same time wanting to do so. Although James was especially adept at expressing his feelings and thoughts once he felt safe enough to do so, this ability obviously has not been present in many other such youngsters.

In meeting for the first time with a bully, I try to give them an experience of an adult (me) that is unlike all the other adults with whom they have had to deal. Teachers, parents, and school administrators may understandably take the approach of finding out the facts of what happened in a bullying situation, making this their primary task. Although it is necessary to do so, a therapist is not (nor should be) bound only to this goal. I do not want the child to view me as a facsimile of the other adults he or she may have dealt with already. How do I do this? How do I differentiate myself from the rest of the interested parties?

It has been my experience that many of these children and teenagers approach meeting with me by trying to maintain a nearly impenetrable stance. James, for example, fell asleep in the early sessions of his treatment, but the stance of resistance can take many different forms. I have encountered the full range of protest behaviors, from children refusing to enter the room, to those who manhandled objects and broke them, to those who cursed me out. I have had to remind myself on several occasions that although this behavior is very disconcerting, it is a vital communication from the child. I am being tested. How I respond at this early juncture will dictate, to a very large degree, how the treatment will unfold. When James refused to enter my office and hid in his parent's car, I couldn't help but experience some of the helplessness he felt. Just as he felt he could not impact his world in a constructive sense, I felt the exact same way in that situation. I also felt embarrassed in front of his mother, who watched as I was unable to resolve this situation. I realized that this embarrassment is probably her experience of herself in so many situations when she is unable to ameliorate her son's behavior. James was letting me know how his attempts to manage his life were not working at all. As I got to know James and his parents, this hunch was confirmed several times over. It also made me think how critical it was to maintain an empathic stance, no matter what James did—which is what I felt all along that he so sorely needed from me—and his seeing if I could indeed deliver.

When I meet with bullies, I very often decide to "change things up," to behave in an unexpected way. Instead of questioning them about their bullying incidents, I ask about their interests and achievements. I find that not only does this help to put them at ease, but it also communicates that I see them as more than a bully or problem child. I want to look beyond their difficulties in attempting to help them acknowledge and share their sense of competency. Many of these children are so out of touch with that dimension of themselves, and their behavior only serves to distance them and others from it. Their self-worth has been marginalized repeatedly. In working with James, I let his natural capabilities rise to the forefront and be expressed, especially in trying to establish an alliance with him. Through his expertise in using the Pokémon cards or playing Mad Libs, James was demonstrating that he indeed was capable of doing things well. It is likely that other adults in his life had not taken the time to engage with James in this way. Although the

bully's need to dominate and control peers is something that certainly needs to be addressed, in dealing with the bullies I have treated, I have tried to broaden the focus of our work together. These children need the opportunity to experience how to connect with others by seeing that they have something worthwhile to offer. Play therapists can help bullies discover and acknowledge their inherent worth.

In working in a school setting the occurrence of bullying behavior needs to be managed within an organizational context. Very often administrators and teachers demand quick results and some assurances that the bully in question has learned his or her lesson and will not engage in this behavior again. In an era of zero tolerance for bullying and other maladaptive behaviors in schools, the student accused of bullying may be suspended automatically if deemed guilty, and this suspension will certainly impact the level of cooperation he may offer school counselors. In this instance there is little else that can be done but to assure the student that I will certainly be available upon his or her return. In a move that very often surprises a student who is suspended due to bullying behavior, I have checked in with him or her by calling the student at home and using the call to remind him or her of my interest and availability, paving the way for follow-up when the student returns.

Helping the bully adjust to the school environment following his or her return is another area that needs to be addressed. I will very often meet with other students who have been impacted by the bully and prepare them for the student's return by listening to their concerns and trying to identify how these can be realistically addressed at school. In my role of school psychologist I have often brokered agreements between bully and victim to help them achieve a workable detente with each other. The results have been constructive in reducing the likelihood of the bullying behavior continuing, and the approach teaches all parties that here is an alternative to working out their differences.

Helping a child to realize that he or she can reach out for help and feel safe, secure, and accepted, when that experience has been denied or minimized, remains the goal. Although not always successful in doing so, we owe it to these children to try to help them experience this level of acceptance that is so foreign to them and to help them learn to trust not only the play therapist but the world at large.

REFERENCES

Banks, R. (1997). Bullying in schools. *ERIC Digest*, pp. 97–17.

Barboza, G. E., Schiamberg, L. B., Oehmke, J., Korzeniewski, S. J., Post, L. A., & Heraux, C. G. (2009). Individual characteristics and the multiple contexts of adolescent bullying: An ecological perspective. *Journal of Youth and Adolescence, 38*, 101–121.

Bazelon, E. (2013). *Sticks and stones: Defeating the culture of bullying and rediscovering the power of character and empathy.* New York: Random House.

Beaty, L. A., & Alexeyev, E. B. (2008). The problem of school bullies: What the research tells us. *Adolescence, 43*(169), 1–11.

Bradshaw, C. P., Sawyer, A. L., & O'Brennan, L. M. (2009). A social disorganization perspective on bullying-related attitudes and behaviors: The influence of social context. *American Journal of Community Psychology, 43*, 204–220.

Brooks, R., & Goldstein, S. (2001). *Raising resilient children.* Chicago: Contemporary Books.

Bullying Statistics 2010. (2010). Retrieved from *www.bullyingstatistics.org/content/bullying-statistics-2010.html*.

Carlson, L. W., & Cornell, D. G. (2008). Differences between persistent and desistent middle school bullies. *School Psychology International, 29*, 442–450.

Carlyle, K. E., & Steinman, K. L. (2007). Demographic differences in the prevalence, co-occurrence, and correlates of adolescent bullying in school. *Journal of School Health, 77*, 623–629.

Centers for Disease Control and Prevention. (2011, April 22). Bullying among middle and high school students—Massachusetts, 2009. *Morbidity and Mortality Weekly Report, 60*, 165–171.

Christie-Mizell, C. (2003). Bullying: The consequences of interparental discord and child's self-concept. *Family Process, 42*, 237–251.

Dake, J. A., Price, J. H., & Telljohann, S. K. (2003). The nature and extent of bullying at school. *Journal of School Health, 73*, 173–180.

Espelage, D. L., Bosworth, K., & Simon, T. R. (2000). Examining the social context of bullying behaviors in early adolescence. *Journal of Counseling and Development, 78*, 326–333.

Espelage, D. L., & Holt, M. K. (2007). Dating violence and sexual harassment across the bully-victim continuum among middle and high school students. *Journal of Youth and Adolescence, 36*, 799–811.

Fisher, P., Grietmeyer, T., Pollezek, F., & Frey, D. (2006). The unresponsive bystander: Are bystanders more responsive in dangerous emergencies? *European Journal of Social Psychology, 36*, 267–278,

Fitzpatrick, K. M., Dulin, A. J., & Piko, B. F. (2007). Not just pushing and shoving: School bullying among African American adolescents. *Journal of School Health, 77*, 16–22.

Flescher Peskin, M., Tortolero, S. R., & Markham, C. M. (2006). Bullying and victimization among black and Hispanic adolescents. *Adolescence, 41*, 467–484.

Forero, R., McClellan, L., Rissel, C., & Bauman, A. (1999). Bullying behavior and psychosocial health among school students in New South Wales, Australia: Cross-sectional survey. *British Medical Journal, 319*, 344–348.

Georgiou, S. N., & Fanti, K. A. (2010). A transactional model of bullying and victimization. *Social Psychology of Education, 13*, 295–311.

Gini, G., & Pozzoli, T. (2006). The role of masculinity in children's bullying. Retrieved from *www.ingentaconnect.com*.

Gordon, S. (2013). Six consequences bully-victims experience. Retrieved from *http://bullying.about.com*.

Harris, S., & Petrie, G. (2002). A study of bullying in the middle school. *National Association of Secondary School Principals Bulletin, 86*(633), 42–53.

Hazler, R., Carney, J., & Granger, D. (2006). Integrating biological measures into the study of bullying. *Journal of Counseling and Development, 84*, 298–307.

Holt, M. K., & Espelage, D. L. (2007). Perceived social support among bullies, victims, and bully-vicitms. *Journal of Youth and Adolescence, 36*, 984–994.

Isolan, L., Salum, G., Osowksi, A., Hartmann, G., & Manfro, G. (2013). Victims and bully-victims but not bullies are groups associated with anxiety symptomatology among Brazilian children and adolescents. *European Child and Adolescent Psychiatry, 22*, 641–648.

Klein, J. (2012). *The bully society.* New York: New York University Press.

Menesini, E., Modena, M., & Tani, F. (2009). Bullying and victimization in adolescence: Concurrent and stable roles and psychological health symptoms. *Journal of Genetic Psychology, 170*, 115–133.

Mouttapa, M., Valente, T., Gallaher, P., Rohrbach, L. A., & Unger, J. B. (2004). Social network predictors of bullying. *Adolescence, 39*, 315–335.

Nansel, T. R., Overpeck, M., Pilla, R., Ruan, J., Simons-Morton, B., & Scheidt, P. (2001). Bullying behaviors among U.S. youth: Prevalence and association with psychosocial adjustment. *Journal of American Medical Association, 285*, 2094–2100.

Natvig, G. K., Albrektsen, G., & Qvarnstrom, U. (2001). School-related stress experience as a risk factor for bullying behavior. *Journal of Youth and Adolescence, 30*, 561–575.

Pontzer, D. (2010). A theoretical test of bullying behavior: Parenting, personality, and the bully/victim relationship. *Journal of Family Violence, 25*, 259–273.

Salmivalli, C. (1999). Participant role approach to school bullying: Implications for intervention. *Journal of Adolescence, 22*, 453–459.

Schwartz, D., Proctor, L., & Chein, D. (2001). *Peer harassment in school: The plight of the vulnerable and victimized.* New York: Guilford Press.

Shetgiri, R., Lin, H., Avila, R., & Flores, G. (2012). Parental characteristics associated with bullying perpetration in U.S. children aged 10–17 years. *American Journal of Public Health, 102*, 2280–2286.

Stelios, G. N. (2008). Parental style and child bullying and victimization at school. *Social Psychology of Education: An International Journal, 11*, 213–227.

Van Hoof, A., Raajmakers, Q. A., Van Beck, Y., Hale, W. W., III, & Aleva, L. (2008). A multimediation model on the relations of bullying victimization, identity, and family with adolescent depressive symptoms. *Journal of Youth Adolescence, 37*, 772–782.

Vaughn, M. G., Fu, Q., Bender, K., DeLisi, M., Beaver, K. M., Perron, B. E., et al. (2010). Psychiatric correlates of bullying in the United States: Findings from a national sample. Retrieved from *www.ncbi.nlm.nih.gov/pubmed/20177967.*

Wolke, D., Woods, S., Stanford, K., & Schulz, H. (2001). Bullying and victimization of primary school children in England and Germany: Prevalence and school factors. *British Journal of Psychology, 92*, 673–696.

Yang, S., Stewart, R., Kim, J., Kim, S., & Shin, I. (2013). Differences in predictor of traditional and cyber-bullying: A 2-year longitudinal study in Korean school children. *European Child and Adolescent Psychiatry, 22*, 309–318.

CHAPTER 17

Child-Centered Play Therapy and School-Based Problems

Angela I. Sheely-Moore
Peggy L. Ceballos

The existence of mental health problems during childhood is a strong indicator of mental health problems later in life (Richard & Abbott, 2009). This statement is alarming in light of statistics that indicate between 13 and 20% of children experience mental health problems on an annual basis (National Research Council and Institute of Medicine, 2009). Langley, Santiago, Rodríguez, and Zelaya (2013) reported that approximately 20–50% of children are victims of traumatic events. Furthermore, suicide, which often results from the lack of attention to mental health issues, was the third leading cause of death for individuals between the ages of 10 and 14 (Centers for Disease Control and Prevention, 2011).

Researchers highlighted the fact that the prevalence of mental health problems among children and adolescents increases for immigrant youth and those living in impoverished urban communities (Alicea, Pardo, Conover, Gopalan, & McKay, 2012; Langley et al., 2013). According to Eisenberg, Golberstein, and Hunt (2009), the lack of immediate intervention to address mental health problems has dire results on children's productivity at school. Furthermore, Eisenberg and colleagues noted the deleterious impact of this lack of productivity on employment and income in adulthood. Despite these statistics, approximately 20% of children experiencing mental health problems do receive the help they need (Kataoka, Zhang, & Wells, 2002). Researchers and professional organizations have called for school personnel to respond proactively by offering high-quality mental health interventions (American Academy of Pediatrics, 2004; Galassi & Akos, 2007; National Association of School Nurses, 2008; National Organization of School Psychologists, 2012).

The critical need to address mental health issues in the schools to promote academic achievement is recognized in comprehensive school-based mental health services, such as the American School Counseling Association's (ASCA; 2012) National Model. This model serves as a framework for professional school counselors to respond proactively to the needs of all students through the implementation of a comprehensive school counseling program. The ASCA National Model delineates a systemic and systematic approach to address the career, academic, and social–emotional needs of all students. These intersecting developmental aspects are addressed through a delivery system that targets students and stakeholders (e.g., teachers, administrators, parents) to facilitate academic success for all children (American School Counseling Association, 2012). The need for developmentally appropriate services, such as play therapy and expressive arts, seems critical in the overall development of students.

Vernon (2004) recommended therapeutic interventions using nonverbal means of communication as developmentally appropriate when working in schools. Child-centered play therapy (CCPT) is widely accepted as an effective and developmentally appropriate therapeutic modality for young children (Bratton, Ray, & Landreth, 2008). Many studies have been conducted that indicate the effectiveness of CCPT in treating children's behavioral problems in the schools with culturally diverse populations (e.g., Blanco & Ray, 2011; Bratton et al., 2013; Cochran, Cochran, Nordling, McAdam, & Miller, 2010; Garza & Bratton, 2005; Ray, Blanco, Sullivan, & Holliman, 2009; Schumann, 2005). Furthermore, parents who are trained in CCPT can become effective therapeutic agents in their children's lives (Ceballos & Bratton, 2010; Garza, Kinsworthy, & Watts, 2009; Sheely-Moore & Bratton, 2010). Scholars also recommended the use of expressive arts, based on CCPT tenets and principles, to meet and address the developmental needs of adolescents in various mental health settings, including schools (Bratton, Ceballos, & Ferebee, 2009). Despite the limited research conducted with adolescents using expressive arts, promising results of the impact of this modality are apparent (Flahive & Ray, 2007; Packman & Bratton, 2003; Paone, Packman, Maddux, & Rothman, 2008; Shen & Armstrong, 2008).

CCPT and Research

Due to licensure and credentialing standards, mental health professionals working in schools (e.g., school counselors, school psychologists, social workers) are charged to implement empirically supported inventions with students (Bratton, 2010). In fact, professional school counselors not only are faced with the implementation of empirically based services, but also are challenged to provide empirical support in assessing the impact of their services and programs, thus demonstrating accountability (American School Counseling Association, 2012). Therefore, it behooves school mental health professionals to identify developmentally appropriate and responsive treatment modalities with empirical support to demonstrate the promotion of student success.

Landreth, Ray, and Bratton (2009) identified CCPT as having "the longest history of use and the strongest research support" (p. 282), with a total of 84 school-based, play therapy outcome studies conducted since the early 1940s (Bratton, 2010). As indicated previously, many research studies have been conducted in the schools that demonstrate the effectiveness of CCPT for a variety of presenting issues across diverse populations at the elementary school level, as well as emerging studies conducted at the secondary school level using expressive arts. With an emphasis on the therapeutic relationship as the primary change agent and based on the innate human tendency toward positive growth and development (Landreth, 2012), the modalities of CCPT and expressive arts serve to meet the unique developmental considerations of school-age children and adolescents.

Hess, Magnuson, and Beeler (2012) described the cognitive development of children and adolescents to be, in certain ways, "highly distinct from adults" (p. 52). Specifically, children under the age of 12 have a tendency to structure information in a concrete manner, rather than through abstract thought (Piaget, 1962). Even when the stage of formal operations begins approximately at the age of 13, the ability of secondary-school-age students to use logical thought and deductive reasoning cannot be assumed to be at its peak during the teen years (Piaget, 1962). Hence, the use of play and play-based materials serves as a bridge for children and adolescents to express themselves fully, without the necessity of abstract thinking (Landreth, 2012). In addition to using play in therapy and expressive arts as culturally appropriate and responsive mediums of communication for children and adolescents, this humanistic approach serves to enhance the potentiality of the human experience emotionally, socially, personally, and cognitively, to name a few (Berk, 2003; Landreth, 2012; Schaefer & DiGeronimo, 2000).

Based on the humanistic framework of Rogers's (1961) person-centered counseling, the development of CCPT with children was the early work of Virginia Axline (1969), along with additional contemporary contributors to this approach, including Landreth (2012). Despite the critical use of toys and play-based materials to facilitate a wide range of self-expression, toys and the playroom itself remain secondary to the therapeutic alliance developed between practitioner and child (Landreth, 2012). Rather, it is the practitioners' communication of empathy, unconditional positive regard, and genuineness that serves to enhance the inherent tendency for growth and maturation (Fall, Holden, & Marquis, 2010). Axline (1969) described eight basic principles to guide practitioners in their work with children. Specifically, therapists should (1) develop good rapport with the child; (2) accept where the child is at in the moment; (3) communicate a sense of freedom for the child to express self completely; (4) acknowledge and validate the child's emotional state; (5) believe in the child's innate capacity to solve problems; (6) allow the child to lead the session; (7) remain patient with the pace of the child's therapeutic progress; and (8) set limits only

when necessary (pp. 73–74). We propose that these tenets can be easily transferred to work with adolescents as well.

The Use of Expressive Arts

Slavson and Redl (1944) were the first scholars to recommend the need for developmentally appropriate materials and activities in therapeutic interventions when working with adolescents. Since then, several authors have suggested adapting play therapy through the use of expressive art activities to meet the needs of adolescents experiencing mental health problems (Draper, Ritter, & Willingham, 2003; Finn, 2003; Flahive & Ray, 2007; Ginott, 1994; Packman & Bratton, 2003; Paone et al., 2008; Shen, 2007; Veach & Gladding, 2007). Using expressive art materials as a medium of communication for adolescents can lead to their increased self-awareness and, ultimately, to positive change (Knill, Levine, & Levine, 2005; Shen & Armstrong, 2008). Although expressive art materials can be used for many theoretical orientations, in alignment with CCPT tenets, we propose the use of expressive arts within a humanistic perspective.

According to Corey (2005), a humanistic perspective is based on "respect for the client's subjective experience and a trust in the capacity of the client to make positive and constructive conscious choices" (p. 166). Hence, Rogers's (1961) core conditions of the therapeutic relationship remains the vehicle for change, not expressive art materials or the activities utilized in therapy. Additionally, providing self-directed activities serves to meet the developmental needs for autonomy and control during the adolescent years (Bratton, Ceballos, et al., 2009). Gil (1994) suggested a combination of unstructured and structured time during the therapeutic process as beneficial. In response, the adaptation of CCPT for adolescents centers on (1) adjusting the medium of communication to expressive art materials, and (2) encouraging practitioners to remain flexible in incorporating structured activities to reduce adolescents' anxiety in the therapeutic process while giving them opportunities to engage in self-direction (Bratton, Ceballos, et al., 2009). Art mediums that can be used with adolescents include sandtrays, clay, collages, story creation, music, and musical instruments (Bratton, Ceballos, et al., 2009; Gladding, 2005; Malchiodi, 2002; Oaklander, 1988).

CCPT and Expressive Arts: Strategies and Techniques

Using the medium of play and expressive arts in therapy provides children and adolescents with opportunities to express themselves fully, without the need for verbalization. Although verbalization is neither emphasized nor encouraged, both verbal and nonverbal skills are necessary in CCPT and strongly recommended when using expressive arts. In fact, the need to demonstrate nonverbal skills is perhaps even more critical when working with children under the age of 12, due to the developmental emphasis on concrete understanding (Piaget, 1962). Hence, it is critical to demonstrate attentiveness to students' actions through an open-seated posture and to remain connected as they move about the play area by following with one's "nose and toes" (Landreth, 2012, p. 190). Empathic understanding is communicated nonverbally by matching one's tone of voice, facial expression, body posture, and vocal encouragers (e.g., "Hmmm!) with that of the student (Landreth, 2012). According to Landreth (2012), this "way of being" (p. 190) serves to communicate the following message: "I am doing my very best to see and understand the world through *your* eyes" (p. 190). This message also serves as the foundation for verbal responses in CCPT and expressive arts. Based on the essential skills discussed in seminal works on CCPT (Bratton, Ray, Edwards, & Landreth, 2009; Landreth,

2012; Landreth et al., 2009), we have identified four broad categories that encompass these critical skills when working with children and adolescents: (1) responding to nonverbal behaviors, (2) validating responses, (3) empowering responses, and (4) providing relationship-based responses.

Responding to Nonverbal Behaviors (Tracking)

This basic skill involves the recognition and communication of students' play behaviors without judgment, guidance, or interpretation. Rather, the purpose of tracking is to communicate attentiveness and genuine interest in a student's actions (Landreth, 2012). For example, upon entering the playroom for the first time, second grader Maria looks around and immediately grabs the baby-doll. The practitioner might say, "You picked that up" or "You got that one." For the adolescent having difficulty starting the creation of a collage, the school counselor might say, "You're having a hard time deciding where to begin." Tracking should be used with less frequency when working with adolescents, due to the self-conscious nature typically demonstrated in this developmental phase (Sprenger, 2008).

Validating Responses

A few therapeutic skills used with adults can also be applied to children and adolescents, such as reflecting content and feelings. These responses serve to acknowledge and validate children's communication of their experience, which, in turn, promotes self-understanding and self-acceptance (Landreth, 2012). For example, after Mike talks about multiple school- and home-related tasks he has to accomplish for the day, the practitioner may say, "You have a lot of things to do today."

Because adolescents vacillate between being verbal and nonverbal (Bratton, Ceballos, et al., 2009), mental health practitioners use validating responses in the absence of tracking. For example, consider the adolescent who shares details about her parents' divorce as she's shaping a heart out of clay and says, "I wish they could fix things." The practitioner can validate the adolescent's affective experience by saying, "You feel powerless because you cannot make things go back the way they used to be." Note that nonverbal understanding of the adolescent's sense of helplessness can also be reflected in the practitioner's tone of voice and facial expression.

Empowering Responses

In alignment with the Rogerian tenet of the innate capacity to grow in a positive, forward-moving direction (Rogers, 1961), many CCPT skills serve to promote what already exists within the individual, regardless of age. Empowering responses (returning responsibility, facilitating creativity, and esteem building) in CCPT promote self-direction, self-creativity, and self-esteem (Landreth, 2012). When the child asks what toy to play with next, returning responsibility and promoting self-direction could be conveyed by the words "In here, that's for you to decide" or "You can pick." Another example: In the absence of paper towels, a child removes watercolor paint off her fingers with construction paper. The practitioner's response to this creative solution might include "You figured out a way to get that off" or "Ah! You found a way to get rid of that paint." Self-esteem building responses highlight the knowledge base of children and can include statements such as "You know exactly what you need to build that castle" or "You know a lot about dinosaurs."

Granting adolescents the power to decide which activity to choose during unstructured activity time is important as well, especially when considering the developmental need for independence (Erikson, 1982). Returning responsibility to an adolescent can be verbalized with the following statement: "You can decide what you want to do for the remaining 15 minutes left in our session today." Self-esteem responses are therapeutically beneficial for facilitating adolescents' sense of worth. For example, the practitioner can say "You feel proud about that" to an adolescent who boasted about the contents of his collage.

Relationship-Based Responses

Of the three components Axline (1969) identified as the "most favorable conditions" (p. 16) for cultivating growth and development, the therapeutic relationship is paramount. Because the relationship between student-client and practitioner represents a microcosm of larger systems in the child's world, it follows that critical skills are needed to promote and enhance this dynamic. Two CCPT skills serve to meet these goals: (1) facilitating the relationship and (2) setting limits. Responding to student-initiated verbal and nonverbal interactions with the practitioner serves to model effective communication (Landreth et al., 2009). An example of facilitating the relationship: The child draws a picture and then invites the practitioner to draw a house on the same piece of paper. The practitioner may respond in the following manner: "You want us to do this together." With an adolescent, the practitioner can say, "You want this task to be a joint effort," after being invited to join the student in creating a sandtray.

Providing children with opportunities to engage in prosocial behaviors through self-direction is one of the main objectives of the limit-setting skill. Limit setting is deemed necessary to ensure the physical and psychological safety of the child, as well as to protect play-based materials (Landreth et al., 2009). The ACT method of limit setting consists of three steps: (1) acknowledging the child's desire or emotional state; (2) communicating the limit in a firm, yet calm, tone; and (3) targeting a socially appropriate alternative (Landreth, 2012). For example, if the child attempts to paint the wall, the practitioner should respond, using each component of the ACT method:

- Step 1: "I know you want to paint that wall."
- Step 2: "But the wall is not for painting."
- Step 3: "You can choose to use the art easel to paint or you can choose to paint on the egg carton."

Due to adolescents' capacity to think in more abstract terms than younger children (Piaget, 1977), the last step of the ACT method can be done collaboratively. That is, given the developmental need to gain independence from adults (Erikson, 1982), students can be invited to brainstorm alternatives to express feelings in a socially acceptable manner. For example, a practitioner may say something like the following: "You are angry, but the sandtray miniatures are not for breaking. What other ideas do you have in mind so that you could express your anger right now, without damaging the items?"

Specific Considerations When Using Expressive Arts

The following guidelines are recommended when using structured activities based on a humanistic framework such as CCPT: (1) Introduce structured activities only as a suggestion and allow students to make the final decision; (2) use structured activities at the start of the session and grant students unstructured time at the end of the session to engage in a self-directed activity; and (3) remain flexible when adolescents communicate in both verbal and nonverbal ways. School mental health professionals should base the selection of structured activities, as well as the balance between structured and unstructured time, on their clinical assessment of students' needs (Bratton, Ceballos, et al., 2009). For example, the practitioner might recommend a structured activity to facilitate self-expression for students experiencing high anxiety in the use of expressive arts (e.g., "Let me know if you are up to trying a new activity using this sandtray to represent your world").

According to Landgarten (1987), a relationship exists between art modalities and clients' level of control over their creations, with some mediums bringing more unconscious feelings to the surface. Landgarten explained the impact of selected art media on clients' levels of self-expression, defensiveness, and affective state. Heeding Landgarten's analysis, school mental health practitioners should exercise caution when introducing art media with adolescents by assessing the degree of safety within the therapeutic alliance, as well as the emotional readiness of the student to use specific art mediums. Bratton, Ceballos, and colleagues (2009) provided an overview of the various art materials available for use in working with adolescents, using a continuum format based on the degree of control over the selected medium. Examples of mediums on this chart include color pencils, puppets, and sandtray miniatures (Bratton, Ceballos, et al., 2009).

Practitioners should be mindful of the timing of the type of skills used during self-directed activities in a session and avoid disrupting the flow of the therapeutic process for those activities the practitioner recommends for the student. During self-directed time in an expressive art session, school mental health practitioners should use the skill of tracking as the student works on creating a product out of the materials. In contrast, when the activity is recommended by the practitioner, it is important to provide the student self-reflective time while completing the activity (Bratton, Ceballos, et al., 2009). As a witness to the student's creation, the practitioner remains silent throughout the activity and waits to process the creation upon completion. For example, the practitioner might say: "You can use the sandtray to represent your world. I will sit here quietly as you work. Once you're finished, together we can process what you did." Avoiding the use of tracking during this creation time allows students to immerse themselves fully in the task at hand, as well as providing an opportunity to engage in self-awareness, using the medium to express their inner selves.

According to Bratton, Ceballos, and Sheely (2008), four levels of processing can be used to explore clients' finished creations, with each successive level requiring higher emotional/psychological safety and an increased ability to engage in abstract thinking. The following overview provides a brief introduction to each processing level, along with an example:

- Level 1: Invite students to share their creations (e.g., "Tell me about your collage").
- Level 2: Share your impressions of the student's creation (e.g., "I noticed it took you a while to find an object to place in the middle of the collage, but you seemed confident to place this picture of the highway road with cars in the right-hand corner").
- Level 3: Invite the student to enter the metaphor (e.g., "I wonder where would you be going if you could imagine driving one of these cars in the picture").
- Level 4: Ask the student to relate to the creation (e.g., "This picture of the highway seems to be very significant to you—I wonder how you are relating to it").

Application of CCPT and Expressive Arts in the Schools

Working in the school setting provides mental health professionals the unique opportunity to work collaboratively with administrators, teachers, staff, and parents to promote student success. Bronfenbrenner's (1979) social–ecological framework provides a clear blueprint of the interconnecting spheres of influence in a child's world. It is impossible for mental health professionals to address all presenting needs of

the entire school body; hence the need for shared accountability among key stakeholders in school, home, and community is necessary to the success of prevention, intervention, and postvention counseling strategies, including the implementation of CCPT-based services.

In a survey of 239 elementary and secondary school counselors, Shen (2008) identified three barriers to implementing play therapy: lack of training, time, and budget constraints. Ebrahim, Steen, and Paradise's (2012) study of 359 elementary school counselors echoed Shen's findings. Frameworks to provide comprehensive mental health services for children in the schools, such as the ASCA National Model (American School Counseling Association, 2012), could serve as potential aids in overcoming such barriers. Specifically, school mental health professionals can plan to engage in the following actions to bring CCPT-based services to fruition: (1) increase knowledge base of CCPT and expressive arts, (2) establish university–school partnerships, and (3) explore funding options.

Increase and Disseminate Knowledge Base of CCPT and Expressive Arts

With limited (if any) funding provided to mental health professionals working in the schools, these practitioners are challenged to locate affordable CCPT and expressive arts training and supervised experience. Despite the monetary costs, specialized skills and experience to conduct CCPT and expressive arts therapy are necessary, regardless of work setting. Practitioners working in the schools have several options to consider when increasing their knowledge base for these humanistic modalities. First, if enrolling in a graduate-level play therapy or expressive arts course is not feasible, consider the possibility of auditing a course. Traditionally, auditing a course provides the opportunity to attend class sessions without completing course assignments. For more short-term training opportunities, the Association for Play Therapy's (APT; *www.a4pt.org*) website provides a clearinghouse of training opportunities at the local, state, and national levels, ranging from conferences to webinars, which accommodate a wide range of monetary budgets.

Gaining this knowledge base is the first step when working within various systems in the daily lives of children and adolescents; it is just as important to disseminate learned information to administrators, teachers, school staff, and parents, as well as students. A basic introduction to CCPT tenets, as well as highlighting the impact of this modality on student success, could promote better "buy-in" with key stakeholders to provide support for play therapy-based services in the schools.

Establishing University–School Partnerships

In a review of play therapy studies conducted at the elementary level, Ebrahim and colleagues (2012) noted that the majority were conducted with outsiders who came into the schools to provide play therapy services. Shared responsibilities with community members could alleviate the various tasks school mental health professionals are charged to accomplish. Specifically, play therapists from local mental health agencies could opt to provide pro bono Child–Parent Relationship Therapy (CPRT) and Child Teacher Relationship Training (CTRT) training to teachers and parents at the school, or within their respective agencies. School-based practitioners can also dialogue with university educators specializing in play therapy and expressive arts to explore the possibility of serving as a clinical site placement for master's and doctoral-level students in mental health fields (e.g., counseling, school psychology, social work) to provide play-based services. Note that it is imperative that practitioners in the schools who are interested in this option meet required criteria from graduate training programs to serve in the role as site supervisor; thus, the need for training and supervision for practitioners is paramount.

Exploring Sources of Funding

Locating monetary supports to obtain play-based materials can be burdensome, leaving many school practitioners using their own funds to furnish the play area. In fact, the majority of survey respondents, comprised of elementary school counselors, reported using their own money to purchase play therapy equipment (Ebrahim et al., 2012). Requesting donated toys and materials from school personnel, parents, and community organizations is another option available to reduce monetary costs. Working collaboratively with school and community leaders to identify and apply for grants would also serve to reduce the amount of additional tasks for school practitioners (Sheely-Moore & Ceballos, 2011).

Necessary Tools and Logistics

The next step in overcoming the challenges of using play therapy and expressive arts in the schools is obtaining the necessary equipment to conduct actual sessions. Landreth (2012) recommended a list of traditional play items to include within a portable play kit for those located in settings where space availability is limited, such as schools. Bratton, Ceballos, and colleagues (2008) provided a comprehensive list of developmentally appropriate play-based items that can be used with adolescents. It is critical for school mental health professionals to include toys and materials that reflect the world of their student body. Cultural considerations to keep in mind when furnishing the play area include toys and items that reflect various ethnicities, countries of origin, socioeconomic status, geographical location, ability status, to name a few.

Landreth (2012) identified three broad categories of toys to include in a traditional play area: real-life toys and aggressive-release toys, as well as creative- and emotional-release toys. These categories are applicable for adolescents as well, along with the inclusion of expressive-arts-based mediums such as clay, sandtray, and collages. With many school districts implementing "zero tolerance" for violence in the schools, there is an increased likelihood of school administrators disallowing specific toy items (e.g., dart gun, rubber knife) in the play area. When faced with this issue, providing a rationale of granting students the ability to learn how to channel feelings in a constructive, positive manner—within the safety of a therapeutic relationship—is imperative. However, there is no guarantee that such an explanation will overcome this challenge. In this case, it is important to know that children will find creative strategies in efforts to meet their needs, despite the absence of specific toys and materials.

Clinical Case Examples

With an emphasis on the child directing the play or the adolescent leading an activity, it is impossible for practitioners to "plan" ahead with a specific response for any given situation. Rather, in being fully attuned to each student's world, the timing of therapeutic responses occurs in the here and now, based on the student's actions and verbalizations. The following two case examples demonstrate skills used in CCPT and expressive arts during three different phases of treatment: beginning, middle, and end. The first case example features a 5-year-old kindergarten student, followed by another example using expressive arts with a 14-year-old, 10th-grade student. Note that the following case examples are not based on actual clients.

Case 1

A recent transfer halfway into the academic school year, 5-year-old Tomer began the first days at his new school with a rough start. From the moment he was dropped off at school, Tomer made it clear he did not want to be there. His father would have to carry him into the classroom, as Tomer refused to walk. Due to his father's work schedule, Mr. Khan did not have the luxury to stay with him for more than 10 minutes in the classroom, which left Tomer screaming and throwing objects in anger at his father's departure. Both Mr. Khan and Tomer's teacher, Mr. Sayo, agreed that something needed to be done to help Tomer transition to his new school. Hence, they both went to speak to the school psychologist for assistance. As a result of the consultation, all parties were in agreement to start play therapy sessions to support Tomer.

Beginning Phase

The school psychologist arrived at the classroom prior to Tomer's morning arrival to introduce herself and take him to the playroom. Mr. Khan followed through with the school psychologist's request the night before by reading a developmentally appropriate story to his son about going to his first play session. Hence, Tomer's typical outburst in the morning was somewhat abated as he was curious about the playroom. The school psychologist bent down on her knees to be at Tomer's level prior to introducing herself and announced that it was time to go to the playroom. Mr. Khan followed his son and the school psychologist halfway to the playroom before he exited the school building—as Tomer seemed preoccupied wondering what kinds of toys were available in the playroom.

Upon arriving in the playroom, the school psychologist shared the following statement with Tomer: "Tomer, this is our playroom and in here you can play with all of the toys in many of the ways you'd like." From there, the school psychologist sat down in the chair and began to observe Tomer's actions. Tomer's eyes lit up and he immediately ran to the blocks. He stopped abruptly to look back at the school psychologist and asked, "Can I really play with these?" The psychologist responded, "In here, you can decide." The first session continued with Tomer asking "permission" to play with the toys as the school psychologist used the skill of returning responsibility. At one point in the initial session, Tomer began to identify the colors of the rainbow, to which the psychologist responded, "You know exactly what colors make a rainbow."

Middle Phase

The psychologist established a rapport based on acceptance, care, and genuineness (Rogers, 1961), along with her CCPT skills. In response, Tomer's confidence level increased in the playroom as evidenced by his self-directive play, as he no longer needed to ask for permission from the psychologist. Furthermore, Tomer began to expand his range of affect to include bouts of aggression toward various toy objects (e.g., Bop Bag, dinosaurs, toy soldiers). The psychologist validated his expressed emotion by stating, "You're angry at that." At times, the psychologist used the ACT method to ensure the safety of Tomer and herself, as well as the toys. For instance, Tomer planned to create a bad storm by throwing blocks toward the psychologist. To prevent the possibility of his guilt feelings as well as protecting her own safety (Landreth, 2012), the psychologist used the ACT method. In a calm, yet firm, tone of voice, she said, "Tomer, I know you want to throw those blocks at me. But I am not for throwing blocks at. You can choose to throw them on the floor or on the bean bag chair." Tomer's limit-testing behaviors continued during the midpoint of his therapeutic sessions, giving him the opportunity to practice engaging in self-control and selecting a socially appropriate alternative with which to release his desires and emotions. The results were observed in the classroom, as both the teacher and Mr. Khan reported a decline in his morning "outbursts." Furthermore, Tomer's teacher,

Mr. Sayo, reported Tomer's eagerness to serve as a helper in the classroom.

Ending Phase

Based on Tomer's progress from being carried into the classroom to walking to class in the mornings, the school psychologist consulted with Tomer, as well as Mr. Khan and Mr. Sayo, to plan for termination. As a reminder of the impending end of the therapeutic sessions, the school psychologist created a calendar for Tomer so that he could keep track of how many play sessions remained. During the final sessions, Tomer invited the psychologist into his play on a consistent basis. Tomer requested her help to make dinner, to take care of the baby, and to play musical instruments together. During these actions, the school psychologist used relationship-building skills such as, "You want me to help you with making that soup" or "We're taking care of the baby together." During the last session, Tomer drew a picture of him and the psychologist walking hand in hand to the playroom, to which she responded, "You made this picture just for me."

Case 2

Tenth-grade English teacher Ms. Sanders referred 14-year-old Jennifer to the school counselor for behavioral and academic concerns. Jennifer was known to her teachers as a highly sociable straight-A student who participated in class and in many extracurricular activities. Within the last 2 months, however, Jennifer's teachers noticed a shift in her behaviors: She was sad, withdrawn, and less participatory during class. Ms. Sanders disclosed to the school counselor that Jennifer's parents had recently filed for a divorce. Ms. Sanders also noticed a significant decline in Jennifer's academic performance and feared that she might fail the majority of her classes this term. Sharing the teacher's concerns, Jennifer's parents agreed for their daughter to receive school counseling services. After Ms. Sanders shared her concern to Jennifer, she agreed to meet with the school counselor to assist her during this life change.

Beginning Phase

A collage was used during the initial stages of counseling to give Jennifer an opportunity to describe herself in a nonthreatening manner, and without the need for verbalization. The practitioner introduced the activity, directing Jennifer to use available materials on the table (e.g., magazines, markers, colored pencils) to represent herself. With this activity spanning across three sessions, Jennifer was also invited to bring in personal pictures from home to include in the collage. While working on the collage, the counselor used CCPT-based skills to reflect Jennifer's verbalizations and nonverbal actions to facilitate her self-awareness and further develop the therapeutic relationship. For instance, when Jennifer ripped a photograph of the picture of her parents into two separate ones, the practitioner stated, "You adjusted the photo to represent how you see them now." Jennifer responded, "Yeah, I can't do anything about it," to which the practitioner replied, "You feel powerless now."

Upon completion of the activity, the school counselor used the first level of processing skills by asking Jennifer to share her creation. She explained how the collage is divided in half, with each section representing one of her parents, and her feeling stuck in the middle. Jennifer continued to express feelings of embarrassment about her parents' divorce and anger over the impact of this breakup on her life.

Middle Phase

At this stage, Jennifer was given the opportunity to select the medium of choice by the use of the following prompt: "Jennifer, you can choose to use any of the materials you see on the table [or designated area] to tell me more about yourself." At this point, Jennifer selected the sandtray. When using the sandtray, students are able to select various miniatures to represent their perceptions and feelings about their lives. Jennifer began by drawing a line in the middle of the sandtray, similar to the collage she had completed. The first completed sandtray included an array of aggressive animals that represented her mother, father, and herself. There was also a barrage of objects (e.g., bushes, fences, cars, buildings) used to divide the tray into separate sections. Jennifer continued to use this modality for three more sessions.

Jennifer was given the option to discuss as much or as little as she wanted about what she had created in her various sandtrays. As the school counselor used validation-based responses, Jennifer started to talk more openly about her current behavior. In subsequent sandtrays, Jennifer shifted her focus from the divorce itself to representing her recent behavioral and emotional reactions to the divorce. Different levels of processing were used with Jennifer as she worked on the creation of various sandtrays. For example, during the first sandtray, the counselor used the second level of processing skill when sharing her observations with Jennifer: "You placed a lot of divisions in your sandtray; it seems that it would be hard to integrate all the different parts together." A more advanced level of processing skills was used in a later sandtray when the counselor stated, "Your sandtrays are more integrated now with fewer barriers. I wonder if this change is a reflection of how you are feeling."

Through processing her sandtrays, Jennifer gained self-awareness into her reason for withdrawing from friends (i.e., due to her embarrassment). Jennifer also realized how much she wanted to "fix things" between her parents. These insights allowed Jennifer to shift her focus again; she began constructing sandtrays that emphasized how she wanted to be viewed in the school, rather than her parents' divorce. This shift was apparent in the trays as the number of barriers decreased. In addition, Jennifer began to replace aggressive animals with miniature people to represent members of her family—an indication of her ability to cope with anger in healthier ways.

The school counselor also consulted with Ms. Sanders to obtain an update on Jennifer's behaviors and grades. Given the positive feedback of Jennifer "getting back to her old self," the counselor began the process of individual counseling for termination, with the suggestion that Jennifer join a school-based divorce group.

Ending Phase

Jennifer agreed to create a storybook about her life as her final expressive art activity. The counselor introduced this storytelling activity by giving the following simple directive to Jennifer: "I'd like you to create a story with a beginning, middle, and end." Similar to the collage, Jennifer used pictures and words cut out from magazines and family photos, as well as markers to provide the content of the story.

The story began with a description of her current situation, with the middle segment focusing on the peer support she was receiving during her parents' divorce. The story concluded with Jennifer's future desires, which included being happy with, and for, each of her parents, as well as working to improve her grades in order to attend the college of her dreams. Although sadness and loneliness were noted themes in her story, these feelings were more manageable and less dominant than in prior sessions. At this time, the school counselor used self-esteem responses such as "You're proud about your plans to go to college" and "You enjoyed the way you ended the story." These responses promoted Jennifer's self-confidence and sense of progress throughout the counseling. Following individual counseling, Jennifer decided to join the divorce group for continued support.

Conclusion

Meeting the developmental needs of children and adolescents through play therapy and expressive arts serves to promote optimal functioning and well-being (Landreth, 2012). With the overwhelming numbers of underserved children experiencing mental health problems (Kataoka et al., 2002), it behooves practitioners working in the schools to respond proactively to ameliorate long-term deleterious effects of nontreatment (Eisenberg et al., 2009). Mental health professionals working in the schools have a unique opportunity to collaborate with various stakeholders to promote student success. Using developmentally appropriate play-based materials, each troubled child can begin the journey to healing with an empathic, genuine practitioner communicating unconditional positive regard along the way (Rogers, 1961). The use of play therapy and the expressive arts provides a powerful way to optimize healthy functioning and development for school-age children and adolescents, on their own terms and in their own language.

REFERENCES

Alicea, S., Pardo, G., Conover, K., Gopalan, G., & McKay, M. (2012). Step-up: Promoting youth mental health and development in inner-city high schools. *Clinical Social Work Journal, 40,* 175–186.

American Academy of Pediatrics, Committee on School Health. (2004). Policy statement: School-based mental health services. *Pediatrics, 113*(6), 1839–1845.

American School Counseling Association. (2012). *The ASCA National Model: A framework for school counseling programs* (3rd ed.). Alexandria, VA: Author.

Axline, V. (1969). *Play therapy.* Boston: Houghton-Mifflin.

Berk, L. E. (2003). *Child development* (6th ed.). Boston: A & B.

Blanco, P., & Ray, D. (2011). Play therapy in elementary schools: A best practice for improving academic achievement. *Journal of Counseling and Development, 89*(2), 235–243.

Bratton, S. C. (2010). Meeting the early mental health needs of children though school-based play therapy: A review of outcome research. In A. A. Drewes & C. E. Schaefer (Eds.), *School-based play therapy* (2nd ed., pp. 17–58). Hoboken, NJ: Wiley.

Bratton, S. C., Ceballos, P., & Ferebee, K. (2009). Integration of structured expressive activities within a humanistic group play therapy format for preadolescents. *Journal for Specialists in Group Work, 34*(3), 251–275.

Bratton, S. C., Ceballos, P., & Sheely, A. (2008). Expressive arts in a humanistic approach to play therapy supervision: Facilitating therapist self-awareness. In A. A. Drewes & J. Mullen (Eds.), *Supervision can be playful: Techniques for child and play therapist supervisors* (pp. 211–232). Lanham, MD: Aronson.

Bratton, S. C., Ceballos, P. L., Sheely-Moore, A. I., Meany-Walen, K., Pronchenko, Y., & Jones, L. D. (2013). Head Start early mental health intervention: Effects of child-centered play therapy on disruptive behaviors. *International Journal of Play Therapy, 22*(1), 28–42.

Bratton, S. C., Ray, D. C., Edwards, N. A., & Landreth, G. (2009). Child-centered play therapy (CCPT): Theory, research, and practice. *Person-Centered and Experiential Psychotherapies, 8*(4), 266–281.

Bratton, S. C., Ray, D. C., & Landreth, G. (2008). Play therapy. In A. Gross & M. Hersen (Eds.), *Handbook of clinical psychology: Vol. 2. Children and adolescents* (pp. 577–625). New York: Wiley.

Bronfenbrenner, U. (1979). *The ecology of human development: Experiments by nature and design.* Cambridge, MA: Harvard University Press.

Ceballos, P., & Bratton, S. C. (2010). Empowering Latino families: A culturally-responsive intervention for low-income immigrant Latino parents and their children identified with academic and behavioral concerns. *Psychology in the Schools, 47*(8), 761–775.

Centers for Disease Control and Prevention. (2011). Suicidal thoughts and behaviors among adults aged ≥18 years—United States, 2008–2009. Retrieved from *www.cdc.gov/mmwr/preview/mmwrhtml/ss6013a1.htm*.

Cochran, J. L., Cochran, N. H., Nordling, W. J., McAdam, A., & Miller, D. T. (2010). Two case studies of child-centered play therapy for children referred with highly disruptive behavior. *International Journal of Play Therapy, 19*, 130–143.

Corey, G. (2005). *Theory and practice of counseling psychotherapy* (7th ed.). Belmont, CA: Thomson.

Draper, K., Ritter, K. B., & Willingham, E. U. (2003). Sand tray group counseling with adolescents. *Journal for Specialists in Group Work, 28*, 244–260.

Ebrahim, C., Steen, R. L., Paradise, L. (2012). Overcoming school counselors' barriers to play therapy. *International Journal of Play Therapy, 21*(4), 202–214.

Eisenberg, D., Golberstein, E., & Hunt, J. B. (2009). Mental health and academic success in college. *B.E. Journal of Economic Analysis and Policy, 9*(1), 1–35.

Erikson, E. (1982). *The life cycle completed.* New York: Norton.

Fall, K., Holden, J., & Marquis, A. (2010). *Theoretical models of counseling and psychotherapy* (2nd ed.). New York: Brunner-Routledge.

Finn, C. A. (2003). Helping students cope with loss: Incorporating art into group counseling. *Journal for Specialists in Group Work, 28*, 155–165.

Flahive, M. W., & Ray, D. (2007). Effects of group sandtray therapy with preadolescents. *Journal for Specialists in Group Work, 32*, 362–382.

Galassi, J. P., & Akos, P. (2007). *Strengths-based school counseling: Promoting student development and achievement.* Mahwah, NJ: Erlbaum.

Garza, Y., & Bratton, S. (2005). School-based child-centered play therapy with Hispanic children: Outcomes and cultural considerations. *International Journal of Play Therapy, 14*, 51–79.

Garza, Y., Kinsworthy, S., & Watts, R. E. (2009). Child–parent relationship training as experienced by Hispanic parents: A phenomenological study. *International Journal of Play Therapy, 18*(4), 217–228.

Gil, E. (1994). *Play in family therapy.* New York: Guilford Press.

Ginott, H. G. (1994). *Group psychotherapy with children: The theory and practice of play therapy.* Northvale, NJ: Jason Aronson.

Gladding, S. T. (2005). *Counseling as an art: The creative arts in counseling.* Alexandria, VA: American Counseling Association.

Hess, R. S., Magnuson, S., & Beeler, L. (2012). *Counseling children and adolescents in schools.* Thousand Oaks, CA: Sage.

Kataoka, S. H., Zhang, L., & Wells, K. B. (2002). Unmet need for mental health care among U.S. children: Variation by ethnicity and insurance status. *American Journal of Psychiatry, 159*(9), 1548–1555.

Knill, P. J., Levine, E. G., & Levine, S. K. (2005). *Principles and practice of expressive arts therapy: Towards a therapeutic aesthetics.* London: Jessica Kingsley.

Landgarten, H. B. (1987). *Family art psychotherapy: A clinical guide and casebook.* New York: Brunner/Mazel.

Landreth, G. L. (1993). Child-centered play therapy. *Elementary School Guidance and Counseling, 38,* 17–29.

Landreth, G. L. (2012). *Play therapy: The art of the relationship* (3rd ed.). New York: Routledge.

Landreth, G. L., Ray, D., & Bratton, S. (2009). Play therapy in elementary schools. *Psychology in the Schools, 46*(3), 281–289.

Langley, A., Santiago, C. D., Rodríguez, A., & Zelaya, J. (2013). Improving implementation of mental health services for trauma in multicultural elementary schools: Stakeholder perspectives on parent and educator engagement. *Journal of Behavioral Health Services and Research, 40*(3), 247–262.

Malchiodi, C. A. (2002). *The soul's palette: Drawing on art's transformative powers for healing and well-being.* Boston: Shambhala.

National Association of School Nurses. (2008). Position statement: Mental health of students. Retrieved from *www.nasn.org/PolicyAdvocacy/PositionPapersandReports/NASNPositionStatementsFullView/tabid/462/smid/824/ArticleID/36/Default.aspx.*

National Organization of School Psychologists. (2012). Research on the relationship between mental health and academic achievement. Retrieved from *www.nasponline.org/advocacy/Academic-MentalHealthLinks.pdf.*

National Research Council and Institute of Medicine. (2009). Preventing mental, emotional, and behavioral disorders among young people: Progress and possibilities. Retrieved from *www.whyy.org/news/sci20090302Mentalprepub.pdf.*

Oaklander, V. (1988). *Windows to our children.* Highland, NY: Center for Gestalt Development.

Packman, J., & Bratton, S. (2003). A school-based group play/activity therapy intervention with learning disabled preadolescents exhibiting behavior problems. *International Journal of Play Therapy, 12,* 7–29.

Paone, T., Packman, J., Maddux, C., & Rothman, T. (2008). A school-based group activity therapy intervention with at-risk high school students as it relates to their moral reasoning. *International Journal of Play Therapy, 17,* 122–137.

Piaget, J. (1962). *Play, dreams, and imitation in childhood.* New York: Routledge.

Piaget, J. (1977). *The development of thought: Equilibration of cognitive structures.* New York: Viking Press.

Ray, D. C., Blanco, P. J., Sullivan, J. M., & Holliman, R. (2009). An exploratory study of child-centered play therapy with aggressive children. *International Journal of Play Therapy, 18,* 162–175.

Richards, M., & Abbott, R. (2009). Childhood mental health and adult life chances in postwar Britain: Insights from three national birth cohort studies. Retrieved from *www.centreformentalhealth.org.uk/pdfs/life_chances_report.pdf.*

Rogers, C. R. (1961). *On becoming a person: A therapist's view of psychotherapy.* Boston: Houghton Mifflin.

Schaefer, C. E., & DiGeronimo, T. F. (2000). *Ages and stages: A parent's guide to normal childhood development.* New York: Wiley.

Schumann, B. (2005). Effects of child-centered play therapy and curriculum-based small-group guidance on the behaviors of children referred for aggression in an elementary school setting (Doctoral dissertation, University of North Texas, 2004). *Dissertation Abstracts International, 65,* 4476.

Sheely-Moore, A., & Bratton, S. (2010). A strengths-based parenting intervention with low-income African American families. *Professional School Counseling, 13*(3), 175–183.

Sheely-Moore, A., & Ceballos, P. (2011). Empowering Head Start African American and Latino families: Promoting strengths-based parenting characteristics through Child–Parent Relationship Training—an evidence-based group parenting program. *National Head Start Association Dialog: A Research-to-Practice Journal for the Early Intervention Field, 14,* 41–53.

Shen, Y. (2007). Developmental model using Gestalt play versus cognitive-verbal group with Chinese adolescents: Effects on strengths and adjustment enhancement. *Journal of Specialists in Group Work, 32*, 285–305.

Shen, Y. (2008). Reasons for school counselors' use or nonuse of play therapy: An exploratory study. *Journal of Creativity in Mental Health, 3*(1), 30–43.

Shen, Y., & Armstrong, S. A. (2008). Impact of group sandtray therapy on the self-esteem of young adolescent girls. *Journal of Specialists in Group Work, 33*, 118–137.

Slavson, S., & Redl, F. (1944). Levels and applications of group therapy: Some elements in activity group therapy. *American Journal of Orthopsychiatry, 14*, 579–588.

Sprenger, M. (2008). *The developing brain: Birth to age eight.* Thousand Oaks, CA: Corwin Press.

Veach, L. J., & Gladding, S. T. (2007). Using creative group techniques in high schools. *Journal of Specialists in Group Work, 32*(1), 71–81.

Vernon, A. (2009). *Counseling children and adolescents* (4th ed.). Denver, CO: Love.

CHAPTER 18

Trauma Narratives with Children in Foster Care

INDIVIDUAL AND GROUP PLAY THERAPY

David A. Crenshaw
Kathleen S. Tillman

Children are typically removed from their homes and placed into the foster care system as a result of being severely abused and/or neglected by their primary caregivers (Pew Commission on Children in Foster Care, 2003). In the United States, out of all cases investigated by child protective services, more than 75% of children were neglected, more than 15% of children were physically abused, and just under 10% were sexually abused. In 2011, there were approximately 400,540 children in the foster care system, a substantial number of children in the United States (Child Welfare Information Gateway, 2011).

In addition to experiencing traumatic events at the hands of their caregivers, these children are particularly vulnerable for further trauma as a result of removal from the home and frequent changes in their environments (Jones Harden, 2004; Leslie et al., 2005; Vig, Chinitz, & Schulman, 2005). This combination of abuse and/or neglect and removal from caregivers can negatively affect the mental health of children in the foster care system (Dozier, Albus, Fisher, & Sepulveda, 2002; Schneider & Phares, 2005). For example, up to 80% of children in the foster care system have at least one psychological disorder (Stahmer et al., 2005). As a result of being traumatized in so many ways, children in foster care are left feeling afraid and confused and are particularly vulnerable to the development of posttraumatic stress disorder (PTSD) (Racusin, Maerlender, Sengupta, Isquith, & Straus, 2005). These children experience staggering rates of PTSD, with 60% of sexually abused children diagnosed with PTSD, 42% of physically abused children diagnosed with PTSD, and an additional 18% of children in foster care who had experienced neither physical nor sexual abuse diagnosed with PTSD (Dubner & Motta, 1999).

Children in foster care have been removed from their homes often under circumstances that were, at the least, stressful, if not traumatic (Webb, 2007). Some children are removed quite suddenly by child protective services (CPS) because of violence or neglect in the home and/or substance abuse by one or both parents. A recent survey of placements by CPS to the Group Emergency Foster Care (GEFC) program at the Children's Home of Poughkeepsie (CHP) revealed that the 20 most recent admissions were related to substance abuse by one or more parent. The GEFC is one of several foster care programs at CHP, a nonprofit child care agency founded in 1847. Other reasons for CPS emergency removal include incarceration of one or more parents; psychiatric hospitalization of a parent, and chronic illness or death of a parent. Children's exposure to violence may take various forms, including witnessing or being victimized by verbal, physical, or sexual violence and sometimes a combination of these.

These children often encounter a range of providers, including county social workers, community-based mental health therapists, psychiatrists, and school-based support teams. Unfortunately, the organizations working on behalf of children in foster care are overburdened and strive to address their primary charge for services. This workload often leaves staff so busy that they do not find the time to coordinate care or do not see coordination of care as their role for youngsters in the foster care system. With these kids, in particular, it is vitally important for mental health professionals and school personnel to communicate with one another about the strengths, and also the triggers, for these youngsters. The more information that we can gather about these youth, the more comprehensive and coordinated the interventions for them can be. It is important for these teams to meet regularly and frequently so that they can develop therapeutic goals that can be achieved in multiple areas of the child's life. For example, a community mental health provider may be working on helping the child identify triggers and utilize healthy coping skills. If this therapist communicated with the social worker, the child's foster family, and the child's school, all of these newly learned skills could be utilized

and positively reinforced in various milieus, thereby fostering even greater success for the child.

Additionally, it is vitally important for mental health providers and individuals who interact with children in the foster care system to seek out supervision and consultation from one another. It not only benefits the child for a team of providers to work together, but it also benefits the providers. When a clinician is feeling overwhelmed or stressed by a particular child or situation, talking about the situation with a colleague can help the clinician challenge negative thinking, develop new perspectives, and try new ideas. Also, when team members work together, they are able to present a united front and to remain calm and consistent for the children, while also supporting one another. All of these efforts promote self-care for clinicians and stability and the best care possible for children in foster care.

Theory and Research

One way that therapists can best support these children is by helping them process their traumatic experiences through the sensitive and attuned creation of a trauma narrative that captures the experience of what happened to them (Amir, Strafford, Freshman, & Foa, 1998; Cohen, Mannarino, & Deblinger, 2012; Cohen, Mannarino, Kleithermes, & Murray, 2012; Cohen, Mannarino, & Murray, 2011; Gidron et al., 2002; Pennebaker & Susman, 1988; also see Badenoch & Kestly, Chapter 36, this volume). A trauma narrative is essentially a story that children tell about their experiences with traumatic event(s) (e.g., abuse, neglect, and/or removal from the home). This record of what has occurred empowers the child to express thoughts and feelings without judgment while allowing the therapist to gently challenge harmful thinking that the child may have developed in response to the trauma. The purpose of creating this narrative is to help the child create a less harmful, more integrated, and healthy account of experiences (Cohen, Mannarino, & Deblinger, 2006). Trauma narratives have been found to help children reduce anxiety and decrease abuse-related fear, while also reducing the abuse-specific distress that parents experience (Deblinger, Mannarino, Cohen, Runyon, & Steer, 2011).

Trauma narratives help the child convey his or her story in verbal, written, or artistic forms (National Child Traumatic Stress Network, 2007): "[It] is often a difficult process for children to reach the point where they are able to tell the story of a traumatic event, but when they are ready, the telling enables them to master painful feelings about the event and to resolve the impact the event has on their life" (p. 1). In order to help young children feel more at ease when expressing their perceptions of traumatic experiences, clinicians can use children's primary language of play when creating the trauma narrative. Clinicians can use several different play-based modalities to assist children with what can be a very difficult process: creating the trauma narrative. Sandplay, puppet shows, art activities, song writing, and book creation are examples of play-based approaches that can be used, depending on their developmental levels, in both individual and group play therapy to assist children in the creation of their narratives. It is imperative to never lose sight of the therapist's role in facilitating the child's telling of his or her story, but it is also imperative to bear in mind that it is the *child's* story, not the therapist's. The trauma narrative is not co-created with the therapist; it is strictly the child's. The therapist's role is to help children find developmentally and trauma-informed language to enable them to create a cohesive story that gives expression, meaning, and perspective to their lived experiences.

In addition to the stressful family context leading up to the removal, they frequently experience the removal itself as traumatic. We have witnessed the vivid recall of narratives related to the removal years later and were astonished at how emotionally riveting and binding these narratives are even in these significantly delayed disclosures. This discovery has made us more sensitive as clinicians to the psychological cost and burden that results from children carrying internally, sometimes for years, these heart-wrenching narratives until someone finally asks them to tell the story of their removal from home. Most children in foster care, unless quite young, will never forget the day, if not the exact moment, the removal from their home happened. Since we now know there is a precortical memory system that records memories during the preverbal period, we also know that younger children carry the terror of that moment in the form of one or more of the following: visual, auditory, olfactory, sensory, motor, tactile, kinesthetic, and/or visceral memories. Memories from the preverbal period can't usually be recalled consciously or verbally, but certain cues or reminders can trigger them, and they can be acted out behaviorally (Gaensbauer, 2011; Green, Crenshaw, & Kolos, 2010).

Facilitation of Trauma Narratives in Foster Care and Residential Treatment

The Sanctuary Model

Due to our understanding of how the original memories can be buried, often by fear, shame, and neglect of their central importance by their subsequent caregivers, CHP has addressed this clinically cogent issue in multiple ways. All staff members at CHP are trained extensively in a trauma-informed treatment model—the sanctuary model—developed by Sandra Bloom (2000). The education of our staff, including all support and maintenance staff, ensures that everyone on campus working with the children shares a basic knowledge, framework, and language with which to understand and communicate in helpful ways with and about children with histories of trauma.

The training begins with an intensive 3-day focus on trauma and how it impacts children and is followed up regularly with additional trauma-informed training.

Individual Play Therapy: A Developmentally Sensitive Approach

Since 2008, play therapy, a developmentally sensitive intervention for children 7 years and younger (in the case of traumatized children, even adolescents will sometimes need the safety and distance permitted in symbolic play), has been offered to children at CHP whose needs call for an individual approach. Many young children are unable to share their trauma story verbally but are adept at playing it out or depicting it artistically through drawings and artwork. Other children as young as 2 years of age are able to make pictures depicting the trauma events in sandplay therapy.

Empirical research reveals that individuals whose trauma memories are more organized and coherent are less likely to develop PTSD (Dorsey & Deblinger, 2012). Play therapy offers many opportunities to work safely with trauma memories that are triggered in the playroom or brought into the play therapy room by a child haunted by such memories or intrusive images. The play scenarios of preschool children recently and suddenly removed from their homes integrate key components of the empirically supported trauma-focused cognitive-behavioral therapy (TF-CBT) model (Cohen, Mannarino, & Deblinger, 2012). Playing out the violent or terrifying scenes these children witnessed in their homes allows for their safe, gradual exposure to the distressing images and vivid memories that are typically central in PTSD symptoms. Since the children are initiating the play scenes, they are in charge and in control—which is so important for children whose lives have been chaotic and out of control. When children get too anxious in the course of playing out the events, they typically break off the play or rapidly shift to something else that is safer. In the process the children learn to pace and self-regulate—extremely important skills, since the common denominator for nearly all of the children with complex PTSD is the poor ability to regulate their emotions.

Group Play Therapy Approaches

Preschool Play Therapy Group

A preschool play therapy group for children admitted to our GEFC program was begun in the summer of 2012 and has become a fixture in the services offered to the children. Toddlers and preschoolers (3–5 years) rely extensively on play to share their feelings and perceptions, even if language is available to them, because play is the more natural and available means of expression for this age group. Play, because of its natural, anxiety-allaying properties, also becomes a safer means of communicating about threatening parts of their world.

It is Wednesday morning at CHP. The interns and I (Crenshaw) gather at 10:30 A.M., as we do each week to plan our group play therapy session with children in our GEFC program. We discuss the common themes in the play of each of the children and how we can help them create their trauma narratives in play and artwork, the only viable languages of these preschool children. 11:00 A.M. arrives and so do the children. We gather them in a circle for the opening rituals. When the free play begins, Ben, age 4, goes to the sandtray and places the army men and tanks in the sand. The two sides begin to battle, and then an earthquake hits and buries the tanks and army men. Allen, age 3, takes over in the sandtray, where he has two muscle men fighting it out. He then puts some wine bottles in the middle of the sandtray. After that he breaks off his sandplay and goes to the drama center.

Another child, Mike, age 5, wants to make a picture in the sand. He uses two wrestling figures and a miniature that looks like Elvis with a guitar. He sends the Elvis figure to fight—and defeat—the two wrestlers. Not only do the wrestlers lose but they are dead, and Mike buries them under the sand. Mike then moves to the family playhouse. He takes everything out of the house—all the people and the furniture—and says that the family is moving. He continues with his narrative by saying that "the next house has no toys." A 4-year-old, Rita, in the group for the first time, takes everything off the shelves and dumps the huge supply of miniatures in a disorganized pile in the sandtray, apparently reflecting the chaos that her life has been so far. Each child, in his or her own way, is telling his or her story in the only way possible: by creating the trauma narrative in the language of play, the only language the child can reliably use to share the pain of his or her inner world.

We have conducted the weekly preschool play therapy group in GEFC regularly since the summer of 2012, except for brief breaks for fine-tuning and recalibrating. Usually these breaks take place during transitions related to colleges and universities because the groups are facilitated by me and psychology and social work students from area colleges and universities.

Although the group has met regularly, there are frequent changes in the toddlers and preschoolers who attend. It is important that we use a brief and highly focused model of intervention because the program has an intended stay of 30 days or less. Many, though not all, of the children are placed within the 30-day period in foster homes. Since CPS typically brings the children to GEFC, rarely are they returned to the family they were living with prior to removal. If the family of removal was their biological parent(s), there is a long road back before CPS would return the child to the home. The parent(s) would first be required to successfully complete a number of programs, including several of the following: therapy, parenting classes, child abuse prevention programs, drug treatment and/or rehabilitation, and in some cases, family therapy. If removed from a foster home because the child was not safe or too disruptive, it would be highly unlikely that the child would return to that home in the near future. All the young children in the group, some less than 2 years of age, share the common background of recent, sudden removal from their home.

Removal from home can be a traumatic experience for young children especially when unexpected and not understood. Three years ago our clinical staff at CHP began collecting narratives of removal from our older children and were astonished at how vivid and emotionally riveting they were, even when the story of removal was told years later. In our weekly clinical seminars we engaged in extensive discussions of how the children in out-of-home placements carry these powerful narratives within and are rarely asked to share them. As clinicians we became more sensitive to the idea that the *trauma narrative*, as Cohen, Mannarino, and Deblinger (2012) pointed out, for children who experience ongoing trauma or complex trauma is really a case of a *life narrative* rather than a story of discrete trauma events. Many a child in foster care, and especially in residential treatment, experience life as a continuous horror story, a nightmare that never ends. One essential part of that life narrative is the emotional story of removal from home(s). An example from a 5-year-old: "My mom was lying on the floor. I don't know if she was dead or not. A neighbor called the police. An ambulance took my mom. I don't know if she is still there. I don't know if she is dead. I came here [CHP] with a lady in a white car." Some children in foster care have been removed from as many as 22 placements, as documented in a case of an older adolescent who was placed in our GEFC program. In such extreme cases, the concept of a life narrative, as outlined by Cohen and colleagues, takes on new meaning.

Children in the preschool play group make pictures in the sand of a small turtle looking futilely for its mother; play out puppet stories where the mother has left—the word is that she is in New York City, but no one knows for sure. In the family playhouse violent scenes are enacted where the furniture goes flying and the people get knocked over. Some of these play scenes allow for a directed intervention that presents an alternative scenario intended to challenge some of the cognitive distortions common to these children (Dorsey & Deblinger, 2012). In one example, the play therapist, in the form of a fireman, arrives on the scene and states emphatically, "These children are not safe. We must take them to a place where they will be safe from harm." The children are then removed and taken to a "safe home for children." When the children arrive at the safe home, the fireman addresses the children again with strong affect: "You children have done nothing wrong. You were brought here because this is a safe home for children."

Sensitive statements of attunement are used to help empathize with the frightened and bewildered children, some less than 2 years of age. The play therapist might say: "It is so hard to be away from your family, from your mommy [sometimes Daddy, too], but your mommy needs help with her problems before she can take care of you and keep you safe." We emphasize to the children that "we are not your family, we are not your home, and we know you miss your mommy and your home, but we will do our best to take good care of you and to keep you safe until your mommy gets the help she needs to stop drinking [or to stop using drugs, or stop getting into violent fights] so that she can take care of you and keep you safe." This kind of cognitive work is an essential part of evidence-based TF-CBT (Cohen, Mannarino, & Deblinger, 2012). The cognitive work is woven into the play scenarios produced by the children in a developmentally appropriate and sensitive way to therapeutically communicate with them. The goal is to enhance their capacity to develop a cohesive trauma narrative and to gain the meaning and perspective that are so elusive for young children, unless created in their natural language of play.

"Mommy and Me" Group

In 2010, CHP opened a Young Mothers' Program (YMP). Many of the high-risk expectant mothers, and those who already have delivered their babies, have expressed the conviction that they don't want their babies to ever be taken away from them or placed in foster care. As a result, what the young mothers refer to as the "Mommy and Me" group began in the fall of 2012. The purpose was to create a relaxed, comfortable, and safe context in which the mothers could engage in playful interactions with their babies to increase bonding and strengthen attachment.

The Mommy and Me group, co-led by my colleague Stephanie Carnes (social worker for the YMP) and me, has gone through three phases since it began. Since many of the young women had come into foster care as a result of intervention by CPS, it is not surprising that there was a significant lack of trust and a fear that the group leaders were there to judge or evaluate them. During this first phase of *mistrust and apprehension*, the young mothers sat in chairs or on the sofa, but some of them did put their babies down on the blanket in the playroom to play with the group leaders. Not only did the young mothers not sit on the play mat with their babies, but they were also quite hesitant to engage with their babies and the other young mothers. In the second phase of *tentative exploration*, some of the mothers joined their babies on the floor and began to engage in playful interactions with their own babies and the other babies in the room. During the third phase of *active engagement*, the mothers not only engaged with their babies and the other babies in a playful manner but also began to bond with each other and share some of their concerns as young mothers in foster care.

Issues that spontaneously arose in the group discussions were concerns about monitoring and scrutiny by CPS, including fears of their babies being removed from their care and wanting to protect their babies from violent partners both now and in the future. The latter was an especially pertinent issue for the majority of the young mothers who were involved currently, or in the past, in relationships involving intimate partner violence. In the beginning of this third phase, a group trauma narrative began to evolve, although denial and minimization on the part of the adolescent mothers was still evident, especially among those still involved in abusive, violent relationships. This limited the therapeutic value of the collective narrative for some of the mothers. Noteworthy is that they could discuss such sensitive issues at all, since they began the group with significant mistrust toward the group leaders and each other.

The late Walter Bonime (1989), a highly acclaimed psychoanalyst, explained that an active declaration of trust from those whose sense of trust has been badly damaged is a monumental breakthrough and a significant step in the healing process. In the third phase of the group with the greater trust that was established, the group leaders were able to incorporate psychoeducation, including the attachment and bonding processes. We attribute the modeling of playful interactions with the babies in the first phase, and the facilitation and encouragement of the mothers' play with their babies and the other babies in the group in the second phase, with the dramatic increase in trust that allowed the work of increased disclosure and sharing in the third phase to take place.

Sibling Play Groups

In recognition of how important sibling bonds are to children removed from their families, a number of sibling groups have been treated in play therapy with the goals of strengthening and reinforcing the sibling ties as well as facilitating the creation of the shared trauma narrative in the supportive context of the sibling group. In one family, a total of seven siblings were treated together in a home leased and staffed just for this purpose by CHP.

Family Therapy and Family Play Therapy

Cognizant of how crucial it is to work closely with parents who sincerely want their children to return home, family therapy has also been an important part of the services offered. In the case of the seven children, the family therapy extended for 3½ years due to the severity of the trauma experienced by the children and their mother. When the family consists of preschool children, the work may take the form of family play therapy (Gil, 1994).

Clinical Considerations in Using Play Therapy with Complex Trauma

Although not included in the fifth edition of the *Diagnostic and Statistical Manual of Mental Disorders* (DSM-5; American Psychiatric Association, 2013) as an official diagnosis, many clinicians recognize the value of the concept of complex trauma that has been proposed to describe the effects of repeated childhood abuse and other chronic stressors, as compared to single-event trauma (Courtois & Ford, 2009). A high percentage of children in foster care, especially those in residential treatment centers, would meet the criteria for complex trauma. The Adverse Childhood Experiences (ACE) studies (Filitti et al., 1998) have shown that not only the mental health but also the physical health of children exposed to multiple adverse events can be adversely impacted. The study focused on adverse childhood experiences such as physical and/or sexual abuse, neglect, substance abuse or incarceration of a parent, major psychiatric disorder in a parent, and separation or divorce. The critical threshold in the research appears to be four or more adverse childhood events: Those children exposed to four or more adverse events were at significantly higher risk for poor mental and physical health outcomes in adult life, including longevity—on average 10 years shorter (Filitti et al., 1998). An internal, unpublished survey (Crenshaw &

Alstadt, 2011) of the CHP's last 100 admissions in 2010 indicated that 87% of children and adolescents had experienced four or more of the seven risk factors, with some youth exposed to all seven. Children with such childhood histories often suffer from complex trauma because the high degree of exposure to risk factors would ordinarily overwhelm even the best of coping and resilience within the child. There will, of course, be exceptions. There are some children with such harsh beginnings in life who do not show signs of PTSD, let alone complex trauma. Resilience is remarkable to behold in such clinical populations.

Strategies and Techniques

Modifications of TF-CBT for Complex and Ongoing Trauma

Recently there has been a growing recognition in the field that children in foster care (Dorsey & Deblinger, 2012)—especially those children in residential treatment (Cohen, Mannarino, & Navarro, 2012), children with complex trauma (Cohen, Mannarino, Kliethermes, et al., 2012), and children with ongoing trauma (Cohen et al., 2011)—require modifications in the empirically supported TF-CBT protocols. The modifications take the form of changing the proportion of time devoted to different components of the protocol and extending the length of the treatment, a refreshing change that I (Crenshaw) have advocated for (Crenshaw, 2006, pp. 35–36; Crenshaw & Garbarino, 2008, pp. 85–86). Treating youth with complex trauma, for example, requires devoting proportionally more time to coping skills and establishing safety than the original model entailed (Cohen, Mannarino, Kliethermes, et al., 2012). Titrating the gradual exposure to the trauma themes and material was also recommended for youth with complex trauma, as was extending the consolidation and closure phases to address traumatic grief and to allow more time to generalize trust adequately.

I (Crenshaw) remember well a phone conversation I had with Judith Cohen when the 16-session protocol for treating childhood traumatic grief was first published (Cohen & Mannarino, 2004). I was so thrilled that they were doing research on treatment so relevant to those of us who work with child trauma, but I was dismayed that only two sessions in that original protocol were allocated for creating the trauma narrative. My deep respect for the work of Cohen and Mannarino was solidified on that day that I told Judith Cohen that the repeatedly traumatized children I work with could never do a trauma narrative in two sessions. Cohen agreed wholeheartedly and emphasized that there is no substitute for clinical judgment. The difference between treating single-event trauma, what Lenore Terr (1991) called *Type 1 trauma*, and repeated or complex trauma, what Terr called *Type 2 trauma*, is akin to the difference between fighting a forest fire with a garden hose as opposed to helicopters dumping slurry (a mix of water and fire retardant) on the fire from above. Complex, or Type 2 trauma, requires a more comprehensive, complex, and in-depth approach that extends beyond the original protocols developed primarily for single-event trauma.

When working with children who face ongoing traumas, it is of the utmost importance that clinicians emphasize safety (Cohen et al., 2011). It might even be questioned how effective any therapy can be if the child in the present circumstances is unsafe. Safety becomes the priority in such cases and requires communication with a wider social and community network, including family, school, and in many cases child protection agencies and courts (see Shelby & Maltby, Chapter 23, this volume). Clinical experience in foster care has revealed the "parental blinders syndrome," a characterization I (Crenshaw) used to describe what too often happens when parental figures have not faced or resolved their own trauma experiences. Numerous clinical experiences point to the inability of some parents with unresolved trauma to keep their children safe from ongoing trauma because they don't see the danger themselves. They don't see the risk, the perils, the threats to their children because fully confronting those dangers would trigger trauma memories of their own unresolved loss and/or abuse.

One mother, who was repeatedly abused and battered by violent male partners, took no steps to protect her teenage daughter when she became involved with a violent boyfriend despite the fact that she had walked into the room on one occasion when the adolescent boy was holding a knife to her daughter's throat. How can therapy proceed productively without addressing the real and imminent danger in the present resulting from "parental blinders"? For such a mother to effectively protect her daughter in such circumstances, she would need to do her own trauma work so that the "blinders" could be removed. Only then could she see accurately what was happening to her daughter.

During the trauma narrative and processing stage with youth experiencing ongoing trauma, Cohen and colleagues (2011) recommend first making the parents more aware of the extent of the ongoing traumas their children are experiencing. In addition, they recommend working with youth to modify any maladaptive cognitions pertaining to the ongoing traumas. The adolescent girl who was brutally treated by her boyfriend had witnessed repeated violent acts against her mother by her male partners. The girl regarded this violence as normative behavior in romantic relationships. In addition, she had repeatedly witnessed her mother feel guilty about whatever she had supposedly done to provoke the partner, apologize to him, and ultimately take her abusive partner's side. So this young girl came to believe, like her mother, that she didn't deserve to be treated better. It is essential to test, challenge, dispute, and ultimately modify these negative cognitive beliefs.

Finally, youth exposed to chronic or ongoing traumas need to engage in thera-peutic cognitive work to learn how to discriminate between real signs of danger and generalized alarm reactions to trauma reminders. At CHP many of the children who are admitted in an acute trauma state as a result of exposure to violence are unable to sleep at night because they fear the sounds of arguments that so often preceded acts of frightening violence at night in the home. They need help to differentiate between the frightful images of their nightmares and what is real in the waking state. They need lots of help learning *not* to assume that physical violence is coming every time they hear a raised voice. Otherwise they remain in a chronically hyperaroused physiological state, mobilized for danger.

In working with children in foster care, and especially in residential treatment, clinicians will encounter many children with complex trauma. When TF-CBT is modified for complex and ongoing traumas, it is recommended that instead of creating a trauma narrative for each of the multitudinous trauma experiences, the therapist focus the child's attention on a few of the worst ones, and also to look for themes across the trauma experiences and address those themes when creating the trauma narrative.

The Crucial Importance of the Child's Relational World

One of the most compelling features of TF-CBT is its emphasis on involving parents, foster parents, or both in the treatment process. When it is not feasible to include these individuals, one can include caregivers, such as child care workers in residential treatment facilities (Cohen, Mannarino, & Navarro, 2012; Dorsey & Deblinger, 2012). Involving the parents or caregivers is especially critical in foster care and in residential treatment because the frequency and severity of behavior problems among youth in foster care, and even more so in residential care, leave parents, foster parents, and child care workers often baffled, frustrated, and exhausted. Making them allies in the treatment process may not help them develop important parenting skills, but doing so does lend important support to the children and counters the feeling that they are doing the work alone because they are "bad" and entirely to blame for the problems of concern.

The presence of children's relational support system is especially important when creating the trauma narrative, an essential component of TF-CBT, but is also important in one form or another in nearly all trauma-informed approaches to treatment. Family/caregiver support is critically needed when children try to put into words, or play out, the events that previously could not be shared. One caution, however, from our clinical experience: Children will not share the trauma narrative in the presence of the therapist, the parent, the foster parent, child care worker, or caregiver unless convinced that the listener is ready, willing, and able to hear it.

A Creative, Out-of-the-Box Intervention: CHP Facility Dog Program

When foster care placements fail repeatedly, a child ultimately ends up in residential treatment. At that point there may no longer be a biological family to provide a support system for the child or even a place to visit. In some cases (at least for a long time) the child will not consistently trust the child care staff sufficiently to agree to have a child care worker participate in the treatment. In 2010 the CHP began an innovative solution to this problem. The relational support comes in the form of a four-legged animal regarded throughout history as "man's best friend." The CHP Facility Dog Program utilizes service-trained dogs because we want the most highly trained dogs to provide services to our children who have to testify in court, which was the impetus of the program. Rosie, a golden retriever, now deceased, became the first dog in New York court history to be approved by a judge to accompany a 15-year-old in our program on the witness stand when she testified about the sexual abuse she had suf-

fered. Since then we have continued to use only service-trained dogs when needed in the courtroom, and we also regularly utilize them in the therapy room. These dogs have played an immensely valuable role in facilitating the trauma narrative process for children with complex trauma. From an attachment theory perspective, it is not surprising that the children bond more quickly with these calm and loving dogs than with human therapists because it is humans who have typically inflicted the repeated trauma they've suffered The children trust them because they know the dog will not hurt them, judge them, or betray their secrets. The children also learn more quickly to attach to and trust the therapist if the dog is present and clearly attached to the therapist. A clinical example follows.

In one of the most chronic and severe abuse cases I (Crenshaw) have encountered in my career, I worked with a 12-year-old boy who could neither play out nor talk out the worst of the sadistic abuse experiences he had suffered. He was able to approach some of the dark side of his life through artwork that expressed the darkness and hopelessness but not the actual events. He was placed in residential care, and due to his violent and high-risk behavior, including repeated fire setting, he had to be hospitalized for periods as long as 6 months to stabilize his condition and to keep him safe. In family play therapy with the presence of Ivy, our service dog, Roger (fictitious name) was finally able to begin the process of creating his trauma narrative. Lying on the floor under a table next to Ivy with his arm around the dog and his head resting on her, he began to describe events that were as cruel and sadistic as any I've ever heard. In Ivy's presence, Roger continued to process the terror and horror of the abuse he'd suffered repeatedly over a period of years. Roger and his family both firmly believe that he could never have shared these horrific events without the comfort, trust, and safety provided by lying next to Ivy as he shared trauma narratives over a 6-month period.

Clinical Case Example

I (Tillman) worked closely with Michael, an adolescent male placed in familial foster care. When Michael was 15 years old, he was placed in the custody of his maternal aunt after his father received jail time for assaulting his mother and his mother could no longer care for him, due to her own difficulties with substance abuse. Before being removed from the home, Michael witnessed frequent incidents of domestic violence and often physically attempted to stop his father from abusing his mother. When he intervened, Michael became the focus of the abuse and suffered severe injuries at the hands of his father, including broken bones and dislocated joints.

Prior to our first meeting, Michael had never received counseling of any kind. When I went to greet Michael and his aunt in the waiting room, his size immediately stood out to me. Now 17 years old and at least 6 feet tall, Michael was a stocky, African American boy. His aunt brought him for treatment because of his "fits of rage." When Michael became angry, he would destroy property—punching holes in the walls of the family's home, kicking things, breaking tables, and taking drawers out of his dresser and throwing them across the room. Michael's aunt was concerned for her safety and was wondering if he needed to be placed elsewhere.

I spent the first few sessions attempting to get to know Michael. He was quiet and polite, and showed no signs of physical aggression within the confines of the therapy room. I've found that I don't typically witness the level of aggression that families experience in the midst of full-blown disagreements when the child lacks the ability to self-regulate and self-soothe. I did everything imaginable to build rapport, but after three sessions Michael still answered questions and prompts with one-word answers, didn't make eye contact, and appeared to be disengaged.

During our fourth session, Michael asked about the dollhouse sitting directly across

from his chair: "What's that for?" I explained that sometimes it can be difficult for children to talk, so they show me things in the dollhouse, using the people and furniture to act things out. Michael didn't respond verbally, but he slid off of his chair and onto the floor, sitting directly in front of the dollhouse. "I'm going to show you what other kids show you," he said. I simply responded with "okay." Honestly, I was mesmerized. I had a 17-year-old boy sitting on the floor about to play with the dolls in the dollhouse. And with that, his play began.

Michael selected a mother figure, a father figure, and a child figure. He then enacted a terrifying scene in which his father dragged his mother down the stairs while she screamed and cried for help. The boy stood at the top of the stairs watching, not moving. The father then proceeded to kick the mother, who was now lying on the floor, several times, until she stopped screaming and simply whimpered. At that point, the father left the house, and Michael looked at me, saying, "He's leaving to go get some alcohol." Then the boy walked slowly down the stairs to help his mother. He laid her on the couch and got her a drink and some Tylenol. Then the mom told him to leave her alone, that she was okay. So the boy went to his room. He hid in the corner and he cried. Then, very abruptly, Michael turned around, looked at me, and said, "I bet that's what other kids show you, huh?" Until this point I hadn't moved, hadn't tracked behavior, hadn't reflected, hadn't restated, hadn't paraphrased—I hadn't used any basic play therapy skills. I was afraid to startle him, afraid to cause him to feel self-conscious in his play, so I simply observed everything that he did. Still shocked by his play in the dollhouse, I said very little. "The kid in that house must have been pretty scared." Michael stood up and sat back in his chair. "Yup," he replied.

During our next session, before I could say anything, Michael slid onto the floor again and sat in front of the dollhouse. He explained that he was going to show me some other things that kids show me.

He asked if he was right, if kids came in to see me because their parents fight. I told him that they did, that it was difficult for them to talk about such events. When he reached for the figurines this time, I had a plan: I asked if I could watch and talk while he played, and he agreed. This time he selected the same three figurines (mom, dad, and son). Immediately the mother and father were arguing because dinner wasn't ready. The boy suggested that they order a pizza, but his comment went ignored. When this happened, the boy retreated to his room. A few moments later Michael made a loud crashing noise, and the boy came running down the stairs. I reflected that the boy was scared, that he didn't know what had happened. The boy walked in to find his mother lying on the floor, bleeding. The father hit the mother with a frying pan in front of the boy. The boy jumped up and tried to grab the frying pan from his father's hand. The two wrestled, and the boy ended up on the ground, with his father kicking him several times. The boy and the mother were left on the floor as the father stormed out. Michael explained that the mom was hurt badly but that the boy was okay, that he "didn't even cry." I reflected feeling terrified and scared, and Michael quickly interjected with "angry and sad."

A few sessions later, Michael asked if we could record his play to show to other kids whose parents were fighting. I said that recording his play was a great idea, but that we couldn't show other kids because he would be in the video and that would break confidentiality. He said he understood, but he still wanted to record the play for us to watch later. I turned on the camera. He looked directly at the camera and said, "This time things are gonna change." He repeated the exact scene that he had enacted in the previous session—the scene with both mom and son being hurt. But this time, the boy dialed 911 and told them everything that had happened. The police came and they took the mom away in an ambulance. Then they called the boy's aunt to come pick him up. I reflected that the boy stood

up for himself and his mom, that he did his best to help them both, that maybe the boy felt less scared and more proud. Michael just smiled.

A few sessions later his play included themes of interpersonal violence and the boy fighting back against the father. His play also contained themes in which the boy becomes aggressive for no apparent reason. At the end of the session, when he was back sitting in his chair, he asked, "Am I like my dad?" I asked him what he meant, and he talked about how his dad would always scare him and his mom, and that now he scares his aunt and his uncle. He said that he didn't want to be like his dad.

In one of our final sessions, Michael asked if he could record his play to show to his aunt at the end of the session. I was a little worried about what he might act out, so I said "yes" to the recording part and "we'll see" to showing his aunt. His play in this session had a totally different quality to it. Instead of being driven by fear, terror, and helplessness, a whole new experience emerged. Michael selected three figurines (a new figure to be the aunt, a new figure to be the uncle, and the same boy figure). In this scene, the family sat down to dinner and started to argue over the boy's grades. Unlike in previous sessions where the boy would get up and throw or break things, the boy stayed seated at the table. He said that he was trying but was frustrated. The aunt thanked him for staying at the table, and the uncle said that he was proud of the boy. Then they talked about his grades and ways for him to improve his grades. The boy even agreed to let the uncle help him with his homework. At the end, the aunt hugged him and gave him a kiss on the forehead. "I'm done," Michael said as he climbed back into his chair, "now can we show my aunt?" I asked why he wanted to show his aunt the video and he said "'cus that's how things are gonna be now." Clearly, he needed to convey to his aunt that he was trying and that he wanted to make healthier (nonaggressive) choices. So we brought the aunt into the therapy room. She watched the brief video clip, and she cried, and she hugged her nephew. I reflected that Michael must have been feeling proud and loved. He agreed and smiled.

Conclusion

Play therapy, artwork, sandtray, and animal-assisted play therapy allow young children, and sometimes older children, the opportunity to work safely and at their own pace in confronting trauma events or themes in their lives. Not only do young children frequently lack the cognitive and language resources to benefit from language-dependent therapies, but the traumatic events themselves may be encoded in the brain in ways that are hard to access by verbal means. Creating a trauma narrative, or in the case of complex or ongoing trauma, theme-based trauma narratives, is especially challenging in foster care because of the cumulative losses and disrupted attachments experienced by these children, in addition to trauma exposure. Modifications of the evidence-based TF-CBT protocols are discussed in this chapter along with an illustrative case study. The work with this population can be simultaneously discouraging and hopeful, heartrending and heartwarming, and frustrating and invigorating. Even if only one child is able to get through the thicket and go on to live a satisfying life, it is enough for us to keep giving our all.

REFERENCES

American Psychiatric Association. (2013). *Diagnostic and statistical manual of mental disorders* (5th ed.). Arlington, VA: Author.

Amir, N., Strafford, J., Freshman M. S., & Foa, E. B. (1998). Relationship between trauma narratives and trauma pathology. *Journal of Traumatic Stress, 11,* 385–392.

Bloom, S. (2000). Creating sanctuary: Healing from systemic abuses of power. *Therapeutic Communities: International Journal for Thera-*

peutic and Supportive Organizations, 21(2), 67–91.

Bonime, W. (1989). *Collaborative psychoanalysis: Anxiety, depression, dreams, and personality change.* Teaneck, NJ: Fairleigh Dickinson University Press.

Child Welfare Information Gateway. (2011). Foster Care Statistics 2011. Retrieved April 15, 2013, from *www.childwelfare.gov/pubs/factsheets/foster.pdf#Page=1&view=Fit.*

Cohen, J. A., & Mannarino, A. P. (2004). Treating childhood traumatic grief. *Journal of Clinical Child and Adolescent Psychology, 33,* 819–833.

Cohen, J. A., Mannarino, A. P., & Deblinger, E. (2006). *Treating trauma and traumatic grief in children and adolescents.* New York: Guilford Press.

Cohen, J. A., Mannarino, A. P., & Deblinger, E. (Eds.). (2012). *Trauma-focused CBT for children and adolescents: Treatment applications.* New York: Guilford Press.

Cohen, J. A., Mannarino, A. P., Kleithermes, M., & Murray, L. K. (2012). Trauma-focused CBT for youth with complex trauma. *Child Abuse and Neglect, 36,* 528–541.

Cohen, J. A., Mannarino, A. P., & Murray, L. K. (2011). Trauma-focused CBT for youth who experience ongoing traumas. *Child Abuse and Neglect, 35,* 637–646.

Cohen, J. A., Mannarino, A. P., & Navarro, D. (2012). Residential treatment. In J. A. Cohen, A. P. Mannarino, & E. Deblinger (Eds.), *Trauma-focused CBT for children and adolescents: Treatment applications* (pp. 73–102). New York: Guilford Press.

Courtois, C. A., & Ford, J. D. (Eds.). (2009). *Treating complex traumatic stress disorders: An evidence-based guide.* New York: Guilford Press.

Crenshaw, D. A. (2006). *Evocative strategies in child and adolescent psychotherapy.* Lanham, MD: Aronson.

Crenshaw, D. A. & Alstadt, C. (2011). *A study of the adverse childhood events (ACES) in the last 100 admissions to the Children's Home of Poughkeepsie.* Unpublished study, Children's Home of Poughkeepsie, Poughkeepsie, NY.

Crenshaw, D. A., & Garbarino, J. (2008). The hidden dimensions: Unspeakable sorrow and buried human potential. In D. A. Crenshaw (Ed.), *Child and adolescent psychotherapy:*

Wounded spirits and healing paths (pp. 79–91). Lanham, MD: Aronson.

Deblinger, E., Mannarino, A. P., Cohen, J. A., Runyon, M. K., & Steer, R. A. (2011). Trauma-focused cognitive behavioral therapy for children: Impact of the trauma narrative and treatment length. *Depression and Anxiety, 28*(1), 67–75.

Dorsey, S., & Deblinger, E. (2012). Children in foster care. In J. A. Cohen, A. P. Mannarino, & E. Deblinger (Eds.), *Trauma-focused CBT for children and adolescents: Treatment applications* (pp. 49–72). New York: Guilford Press.

Dozier, M., Albus, K., Fisher, P. A., & Sepulveda, S. (2002). Interventions for foster parents: Implications for developmental theory. *Developmental and Psychopathology, 14*(4), 843–860.

Dubner, A. E. & Motta, R. W. (1999). Sexually and physically abused foster care children and posttraumatic stress disorder. *Journal of Consulting and Clinical Psychology, 67,* 367–373.

Felitti, V. J., Anda, R. F., Nordenberg, D., Williamson, D. F., Spitz, A. M., Edwards, V., et al. (1998). Relationship of childhood abuse and household dysfunction to many of the leading causes of death in adults: The Adverse Childhood Experiences (ACE) study. *American Journal of Preventive Medicine, 14*(4), 245–258.

Gaensbauer, T. J. (2011). Embodied simulation, mirror neurons, and the reenactment of trauma. *Neuropsychoanalysis, 13,* 91–107.

Gidron, Y., Duncan, E., Lazar, A., Biderman, A., Tandeter, H., & Shvartztman, P. (2002). Effects of guided written disclosure of stressful experiences on clinic visits and symptoms in frequent clinic attenders. *Family Practice, 19,* 161–166.

Gil, E. (1994). *Play in family therapy.* New York: Guilford Press.

Green, E. J., Crenshaw, D. A., & Kolos, A. C. (2010). Counseling children with preverbal trauma. *International Journal of Play Therapy, 19*(2), 95–105.

Jones Harden, B. (2004). Safety and stability for foster children: A developmental perspective. *Future of Children, 14*(1), 30–47.

Leslie, L. K., Gordon, J. N., Lambros, K., Premji, K., Peoples, J., & Gist, K. (2005). Addressing the developmental and mental health needs of young children in foster care. *Journal of Developmental and Behavioral Pediatrics, 26*(2), 140–151.

National Child Traumatic Stress Network. (2007). Trauma-focused cognitive behavioral therapy (TF-CBT). Retrieved June 24, 2013, from *www.nctsn.org/nctsn_assets/pdfs/promising_practices/TF-CBT_fact_sheet_3-20-07.pdf.*

Pennebaker, J. W., & Susman, J. R. (1988). Disclosure of trauma and psychosomatic processes. *Social Science and Medicine, 26,* 327–332.

Pew Commission on Children in Foster Care. (2003). A child's journey through the child welfare system. Retrieved June 15, 2013, from *http://pewfostercare.org/research/docs/journey. pdf.*

Racusin, R., Maerlender, A. C., Sengupta, A., Isquith, P. K., & Straus, M. B. (2005). Community psychiatric practice: Psychosocial treatment of children in foster care: A review. *Community Mental Health Journal, 41*(2), 199–221.

Schneider, K. M., & Phares, V. (2005). Coping with parental loss because of termination of parental rights. *Child Welfare, 84,* 819–842.

Stahmer, A. C., Leslie, L. K., Hurlburt, M., Barth, R. P., Webb, M. B., Landsverk, J., et al. (2005). Developmental and behavioral needs and service use for young children in child welfare. *Pediatrics, 116,* 891–900.

Terr, L. C. (1991). Childhood trauma: An outline and overview. *American Journal of Psychiatry, 148,* 10–19.

Vig, S., Chinitz, S., & Schulman, L. (2005). Young children in foster care: Multiple vulnerabilities and complex service needs. *Infants and Young Children, 18*(2), 147–160.

Webb, N. B. (Ed.). (2007). *Play therapy with children in crisis: A casebook for practitioners* (3rd ed.). New York: Guilford Press.

CHAPTER 19

Play Therapy with Children Experiencing Homelessness

Debbie C. Sturm
Christopher Hill

According to the National Coalition for the Homeless (2009), one in 35 children experience homelessness, meaning that almost 2 million children in the United States are without stable or adequate housing. Homelessness has many faces. Perhaps it is the face of a 6-year-old girl who lives with her parents and baby brother in the dining room of a relative since being evicted 2 months ago. She sees the stress her parents experience as they try to find work and manage the pressures of a host family whose patience is wearing thin. It may be the face of a 9-year-old boy, whose 16-year-old brother and hero is staying in a different shelter with their dad, while he and his mom are in a shelter for women and young children. And it is the face of a 4-year-old girl whose mother is fleeing an abusive relationship and struggling with her own history of depression and substance abuse.

What exactly does it mean to be homeless in the United States today? Although the definition is not standardized, the U.S. Government Accountability Office considers homeless people to be those living on the street or in shelters, without a permanent address. Furthermore, it defines homelessness as those suffering from economic hardship and relegated to living without a permanent residence (Cackley, 2010). We also offer the older McKinney–Vento Homeless Assistance Act of 1987 definition (2001) of homeless children and youth—individuals who lack a fixed, regular, and adequate nighttime residence—which can include:

- Children and youth who are sharing the housing of other persons due to loss of housing, economic hardship, or a similar reason;
- Children who may be living in motels, hotels, trailer parks, shelters, or awaiting foster care placement;
- Children and youth who have a primary nighttime residence that is a public or private place not designed for, or ordinarily used as, a regular sleeping accommodation for human beings;
- Children and youth who are living in cars, parks, public spaces, abandoned buildings, substandard housing, bus or train stations, or similar settings;
- Migratory children who qualify as homeless because they are children who are living in circumstances similar to those listed above.

To expand the picture further, we would also include children who are considered runaways, a portion of the 2 million homeless children in the United States—a group of children whose current status is unknown and may be missing by choice, by abandonment, family rejection, or some involuntary situation (Hammer, Finkelhor, & Sedlak, 2002; National Coalition for the Homeless, 2009).

The road to homelessness is often complex and encompasses a wide variety of factors unique to each family. Issues such as unemployment, underemployment, housing difficulties, substance abuse issues, parental mental health issues, relationship breakdown, and in some cases, choice (Tischler, Redemeyer, & Vostanis, 2007) could lead to homelessness. Each family brings a unique history and a personal constellation of these factors. Experiences with homelessness are often cyclical, resulting in families potentially experiencing homelessness more than once (Thompson, Pollio, Eyrich, Bradbury, & North, 2004). Given this variability, how do we understand the impact of homelessness on the mental health of the children we are serving? According to Buckner (2012) and his historical review of the literature pertaining to homeless children over the past 20 years, homeless children are typically exposed to three different types of risk factors. These include:

1. Risks specifically related to being homeless, such as stressful conditions within a shelter or temporary living situation;
2. Risks that are shared by children from low-income or impoverished families, such as exposure to community violence and safety/security concerns;
3. Risks that all children, regardless of family income or living situation, tend to face, including biological and family system problems.

One of the most important considerations for any clinician working with children and families who are experiencing homelessness is the broad range of within-group differences (Cutuli, Wiik, Herbers, Gunnar, & Masten, 2010). Often, one of the only common denominators a group of homeless children may share is their lack of permanent housing. Buckner (2008) captured this well by stating:

> As an assortment of investigations has indicated, homeless families are not a static and isolated group. They emerge from a broader population of low-income families living in housing and eventually return to this larger group. Because homelessness is but one of many stressors that children living in poverty can experience, it is wise to be mindful of the broader context of poverty in understanding the issues of homeless children. (p. 734)

Comprehensive and historical assessment is critical at all stages of engagement with the child, the family, and the systems within which they are involved. Cutuli and colleagues (2010) also recommend viewing the child and family within a risk and resiliency framework, noting that even amid the challenges faced by families experiencing homelessness, significant strengths and protective factors are also likely to exist.

Physical and Psychological Challenges

Children who are homeless often experience poorer health outcomes than children in more stable housing. Homeless children are more likely to have chronic health conditions, including (but not limited to) respiratory illness, such as asthma or chronic bronchitis, and gastrointestinal complaints, such as stomach pains or disrupted appetite, as well as complications resulting from lack of preventive care, such as regular dental checkups and wellness visits. Moreover, the likelihood of treatment is much lower because homeless families with children have poorer access to affordable care, insurance, doctors, hospitals, or other medical services. The course of an illness may lengthen or result in complications due to the lack of basic needs being met or sufficient treatment being offered (Schwarz, Garrett, Hampsey, & Thompson, 2007).

Furthermore, food insecurity is often a problem for children experiencing homelessness. The U.S. Department of Agriculture defines food insecurity as "limited or uncertain availability of nutritionally adequate and safe foods or limited or uncertain ability to acquire acceptable foods in socially acceptable ways" (Coleman-Jensen, 2013). The idea of acquiring foods in socially acceptable ways—that is, without resorting to emergency food supplies, scavenging, stealing, or other coping strategies—is especially pertinent to children experiencing homelessness. Food insecurity can lead to malnourishment or hunger in this population. Rates of childhood obesity are a problem in the United States, and they are especially problematic for homeless youth. Moreover, the rates of homeless youth with overeating problems may be linked to the inexpensive and low-nutrition food available to them and the very real fear of a return to scarcity (Schwarz et al., 2007). The combination of infrequent and inaccessible health care with less-than-optimal nutrition serves as complicating factors to the overall well-being and development of children experiencing extreme poverty and homelessness. It reminds us as practitioners to always utilize a holistic, developmental, and historical lens when assessing the needs of children and families experiencing homelessness. It is easy to overlook hunger, pain, dehydration, and other physical discomfort if we focus too quickly on psychological and educational symptoms. As we know, they are all so closely intertwined.

Mental Health Implications

While exceptions certainly exist, homelessness is generally accompanied by a number of other well-known developmental risk factors such as low family income, educational or employment barriers for parents, exposure to community violence, and substandard housing (Cutuli et al., 2010). Each of these risk factors tends to share relationships with negative life events—chronic or acute traumas—such as "child maltreatment, parental conflict, domestic violence, parental substance abuse or mental illness, and other risk factors associated with family instability" (Cutuli et al., 2010, p. 831). Much of the research related to the emotional and psychological impact of homelessness on children seems to parallel the research on children raised in extreme poverty (Buckner, 2012; Schmitz, Wagner, & Menke, 2001; Zeisemer, Marcoux, & Manvell, 1994). Although similarities exist, play therapists are cautioned to seek out information clarifying the differences between children in poverty and children in poverty resulting in homelessness. In a study by Ziesemer and colleagues (1994), homeless children were found to be no more at risk of negative academic functioning and problem behavior than nonhomeless children living in poverty. Their conclusion was that homelessness should be viewed as an additional, but not necessarily more damaging, life event along the continuum of stressors experienced by children and families living in poverty.

One of the important considerations of time spent in unstable or frequently changing housing situations is the intensity and duration of the stress experienced directly by the children and indirectly through parental stress. Researchers are exploring the role of elevated cortisol (one of the stress hormones) among children experiencing homelessness. One interesting finding among these children highlighted a difference between children who were experiencing homelessness due to economic distress and those who were experiencing homelessness due to both economic distress and negative life events, such as events resulting in disruptions or threats to the family. Cortisol levels among children with the added negative life events were significantly higher than those with just economic distress (Cutuli et al., 2010), such as temporary homelessness resulting from a job loss or eviction. This seems to underscore the importance of a full assessment of the family system and lifespan stressors prior to beginning treatment. Simply put, homelessness may be the shared experience among a group of children, but the factors leading to homelessness are likely the root of the psychological and mental health issues experienced by the children.

Additional studies serve as reminders to clinicians to consider the mental health status of the accompanying parent. (Most of the available research has been conducted with mothers as participants.) Mothers' mental health status, history of incarceration, and cumulative history of trauma, as well as the child's exposure to trauma were the factors most strongly associated with the child's experience of emotional or mental health problems (Bassuk et al., 1996; Gewirtz, DeGarmo, Plowman, August, & Realmuto, 2009; Harpaz-Rotem, Rosenheck, & Desai, 2006). Early studies (Tischler, Karim, Rustall, Gregory, & Vostanis, 2004; Vostanis, Cumella, Briscoe, & Oyebode, 1996) found the most common causes of homelessness among children who entered shelters with their mothers were relationship breakdown and domestic violence. Children who were exposed to violence or traumatic life events prior to coming to the shelter had higher incidences of depression and anxiety (Harpaz-Rotem et al., 2006).

Given the relationship between a child's well-being and parental mental health, it is encouraging to know that mothers in supportive or temporary housing, wherein mental health services are offered, tend to utilize those services at high rates (Park, Fertig, & Allison, 2011). Women who experience relationship breakdown and domestic violence also report difficulty in confiding in family and friends and a general lack of a support system. In shelters providing supportive services, mothers reported feeling a greater sense of connection and efficacy in their problem-solving efforts (Karim, Tischler, & Gregory, 2006).

Keep in mind that children are often separated from one or both of their primary caregivers during periods of homelessness. Women who are struggling with violent or dangerous relationships, with addiction or dependence, or serious psychiatric issues may temporarily lose the care of their children through child protective services action. Parents, regardless of gender, may choose to place their children with friends or family members while they seek help for their problems. These children still fall under the federal definition of homelessness even though they are in private residences. Although kinship caregiving can be a stable option for many families, for just as many families it can be accompanied by problems that compound the difficulty of separation, such as strained family relationships, exposure to risk factors such as abuse or neglect, and relatives who may seek to keep the family members apart (Barrow & Lawinski, 2009). These are all additional stressors that may impact the mental health and academic functioning of the child.

Clinicians will also want to consider the patterns of separation that may occur within a family. Twenty-five percent of women in a New York homeless shelter reported being separated from a minor child at least once (Cowal, Shinn, Weitzman, Stojanovic, & Labay, 2002) and nearly one-third of all women entering the shelter reported entering without their children (Dotson, 2011). Their experiences differed based on whether their children were absent due to voluntary or involuntary placements. Voluntary placements, such as placing children with a friend or relative, afforded the mother more choice and agency over the safety and well-being of her children. Involuntary placements tend to involve some type of removal due to safety concerns for the children. According to Dotson (2011), the primary factors influencing the likelihood of children being separated from their mothers during homelessness are domestic violence, substance abuse, and mental illness. Many of the women who were in the shelter with their children seemed to present with low occurrences of domestic violence, substance abuse, or mental illness, higher awareness of the challenges in their current situation, and greater coping skills. This overview serves as a reminder to play therapists to be mindful of the role of these factors, how they relate to the family's separation or togetherness, and how to assess for risk factors and strengths.

In addition, some families who go to shelters find that family shelters often exclude men and/or adolescent/teenage boys. It is not uncommon to see siblings separated or to work with a young child whose male teenage brother is at a male-only shelter or placed in a foster home. No studies were identified that clearly explored the factors relating to family separation while in homeless shelters; however, clinicians should be aware this kind of separation does occur and become curious about the impact of this additional separation and ambiguity on the child (Barrow & Lawinski, 2009). Always ask, "Who *isn't* here?"

Finally, one of the factors that seem to be unique to children who are homeless, particularly in the way it impacts their psychological and educational functioning, is the actual quality and condition of the shelter or other temporary living conditions (Buckner, 2008). Behavioral problems, feelings of safety (or lack thereof), family interaction, and the overarching unknown can all be influenced by the shelter or housing environment. Clinicians want to take the time to understand the culture within the shelter or organization and explore children's perceptions of their stay in order to properly assess the factors that may be impacting their well-being.

Executive Functioning

Extreme stress and adversity, particularly among families with few resources and limited support systems, can have a nega-

tive impact on a child's executive functioning (EF). Performance of cognitive tasks, particularly those that require children to pay attention closely, remember details and instructions, move from one task to another, and deliver expected responses can be slowed or compromised (Masten et al., 2012).

A study comparing the differences between social skills and behavior problems among preschoolers in a Head Start program yielded no differences between homeless and housed children when it came to social skills at entry into the program or at the 6-month mark (Koblinsky, Gordon, & Anderson, 2000). This finding supported results from a prior study (DiBiase & Waddell, 1995) that also found no difference in the two groups. The researchers concluded that, although the Head Start children as a whole experienced some *social skills* differences from the typical preschool population, these differences are likely attributable to poverty, not homelessness. However, when they examined *behavior* problems, significant differences did emerge. Also consistent with the DiBiase and Waddell (1995) study, researchers found that the disorganized and stressful condition of homelessness resulted in more immature, stubborn, and hyperactive behavior, along with higher rates of anxious or depressed behaviors.

Researchers have examined the impact of homelessness on EF among preschool and elementary school children and determined that it is far more likely that the adverse conditions precipitating homelessness are a better predictor or stronger influence on EF skills (Masten et al., 2012). In addition, the plasticity of skills associated with EF (e.g., planning, attention, problem solving, verbal reasoning, inhibition, mental flexibility) is a reminder that effective interventions within the schools in a consistent and timely manner can greatly lower the risk of longer-term EF impairment and can strengthen protective factors.

Finally, children in the care of a homeless mother or a mother at risk of becoming homeless were less likely to be enrolled in school, and those who were enrolled had higher incidences of truancy and tardiness (Harpaz-Rotem et al., 2006). This is also a good opportunity to keep in mind the mediating factors available through compliance with the McKinney–Vento Act. That act, influenced by an Illinois statute aimed at protecting homeless children and providing access to consistency in their educational setting, expanded the definition of homeless children to include "individuals who lack a fixed, regular, and adequate nighttime residence." In addition to broadening the definition, the McKinney–Vento Act ensures homeless children transportation to and from school free of charge, allowing children to attend their school of origin (the school they attended when they first became homeless) regardless of what district the family resides in. The act also requires schools to register homeless children even if they lack normally required documents, such as immunization records or proof of residence. Local school districts must appoint local education liaisons to ensure that school staff are aware of these rights, to provide public notice to homeless families (at shelters and schools), and to facilitate access to school and transportation services. What this act means with regard to the impact of homelessness on academic performance is that school districts must have systems in place to better identify children who are at risk. Early identification and intervention are central to mitigating the negative effects of unstable living situations on academic performance and cognitive development.

Assessment and Psychometrics

As suggested in this chapter, it is important for clinicians to engage in an assessment process that is holistic, client-centered, developmental, historical, and inclusive of the family milieu. Ideally, the multidomain assessment begins at intake in order to di-

agnose and locate the appropriate services for the individual. The psychosocial assessment consists of a multitiered compartmentalization of domains, including mental health status, medical problems, education level, family background, criminal history, past substance abuse, and spiritual or cultural concerns. Furthermore, a review of the domains allows for the individual to be assessed in a holistic manner, whereby the assessor is able to provide immediate feedback, counseling, or a link to services as necessary. Moreover, the assessment allows for the client's voice to be heard over the din of the clinical jargon that often monopolizes the clinical process. Best practices include the client's presenting strengths, coping skills, or mechanisms of survival. Although negative aspects of the lifespan are reviewed, they are described in the positive, healing light of possible change and are not used to blame or condemn the individual (Johnson, 2010; McQuaid et al., 2012).

The initial psychosocial focus is helpful not only in the assessment of needs and monitoring the progress of the client, but also in informing the larger system about the needs of the children and families being served (Johnson, 2010). Play therapists may consider using broad-spectrum rating scales for assessing the behaviors and emotions of children, such as the Behavioral Assessment System for Children–Second Edition (BASC-2) and the Beck Youth Inventories for Children and Adolescents. These instruments are recognized as excellent tools for children who have experienced trauma, behavioral issues, and/or symptoms consistent with DSM-5 diagnoses.

Clinical Approaches

As we reflect on some of the known potential issues experienced by children who are homeless, a clearer picture begins to emerge with regard to treatment options involving play therapy. Baggerly and Jenkins (2009) provided a good reminder that homeless children, highly influenced by acute and chronic traumas associated with abuse, neglect, family disruption, substance abuse, family violence, and poverty, are subject to interruptions in both neurodevelopment and attachment. We are also reminded that these children often experience loss or significant and often ambiguous disruption of important relationships, such as those with grandparents, teachers, friends, other significant relatives, and sometimes even siblings (National Coalition for the Homeless, 2007). The therapeutic relationship can be a wonderful vehicle for understanding the child's uniquely personal experience with the trauma, loss, and instability, and also a place to help heal and form new and renewed attachments. We now consider several approaches to play therapy with this population that have been supported by the literature.

Child-Centered Play

Several studies over the past decade support the use of child-centered play therapy (CCPT) with elementary school-age children who are experiencing homelessness (Baggerly, 2003, 2004; Baggerly & Borkowski, 2004). Specifically, CCPT is defined as

> a dynamic interpersonal relationship between a child and a therapist trained in play therapy procedures who provides selected play materials and facilitates the development of a safe relationship for the child to fully express and explore self (feelings, thoughts, experiences, and behaviors) through play, the child's natural medium of communication, for optimal growth and development. (Landreth, 2002, p. 16)

The primary value system underlying child-centered play considers the child to be an expert on his or her own experience as well as a guide in his or her own healing. By allowing the play to be directed, crafted, and expressed in the way of the child, rather than through the direction of

the therapist, child-centered play practitioners demonstrate their belief and trust that the child's truest expression and healing are possible. These factors are central, in so many ways, to the issues faced by children experiencing homelessness.

In a specific study implementing CCPT interventions with children who are homeless, Baggerly and Jenkins (2009) sought to understand whether or not this approach would have an effect on developmental strands and diagnostic profiles of these children. Results from their work indicated that participants who received CCPT demonstrated an increase in self-control in the classroom and an overall higher ability to internalize control, characterized by feeling more emotionally secure, responding to limits more positively, and responding more constructively to others. Overall, children who participated in CCPT had decreased reports of classroom behavior problems and also showed positive trends toward reduction in avoidance or rejection of attachment, less negativity toward self and others, and a more developed or secure sense of self. Although the researchers were clear to identify the limitations of their study, particularly the limited sample size and the fact that the children received 14 sessions rather than the recommended 32, this study can be viewed as one that supports clinicians using CCPT with children who are homeless and indicates that doing so within a school setting can have a positive impact in the classroom as well.

Sibling Play

Reflecting on some of the challenges faced by families without permanent housing, a few points emerge to support sibling play as an important tool. First is the realization that children may be separated from their siblings due to their age, possibly having a different biological parent, or because of restrictions placed within the temporary housing situations. Creating opportunities for the children to be together in the context of a play therapy environment gives them a safe place in which to navigate their relationship and to maintain the sibling bond in the midst of other changes and separations. For children who are housed together, clinicians are able to create a cooperative context within which siblings can influence each other with regard to self-control, verbalizing feelings, and playing through the themes of their relationship and the shared struggles they have experienced with family and economic instability (Hunter, 1993). And, by increasing the connection between the siblings, parents—who may or may not be in a position to seek help themselves—experience lower levels of stress as family conflict decreases and cooperation increases. As Hunter (1993) states, "Empowering siblings to accept and nurture each other can help to counteract isolation and interrupt destructive intergenerational cycles" (p. 69). Any opportunity for sibling play, whether in a school setting, clinic, or temporary housing setting, contributes to the strength and resiliency of the whole family.

Filial Therapy

The typical length of stay for families in shelters is anything but typical and is highly dependent on the situation, the resources available, the parameters or conditions of the specific organization, and the factors influencing homelessness. Regardless, time spent in the shelter requires families to adapt to the new system, navigate shared spaces, and adjust to new rules and relationship dynamics. The adjustment influences important family rituals such as meals, play, and leisure time (Ray, 2006). Therefore, traditional parent–child roles during mealtime, family time, or leisure/playtime can bump up against expectations. In addition, parent–child dynamics can be complicated by the roles of other parents, children, and professionals in the environment.

Often the stressful events leading up to homelessness and the adjustment to the new temporary living situation can take a toll on the parent–child relationship. Ray's research (2006), along with the research of Wachs (1987) and Vibbert and Bornstein (1989), underscores the importance of maternal socioemotional behaviors as the strongest predictor of the child's socioemotional development, play, and use of language. Additionally, children develop competencies through predictable or trusting supportive routines or activities with significant adults (Ray, 2006; Rovee-Colier & Gulya, 2000). Counselors and other practitioners can advocate for the time and space to help parents connect with their children more effectively. This intervention fosters a feeling of competence in parents, who may already be struggling with their view of themselves as good parents. Practitioners may also need to advocate within the setting for the tools and the physical space conducive to socioemotional playtime separate from the emotionally laden interactions and routines within the larger shelter living space. Simply put: Filial therapy serves both preventive and therapeutic purposes, empowering often disempowered parents to provide safety and structure for their child, even in the most challenging situations.

In studies examining the socioemotional engagement between mothers and their toddlers in shelter environments, Ray (2006) stressed the importance of supporting consistent, positive, and relationship-affirming socioemotional experiences for parents and their children. To put this point plainly in play therapy terms, this research highly supports the use of filial therapy. Filial therapy is the parent–child derivative of CCPT and involves clinicians working with the primary caregiver in order to "facilitate a positive relationship with their child while learning skills to effectively manage children's behaviors" (Kolos, Green, & Crenshaw, 2009, p. 366). This improvement happens primarily through the strengthened and attuned relationship rather than through specific skills training. In their extensive review of the literature, Kolos and colleagues (2009) highlighted that, although the topic of filial therapy with homeless families was largely absent in the literature, filial therapy has shown strong efficacy with families from racial minorities—families with high levels of stress and single-parent living situations. Those characteristics, as we have already discussed, describe families who experience homelessness.

Again, a strong parent–child relationship provides "protection from the negative, long-term outcomes that perpetuate a cycle of homelessness" (Kolos et al., 2009, p. 367) and fosters parents' ability to provide warmth and stability to their children even in times of stress. An increase in the positive bond between parent and child results in a decrease in parental stress and more effective parenting. In turn, effective parenting correlates with decreases in child problem behaviors, a higher ability to mitigate the dangers in high-risk environments, and increases in academic and social skills and success (Kolos et al., 2009).

School-Based Counseling

Schools have a unique opportunity to create a space of stability, routine, and predictability during a time that otherwise may be filled with change and uncertainty (Moore & McArthur, 2011; Nabors & Weist, 2002). Although many children around the country experience absences, tardiness, difficulty with academic performance, and social challenges related to homelessness, the McKinney–Vento Act has minimized the frequency or necessity of children changing schools, and thereby suffering even further socially and academically. School counselors and social workers have an excellent opportunity to help strengthen children's relationships with significant adults, peers, and their own siblings within those school systems. Moore and McArthur (2011) suggested the use of play buddies, play partners, or play groups within the school. These could include:

- Structured or CCPT sessions involving the child and one or more peers who can serve as stable, positive, relationship role models and create space for problem solving and emotional regulation.
- Structured or CCPT sessions with the child and his or her sibling within the same school to help them develop a shared connection to the school environment and the significant caregiving adults.
- Opportunities for structured or semi-structured play groups to facilitate relationship building, problem solving, and sense of connectedness.

Such peer and group play therapy time is helpful for students who remain in their same school yet are experiencing disruption in housing, and they are equally valuable for students who have had to change schools. School-based practitioners can also provide structures and unstructured play designed to help students (1) grieve the loss of their home, the loss of a former school, separation from extended family or siblings and (2) deal with the factors that may have contributed to homelessness, such as domestic violence, economic stressors, parental substance abuse, or parental mental health issues. Peers, particularly those who have successfully navigated some of those issues, can help normalize the experience and serve as unintentional "guides" for the child newly exploring them. In one case study, Baggerly and Borkowski (2004) found that a homeless elementary student who engaged in group play therapy with one play buddy gradually experienced more cooperative play, less attention-seeking behavior, increased collaboration with her play buddy, and more socially appropriate attention seeking within the classroom setting. She also exhibited lower dependency behaviors and higher levels of trust. Although this was just one case study, the implications for group play therapy for homeless children are interesting. Creating a space that provides consistency, stability, and peer/adult supporters can help children anchor to the new school while the family adjusts to the changes in the living situation. As always, any time counselors or other practitioners can reach out and involve parents in this process, the child benefits. And parent–teacher–counselor collaborations are always going to be the most effective means of helping these children within school settings.

Implications for Practitioners

One of the most important prerequisites for clinicians involved in this work is self-reflection to examine personal beliefs and biases related to this population. It would not be uncommon for clinicians—who are, after all, just people—to harbor frustration, anger, or disappointment toward parents who would somehow allow, either through their choices or through their challenges, their children to live in a state of homelessness or transience. Such a belief could easily and quite subtly influence the type of therapy a clinician chooses to conduct and the level of engagement a clinician may seek with a parent.

In addition, it can be just as easy for a clinician to view the homelessness as the "problem," whereas the time spent in the shelter or temporary housing may actually represent security and stability. In families plagued by interpersonal violence, substance abuse, community violence, and extreme poverty, the time spent in a shelter may be the first time in a long time where they have been able to feel safe together. And it may be that the very factors contributing to their current situation are, in fact, the most significant to their therapy. As Ziesemer and colleagues (1994) suggested, clinicians who are working with homeless children and families may need to focus on the short-term experience of homelessness while also addressing the larger implications of poverty and instability on individual, family, and systemic levels. Masten and

colleagues (2012) also reminded us that academic-related issues, such as compromised EF, are as common among homeless children as they are among economically disadvantaged students who experience negative life events and frequent mobility. More and more evidence continues to strengthen the importance of a comprehensive assessment of the child's and family's experience beyond their current state of homelessness.

We were unable to identify research specifically examining counselors' or mental health practitioners' views of homeless children or families; however, Kim (2013), in examining the perceptions of preservice early education teachers, discovered some food for thought. Most of the preservice teachers held deficit perspectives of these children, seeing them as likely to misbehave, be unable to focus, dress poorly, and be delayed in their development. They also expressed concern over how to interact with shelter staff and fears about whether the parent would feel judged by the teacher. However, time spent in the shelter in the context of field experiences resulted in significant shifts in teachers' beliefs and fears. What these shifts mean for mental health practitioners is that we must take the time to visit shelters, talk to the staff, hear the stories of homeless families, read and research the wide range of within-group differences, and put aside assumptions that we may hold. Again, the most effective way to do this?: through exposure and self-reflection.

In essence, clinicians must work to clearly examine their own assumptions about families experiencing homelessness so as not to let those assumptions get in the way of fully understanding the lived experience of their clients. In doing so, clinicians will also be able to uncover the strengths of the family and understand how their relationship dynamics have helped them survive to this point. Most importantly, as research has suggested, one of the most significant factors influencing a child's mental health is the mental health of the parent (Dotson,

2011; Gewirtz et al., 2009). As compelling as the needs of the children may be, there is a tandem need to attend to the well-being of the parent. Inclusion of parents and facilitating their strengths will ultimately benefit the child.

Finally, nearly all of the studies examined highlighting the parallels between children living in poverty and children who become homeless stressed the importance of preventive measures and advocacy. It becomes important as clinicians and as social justice advocates to learn about the populations in your community who are most at risk of future homelessness. And given what we know about the parental factors that often lead to homelessness, it becomes important to also advocate on behalf of parents at risk. Early intervention with these at-risk populations, particularly drawing on CCPT, sibling therapy, and parent–child interaction or filial therapy, can do so much to strengthen families and build the protective factors that are critical for navigating economic and residential instability.

Clinical Case Example

A teacher at a nearby elementary school has noticed significant changes in concentration, timely completion of assignments, and general interest during classroom time by 7-year-old Kenny. She has also noticed an increasing cough as well as more days tardy or absent than earlier in the school year. Upon reaching out to Kenny's mother, the teacher learned that the family had recently moved into a shelter. For Mychelle, Kenny's mom, homelessness started with abuse. She is 26 years old, married, and now the single mother of three. All three children, the oldest of whom is Kenny, witnessed the physical abuse and frequently went to sleep to the sounds of arguments. After 6 years, it finally became too much. Concerned for the safety of her children, Mychelle fled to a domestic violence shelter and later to the small basement bedroom of a friend. When tensions grew between Mychelle and her friend, another move was necessary.

This time Mychelle and her family found refuge in a temporary family shelter. Soon after arriving, Kenny developed an unremitting cough that went untreated because the family was without health insurance. A Good Samaritan in the shelter connected the family with free medical care and Kenny was diagnosed with asthma. The physician, who was attuned to the challenges presented by this family, also became concerned about the depression and anxiety that seemed present for both Mychelle and Kenny as well as the trauma that Mychelle had experienced in her abusive marriage. Mychelle shared this concern with Kenny's teacher, and the teacher suggested Mychelle and Kenny meet with Michael, a local counselor.

During the initial intake with Kenny and his mom, Michael, a clinician specializing in play therapy, quickly realized that the experience of homelessness had taken a toll on Kenny's physical and emotional health. Asthma triggers had been pervasive in the basement room and now in the shelter environment. Coughing and breathing difficulties limited his ability to play, talk, and sleep comfortably. Mychelle's homelessness, her financial situation, and her worries about her younger children made it difficult for her to access the services needed to address Kenny's health to the extent she wanted. She also felt that she was failing her children.

The impact of years of domestic violence had also left a lasting impression on Kenny. He felt insecure in the shelter, often awakened by the typical noises present in a busy building, and not easily trusting the other parents and shelter staff. The only true stability has been his ability to remain in his same elementary school with his same classroom teacher. He loved his teacher but worried that he was disappointing her and that she would not like him anymore.

In addition to the psychosocial intake, Michael administered the Beck Youth Inventory to Kenny and noticed that signs of both depression and anxiety were strongly represented in the results. He recommended weekly play therapy sessions to Mychelle, who responded with concern. Transportation to the session was complicated to arrange and the evening hours at the shelter were full of duties, such as shared mealtimes and family activities that she thought were important. She also expressed a need to be as present as possible for her other two children who were having their own difficulties adjusting to all the changes.

Michael felt compelled to help them and was able to recognize all the barriers facing this family. He agreed to consult with his colleagues and with the shelter to see if there were other alternatives.

One of the significant concerns that emerged as Michael consulted with his other colleagues—all of whom typically worked with children and families and had, at various times, encountered families experiencing homelessness—was the need to meet these families wherever they are, literally and figuratively. The barriers with regard to time, transportation, finances, stable schedules, and consistent living situations were huge, and the counselors did not want to compound the complexity of the situation. They were also acutely aware of the importance of fostering a strong parent–child relationship as well as a sense of safety and security among the children. Together they approached the directors of the shelter about developing a support group and opportunities for both filial and sibling play therapy sessions.

Whenever possible, counselors should seize the opportunity to collaborate with their partners in the community. As Michael and his colleagues soon realized, the pairing of the different perspectives can open the door to countless ideas on how to best serve children and families. They worked to clarify such questions as these:

What does *temporary* mean in relation to the shelter?

Are there conditions to remaining in the shelter?

Are there members of the family or children, due to age, that are not able to stay there?

How are rules, chores, and other duties divided?

What degree of privacy and autonomy do families have?

What facilities are available for quiet family time, meal preparation and shared meals, counseling or other support services for adults and children?

To what extent are issues around employment, transportation, general safety and security, and transitions addressed?

Ultimately, thanks to the genuine sharing by Kenny and Mychelle and the thoughtful referral by his teacher, Michael and his colleagues opened up a discussion with the temporary shelter staff that allowed for the development of a small pilot program. This included structured play for the children as well as filial play with parents and their children. It also allowed for a therapist who could work in a group setting specifically to meet the needs of the mothers, many of whom were experiencing mental health issues and trauma histories. The group included parenting skills, coping skills, mindfulness practices, and supportive care. Everyone remained realistic as to the challenges: the ever-changing population, the complexity of issues and varying family dynamics, and the challenges of merging multiple systems. Their long-term goal became sustaining the current partnership and involving additional parties—such as Kenny's elementary school and the physician at the free clinic who was so sensitive to Mychelle's limited financial means. As mentioned throughout this chapter, working with children and families experiencing homelessness is a complex undertaking that requires clinicians to think holistically and interprofessionally as they reverently witness and work with the unique and complex story of each family.

REFERENCES

Baggerly, J. N. (2003). Child-centered play therapy with children who are homeless: Perspective and procedures. *International Journal of Play Therapy, 12,* 87–106.

Baggerly, J. N. (2004). The effects of child-centered group play on self-concept, depression, and anxiety of children who are homeless. *International Journal of Play Therapy, 13,* 31–51.

Baggerly, J. N., & Borkowski, T. (2004). Applying the ASCA National Model to elementary school students who are homeless: A case study. *Professional School Counseling, 8*(2), 116–123.

Baggerly, J. N., & Jenkins, W. W. (2009). The effectiveness of child-centered play therapy on developmental and diagnostic factors in children who are homeless. *International Journal of Play Therapy, 18*(1), 45–55.

Barrow, S. M., & Lawinski, T. (2009). Contexts of mother–child separations in homeless families. *Analysis of Social Issues and Public Policy, 9*(1), 157–176.

Buckner, J. C. (2008). Understanding the impact of homelessness on children: Challenges and future research directions. *American Behavioral Scientist, 51,* 721–736.

Buckner, J. C. (2012). Education research on homeless and housed children living in poverty: Comments on Masten, Fantuzzo, Herbers, and Voight. *Educational Researcher, 41*(9), 403–407.

Cackley, A. (2010). *Homelessness: A common vocabulary could help agencies collaborate and collect more consistent data* (Report to congressional requesters [GAO-10-702]). Washington, DC: U.S. Government Accountability Office.

Coleman-Jensen, A. (2013). Food security in the U.S. Retrieved from *www.ers.usda.gov/topics/food-nutrition-assistance/food-security-in-the-us/measurement.aspx.*

Cowal, K., Shinn, M., Weitzman, B., Stojanovic, D., & Labay, I. (2002). Mother–child separations among homeless and housed families receiving public assistance in New York City. *American Journal of Community Psychology, 30,* 711–730.

Cutuli, J. J., Wiik, K. L., Herbers, J. E., Gunnar, M. R., & Masten, A. S. (2010). Cortisol function among early school-aged homeless children. *Psychoneuroendocrinology, 35,* 833–845.

DiBiase, R., & Waddell, S. (1995). Some effects of homelessness on the psychological functioning of preschoolers. *Journal of Abnormal Child Psychology, 23,* 783–792.

Dotson, H. M. (2011). Homeless women, parents, and children: A triangulation approach analyzing factors influencing homelessness and child separation. *Journal of Poverty, 15,* 241–258.

Gewirtz, A. H., DeGarmo, D. S., Plowman, E., August, G., & Realmuto, G. (2009). Parenting, parental mental health, and child functioning in families residing in supportive housing. *American Journal of Orthopsychiatry, 79*(3), 336–347.

Hammer, H., Finkelhor, D., & Sedlak, A. (2002). *Runaway/thrownaway children: National estimates and characteristics.* Washington, DC: U.S. Department of Justice, Office of Justice Programs, Office of Juvenile Justice and Delinquency Prevention.

Harpaz-Rotem, I., Rosenheck, R. A., & Desai, R. (2006). The mental health of children exposed to maternal mental illness and homelessness. *Community Mental Health Journal, 42*(5), 437–448.

Hunter, L. B. (1993). Sibling play therapy with homeless children: An opportunity in the crisis. *Child Welfare League of America, 27,* 65–75.

Johnson, D. L. (2010). *A compendium of psychosocial measures: Assessment of people with serious mental illnesses in the community.* New York: Springer.

Karim, K., Tischler, V., & Gregory, P. (2006). Homeless children and parents: Short-term mental health outcome. *International Journal of Social Psychiatry, 52*(5), 447–458.

Kim, J. (2013). Confronting invisibility: Early childhood pre-service teachers' beliefs toward homeless children. *Early Childhood Education, 41,* 161–169.

Koblinsky, S. A., Gordon, A. L., & Anderson, E. A. (2000). Changes in the social skills and behavior problems of homeless and housed children during the preschool year. *Early Education and Development, 11*(3), 321–338.

Kolos, A. C., Green, E. J., & Crenshaw, D. A. (2009). Conducting filial therapy with homeless parents. *American Journal of Orthopsychiatry, 79*(3), 366–374.

Landreth, G. L. (2002). *Play therapy: The art of the relationship* (2nd ed.). New York: Brunner-Routledge.

Masten, M. S., Herbers, J. E., Desjardins, D., Cutuli, J. J., McCormick, C. M., Sapienza, J., et al. (2012). Executive function skills and school success in young children experiencing homelessness. *Educational Researcher, 41,* 375–384.

McKinney–Vento Homeless Assistance Act of 1987, 42 USC § 11431 et seq. (2001). Retrieved August 17, 2013, from *www.nationalhomeless. org/publications/facts/McKinney.pdf.*

McQuaid, J. R., Marx, B. P., Rosen, M. I., Bufka, L. F., Tenhula, W., Cook, H., et al. (2012). Mental health assessment in rehabilitation research. *Journal of Rehabilitation Research and Development, 49*(1), 121–137.

Moore, T., & McArthur, M. (2011). Good for kids: Children who have been homeless talk about school. *Australian Journal of Education, 55,* 147–160.

Nabors, L. A., & Weist, M. D. (2002). School mental health services with homeless children. *Journal of School Health, 72*(7), 269.

National Coalition for the Homeless. (2007). Why are people homeless? NCH Fact Sheet #1. Retrieved September 1, 2013, from *ww.nationalhomeless/org/publications/facts/ Why.pdf.*

National Coalition for the Homeless. (2009). How many people experience homelessness? NCH Fact Sheet #1. Retrieved October 4, 2013, from *www.nationalhomeless.org/fact-sheets/How_Many.html.*

Park, J. M., Fertig, A. R., & Allison, P. D. (2011). Physical and mental health, cognitive development, and health care use by housing status of low-income young children in 20 American cities: A prospective cohort study. *American Journal of Public Health, 38,* 421–432.

Ray, S. A. (2006). Mother–toddler interactions during child-focused activity in transitional housing. *Occupational Therapy in Health Care, 20,* 81–97.

Rovee-Collier, C., & Gulya, M. (2000). Infant memory: Cues, contexts, categories, and lists. In D. L. Medin (Ed.), *The psychology of learning and motivation* (pp. 1–46). San Diego, CA: Academic Press.

Schmitz, C., Wagner, J., & Menke, E. (2001). The interconnection of childhood poverty and homelessness: Negative impact/points of access. *Families in Society, 82*(1), 69–77.

Schwarz, K. B., Garrett, B., Hampsey, J., & Thompson, D. (2007). High prevalence of overweight and obesity in homeless Baltimore children and their caregivers: A pilot study. *Clinical Nutrition and Obesity, 9*(1), 48.

Thompson, S. J., Pollio, D. E., Eyrich, K., Bradbury, E., & North, C. S. (2004). Successfully exiting homelessness: Experiences of formerly homeless mentally ill individuals. *Evaluation and Program Planning, 27*(4), 423–431.

Tischler, V., Karim, K., Rustall, S., Gregory, P., & Vostanis, P. (2004). A family support service for homeless children and parents: Users' perspectives and characteristics. *Health and Social Care in the Community, 12*(4), 327–335.

Tischler, V., Redemeyer, A., & Vostanis, P. (2007). Mothers experiencing homelessness: Mental health, support, and social care needs. *Health and Social Care in the Community, 15*(3), 246–253.

Vibbert, M., & Bornstein, M. (1989). Specific associations between domain of mother–child interaction and toddler referential language and pretense play. *Infant Behavior and Development, 12,* 163–189.

Vostanis, P., Cumella, S., Briscoe, J., & Oyebode, F. (1996). A survey of psychosocial characteristics of homeless families. *European Journal of Psychiatry, 10*(2), 108–117.

Wachs, T. D. (1987). Specificity of environmental action as manifest in environmental correlates of mastery motivation. *Developmental Psychology, 23,* 782–790.

Zeisemer, C., Marcoux, L., & Manvell, B. (1994). Homeless children: Are they different from other low-income children? *Social Work, 39*(6), 658–668.

CHAPTER 20

Play Therapy with Children of Divorce

A PRESCRIPTIVE APPROACH

Sueann Kenney-Noziska
Liana Lowenstein

Divorce is a chaotic experience that sets off a domino effect for families and typically involves a series of transitions and emotional distress. Rather than considering divorce a single event, emerging perspectives conceptualize divorce as a process involving a number of family transitions (Amato, 2010). Family members are dealing with a range of emotions and issues, including grief, sadness, loss, anger, establishing new relationships, learning new roles in the family system, and establishing new communication patterns. It is not uncommon for children to receive therapy during the divorce process. Play therapy is perhaps the most developmentally appropriate modality for children. Play helps to engage children in treatment; create a safe, therapeutic environment; facilitate communication between therapist and child; assess the child and family's treatment needs; and help address treatment goals.

This chapter focuses on using a prescriptive play therapy approach with families experiencing separation and divorce. A prescriptive theoretical play therapy model emphasizes the creation of a tailor-made treatment plan based on selecting and matching play therapy approaches and interventions that are supported in the literature and research as being effective for a particular symptom, issue, or problem. This prescriptive approach is particularly important for cases of divorce because the impact of the divorce will vary from individual to individual.

The play therapy interventions described in this chapter aim to address the most common treatment domains for children of divorce. Complexities related to special issues such as alienation, intimate partner violence, or allegations of child sexual abuse may also need to be addressed with some families, and the reader is encouraged to obtain additional resources to treat those complicated factors.

Clinical Considerations

A comprehensive, ongoing assessment will aid the play therapist in effective treatment planning and intervention. This is particularly crucial when using a prescriptive play therapy approach as this approach is based on a comprehensive assessment of individual needs (Gil & Shaw, 2009). Since many children and adolescents experiencing divorce display symptoms of anxiety, depression, and low self-esteem (Amato, 2001), using standardized assessment measures and questionnaires can facilitate an understanding of various symptoms. However, general standardized measures of well-being may overlook or minimize many of the subtler consequences for children of divorce, as this population appears to experience levels of distress related to being forced to take on adult responsibilities, feeling lonely, experiencing family events and holidays as stressful, and feeling torn between their mother's and father's households (Amato, 2010). Since these factors are not typically accounted for by most standardized measures, questionnaires specific to divorce, such as the Perceptions of Children Towards Parental Divorce Scale (Kurdek & Berg, 1987) or the Divorce Adjustment Inventory—Revised (DAI-R; Portes, Smith, & Brown, 2000), may be more appropriate measures.

Working with families of divorce involves multiple considerations and collaboration with other professionals during assessment and treatment. In addition to clinical interventions, the use of play therapy in cases of divorce may be more effective if utilized with additional supports such as mediation and parent coordination. Mediation, which emphasizes conflict reduction between the divorcing parents, may result in overall stress reduction because parental conflict is typically a primary stressor for children and the family system. Parent coordination or coparenting, which promotes the best interests of children by reducing parental conflict and litigation, strives to assist parents in developing, implementing, and complying with a parenting plan, making timely decisions consistent with children's developmental and psychological needs, and reducing the level of conflict.

Custody recommendations are also important and can significantly impact treatment. These recommendations vary considerably and are generally defined clearly in a court order or in the divorce decree. When the parents are legally divorced, best practice from a legal standpoint is for the treating therapist to obtain a current copy of the divorce decree and all modifications prior to commencing treatment (Bernstein & Hartsell, 2004). If a therapist is in doubt or unclear about any portion of these documents, he or she should have an attorney interpret the court order (Remley & Herlihy, 2010).

The current trend in custody emphasizes a more equal custody-sharing arrangement as, barring dangerous/unsafe conditions, most children appear to benefit from having a positive relationship with, and regular access to, both parents. Given that this type of custody plan may be a challenge in the midst of divorce, collaborative practice, a voluntary dispute resolution process, may serve beneficial for families. Collaborative practice provides an approach that supports parents in resolving legal disputes without judges, magistrates, or court personnel. The International Academy of Collaborative Professionals (IACP), comprised of attorneys, judges, mental health practitioners, and financial experts, is an organization that encourages this type of partnership to reduce overall conflict, negotiate acceptable resolutions, and facilitate open communication.

Given potential legal complications in families of divorce, documentation throughout treatment is critical (Bernstein & Hartsell, 2004). When parents are in conflict with one another, the therapist must maintain a professional role, ensure that boundaries are in place, and clearly define the role and scope of his or her services. Prior to accepting the child or adolescent as a client, it is the therapist's responsibility to understand the laws in his or her jurisdiction as they pertain to parental rights in divorce. Informed consent, the role of the therapist, and all rights and obligations should be explicitly stated in the therapist's consent forms and should additionally be discussed during the intake with both parents (Bernstein & Hartsell, 2004).

Research and Theory

Review of Research on Divorce

Despite the high incidence of divorce in our society, there remains little rigorous research delineating the impact of divorce on children and adolescents (Barczak et al., 2010). The research that is available has inconsistent findings. For example, research from Wallerstein and Lewis (2004) suggests that divorce results in lasting psychological problems for children, with damage attributed to the divorce itself versus issues related to the parents or the conflict of the marriage. Other research findings indicate that children from divorced families have similar adjustments to children from typical intact families in situations in which the divorce is associated with children moving into a less stressful situation (Gordon, 2005). Still other research suggests that, following divorce, children have more symptoms than those in high-conflict nondivorced families, but, as the children adapt to the new divorced situation, the pattern of differences reverses (Barczak et al., 2010).

Outcomes regarding the effects of divorce on children and adolescents vary considerably. Children with divorced parents compared with children with continuously married parents score lower on a variety of emotional, behavioral, social, health, and academic outcomes (Amato, 2010). Divorce that occurs early in a child's life has been associated with both internalizing and externalizing behaviors (Barczak et al., 2010), whereas divorce that occurs later in the child's life is associated with poor academic performance (Barczak et al., 2010). Based on these findings, interventions that target the remediation and prevention of

internalization and externalization may be appropriate for the former population, and interventions that emphasize academic achievement for the latter. However, the clinician must be aware that low academic performance may be how distress related to divorce (e.g., poor concentration, anxiety) manifests at any age.

The impact of divorce also appears to be influenced by the age and gender of the child. In adolescents, divorce has been associated with internalizing disorders, externalizing disorders, nonalcoholic substance use, and/or alcohol consumption (Barczak et al., 2010). Boys and girls often react to divorce differently and thus have different treatment needs. Conduct disorders have been linked to adolescent males, whereas increased depression is more common for adolescent females (DeLucia-Waack, 2011). A recent study by Majzub and Mansor (2012) suggests that adolescents' perceptions of divorce can be both positive and negative, with no significant differences in perception according to gender. The quality of the parental pre- and postdivorce relationship is one of the most important overall factors in determining whether or not subsequent delayed effects of divorce on children and adolescents will occur (Barczak et al., 2010).

Pathways that lead to outcomes specific to children and adolescents confronting divorce are not well understood but are believed to be influenced not only by risk factors, but also by individual, family, and extrafamilial protective factors (Pedro-Carroll & Jones, 2005). Individual protective factors include a realistic appraisal of control and accurate attributions. Family protective factors include protection from interparental conflict and the overall psychological well-being of the parents. Protective factors from outside the family include supportive relationships with positive adult role models and a strong support network.

Although negative short- and long-term effects of divorce are well documented in the research and literature, many children experience distress as a result of divorce but the majority do not appear to suffer long-term adjustment problems (DeLucia-Waack, 2011). Additionally, some research suggests that divorce can bring benefits, in particular, in research that uses comparison groups, controls for selection bias, measures marital adjustment carefully, and takes domestic violence into account (Rutter, 2009). In other words, the impact of the divorce depends on what it is being compared to. Furthermore, despite conflicting findings and information, there is a consensus that resilience characterizes some children of divorce (Rutter, 2009).

Best-Practice Guidelines for Court-Involved Therapy

Best-practice guidelines for therapists providing mental health services to families going through court-involved therapy in the family court have been established by the Association of Family and Conciliation Courts (2010). Specifically, these guidelines are intended to aid the therapist's understanding of how the legal system impacts treatment and to provide guidance to others regarding the practitioner's roles and responsibilities. These guidelines, based on relevant research and ethical standards, provide a concise resource for understanding mental health treatment in the context of the law. Underscoring the complexity of therapy when the family court is involved, this framework aids in balancing boundaries, roles, confidentiality, and professional objectivity while protecting the sanctity of the child's treatment.

Integrative Play Therapy

Integrative play therapy—the blending together of various play therapy theories and techniques—is applicable to a variety of disorders and may create a best fit for treatment needs (Drewes, 2011). From an integrative perspective, the emphasis is on clinical utility versus theoretical consistency (Seymour, 2011). Given the diversity of clin-

ical profiles addressed in cases of divorce, an integrative approach may be appropriate. Indeed, the play therapy field appears to be evolving from allegiance to one particular model of play therapy to a "client-focused theoretical approach" tailored to the individual needs of the client (Kenney-Noziska, Schaefer, & Homeyer, 2012).

According to the Substance Abuse and Mental Health Services Administration's National Registry of Evidence-Based Programs and Practices (SAMHSA's NREPP), cognitive-behavioral therapy, child developmental theory, and family systems theory, with an emphasis on parent skill building and education, may be important theoretical constructs to integrate when working with families of divorce. Using a prescriptive play therapy perspective, these approaches can be considered along with current research to formulate a tailor-made treatment plan.

Prescriptive Play Therapy

Norcross (2005) delineates four types of integrative approaches to psychotherapy with one being *technical eclecticism*. This type of integration involves using research to prescriptively select a treatment that is a best fit for an individual client. In the play therapy field, this is referred to as *prescriptive play therapy* and was first defined by Schaefer (2001), with more recent clinical applications described in contemporary play therapy literature by Gil and Shaw (2009) and Schaefer (2011). In cases of divorce, this research-informed method allows the play therapist to select a play therapy approach that has demonstrated effectiveness for a specific symptom or issue (Gil & Shaw, 2009). The literature and research are used to inform the play therapy process. One downside of this approach is the lack of rigorous research regarding the impact of divorce. Nevertheless, a prescriptive approach provides clinical intervention that is individualized yet clinically and empirically grounded.

Strategies and Techniques

Creative, play-based activities, presented within the context of an empathically attuned therapeutic relationship, can engage children and help them safely express their thoughts and feelings. Directive play therapy techniques provide a concrete approach that facilitates open disclosure and guides children closer to specific treatment issues. Bringing children's divorce-specific issues out into the open in a direct but engaging manner lets them know that their problems are not shameful and can be discussed. Below are some examples of structured play therapy techniques for use with children of divorce.

Children benefit from opportunities to clarify divorce-related misconceptions, and appropriately express feelings related to divorce. In the Basketball Game (Lowenstein, 2006) players take turns answering questions when they miss a basket. Topics covered in the game include feelings related to the divorce, reasons parents get divorced, self-blame for the divorce, and healthy coping strategies. The game allows the therapist to prescriptively select and modify question cards to ensure that treatment goals are addressed. The practitioner can play the game along with the child to facilitate playful interaction and model open communication. As the game proceeds, the therapist provides supportive feedback and offers praise when the child takes risks in expressing thoughts and feelings. It is also useful to ask the client to make up a few of his or her own cards to be included in the game. This exercise of creating question cards is projective in nature, and often gives the practitioner added insight into the client (Gil, 1994). There are a variety of ready-made therapeutic board games that can also be used in play therapy sessions to help children address divorce-specific issues, such as Daring Dinosaurs (Pedro-Carroll & Jones, 2005) and Upside Down Divorce (Childswork Childsplay, n.d.).

The purposeful use of books in therapy, known as bibliotherapy, and other storytelling techniques can be particularly effective with children of divorce. If the book or story is relevant to the child's situation, "the child will identify with the character or story, and will have increased understanding and insight after reading the book" (Malchiodi & Ginns-Gruenberg, 2008, p. 168). Books can facilitate discussion of divorce-specific issues, help children realize they are not alone in their feelings and reactions to the divorce, and often answer questions related to complex issues. The therapeutic value of bibliotherapy can be greatly enhanced by using stories as a springboard for further discussion. There is a wide variety of books available on divorce, or the practitioner can write his or her own stories to read to clients.

Children from divorced families may struggle with complex issues such as loyalty conflicts, witnessing parental conflict, or coping with a faraway or absent parent. When children have difficulty openly talking about these painful issues, puppet techniques can be helpful, such as Lowenstein's (2013) Upsetting Situations. This activity includes a variety of scenarios and coping statements for the child to reenact with puppets. Puppet play is used as a displacement technique that is a helpful strategy for children dealing with emotionally laden issues. The purpose of the displacement technique is to represent the child's distress about a situation and alternative ways of coping (Kalter, 1990). Since the success of the intervention will be greatly enhanced by engaging the parents in treatment, the activities in this protocol include handouts that can be discussed in sessions with each parent.

Playful cognitive-behavioral techniques can be a helpful approach with children, particularly when they blame themselves for the divorce. Getting Rid of Guilt (Lowenstein, 2006) is an intervention used to challenge and correct distorted thoughts regarding self-blame. The child is given several cartoons depicting scenarios. In each scenario, there is a child who makes a guilt-ridden statement and another child who responds with an appropriate challenge to that guilty statement. For example, the "guilty" child says, "I made my parents divorce because I was bad." The "helper" child responds, "Nothing you said or did made your parents get a divorce." In another cartoon scenario, the "guilty" child says, "I should have been able to save my parents' marriage." The "helper" child responds, "It's not up to kids to fix their parents' marriage." There are a number of cartoon scenarios for the child to read through, as well as blank cartoons so children can add other scenarios. The activity includes discussion questions to guide the practitioner in effectively processing the child's thoughts and feelings. Thinking Caps (Goodyear-Brown, 2005) is another playful cognitive-behavioral therapy (CBT) activity to help children replace guilt-ridden thoughts with helpful thoughts. Helping children develop accurate attributions for parental problems leads to better adjustment in children (Pedro-Carroll & Alpert-Gillis, 1997; Stolberg & Mahler, 1994).

Directive techniques are not the therapy, merely the tools to facilitate the therapeutic process. As such, underlying any techniques is a core set of skills that determines the practitioner's effectiveness in working with children impacted by divorce. As it is beyond the scope of this chapter to outline these core skills, the reader is encouraged to review additional resources on this topic. Directive interventions should not be used in isolation but integrated into a comprehensive treatment approach, as illustrated in the case example below.

As part of being attuned in the therapeutic relationship, therapists must be mindful that the use of directive interventions may be overwhelming to the child. For this reason play therapists must be flexible in their application of such strategies and may need to consider less directive approaches with certain clients, such as child-centered play therapy (CCPT). Relational components, including empathy, warmth, congruence, and therapeutic presence, offer curative properties for children confronting divorce, and their importance cannot be underemphasized.

Clinical Case Example

Referral Information

Joey, age 7, was an only child referred to play therapy by his mother, Lisa. Joey's parents had separated 6 months prior to the referral. The case was still before the courts with an interim order for joint custody and a shared access schedule. Lisa indicated that her son was in need of therapy to help him cope with the separation. She stated that Joey was having difficulty coping with the marital separation because his father, Dave, was badmouthing her and telling Joey that she was to blame for the divorce. She further indicated that Joey was experiencing frequent stomachaches and was clingy toward her, especially when he returned from visits with his father.

Lisa indicated that she did not want Joey's father to be involved in the therapy as she felt he would undermine the process. Once the therapist explained to her the benefits of both parents' involvement in Joey's therapy, Lisa agreed to ask Dave to call the clinician. When Dave called, the therapist emphasized his important role in helping Joey adjust to the marital breakup and asked for his perception of Joey's post-separation functioning. Dave indicated that Joey was having some trouble dealing with the divorce and blamed these difficulties on Lisa's "overcontrolling" nature.

After several phone calls with each parent to engage them, collect some initial information, explain play therapy and the assessment process, sort out payment details, and convince them of the rationale for them to meet with the therapist together for the initial session, a time was set up to meet.

Engagement and Assessment

In the initial session with Lisa and Dave, it was crucial that the therapist develop a positive rapport with both parents. Remaining neutral while still connecting with each parent can be a challenge when working with families of divorce, yet it is an essential element of effective clinical practice. The therapist conveyed empathy for the stress they were each experiencing and commended them for seeking help for their family.

The therapist explained to Lisa and Dave that play therapy would provide Joey with a safe and neutral therapeutic environment. It was clearly explained that it was not the role of the child's therapist to make recommendations to the court regarding custody/access issues. Both parents signed a form committing to closed counseling. This form was essential in ensuring that the therapist remained disengaged from the custody dispute.

The therapist asked Lisa and Dave to each describe their perception of Joey's current functioning. Each parent blamed the other for Joey's problems and their anger toward one another quickly escalated. Although challenging for the therapist, the volatile interaction demonstrated how hard the situation must be for Joey. In an effort to reduce the tension and to redirect Lisa and Dave to the needs of their son, the therapist asked them to each choose a toy or item from the playroom that represented "a happy, well-adjusted child." Lisa chose a boy on a skateboard from the collection of sandtray figurines, and stated, "I want Joey to be happy and carefree, not to feel stressed by the divorce." Dave picked up the basketball and stated, "I'd like him to have more fun when he's with me." This intervention deescalated their hostility. Moreover, it added an element of playfulness as they explored the playroom and described the symbolic meaning of the toy they chose. The therapist then asked what they could each do to help Joey adjust to the divorce in a healthy way. A fruitful discussion ensued and the therapist commended their ability to identify ways they could each nurture Joey's resilience. The therapist commented that the atmosphere in the session was more relaxed and that Joey would also likely feel better when Mom and Dad were more amicable.

Valuable assessment information was collected in this initial session with the parents that would later inform the treatment plan. Of particular significance, the following information was learned: Lisa and Dave had dated for 7 months, then married after Lisa became pregnant with Joey; the couple bickered often throughout their marriage and were verbally abusive toward each other in Joey's presence; they never fully explained the reason for the separation to Joey, as they did not know what to say; Joey often resists visitation with his father and is clingy with his mother when he returns from his father's; Joey complains of frequent stomachaches, and his teachers describe him as sad and withdrawn.

While exploring their childhood histories, it was noted that both Lisa and Dave had grown up in divorced families. Lisa maintained a close relationship with both her parents when they split up, whereas Dave was raised by his mother after his father abandoned the family shortly after his birth.

To enable each parent to articulate goals for therapy, they were asked, "What would need to happen in therapy to make you think this was a good, helpful idea?" Lisa responded, "To help us understand how Joey is feeling, and to help Joey know that none of this is his fault." Dave said, "Help me and Joey have more fun together because he often cries for his mom when he's with me." The parents were thanked for helping the therapist understand their priority goals for therapy.

Two assessment sessions were conducted with Joey. Each session began with structured play-based engagement and assessment activities, followed by observation of Joey's nondirective play. The first session with Joey focused on rapport building and gathering initial assessment data. Joey was initially nervous and did not make eye contact with the therapist. He became more at ease during a rapport-building game called Rock, Paper, Scissors (Cavett, 2010). The therapist paced the game by initially asking neutral questions, such as, "What's your favorite movie?" Joey played the game enthusiastically, giggled at appropriate times, and cheered when he won a round. Once it was apparent that Joey was engaged and relaxed, the focus of the game shifted to questions that required greater emotional risk-taking:

THERAPIST: What's something that really upsets you?

JOEY: (*in a sad tone*) When Mom and Dad be mean to each other.

THERAPIST: (*Leans closer to Joey.*) I can see that it makes you feel upset when Mom and Dad are mean to each other. Can you tell me more about that—what do Mom and Dad do and say to show they are being mean to each other?

JOEY: They yell and swear. Dad is meaner and even uses the F-word. (*Looks down, face gets flushed.*)

THERAPIST: (*careful to remain neutral and not to make a statement that would emphasize one parent as "meaner"*) It must be very upsetting for you when Mom and Dad are mean to each other. Lots of children who come here have upset feelings like that, and it is my job to help with those upset feelings. We'll do some talking and some playing to help you with your feelings.

The therapist felt it was especially important in this first session with Joey to validate his feelings and clarify the therapist role.

In the second session, Joey came happily into the playroom and asked to play Rock, Paper, Scissors. He played the game with enthusiasm, giggled at appropriate times, maintained eye contact with the therapist, and discussed salient feelings with greater openness. This behavior demonstrated that he felt at ease with the therapist. The therapist utilized an activity (How I Think, Feel, and Behave; Lowenstein, 2006) to assess Joey's feelings, behaviors, and coping strategies. The survey contains 22 statements, and clients are asked to place self-adhesive dots beside the statements that apply to them. The child places more dots beside the statements that are bigger worries. Joey placed the most dots beside the following statements:

- I have more worries since my parents divorced [three dots].
- I sometimes get stomachaches when I feel upset [three dots].
- I think the divorce is my fault [three dots].
- My parents argue a lot [five dots].
- My parents tell me mean things about each other [five dots].
- It's hard going back and forth between two homes [five dots].

Joey provided additional information when the activity was processed, particularly regarding the frequent arguing between his parents both prior to and since his parents' separation. This activity clearly revealed that Joey is experiencing a number of stressors related to the divorce.

An important component of the assessment process is to ascertain the child's perception of him- or herself and family dynamics. The Play Geno-Gram (Goodyear-Brown, 2002) revealed significant information regarding Joey's feelings toward his parents. When asked to choose a toy in the room to be his mom, he excitedly picked up the princess figurine and stated, "She's beautiful!" He had more difficulty choosing an item to represent his father. He finally placed the fire-breathing dragon on the genogram but would not articulate his reason for choosing this toy. For himself he chose a car and stated in a sad tone, "I go in the car a lot, back and forth to Dad's house and to Mom's house." His story also provided rich assessment information: "Once there was a beautiful princess and she was happy until the fire-breathing dragon burned her house down, and then the car drove far away to get away from the fire but then the princess found the car and took it to another house and they went to sleep." When asked if there is any character that he would like to change or replace with another toy, he stated, "Maybe the fire-breathing dragon could be a prince instead and then the princess would like him." The items that Joey chose for the genogram, as well as the story and his responses to the process questions, highlighted a number of salient issues to aid in treatment planning.

Several recurring themes were observed in Joey's nondirective play. He created battle scenes with the army figurines in the sandtray and with the adult male and female dolls in the dollhouse. Themes of loss and abandonment were also evident.

When working with divorced families, it is important to observe the child with each parent to assess issues of competence, cohesion, closeness, and control. Assessment activities provide a window for therapists to observe process and content within family interactions (Gil & Sobol, 2000). The Family Puppet Interview (Gil, 1994) was used to assess Joey's relationship with his mother. The therapist asked Joey and Lisa to each choose a puppet and to use the puppets to tell a story with a beginning, middle, and end. Joey chose the puppy and Lisa selected the kangaroo with, literally, the "joey" in its pouch. During the puppet show, Joey pulled the "joey" puppet from the mother kangaroo's pouch and became very upset when he could not fit the puppy inside the pouch. He threw the puppy across the room, picked up the joey, placed the joey back in the kangaroo's pouch, and proceeded to tell a story about a baby kangaroo who was afraid to be kidnapped so he stayed in his mom's pouch all day and all night. Lisa allowed Joey to direct most of the puppet play, though she did add that the kangaroo hopped around carefully so the joey would not fall out.

Using the Boat Storm Lighthouse Assessment (Post Sprunk, 2010) revealed salient information regarding the relationship between Joey and his father. They were instructed to fill a poster board with one drawing of a boat, a storm, and a lighthouse. They each drew independently with little interaction or collaboration. Joey drew a tiny boat atop a wavy sea, while his father drew a dark sky with storm clouds, torrential rain, and lightning. Dave then added a small lighthouse in the far corner of the poster board. Once the drawing was complete, they were each asked to tell a story about what happened before, during, and after the storm. Dave's story centered on a little boat that capsized during the storm and all the passengers on the boat drowned. Joey recounted that the boat got lost because it was too stormy to see the lighthouse. Both stories contained pessimistic themes and characters lacking in the ability to mobilize inner resources or access external support when faced with danger. During the second part of the session, in which Joey and his father had the opportunity to choose something to play together, Joey enacted a battle scene with the army figurines while Dave sat on the chair and watched Joey in silence.

Feedback Session with the Parents

The therapist met with Lisa and Dave to provide feedback on the assessment, contract for ongoing service, and collaborate to develop a comprehensive treatment plan. The therapist reiterated that therapy was closed to ensure that both parents were clear that the information discussed would not be used in their custody dispute. The strengths of the family members were highlighted, as well as their desire to seek help at this time. When conflict between Lisa and Dave escalated during the session, the therapist interjected, utilizing motivational interviewing strategies (Rosengren,

2009) to evoke change talk. For example: "In what ways do you think your fighting harms Joey?" and "How would things be better if you each changed?" These kinds of questions diffused their anger and brought the discussion back to the development of treatment goals. Lisa and Dave left the session with a clear sense of the direction for therapy and an increased motivation for change.

Treatment Sessions

A prescriptive approach was used in which various models, modalities, and techniques were selected to ensure that treatment goals were addressed. The therapy involved individual sessions with Joey, integrating playful CBT and CCPT, as well as family play therapy and filial therapy sessions with Joey and each of his parents. The therapist met with the parents periodically to provide feedback on Joey's progress, to facilitate their ability to focus on Joey's emotional needs, and to strengthen their parenting skills. Interventions were incorporated into the parent sessions that fit with Pedro-Carroll's emotionally intelligent parenting practices (2010), specifically to help Lisa and Dave establish new family rituals and traditions, maintain household structure and routines, engage in positive parent–child time, and implement strategies to encourage open communication. Lisa and Dave were referred to a parent coordinator to help them foster a more positive coparenting relationship. Each parent also sought the support of an individual therapist. The therapist collaborated closely with the members of the treatment team.

Priority goals for the initial phase of treatment with Joey included addressing divorce-related misconceptions, strengthening healthy coping skills, and expressing emotions related to the divorce. The assessment revealed that Joey was experiencing significant distress related to the divorce, particularly when exposed to parental conflict and when transitioning between two homes. As such, it was important to gear the initial phase of treatment toward teaching him healthy coping skills. Playful deep breathing and progressive muscle relaxation strategies were selected so that Joey would be motivated to practice and implement the techniques. He was taught several different techniques, then given the opportunity to choose the strategy he liked best and to practice this strategy at home each night at bedtime. His parents were enlisted to coach him at home to practice and utilize the coping skills. At first neither parent coached Joey to practice and implement the coping skills, but as they became more engaged and invested in therapy, they began to follow through with homework. Over time, Joey mastered Cookie Breathing (Lowenstein, 2013) and utilized this skill in times of need.

The stress associated with divorce causes a range of feelings that can be difficult for children to understand, identify, and express. Conveying warmth and acceptance and reflecting and validating Joey's feelings helped create an atmosphere of safety and trust. A number of therapeutic games were utilized as a safe way for Joey to emotionally connect with the therapist and to support his expression of overwhelming thoughts and feelings. Joey particularly enjoyed playing Feelings Hide and Seek (Noziska, 2008). In this therapeutic version of the popular childhood game hide-and-seek, instead of having people hide, the therapist hides cards with various feeling words around the room for the child to find and then discuss. Below is an excerpt from the game:

JOEY: (*enthusiastically searches the playroom and finally finds the "sad" emotion card hidden under a teacup*) I felt sad when Mom and Dad split up and we had to move. Now I never get to see my friends.

THERAPIST: Lots of things changed in your life when Mom and Dad split up. You had to move and now you feel sad because you really miss your friends.

JOEY: Yeah, and I hardly have any friends at my new school. (*looks down, gets quiet for a moment*) Maybe I can go visit my friends sometime.

THERAPIST: It can be really hard to move and to make new friends. The divorce has been really tough on you.

JOEY: (*Starts to search for another emotion card.*)

THERAPIST: [I respect Joey's need to move on with the game and decide not to process further at this time.]

The game proceeds and Joey engages in meaningful interchanges with the therapist regarding his feelings. The therapist notes Joey's social isolation as an issue to process further in later sessions.

Several divorce-specific books were read to Joey to normalize and validate his feelings. He seemed to especially relate to the book, *My Parents Are Divorced, My Elbows Have Nicknames, and Other Facts about Me* (Cochrane, 2009). The books were used as a springboard to engage Joey in further discussion about his feelings related to the divorce.

A critical treatment goal was to help Joey have a more balanced and positive relationship with both parents. Filial therapy was integrated into sessions with Joey and his father to enhance this parent–child relationship. Progress was initially slow because Dave blamed Lisa for his distant relationship with Joey. However, as therapy progressed, Dave began to see that his ability to provide a more nurturing environment for his son resulted in a closer relationship. Joey reported more positive feelings about visits with his father, which further substantiated the progress made in the father–son relationship. Filial sessions were also conducted with Joey and his mother to help Lisa implement consistent limits.

Sessions with the parenting coordinator helped Lisa and Dave better support each other's parenting role, which was an essential factor to the success of clinical work

with the family. In individual therapy, Dave explored his estranged relationship with his father, which fueled his motivation to work on a closer bond with Joey.

A pivotal time with this family came prior to summer holiday. Joey was anxious about spending a week away with his father. Lisa wanted the therapist to intervene to stop this visit because she felt that Joey was not ready for so much time away from her. The therapist met with both parents to discuss the matter and emphasized that it is not the role of the child's therapist to make recommendations regarding visitation issues. When Lisa expressed anger toward the therapist for not stopping the visit, the therapist validated her concern for Joey and redirected the focus to the benefits of Joey spending positive, high-quality time with each parent. The therapist facilitated a discussion about how each parent could support Joey prior to and during this extended visit with his father. As well, a session with Joey reinforced his use of coping skills learned in prior sessions so he could manage his anxiety. A conjoint session between Joey and his father provided additional support. When he returned from the vacation with his father, Joey reported to the therapist that he'd had a good time, and he proudly said that he used Cookie Breathing several times during the vacation to ease his anxiety.

It is common for children to blame themselves for the divorce. Joey revealed in the assessment and in subsequent sessions that he felt the divorce was his fault because his parents often had arguments about him. Several interventions were implemented to eliminate Joey's feelings of self-blame for the divorce. The book *Was It the Chocolate Pudding?* (Levins & Langdo, 2005) was read and discussed. Joey identified with the main character, and the story helped him to identify his own feelings of self-blame for the divorce. The therapist adapted a playful cognitive-behavioral technique, Getting Rid of Guilt (Lowenstein, 2006), and had Joey reenact the scenarios with puppets. He then created his own puppet show depicting a "helper" puppet challenging and correcting the guilt-ridden puppet. The puppet show was videotaped and a "movie premiere" was held with each of his parents—with popcorn. The therapist met with the parents ahead of time to prompt them to respond appropriately in the session. Dave praised Joey's efforts on the movie and joked that he should be nominated for an academy award. It was a funny and poignant moment and evidence of how far this father and son had come.

As mentioned above, conflict between parents in front of their children, especially around issues related to the children, is associated with a number of psychological problems. A key treatment goal for this family was for Lisa and Dave to learn conflict resolution skills, and most importantly, to reduce their level of conflict in the presence of their son. Lisa and Dave worked on this goal with their parenting coordinator. Concurrently, the therapist helped Joey express his emotional distress related to the parental conflict. Listening and validating his feelings helped Joey express his painful emotions within the safety of the therapeutic milieu. The therapist's use of facilitative responses when Joey reenacted battle scenes in his nondirective play helped Joey express his internal distress.

Conclusion of the Case

Reports from Joey, Lisa, and Dave, coupled with clinical observations, indicated that Joey had achieved the goals set out in the treatment plan. In sessions with Lisa and Dave, they were more respectful toward each other and better able to put Joey's needs ahead of their own anger. Joey's nondirective play also revealed that significant progress had been made; the aggressive battle scenes and themes of loss/abandonment had diminished.

Children of divorce have a history of prior losses and difficult goodbyes. Termination with these children, therefore, is a unique opportunity for the play therapist to provide the client with a new experience of loss—one for which the client is appropriately prepared, and one that is embedded with positive messages. Goals for Joey's ending phase of play therapy included reviewing what he had learned over the course of treatment, processing his feelings about ending therapy, and providing him with a positive goodbye experience. During the activity Sands from Our Time (Behzad, 2011), in which Joey was instructed to pour colored sand into a container and identify progress made in therapy, he stated, "I learned the divorce was not my fault, and I can do Cookie Breathing when I feel upset." The therapist reinforced Joey's progress by offering specific examples of his therapeutic achievements.

A special celebration was conducted during the last session, which included a gift-giving activity, What I Learned Layered Gift (Lowenstein, 2008), as well as a letter from the therapist highlighting Joey's therapeutic gains. This gift and letter were transitional objects for Joey, reminding him of his experience in sessions and a permanent connection to therapy. Moreover, the healing messages in the letter provided a reminder that he is cared for, which strengthened his self-worth.

Postdivorce therapy included periodic check-ins. Things continued to go well, though Joey and his parents needed therapeutic support when Dave became involved in a serious intimate relationship. With guidance, the family was able to appropriately manage this transition.

Conclusion

Although reactions to divorce vary, it is clear that divorce transforms families. Therapy may help families through this process as they establish a new, two-home existence. The focus of treatment should always be the best interest of the child's psychological welfare.

Children and adolescents experiencing divorce are a heterogeneous population. Play therapists may encounter individuals with mild distress all the way to those with severe symptomology. In cases of divorce, a prescriptive approach supports practitioners in creating a tailor-made treatment plan for the diverse needs of this population. The use of play therapy engages children and results in more successful treatment outcomes. Regardless of which type of interventions and approaches are utilized, it is important that play therapy be employed in conjunction with supplementary interventions such as mediation, parenting coordination, or other clinically indicated services.

Gaps in the research and literature regarding the impact of divorce, factors that serve as risk versus protective factors, and rigorous scientific studies for well-established or probably efficacious treatment protocols clearly exist. Closing these gaps will likely serve to improve overall service delivery and may aid the work of play therapists who rely on research to select the best interventions for children, adolescents, and families confronting divorce.

REFERENCES

Amato, P. R. (2001). Children of divorce in the 1990s: An update of the Amato and Keith (1991) meta-analysis. *Journal of Family Psychology, 15*, 355–370.

Amato, P. R. (2010). Research on divorce: Continuing trends and new developments. *Journal of Marriage and Family, 72*, 650–666.

Association of Family and Conciliation Courts. (2010). *Guidelines for court-involved therapy.* Madison, WI: Author.

Barczak, B., Miller, T. W., Veltkamp, L. J., Barczak, S., Hall, C., & Kraus, R. (2010). Transitioning: The impact of divorce on children throughout the life cycle. In T. W. Miller (Ed.), *Handbook of stressful transitions across the lifespan* (pp. 185–215). New York: Springer-Verlag.

Behzad, S. (2011). Sands from our time. In L.

Lowenstein (Ed.), *Assessment and treatment activities for children, adolescents, and families: Volume 3. Practitioners share their most effective techniques* (pp. 185–186). Toronto: Champion Press.

Bernstein, B. E., & Hartsell, T. L. (2004). *The portable lawyer for mental health professionals: An A–Z guide to protecting your clients, your practice, and yourself* (2nd ed.). Hoboken, NJ: Wiley.

Cavett, A. (2010). *Structured play-based interventions for engaging children in therapy.* West Conshohocken, PA: Infinity Publishing.

Children's Institute. (n.d.). Daring dinosaurs board game. Available at *childrensinstitute.net.*

Childswork Childsplay. (n.d.). Upside down divorce game. Available at *www.childswork.com/The-Upside-Down-Divorce-Board-Game.*

Cochrane, B. (2009). *My parents are divorced, my elbows have nicknames, and other facts about me.* New York: HarperCollins.

DeLucia-Waack, J. L. (2011). Children of divorce groups. In G. L. Greif & P. H. Ephross (Eds.), *Group work with populations at risk* (pp. 93–114). New York: Oxford University Press.

Drewes, A. A. (2011). Integrating play therapy theories into practice. In A. A. Drewes, S. C. Bratton, & C. E. Schaefer (Eds.), *Integrative play therapy* (pp. 21–35). New York: Wiley.

Gil, E. (1994). *Play in family therapy.* New York: Guilford Press.

Gil, E., & Shaw, J. A. (2009). Prescriptive play therapy. In K. J. O'Connor & L. D. Braverman (Eds.), *Play therapy theory and practice: Comparing theories and techniques* (2nd ed., pp. 451–487). New York: Wiley.

Gil, E., & Sobol, B. (2000). Engaging families in therapeutic play. In C. E. Bailey (Ed.), *Children in therapy: Using the family as a resource.* New York: Norton.

Goodyear-Brown, P. (2002). *Digging for buried treasure: 52 prop-based play therapy techniques.* Nashville, TN: Sundog, Ltd.

Goodyear-Brown, P. (2005). *Digging for buried treasure: 52 more prop-based play therapy techniques.* Nashville, TN: Sundog, Ltd.

Kalter, N. (1990). *Growing up with divorce.* New York: Macmillan.

Kelly, J., & Johnston, J. (2001) The alienated child: A reformulation of parental alienation syndrome. *Family and Conciliation Courts Review, 39*(3), 249–266.

Kenney-Noziska, S. G. (2008). *Techniques–*

techniques–techniques: *Play-based activities for children, adolescents, and families.* West Conshohocken, PA: Infinity Publishing.

Kenney-Noziska, S. G., Schaefer, C. E., & Homeyer, L. E. (2012). Beyond directive or nondirective: Moving the conversation forward. *International Journal of Play Therapy, 21*(4), 244–252.

Kurdeck, L. A., & Berg, B. (1987). Children's belief about parental divorce scale: Psychometrics, characteristics, and concurrent validity. *Journal of Consulting and Clinical Psychology, 55*, 712–718.

Lowenstein, L. (2006). *Creative interventions for children of divorce.* Toronto: Champion Press.

Lowenstein, L. (Ed.). (2008). *Assessment and treatment activities for children, adolescents, and families: Practitioners share their most effective techniques.* Toronto: Champion Press.

Lowenstein, L. (2013). *Cory helps kids cope with divorce: Playful therapeutic activities for young children.* Toronto: Champion Press.

Majzub, R. M., & Mansor, S. (2012). Perception and adjustment of adolescents towards divorce. *Social and Behavioral Sciences, 46*, 3530–3534.

Malchiodi, C. A. & Ginns-Gruenberg, D. (2008). Trauma, loss, and bibliotherapy: The healing power of stories. In C. A. Malchiodi (Ed.), *Creative interventions with traumatized children* (pp. 167–185). New York: Guilford Press.

Norcross, J. C. (2005). A primer on psychotherapy integration. In. J. C. Norcross & M. R. Goldfried (Eds.), *Handbook of psychotherapy integration* (2nd ed., pp. 10–23). New York: Oxford University Press.

Pedro-Carroll, J. L. (2010). *Putting children first: Proven parenting strategies for helping children thrive through divorce.* New York: Penguin.

Pedro-Carroll, J. L., & Alpert-Gillis, L. J. (1997). Preventive interventions for children of divorce: A developmental model for 5 and 6 year old children. *Journal of Primary Prevention, 18*, 5–23.

Pedro-Carroll, J. L., & Jones, S. H. (2005). A preventive play intervention to foster children's resilience in the aftermath of divorce. In L. A. Reddy, T. M. Files-Hall, & C. E. Schaefer (Eds.), *Empirically based play interventions for children* (pp. 51–75). Washington, DC: American Psychological Association.

Portes, P. R., Smith, T. L., & Brown, J. H. (2000). The Divorce Adjustment Inventory—Revised. *Journal of Divorce and Remarriage, 33*, 93–109.

Post Sprunk, T. (2010). Boat storm lighthouse. In L. Lowenstein (Ed.), *Creative family therapy techniques: Play, art, and expressive therapies to engage children in family sessions* (pp. 12–13). Toronto: Champion Press.

Remley, T. P., & Herlihy, B. (2010). *Ethical, legal, and professional issues in counseling* (3rd ed.). Upper Saddle River, NJ: Merrill.

Rosengren, D. B. (2009). *Building motivational interviewing skills: A practitioner workbook.* New York: Guilford Press.

Rutter, V. E. (2009). Divorce in research vs. divorce in media. *Sociology Compass, 3*(4), 707–720.

Schaefer, C. E. (2001). Prescriptive play therapy. *International Journal of Play Therapy, 10*(2), 57–73.

Schaefer, C. E. (2011). Prescriptive play therapy. In C. E. Schaefer (Ed.), *Foundations of play therapy* (2nd ed., pp. 365–378). Hoboken, NJ: Wiley.

Seymour, J. W. (2011). History of psychotherapy integration & related research. In A. A. Drewes, S. C. Bratton, & C. E. Schaefer (Eds.), *Integrative play therapy* (pp. 3–19). New York: Wiley.

Stolberg, A. L., & Mahler, J. (1994). Enhancing treatment gains in a school-based intervention for children of divorce through skill training, parental involvement, and transfer procedures. *Journal of Consulting and Clinical Psychology, 62*, 147–156.

VanFleet, R. (1994). *Filial therapy: Strengthening parent–child relationships through play.* Sarasota, FL: Professional Resource Press.

Wallerstein, J., & Lewis, J. (2004). The unexpected legacy of divorce. *Psychoanalytic Psychology, 21*, 353–370.

CHAPTER 21

Play Therapy for Children Experiencing Grief and Traumatic Loss

WHAT MATTERS MOST

William Steele

If you don't think what I think, feel what I feel, experience
what I experience and see what I see when I look at myself,
others and the world around me, how can you possibly know
what matters most to me?
   —VOICES OF GRIEVING AND TRAUMATIZED CHILDREN
      (in Steele & Kuban, 2013, p. 3)

The evidence-based sensory intervention model presented in this chapter, SITCAP® (Structured Sensory Interventions for Traumatized Children, Adolescents and Adults), began its development in 1990 at the National Institute for Trauma and Loss in Children (TLC), a nonprofit program of the Starr Global Learning Network. Because trauma generally results in various losses that induce grief in children, it is important that intervention models addressing trauma also address grief. SITCAP uses structured, sensory-based, sequential drawing activities specific to the subjective experience of grief and trauma. Drawings are followed by curious, specifically framed questions to help practitioners enter the world of the iconic, implicit memories and sensations driving grieving and traumatized children's behaviors and symptoms.

We begin by addressing the role of subjectivity in our approach to (1) helping grieving and traumatized children find relief from their experiences, and (2) establishing the rationale for using SITCAP's theme-driven drawing activities to assist children with these experiences whether or not they are the result of grief or trauma. A brief description of SITCAP's evidence-based status and the practice history associated with drawing as a play-based intervention is presented. Case examples are used to illustrate several drawing activities and the way they help children bring us into their subjective worlds to discover what matters most in their efforts to not only survive but also to flourish.

The examples presented also address the following critical considerations and intervention mandates when assisting grieving and traumatized children:

- That we spend time in their world—a world without reason, logic, or language—to describe what they see when they look at themselves, others, and the world around them as a result of their frightening losses and terrifying trauma experiences.

- That if we are to support the primary dictate of trauma-informed care to "do no harm," assigning an appropriate intervention demands that we must first determine how children are experiencing that to which they are exposed.

- That we become curious witnesses to children's subjective experiences in order to present new sensory experiences designed to help them arrive at a cognitive understanding of their lives through a lens of hope, strength, and resilience.

- That we provide grieving and traumatized children with non-word (sensory)-based ways to express and communicate what their worlds are like, and, in so doing, reveal what matters most to each of them.

- That we actively involve children in sensory-based activities related to each of their subjective experiences to help diminish the activation of those experiences as sensory responses to their world, while presenting new experiences that help them arrive at a resilient, strength-based response and view of self, others, and the world.

- That we appreciate that to change unwanted behavior of grieving and traumatized children, we must change the subjective way they experience themselves, others, and the many environments they must navigate daily.

- That our interactions are safe, structured, predictable, and directed by children, but also directed at helping children learn ways to regulate their reactions.

Because today's world is traumatic for so many children, and because traumatized children also experience many losses and subsequent grief, I also examine the core criteria of a trauma-informed approach to treatment regardless of whether children are experiencing grief or trauma and how the processes of SITCAP support these trauma-informed criteria. The chapter ends with a summary of the key concepts of this evidence-based intervention process.

Description of SITCAP: The Subjective World of Grief and Trauma

Over the years I have spent time with children exposed to violent and nonviolent grief- and trauma-inducing situations. What these survivors taught me was that grief and trauma were rarely separate entities, often coexisted, and that symptoms could often be attributed to either grief or trauma. Often I could not immediately differentiate the difference until I had spent time in their world. This being the case, the clinical application dictated that any intervention address both grief and trauma.

Advances in neuroscience clearly support rethinking our understanding of grief and trauma and the interventions we practice. "The five stages of grief, for example, developed by Dr. Kübler-Ross in the late 1960's have been used for years to guide the treatment of grief. Today these stages are axiomatic, no longer reflecting the reality of how grief is experienced and processed" (Steele & Kuban, 2013, p. xvi). What I discovered mattered most to those who were grieving and traumatized were not their symptoms but the ways they were experiencing themselves, others, and the world around them as a result of their experiences. I now refer to this experience as their *subjective world* or their *subjective view*. Clinical application suggests that we, as clinicians, direct our intervention at this subjective world rather than directly at symptoms.

The subjective world of grieving and traumatized children is an implicit world that acts and reacts to the sensations triggered by what is seen, heard, and sensed to be a potential threat (Rothschild, 2000).

Children of grief and trauma are poised to act, not because of what they think, but because of what they sense (Ziegler, 2002). It is a world where hand gestures, facial expressions, tone of voice, physical features, body posturing, and environmental factors become far more important to survival than the cognitive processing of information (Steele, 2003a). It is a world where children struggle to regulate their reactions to what is being sensed as a threat to their safety and well-being. It is a world of "physiological phenomenon rather than a purely psychological one" (Levine & Klein, 2012, p. 5) wherein the body is highly charged (aroused), creating the potential for repeated symptoms. Clinical application therefore dictates that we direct our interventions at restoring these children's sense of safety and empowerment to deactivate their aroused survival responses.

Experience Drives Behavior

We discovered early in our field of psychology that it is this subjective view of self, others, and the world that shapes our private logic (Adler, 1930) and drives our behaviors. For example, if you tell me that you love me and then you betray me, that experience causes me to think differently about you, to distrust you, and to engage behaviors that help me avoid being hurt again. When our losses are significant or our experiences traumatic, we immediately resort to survival behaviors. We see these survival behaviors of fight, flight, and freeze following unresolved or unattended grief and trauma. The subjective world of grief and trauma is one that teaches us that, if we want children's behaviors to change, we must change the way they experience themselves, others, and the world around them, as "learning and changing anything requires building new neural networks by being actively involved in what is being learned" (Fischer, 2012).

To accomplish this fundamental change, the intervention process—in this case theme-driven drawing activities and curiosity-based questions related to the specific theme being addressed—must relate to this subjective world in ways that facilitate the externalization of these memories, sensations, and experiences into a concrete form. This form must be one to which children can relate, explain, reorder as needed, learn from and manage, and ultimately become an agent of change rooted in strength-based and resilience-focused views of themselves, others, and their worlds. The structured drawing processes and activities of SITCAP facilitate this process.

Talk Is Limited in This World

Most importantly, children have taught us what neuroscience confirms: that this cannot be accomplished by word-based efforts alone. Gil (2006) notes that "traumatic events are experienced and stored in the right hemisphere of the brain" (the non-thinking brain) and that "this suggests that allowing children a period of time to access and stimulate the right hemisphere of the brain could eventually activate the necessary functions of the left hemisphere (the thinking brain), which appears to shut down during traumatic experiences" (p. 102). I have found this to be the case with many grieving children as well. Cognitive reframing is certainly important to healing and restoring the natural balance between explicitly left and implicitly right hemispheres, the *thinking* and *feeling* brain (Cohen, Mannarino, & Delinger, 2006). However, until we spend time in the child's subjective world, we cannot possibly know what might be a meaningful reframing, one that fits the context in which the child is experiencing him- or herself and the environment; one that empowers the child to think and behave differently, one the child can accept and internalize as a source of strength and resilience.

Ogden, Minton, and Pain (2006) wrote, "In a psychotherapeutic setting focusing primarily on word-based thinking and narratives can keep therapy at a surface level and trauma may be unresolved" (p. xiv). In the world of grief and trauma our cognitive/explicit processes are no longer in balance with our implicit, nonreasoning survival brain (Fosha, 2000). We respond to what we sense we need to do, not what is reasonable or logical. Therefore it is necessary to apply a clinical intervention that meets grieving and traumatized children where they are living—in their subjective world—a world that does not always respond to reason, logic, and other upper-brain cognitive processes (Schore, 2001; van der Kolk, McFarlane, & Weisaeth, 1996), a world where children struggle and are often unable to identify and verbalize their experiences (Fosha, 2000). Theme-driven drawing activities can allow these children to both identify and express those experiences.

One example of why entering the subjective world of children matters is when we focus on the worries that grieving and traumatized children can experience. "Who will take care of me? What other bad thing is going to happen?" could be the worries of either grieving or traumatized children. We know that both groups of children have similar worries, yet what may be a clinically significant worry for one group is not necessarily significant for the other. We can't really know the intensity of children's worries and what the scope of our intervention needs to be until they literally show us or tell us what will be most meaningful to them, based on how they are experiencing what is happening to them or around them. For example, ask two children exposed to the same incident what worries them the most. One might worry about what other bad things are going to happen, whereas the other worries about their field trip being canceled. Both are exposed to the same situation yet experience it quite differently at a subjective level, thereby re-

vealing to us what will matter most for each one.

To apply appropriate interventions for grieving and traumatized children, we must first determine how children are experiencing their world. Supporting the primary dictate of providing trauma-informed care that avoids retraumatizing (Hodas, 2006) or placing children at risk requires that we also avoid treatment assumptions based on behaviors and symptoms rather than on the ways these children are subjectively experiencing their worlds. The following example supports how SITCAP and its drawing components support the clinically appropriate application of interventions.

Eight-year-old Eric had a thin frame. He was physically assaulted over a 2-year period while in a foster care home. A comprehensive evaluation revealed a number of sensory integration challenges among other trauma-related symptoms. Use of a weighted blanket was recommended as one of the interventions. The weighted blanket technique is designed to help calm an aroused nervous system and reduce anxiety. It is an intervention that has helped many children (Mullen, Champagne, Krishnamurty, Dickson, & Gao, 2008). However, not every intervention fits every child and although helpful to some, that same intervention may be harmful to others. Knowing the subjective ways in which children experience their trauma can help prevent retraumatization.

Eric was repeatedly assaulted by a 160-pound boy who was 6 years older than he. When asked to draw a picture of what that was like, he drew a small circle representing his head and then darkened his entire body to represent the boy who beat him frequently (Figure 21.1). When asked what the worst part of that experience was like, he replied, "He sat on me when he beat me and sometimes laid on me so I could hardly breathe." Using a weighted blanket could potentially place Eric at risk for activation and further trauma. Knowing the subjective ways in which children experience grief and trauma is essential to applying appropriate interventions.

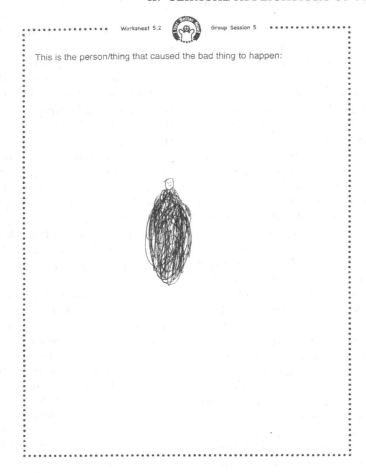

FIGURE 21.1. Eric's drawing. Copyright 1998 by TLC. Reprinted by permission.

A Trauma-Informed, Evidence-Based Drawing Process

The core principle of the SITCAP model is that by providing children with the opportunity to safely revisit and rework the primary subjective experiences of trauma, within the sensory, not cognitive context in which they are experienced, stored, and remembered, PTSD symptoms and grief- and trauma-related mental health reactions can be significantly reduced, the gains sustained, and resilience developed and/or strengthened in ways that support growth.
—STEELE AND KUBAN (2013, p. 7)

SITCAP's drawing process helps children externalize their implicit sensations, iconic memories, and subjective experiences into a concrete form so "they can be encoded and expressed through language" (Steele, 2003b, p. 142). The content of drawings is not interpreted or analyzed. SITCAP's drawing process is structured so that drawing tasks are specific to each subjective experience being addressed. These structured, theme-driven drawing activities allow clinicians to see what children see as they look at themselves, others, and the world around them and what matters most in their world as a result of their exposure to grief- and/or trauma-inducing incidents. Furthermore, this process allows children to externalize their many subjective experiences into a concrete, manageable form and, in doing so, find relief from them, as documented by evidence-based research and practice-based history.

Research- and Evidence-Based Practice History for SITCAP Strategies and Program

Research Base for the Use of Drawings

The primary strategy in the SITCAP process is the use of theme-based drawing activities related to the common subjective experiences of grief and trauma. Drawing activities have been used in play therapy for many years for evaluation purposes, to provide children a medium in which to express what they may not have words to express and to regulate their reactions (Crenshaw & Mordock, 2005; Green, 2009). Byers (1996) noted that numerous studies illustrated the use of drawings in helping children access, reveal, and heal from their traumatic memories. Magwaza, Killian, Peterson, and Pillay (1993) achieved similar results with South African children exposed to community violence. Saigh and Bremner (1999) suggested that "children draw sketches of their stressful experience and verbally repeat the content of their experiences" (p. 370). In response to 9/11, the World Trade Center Children's Mural Project was unveiled on March 19, 2002, and depicted over 3,100 portraits that "served to lessen feelings of isolation and helplessness felt among those children who had difficulty understanding cognitively the complexity of this tragedy" (Berberian, Bryant, & Landsburg, 2003, p. 110).

In the early 1990s Pynoos and Eth (1986) used drawing to interview children and to "identify traumatic imagery, to introduce discussion of the child's individual traumatic experience and to assess the embedded perceptual aspects of the trauma" (p. 379). Gross and Haynes's (1998) research found that children asked to draw included more feelings and sensations and were more descriptive of what had happened than children who were only asked to talk about what had happened.

Evidence-Based Practice History for SITCAP

SITCAP's intervention programs and structured drawing processes for children and youth ages 6–18 are evidence-based programs listed on the California Evidence-Based Clearinghouse for Child Welfare and the Substance Abuse Mental Health Services Administration's (SAMSHA) National Registry of Evidence-Based Programs and Practices. Research outcomes validating SITCAP's value are published in numerous journals and books (Steele & Kuban, 2013; Steele, Kuban, & Raider, 2009; Steele, Raider, Delillo-Storey, Jacobs, & Kuban, 2008). However, many argue that evidence-based research does not necessarily speak to the practical value of an intervention and its usability in different settings with different populations exposed to different situations. SITCAP is not only evidence based but has a 23-year practice history that answers the challenges presented by those who question evidence-based processes and outcomes. Dietrich (2008) suggests that an intervention that has a history of producing repeated and documented desired outcomes, which SITCAP has demonstrated, is evidence of the value of that practice. Following are several additional criteria that also support SITCAP's practice-based value (Steele & Kuban, 2013).

- The intervention has demonstrated, in varied settings such as schools and clinical settings, consistent documented outcomes over time (minimum of 10 years) with varied treatment populations, such as children victimized by violent incidents as well as those exposed to nonviolent, grief-inducing incidents.
- The intervention is practical, meaning

it can be used by most practitioners as a group or individual process, is fairly easy to learn, and is manualized to allow for greater practice fidelity so it can be accurately evaluated and used appropriately.

- The intervention has undergone at least one controlled empirical research study, using an evidence-based research model, and has documented significant reduction of symptoms.
- The intervention is based on well-researched, articulated findings involving neuroscience, resilience, and strength-based research.

A Trauma-Informed Approach for Grieving and Traumatized Children

The National Center for Trauma-Informed Care (2011) has increased the awareness of the prevalence of childhood trauma, its long-term impact when not treated, the compelling need for child care systems to be trauma-informed, and for practices with traumatized children to be guided by the following core criteria of a trauma-informed approach. We add that these criteria be applied to grieving children as well. An entire chapter could be devoted to the ways these criteria are integrated into SITCAP. Here I briefly address the following five criteria and their integration into the SITCAP model (Steele & Malchiodi, 2012).

1. Restore a sense of safety, empowerment, and self-regulation (Bath, 2008; Levine & Klein, 2007).
2. Integrate implicit (right-brain) and explicit (left-brain) processes (Gil, 2006; Langmuir, Kirsh, & Classen, 2012).
3. Apply neurodevelopmentally appropriate interventions (Perry, 2009).
4. Include interventions that respect and support cultural diversity (Boden, Horwood, & Fergusson, 2007).
5. Promote trauma-informed relationships (Bloom & Farragher, 2010).

Safety and Empowerment

Practitioners trained to use SITCAP are reminded that there is no one intervention that fits every situation or every child. Furthermore, in trauma treatment there is no such thing as resistance; either children feel safe or they do not. Our responsibility is to avoid creating further grief or trauma and to help children develop within a safe relationship and intervention process. SITCAP intervention sessions begin and end in a safe place and engage in titrating, regulating, and cushioning the focus on subjective experiences between these safe places. Children are taught that they can say *yes* or *no* to anything we ask them to do or talk about. All drawing activities are completed within an 8″ × 11″ bordered worksheet to further contain the externalization of their sensory experiences and affect. These processes empower them to safely guide clinicians' efforts at their pace and in areas where they feel safest.

Self-Regulation

The above structured processes encourage self-regulation by following a predictable course, empowering the child to stop or continue activities, and by containing the sensory processes in a manageable format. Because our bodies (Rothschild, 2000) and our nervous systems (Levine & Klein, 2007) are activated by intense grief and trauma experiences and reactivated by reminders of those experiences, it is important to teach children how to regulate their reactions. Bessel van der Kolk (2006) concurs with Rothschild's observations: "For therapy to be effective it might be useful to focus on the patient's physical self-experience and increase their self-awareness, rather than focusing exclusively on the meaning that people make of their experience" (p. 13).

SITCAP addresses the body's memories and reactions. For example, children are asked to identify where in their bodies they feel (or felt) the hurt or the fear the most.

They are asked to draw what that hurt or fear might look like. Our curious, theme-specific questions related to that hurt or fear assist them in defining what that experience is like, what it makes them do or not do, what it would say to them if it could talk, what they would say to it if it could listen, and so on. This process is self-regulating in itself. Children also learn in this process how to shift from that hurtful place to their happy, safe place. This shifting, in addition to regulating the focus on their reactions between the safe beginning and ending of every session, reinforces children's self-regulation skills.

Developing a Trauma-Informed Relationship

Regulated processes also support the development of a trauma-informed relationship. Practitioners of SITCAP are taught to be curious, not analytical, because curiosity is the cornerstone of empathy (Smith, 2012) and attunement (Perry, 2009). Fostering a safe and curious relationship helps children feel less alone in their world, whereas a relationship based on analytical interpretations and directions does not. In addition, when our curiosity is directed at *how the child is experiencing* what happened, rather than toward the *factual events* in his or her life, and "when it is conveyed with both affective and reflective features, the child is likely to go with the therapist very deeply into his or her life story and experiences co-regulation of emotions related to what is being explored and the meaning given for those events" (Hughes, 2009, p. 169). This therapeutic stance also supports a relationship that is reciprocal; our curiosity evokes curiosity in children.

Developmentally Appropriate and Culturally Sensitive

SITCAP activities and programs are developmentally appropriate for children/ adolescents between the ages of 6 and 18 years. The focus on subjective experiences remains the same, but the worksheets and activities differ to accommodate different developmental levels. The focus on the subjective experiences of children also allows the intervention to help many diverse populations. Grieving and traumatized children throughout the world experience fear. Fear is fear in any language or culture. SITCAP's structured drawing activities allow children across cultures to use their own cultural symbols and language to safely portray and express the many different ways they are experiencing that fear regardless of language, culture, or customs.

The SITCAP Process: Strategies and Techniques

SITCAP's drawing process helps children externalize their implicit sensations, iconic memories, and subjective experiences into a concrete form so "they can be encoded and expressed through language" (Steele, 2003b, p. 142). The drawing process is structured so tasks are specific to each subjective experience being addressed. In 1990, the National Institute for Trauma and Loss in Children (TLC) listed the following subjective experiences presented by the grieving and traumatized children: fear, terror, worry, hurt, anger, revenge, guilt and shame, feeling unsafe and powerless, and engaging in victim thinking versus survivor/thriver thinking and behaviors (Steele & Raider, 2009). These subjective experiences remain the focus of our structured, developmentally appropriate, evidence-based intervention today.

Drawing allows us to see what children see as they look at themselves, others, and the world around them and what matters most in their world. Gil (2010) wrote, "It [drawing] is congruent with trauma focused play in which children are encouraged to use play in order to externalize their areas of distress; to learn to tolerate and release affect; and to compensate for injuries and create feelings of mastery" (p. 57). It doesn't matter what they draw or how they draw. We do not evaluate or analyze these drawings, only use them as a vehicle for helping children externalize those experiences into a concrete form, making it easier for them to detail what their experiences are like, the meaning they give to them, and what matters most to their healing within the norms and customs of their culture.

Theme-Specific Curious Questions

Initially, being curious is not an easy process for many professionals. In SITCAP training we conduct an activity in which we present participants with a theme-specific question and then ask them to take time in their groups to identify as many questions as possible that could be asked about that theme-specific question. For example, we present the question, "What was the worst part?" Almost immediately we hear participants asking, "The worst part of *what*?" Our response is, "You do not need to know the *what* to help children communicate how they experienced the worst part of what happened." Practitioners tend to be far more focused on the details of what happened than how that child actually experienced what happened. When focusing on details, many faulty assumptions are likely to be made as to what will matter most to that child. TLC's theme-specific questions are open-ended and specific to each subjective experience. Olafson and Kenniston (2008) explain that in creating optimal information-gathering conditions for forensic interviewing, "open-ended questions are the most productive; even reluctant or non-disclosing children respond most fully to open questions" (p. 77).

Following are several of the curious questions we can ask to help children bring us into their world at the time they experienced the worst part of what happened. The questions vary depending on different developmental levels. When working with adolescents, we might ask, "On a scale of 1 to 10, with 10 being as bad as it gets, where would you place your worst part?" When working with younger children, we often use a worksheet with four different-size animals and ask them to color the animal that best shows how small or big the worst part is for them. Additional questions might include:

"Where do you feel the worst part the most in your body?"
"What does the worst part make you do?"
"Is there anyone or anything that brings the worst part back?"
"Is there anyone or anything that makes the worst part go away?"

There is a multitude of additional questions that can help children express how they experienced each of their subjective experiences. However, children will only do so if we remain curious and our curiosity is in direct response to the responses that they provide us. Questions are not fired rapidly, but are related to the context of the responses children provide us. For example, if we hear that there is someone or something that brings the worst part back, remaining curious dictates that we ask such questions as, "What can you tell me about that person that makes the worst part come back?" In children's subjective worlds there are often numerous story lines, characters, and events that make up that one experience. Being curious allows the child to take us deeper and deeper into that experience, often helping us to also arrive at a more meaningful appreciation of what is driving his or her behavior as well as what is going to matter most in our efforts to help.

The reality is that both grieving and traumatized children can experience similar reactions that induce tremendous anxiety, such as nightmares. The difference is how they experience them. For example, the nightmares of grieving children are typically about something happening to someone else or about the person who is no longer with them. In trauma-driven nightmares children are in their own dreams in potential harm's way. "My sister is falling through a dimension and she is being chased and shot at" is a dream that certainly can startle a child awake, yet the child is the observer of what is happening. Although the dream is frightening, as an observer, the child is in a safe place. A trauma-driven dream would be more like this: "I am falling through a dimension and being chased and shot at." This child's experience is far more intense and terrifying because he or she is not safe and feeling powerless. As you read the following case examples, keep in mind that what matters most is providing children with an opportunity to bring us into their world so they are no longer alone in their experience. An equally important part is providing a medium for them—in this case, theme-driven drawing activities—that allows us to see what they see when they look at themselves, others, and the world around them, and the meaning they apply to their view of self and the grieving and traumatized experiences they have endured or continue to experience.

Clinical Case Examples

Communicating the Subjective Experience Bullying

Most agree that bullying can induce tremendous grief and trauma in its victims. Fifteen-year-old Robert was experiencing depression with suicidal ideations. He viewed himself as powerless and useless as he experienced continual bullying by his peers. When asked to draw a picture of what this was like, he provided me with a much greater appreciation for how he is experiencing the bullying, the reason why he has been unable to stop returning to those who were victimizing him, and what mattered most in his efforts to disconnect from those bullying him.

Robert changes the word at the top of the worksheet from *happened* to *happens* to let us know this is still happening. He then divides his drawing (Figure 21.2) into "two worlds." Robert is surrounded by his peers as depicted on the right side of the paper. He writes in some of the mean things they say to him. He says he can leave but always comes back to them. In his "other world" on the left side of the page he draws himself as faintly and as small as possible while others are at the top of the paper. I drew a circle around his self-portrait to indicate that this was Robert. Being curious, I asked him to tell me about the differences between his two drawings. Pointing to his "other world," he says, "Others are there, but it's like they don't ever see me, like I'm invisible." At that point I understand what draws him back to the peers who treat him so badly. When asked what he thinks draws him back to those who are bullying him, he replies, "At least they have fun with me and sometimes let me stay awhile."

This activity allowed Robert to give me a view of his subjective world that he had not previously described or discussed in any detail. Talk always centered on his references to being a loser with his peers and provided little insight as to the fact that being with bullies was less painful than not being with them. His drawing vividly explains what mattered most to him in his efforts to move away from that group of peers: the need to be acknowledged, to belong, and at a deeper level, the need for experiences that changed his view of self and others. Selecting an appropriate focus of intervention that would make sense in his world was made much easier as a result of this one drawing activity.

Releasing the Hurt

Twelve-year-old Emily had been sexually abused by her uncle and cousin while living in their home. The abuse had started at age 5 and continued until she was removed from the home at age 11. Her initial foster

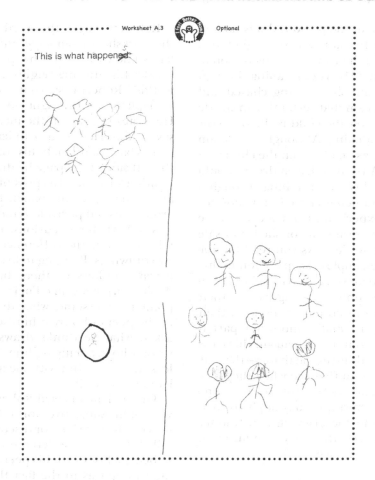

FIGURE 21.2. Robert's drawing. Copyright 1998 by TLC. Reprinted by permission.

placement did not work out. She had been in her current foster home for 6 months when she began SITCAP. Her foster mother described her as "frozen in time." She indicated that Emily rarely talked, made no friends, and was struggling with school. She referred to Emily as a "lethargic, scared little girl." She also indicated she could not remember seeing Emily running around, playing like others her age, and that she had no "animation to her."

SITCAP's fourth session addresses physical and emotional hurt. Emily was asked where she felt that hurt the most in her body when things reminded her of what hap-

pened. She was then asked, using the outline of a body on the worksheet (Figure 21.3), to show us that hurt and what it would look like. She indicated that her stomach felt hollow but also filled with "wavy-like butterflies that wouldn't stop flying." In the facial area she drew clouds and indicated that nothing was right, that she couldn't think, and that her head was "being squeezed tight." She drew arms hanging down because her "arms always hang down." She darkened her feet and indicated they would get stuck and sometimes she could not feel them.

Her entire body had not yet discharged the impact of years of abuse, and her draw-

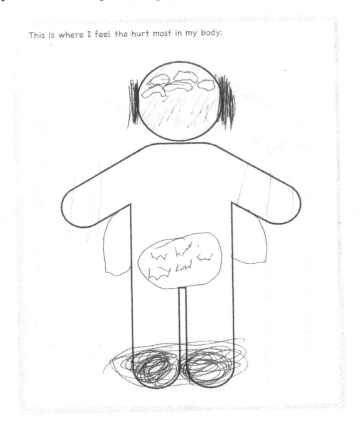

This is where I feel the hurt most in my body:

FIGURE 21.3. Emily's drawing of where she felt hurt. Copyright 1998 by TLC. Reprinted by permission.

ing supported the foster mother's description of Emily as frozen and lethargic. That frozen response had become her protective survival mechanism in a world that was still filled with terror, a world where reason and logic did not matter. Her foster mother was patient, supportive, and nurturing, yet Emily's body was still living as if the present were no different than the past. In the weeks that followed, Emily was introduced to a number of physical activities to help her discover that she could *unfreeze* her body, that her body had lots of energy and strength, and how using her body differently now was changing (regulating) the survival responses to current reminders of that terrifying time in the past.

Then–Now: My Future

Emily made wonderful progress following repeated body resourcing and other drawing activities focusing on her survivor self. One SITCAP activity, titled *My Book Cover* (Figure 21.4), asks children to give their book a title that would let others know how far they have come and where they see themselves in the future. Children are free to then draw on the cover they wish. Emily titled her book *Not Over* and amazingly identified several chapters of her book that covered her abuse and the gains made in SITCAP. The last chapter was titled *Amazing*. Her theme was, "What happened, happened. My life is not over, it is just beginning and I will be amazing."

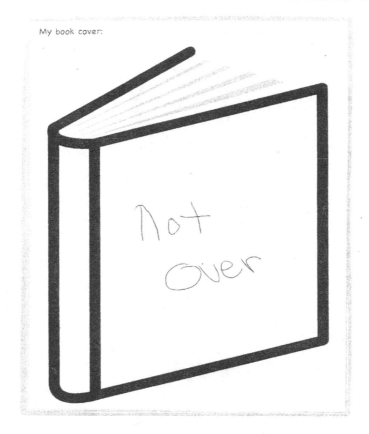

FIGURE 21.4. Emily's book cover. Copyright 1998 by TLC. Reprinted by permission.

Meaningful Reframing

When using drawing with children to help them externalize their subjective experiences into symbolic forms, they often arrive at their own meaningful reframing of their view of self. Alexa, a 12-year-old female, was adopted from an orphanage overseas at the age of 4. Over the years a great deal of conflict had developed between her and her adoptive mother to the point that Alexa would become irrational and physically attack her mother. Alexa was taken from her home shortly after turning 12 as a result of her assaults but also her mother's neglect.

When asked to draw a picture of an angry person, she drew a large angry face. After expressing curiosity about what she could tell us about her drawing, she was then given another worksheet to draw a picture of the person who had caused these bad things to happen to her. She drew a picture of her mother (Figure 21.5). Afterward, when comparing the two drawings, Alexa replied, "I look like her [her mother] when I'm mad—I don't want to be like her."

This one activity became a major transition point in Alexa's life. She compared her drawing of her mother to the previous drawing of an angry person, which she then referenced as herself. The reframing that followed the comparison was immediate. Reaffirming that she was not like her mother and that she had choices she could make to help her manage her anger, now became a positive, strength-based, meaningful reason to change. A number of activities we presented were chosen by her and

This is the person/thing that caused the bad thing to happen:

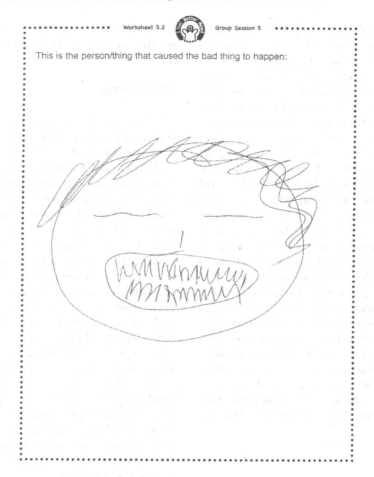

FIGURE 21.5. Alexa's drawing of her mother. Copyright 1998 by TLC. Reprinted by permission.

repeatedly practiced, resulting in a remarkable improvement in the regulation of her anger.

Allowing the Child to Show Us What Matters Most

Children really are the best experts as to what will matter most in their efforts to heal from, and become resilient as a result of, their experiences. When Amber was 8 years old, her mother died of cancer. Amber's behaviors 1 year later could be attributed to grief or trauma depending on the various ways her behaviors were described by her father, her teachers, and the two professionals her father sought help from over the past year. She was presenting significant challenges at home and at school. We know that behaviors can be misleading. We also know that when behaviors are being fueled by an unfulfilled need associated with the subjective ways children experience grief or trauma, attempting to control that behavior can further activate children and lead to additional challenges. Whether Amber's behaviors were grief or trauma driven, what mattered most was empowering her with the opportunity to find a way to meet her needs associated with the subjective ways she was dealing with this significant loss.

To accomplish this empowerment process, Amber was given the opportunity to address all the subjective experiences associated with grief and trauma through drawing. At one point she was asked to draw a picture of the person or thing that caused her mother to die. She drew lines representing the bad "canser sells." She was then asked to draw what she would like to see happen to those bad cells. She drew each cell over again (Figure 21.6) and then turned each of them into bombs and went through the process of lighting and exploding each one until they were dead too. From this point on Amber was a different child. She finished the remaining sessions of SITCAP and, in the months that followed, flourished at home and at school.

By having been given the opportunity to address, through theme-specific drawings, the common subjective experiences of grief or trauma—fears, worries, hurt, regrets, guilt, shame, sadness, feeling unsafe, and, in this example, her anger and sense of powerlessness—she was able to demonstrate through this one drawing activity that she knew, in her subjective world, what she needed in order to feel better.

Conclusion

SITCAP meets the practice criteria as a trauma-informed intervention. It is an evidence-based intervention supported by a 23-year practice-based history and has demonstrated and documented its value with children and adolescents exposed to single and multiple violent and nonviolent grief- and trauma-inducing incidents. Although it is a structured process designed to keep the intervention as safe as possible for children, it also allows children to direct the intervention in areas of their lives and experiences they want their therapist to experience with them, through his or her curiosity, theme-specific questions, and use of specific drawing activities associated with their subjective experiences. It is a process that is directed at restoring a balance among implicit and explicit, sensory and cognitive processes to help children regulate adverse reactions to the posttraumatic sensations, iconic images, and memories from their experiences as well as the ongoing stress in their lives.

SITCAP's use of drawing allows children to show us what they see when they look at themselves and the world around them as a result of their experiences, but also what matters most in helping them to reshape a strength-based, resilient view of self and the world. SITCAP's structured drawing activities related to the subjective experiences of trauma, its curious theme-specific questions, and its trauma-informed practices provide play therapists with yet another approach to meeting the unique challenges that grieving and traumatized children present. A comprehensive detailed description of the SITCAP processes can be found in *Working with Grieving and Traumatized Children and Adolescents: Discovering What Matters Most Through Evidence-Based, Sensory Intervention* (Steele & Kuban, 2013).

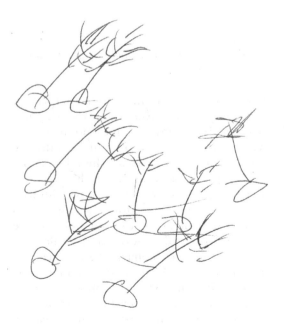

FIGURE 21.6. Amber's drawing of cancer cells.

REFERENCES

Adler, A. (1930). *The problem child.* New York: Putnam.

Bath, H. (2008). The three pillars of trauma-informed care. *Reclaiming Children and Youth, 17*(3), 5.

Berberian, M., Bryant L., & Landsburg, M. (2003). *Interventions with communities affected by mass violence.* New York: Pearson.

Bloom, S. L., & Farragher, B. (2010). *Destroying sanctuary: The crisis in human service delivery systems.* New York: Oxford University Press.

Boden, J. M., Horwood, L. J., & Fergusson, D. M. (2007). Exposure to childhood sexual and physical abuse and subsequent educational achievement outcomes. *Child Abuse and Neglect, 31*(10), 1101–1114.

Byers, J. (1996). Children of the stones: Art therapy interventions in the West Bank. *Art Therapy: Journal of the American Art Therapy Association, 13,* 238–243.

Cohen, J. A., Mannarino, A. P., Deblinger, E. (2006). *Treating trauma and traumatic grief in children and adolescents.* New York: Guilford Press.

Crenshaw, D., & Mordock, J. (2005). *A handbook of play therapy with aggressive children.* Lanham, MD: Rowan & Littlefield.

Dietrich, R. (2008). Evidence-based education: Can we get there from here? *Association for Behavioral Analysis International, 31*(3). Retrieved December 12, 2012, from *www.abainternational.org/ABA/newsletter/vol313/Detrich.asp.*

Fischer, K. (2012). Neuroscience in the classroom: Making Connections, Section 2. Retrieved June 5, 2012, from *www.Learner.org/neuroscience/text.html?dis=u&num=05&Sec=02.*

Fosha, D. (2000). *The transforming power of affect: A model of accelerated change.* New York: Basic Books.

Gil, E. (2006). *Helping abused and traumatized children: Integrating directive and nondirective approaches.* New York: Guilford Press.

Gil, E. (Ed.). (2010). *Working with children to heal interpersonal trauma: The power of play.* New York: Guilford Press.

Green, E. (2009). Jungian analytical play therapy. In J. O'Connor & L. D. Braverman (Eds.), *Theory and practice: Comparing theories and techniques* (2nd ed., pp. 83–122). Hoboken, NJ: Wiley.

Gross, J., & Haynes, H. (1998). Drawing facilitates children's verbal reports of emotionally laden events. *Journal of Experimental Psychology, 4,* 163–179.

Hodas, G. (2006). Responding to childhood trauma. Retrieved January 15, 2012, from *www.nasmhpd.org/general_files/publications/ntac_ pubs/Responding to Childhood Trauma-Hodas.pdf.*

Hughes, R. (2009). Attachment focused treatment for children. In M. Kerman (Ed.), *Clinical pearls of wisdom* (pp. 169–181). New York: Norton.

Langmuir, J., Kirsch, S., & Classen, C. (2012). A pilot study of body-oriented group psychotherapy: Adapting sensorimotor psychotherapy for the group treatment of trauma. *Psychological Trauma: Theory, Research, Practice, and Policy, 4*(2), 214–220.

Levine, P. A., & Klein, M. (2007). *Trauma through a child's eyes: Awakening the ordinary miracle of healing.* Berkeley, CA: North Atlantic Books.

Levine, P. A., & Klein, M. (2012). Establishing safety through self-regulation. In W. Steele & C. Malchiodi (Ed.), *Trauma informed practices with children and adolescents* (pp. 75–97). New York: Routledge/Taylor & Francis.

Magwaza, A., Killian, B., Peterson, I., & Pillay, Y. (1993). The effects of chronic stress on preschool children living in South African townships. *Child Abuse and Neglect, 17,* 795–803.

Mullen, B., Champagne, T., Krishnamurty, S. L., Dickson, D., & Gao, R. (2008). Exploring the safety and therapeutic effects of deep pressure stimulation using a weighted blanket. *Occupational Therapy in Mental Health, 24,* 1.

National Center for Trauma-Informed Care. (2011). What's trauma-informed care? Retrieved June 30, 2011, from *www.samhsa.gov/nctic/trauma.asp.*

Ogden, P., Minton, K., & Pain, C. (2006). *Trauma and the body: A sensorimotor approach to psychotherapy.* New York: Norton.

Olafson, E., & Kenniston, J. (2008). Obtaining information from children in the justice system. *Juvenile and Family Court Journal, 59*(4), 71–89.

Perry, B. (2009). Examining child maltreatment through a neurodevelopmental lens: Clinical applications of the neurosequential model of therapeutics. *Journal of Loss and Trauma, 14*(4), 16.

Pynoos, R., & Eth, S. (1986). Witness to violence: The child interview. *Journal of the American Academy of Child Psychiatry, 25,* 306–319.

Rothschild, B. (2000). *The body remembers: The psychophysiology of trauma and trauma treatment.* New York: Norton.

Saigh, P., & Bremner, J. (1999). *Posttraumatic stress disorder.* Boston: Allyn & Bacon.

Schore, A. (2001). The effects of a secure attachment relationship on right-brain development, affect regulation, and infant mental health. *Infant Mental Health Journal, 22*(1–2), 7–66.

Smith, J. (2012). *Integrative psychotherapy.* Retrieved March 6, 2012, from *www.psytx.com/03sessions.html.*

Steele, W. (2003a). Helping traumatized children. In S. L. A. Strausner & N. K. Philips (Eds.), *Understanding mass violence: A social work perspective* (pp. 41–56). New York: Allyn & Bacon.

Steele, W. (2003b). Using drawing in short-term trauma resolution. In C. A. Malchiodi (Ed.), *Handbook of art therapy* (pp. 139–151). New York: Guilford Press.

Steele, W., & Kuban, C. (2013). *Working with grieving and traumatized children and adolescents: Discovering what matters most through evidence-based, sensory interventions.* Hoboken, NJ: Wiley.

Steele, W., Kuban, C., & Raider, L. M. (2009). Connections, continuity, dignity, opportunities model: Follow-up of children who completed the I Feel Better Now! Trauma Intervention Program. *School Social Work Journal, 33*(2), 98–111.

Steele W., & Malchiodi, C. A. (2012). *Trauma-informed practices for children and adolescents.* New York: Routledge/Taylor & Francis Group.

Steele, W., & Raider, M. (2009). *Structured sensory interventions for children, adolescents and parents (SITCAP)* (rev. ed.). New York: Edwin Mellen Press.

Steele, W., Raider, M., Delillo-Storey, M., Jacobs, J., & Kuban, C. (2008). Structured sensory therapy (SITCAP-ART) for traumatized adjudicated adolescents in residential treatment. *Residential Treatment for Children and Youth, 25*(2), 167–185.

van der Kolk, B. A. (2006). Clinical implications of neuroscience research in PTSD. *Annals: New York Academy of Sciences, 1,* 1–17.

van der Kolk, B. A., McFarlane, A. C., & Weisaeth, L. (Eds.). (1996). *Traumatic stress: The effects of overwhelming experience on mind, body, and society.* New York: Guilford Press.

Ziegler, D. (2002). *Traumatic experience and the brain: A handbook for understanding and treating those traumatized as children.* Phoenix, AZ: Acacia.

CHAPTER 22

Jungian Analytical Play Therapy with a Sexually Abused Child

J. P. Lilly

It is my hope to provide some fluidity to the process by which a therapist employing Jungian analytical play therapy (JAPT) approaches a case. As the "lead mechanic" for JAPT, I consider this chapter as the "operator's manual" for this approach. To that end, I utilize a structured form I created—the "Analytical Play Therapy Session Review Form" (Figure 22.1)—to clinically track a session from a JAPT perspective. I have found this form to be useful in explaining the things that the JAPT therapist looks for during a session. My hope is that it serves to synthesize the theory and the practical application of this approach.

Clinical Approach

In starting a new case, I meet with the parents and generate a three-generational genogram. Jung carved the way for a deeper look at family systems and the influence that parents have on their children. As early as

Definitions for several Jungian terms used in this chapter can be found in Chapter 4.

1939, Jung wrote, "If there is anything that we wish to change in the child, we should first examine it and see whether it is not something that could better be changed in ourselves" (1971, p. 285), and two decades later, "The most powerful effects upon children do not come from the conscious state of the parents, but from their unconscious background" (1954, para. 84). Jung carved the way for a deeper look at family systems and the influence that parents have on their children. It is a necessary chore of the JAPT therapist to poke around and see what unfinished business there is in the multigenerational system from which the child has come.

Later, in family systems theory, terms such as *legacy* and *revolving slates* were used to explain the dynamic of how these unresolved issues are passed down (Boszormenyi-Nagy & Ulrich, 1981). Children are greatly affected and influenced by the *unconscious* of those who have gone before them. Many times it is the child who will pick up the unresolved issues of the parents or grandparents and act them out. Sometimes these unresolved issues are "secrets" kept within the family consciousness, but unconsciously

Date _____ Session Number _____ Child's Name _____

Stages

Acclimation time _____

Exploration time _____

Working time _____

Resolution time _____

Play Types   **Dynamics**
  Isolative   Compensatory
  Parallel   Confirmational
  Associative   Neutral/disengaged
  Cooperative
  Collaborative
  Competitive
  Combative

Physical Aspects
  Eye contact
  Body posture
  Physical distance
  Spatial relationship in play
  Verbalizations
  Places used in the room
  Symbolic value of toys engaged

Archetypes Awakened/Major Themes: **Soft Hypotheses**
Engagement/Deintegration/Reintegration

Interactive Strategies Used by the Therapist
  Affect identification
  Cognitive identification
  Behavioral tracking
  Transcendent function
  Containment/limit setting
  Testing soft hypotheses
  Nondirective strategies
  Unconscious connectedness
  Therapist awareness

Sequencing and Tracking

Activity   Time   Stage/Theme   Soft Hypothesis

FIGURE 22.1. Analytical Play Therapy Session Review Form.

they are passed onto the children. Only by conducting a thorough history of the family system can the JAPT therapist achieve some sense of understanding of what might be happening with the outwardly manifested symptoms of a child in relationship to the system dynamics.

Let's now work our way through the analytical form how the JAPT therapist perceives and organizes material that occurs in a typical play therapy session.

The review form begins with the date of the session, the number of the session, and the name of the child. I view the date as important for my own growth and understanding as I continue to evolve as a clinician and as a person, so this gives me some reference to where I was emotionally and psychologically. Given a point of reference to the date can help me assess where my own growth and development as a clinician was at that time, as well as point out to me any issues with which I was dealing. The session number is important so that I can reference it in relation to the stages the child experienced during the session. If the child is in his or her eighth or ninth session and is still acclimating to the room and to the therapeutic relationship, then I need to investigate further to see if there is something I am doing to impede the process of therapy for that child or if the home environment is contributing to the child's lack of progress. The child's name is attached here for obvious reasons.

Stages

The next piece of information that is useful to me as a JAPT therapist is to note the stages of play therapy experienced by the child during our session. The stages are not linear to the JAPT therapist, but can be accessed at any time by the child during the play therapy session. I also mark on the "time" space how many times the child entered that particular stage. The key dynamic behind the child shifting from one stage to the other is that of ego deintegra-

tion and ego integration. It is typical for children to enter the working stage to confront difficult material and experience ego deintegration. Given that this encounter requires a markedly strenuous effort, it is also typical for children to then regress to a less taxing stage to reintegrate. In one case with which I was working, the child had a difficult confrontation with some powerful material, causing her to deintegrate substantially. Instinctively, she regressed to another task over which she was a master: reciting her ABCs. This return to an undertaking she had mastered reintegrated her enough to venture two more confrontations with the overwhelming material. The key dynamic that establishes on which stage the child lands is determined by ego deintegration and ego reintegration.

For the sake of simplicity, I have chosen to identify only four stages in the play therapy process. The stages can be viewed on a continuum of engagement. In the *acclimation stage* of play the child works to gain a sense of safety, of *temenos*, in the room and with the therapist. The child is not actively engaged with any symbolic material; first she is focused on creating a safe environment in which she can engage the material for which she is attending therapy. Typical behaviors in this stage include avoiding eye contact with the therapist, stressed verbalizations, shaky voice, asking lots of questions about the room and the therapist, keeping physical distance from the therapist, turning one's back to the therapist, limited physical movement, and avoidance of engaging with the toys.

Typical play types include isolative and parallel play. In *isolative play* the child separates himself from the therapist physically and engages in play alone, clearly not allowing the therapist to either see or be part of his play. *Parallel play* refers to the child and the therapist doing the same activity, but separately. The child might say, "These are my blocks—you go over there and play with the sand, and I'll stay here." The therapist's strategy here is the creation of a safe place for the child, a *temenos*. The therapist needs to avoid too many verbalizations that can prove to be ego deintegrating for the child and are an impediment to the development of the child's safety. The therapist also must avoid any attempts to "speed" along the process of therapy.

The central dynamic of the next stage is the *exploratory stage*. The central dynamic in this stage is that the child is beginning to allow herself to be "drawn" to certain toys (symbols) in the play therapy room. Typical behaviors in this stage of play therapy demonstrated by the child include touching and picking up toys without developing any play theme with them; beginning to relax, as she shifts her focus from solely monitoring her safety in relationship to the therapist and the room; checking out the function of the toys, how they work, what the toys are called (may ask questions about specific toys); and behaving in ways that foreshadow work that is to come. Play types here include isolative, parallel, and associative. *Associative play* refers to the parallel play with the same objects. The child gives the therapist some blocks to play with, but the child continues to play by herself, separately from the therapist.

As the child moves through the exploration play stage, and begins to move toward the working stage, there is a demonstrative change in the child's work. Where his or her work had centered on being safe in the play therapy room and creating *temenos*, at the end of the exploration stage different play behaviors begin to emerge. Some of these typical behaviors from children at the later stages of the exploration stage can include more frequent eye contact with the therapist (culture-dependent), more open and engaging body posture with the therapist, less physical distance between the child and the therapist; the spatial relationship during the child's play is lessened and is more open to viewing by the therapist; verbalizations by the child are more related to play materials and the play therapist; and

play themes begin to emerge as the toys are given a specific theme and purpose.

The dynamics in the working stage begin to emerge in the late stages of the exploration stage. Compensatory dynamics (acting out the opposite of his complex—the weak becomes strong) and confirmational dynamics (acting out his experience in a similar manner to the complex) are witnessed by the therapist. While the therapist is keenly aware that these dynamics of play are emerging, there is not a defined strategy to the child's implementation of this kind of play. The play themes are sporadic, disjointed, and do not create a cohesive linear track that can be followed easily. These types of play often seem unorganized and fragmented, but careful analysis of the play reveals bits and pieces of the work that is yet to come. The therapist's strategies include tracking behavior first, identifying cognitions second, attending to affect last, introduction of soft hypotheses, and keen physical and psychological attention to the process. Caution should be taken against making premature interpretations, as doing so could severely damage the *temenos* of the therapeutic container. The therapist must always stay within the metaphorical content that the child is presenting and remain aware of his emotional reactions to any of the toys the child engages.

The next stage is the *working stage*. Typical behaviors include all of those listed in Figure 22.1 plus the addition of cooperative play, collaborative play, competitive play, and combative play. All of these play types can include the therapist or the child may act out the theme with toys in the room. *Cooperative play* begins to use the therapist to complete a joint task. The child might say, "Okay, you do this, then I'll do that." This form of play requires both parties to agree to act a certain way with one another. The implications for trust here are obvious. *Competitive play* is just that: There is a competition between the therapist and the child, or the child has two objects competing against one another (e.g., two boats racing in the water). In *combative play*, as in competitive play, either the therapist is the child's opponent, or the child acts out this play type with two toys. There is an intensity to the engagement of play here. Strong affect, both positive and negative, accompanies the play. Physical movement around the room is unbridled. Transference is powerful and can be placed on anything in the room. New archetypal material is generated and created within the play—something is found, overcome, changed, etc. Ego deintegration is a certainty as the child struggles through this heroic battle. The therapist is vigilant in attending to the full spectrum of the child's experience: behaviors, cognitions, and emotions. The therapist tests soft hypotheses for clarity and to track any emergence of the transcendent function. The primary roles of the therapist are engaged: interpreter, witness, and container.

The final stage of play therapy in this model is *resolution*. The child has completed the heroic journey, engaged complex material, created new scripts and schemas, and established a meaningful integration of the opposites that represented imbalance in the psyche. As in Joseph Campbell's (1949) *Hero with a Thousand Faces*, a critical step in the journey of the hero is to return to "celebrate" his or her victory. Resolution resonates with victory. There is no need for further engagement, so the probability of deintegration is nearly eliminated. All play types may occur, but there is a marked absence of intense emotion, and the play feels more like normal childlike play. There are no compensatory or confirmational dynamics. The child's movement is unbridled, but not driven by any internal force. The therapist makes no attempt to "recap" the child's progress or therapeutic journey because to do so would be disrespectful to the path of healing. I personally *love* this stage, as it is the only time that I get to truly play with the child in the joy he or she has recovered.

Play Types and Dynamics

Listed to the side of the play types are the *dynamics* associated with the play. The dynamic associated with the play type is most important to determining *engagement*. The compensatory or confirmational nature of the child's play is determined by the toys with which the child plays, the play theme, and their relationship to the complex with which the child presented for treatment. These dynamics are easily identified in children whose complexes have been determined. It can be a little bit complicated to determine which dynamic is actually being forwarded by the child, but with the judicious use of soft hypotheses, these dynamics can be understood more deeply and fully.

For example, let's take a female child who presents with a "victim" complex following an overwhelming experience of abuse. *Temenos* has been established, and the child has acclimated to the room. The child is ready to work by engaging with her unconscious material. She grabs the play hammer from the shelf. The hammer can represent many different things depending on the use of it. The child takes the hammer and begins bashing one of the predator animals on the shelf. The soft hypothesis could be formulated that the child is engaging in a compensatory play theme to compensate her feeling of victimization, and by acting out this play theme, moves closer toward a meaningful integration of her own power. A soft hypothesis regarding this dynamic might sound like this: "You took that hammer and smashed that mean thing right there. You looked pretty powerful doing that." My position would be to track the behavior, but also to address the compensatory part of the child's complex by amplifying and personalizing it, making it specific to her.

Conversely, if the child did the same play theme with the same toys, she could be projecting her own experience specifically on to the animal she destroyed. This dynamic of the play behavior would "confirm" her experience and would require a different response. My response would be along the lines of, "Boy, that thing sure took a beating. I bet it feels pretty sad right now." Any emotional response from the child is noted and is directed to the child through the metaphorical content presented. The JAPT therapist is vigilant in witnessing the emotions demonstrated by the child, and the level of ego deintegration in the child directs the therapist's feedback to ensure that *temenos* is maintained.

In each case noted above, the child always has the ability to refute the hypothesis, ignore the therapist's hypothesis altogether, or correct the therapist. My goal as a JAPT therapist is to hold at least three soft hypotheses about a child's play behavior at a time—so that means that I'm either right only one time out of three, or wrong three out of three. It is our belief that this kind of analytical attitude fosters the unconscious connection between child and therapist and facilitates the emergence of the Healer. My personal belief is that my unconscious resonance with the child's inner Healer is critical in the child's therapeutic process and, that by holding deep hypotheses regarding the child's play, the Healer "recognizes" the healing power of the play therapy room, the archetypal material, and the intent of the therapist to understand things on the deepest of levels.

Play that is compensatory or confirmational in nature is naturally "engaged" play. Because these dynamics of play deal specifically with complex, and therefore intense, emotions, it is relatively easy to see when a child has engaged on this level. The first two play types, isolative and parallel, are often disengaged with complex material and don't carry the intensity of emotion. This is the "neutral or disengaged" play dynamic, and simply indicates that the child is engaged in work that is not specific to a complex.

Physical Aspects

The next section of the review sheet deals with the physical aspects of the child in the play therapy room. I have embedded these physical aspects of the child's play in the Stages section of this chapter. These aspects are important to note, and there is even theory that children tend to perform certain parts of their work in specific areas of the play therapy room. The JAPT therapist feels the freedom to move around the room so long as *temenos* is maintained for the child. I generally ask permission to move closer to the child, or, if the child is in a very deep level of play, I will simply announce my movement so as not to break the continuity of his or her work.

Archetypes Awakened/Major Themes

The next section of the review form considers the content of the material used by the child and the themes presented. The JAPT therapist is familiar with the different symbolic representations of the toys in his or her play therapy room. It is absolutely essential to understand the symbolic meaning of our toys, as well as to incorporate a cultural sensitivity to expand the possible meaning of the toys. For example, whereas an owl might be seen as a symbol of wisdom to the Western world, for some of the American Indian children I treat, it is a symbol of death. It is incumbent on the JAPT therapist to know these important differences and to be prepared to understand these toys in different cultural contexts.

Not only do many of the toys have multiple meanings unconsciously and culturally, the JAPT therapist is sensitive to the fact that the child may have a different interpretation of the symbol as well. Children also have a personal unconscious they bring into therapy sessions, and it is important for the JAPT therapist to understand that a child's meaning of the toy may run in a very different direction than that listed in a symbol dictionary. We are also sensitive to the cultural aspects of the animals we place in our play therapy rooms. I remember working with one child of African American descent who had been adopted by a European American family. I was conducting filial play therapy with the young boy and his adoptive mother. He compiled a family constellation on the floor, using different animals to represent different individuals in his adoptive family. He chose a zebra to represent himself. I wouldn't have been smart enough to pick that animal for him, but he was brilliant to select the appropriate one for himself.

To make sense of the work of the child, the JAPT therapist now takes into consideration (1) the age of the child and responds on his or her cognitive level, (2) which session the child is attending, (3) what stages he or she is working in, and (4) the play types represented, with each of their associated dynamics. The JAPT therapist does this by witnessing how the archetypal material is manifested through the themes of the child's play. With each passing play theme, the JAPT therapist is creating and holding *soft hypotheses* in order to deepen his or her understanding of the child's psyche, and to create an environment in which the inner Healer can emerge. It is an awful lot to keep track of; my favorite way to synthesize a session is to refresh my memory of the different play activities when I clean up the room after the child has left.

Interactive Strategies

The next section of the form deals with the interactive strategies used by the therapist. In this self-evaluation, the JAPT therapist assesses and evaluates his or her levels of interaction with the child during the session. Behavioral tracking, cognitive identification, and affect identification have already been addressed in this text, so it is not repeated here. The issue of "transcendent function" has also been addressed, as well as the role of the JAPT therapist in assisting the child in bringing unconscious material into consciousness. The JAPT therapist maintains a series of soft hypotheses about a child's play theme and uses careful, nonintrusive statements to reflect the dynamics of the child's play in relation to the conscious ego strength of the child. The JAPT therapist serves as a bridge between the child's unconscious material and his or her defended or chaotic conscious ego. The process by which the JAPT therapist bridges this gap is the "art" of therapy and the seat of true transformation.

The next item listed under the interactive strategies is that of containment and limit setting. The JAPT therapist uses this strategy to preserve and maintain *temenos* in the play therapy room. The play themes of a child with very weak ego defenses can be chaotic and feel crazy, like nonsensical random play. There is no direct connection between the child's play and complex material, and the energy driving the play is pure, unbridled unconscious material. During these times, to restore and preserve *temenos*, it is necessary for the JAPT therapist to "create" order. Limit setting requires stating and enforcing rules for safety. For example, the therapist might simply state to the child, "I understand why you might feel that you need to do "X behavior," and that is not for doing in the play therapy room. If you choose to continue to do "X behavior," then you will choose to not play with that for the remainder of our time together today. It will be here next time for you to play with." This will sound very familiar to child-centered play therapists, as wonderfully explained in Landreth's (2002) book. The only difference is that the JAPT therapist implies in the first part of the statement that he or she understands why the child needs to engage in the play theme. This message is a direct statement to the child's unconscious and this verbal and conscious communication is vital to creating and maintaining an active relationship with that part of the child's psyche.

Testing soft hypotheses is worth reviewing from a JAPT therapist perspective. We need to examine the content of our feedback for the following: (1) appropriateness in relation to the cognitive development of the child; (2) that the hypothesis holds a connection between the child's conscious ego and the child's unconscious, and that it is specifically related to complex material; and (3) that the verbalized hypothesis does not intrude with the flow of the child's play and cause ego deintegration. Ego deintegration is controlled by the child, not by the therapist. If the therapist's soft hypothesis causes ego deintegration for the child, then the therapist needs to first examine if it was something in him or her that created that deintegration, or if it was simply the nature of the material being engaged. This point speaks to the last item listed in this part of the form—that of therapist awareness. The JAPT therapist has to be vigilant in maintaining awareness of his or her own psychological and emotional state. As noted by Peery (2003), the therapist must maintain "her ego awareness to notice what is going on in the play, and what is going on between her and the patient" (p. 42). It is important for the JAPT therapist to keep one foot securely on the shore as he or she and the child begin wandering into the unconscious regions of the child's psyche.

Nondirective strategies and *unconscious connectedness* refer to the silent space between the child and the therapist. Nondirective strategies encompass accompanying the child into the *nigredo* (dark places of ego consciousness) of their work. The JAPT therapist respects the darkness of the work that needs to be done. Honoring the child's work requires the JAPT therapist to support the child's work while ensuring that the child is not in danger of hurting him- or herself or the therapist. *Unconscious connectedness* refers to the therapist's ability to enter the child's play from both a conscious

and unconscious level. Consciously, the JAPT therapist stays connected to what he or she does, thinks, and feels in the process of the child's play. While maintaining this awareness, the JAPT therapist is also keenly aware that there are powerful dynamics that cannot be seen stirring in the child. There have been times when I, while working with abused children, have felt scared even when there was nothing happening in the play on a conscious level that would solicit this emotion. Strange as it may sound, JAPT therapists are aware of these feelings and note them as empirical manifestations of the unconscious energy emerging from the child's psyche.

Sequencing and Tracking

The final page on the review form is a tracking sheet that can be used to create a fluid, linear review of the play therapy session. The sequencing is important so that the levels of deintegration and reintegration can be effectively followed. The *activity* refers to the items with which the child played. The *time category* is to track how much time the child spent on each activity. The *stage* refers to the stage the child was experiencing when engaged in the play activity, and the theme that was present. Noting the theme is important to delineate how the play activity engages with the child's unconscious material. Making sense of the child's play and connecting the play items and play themes to complex material is one of the primary tasks of the JAPT therapist. Writing down and noting the soft hypothesis regarding the play activity, as it is connected to the child's complex energy, is another of the primary tasks of the JAPT therapist.

This "operator's manual" is intended to assist the play therapist not familiar with JAPT theory and provide some structure by which one might view a play therapy session from this perspective. This review form is far from comprehensive, but hopefully it provides some structure to the often esoteric and nebulous nature of JAPT.

Clinical Case Example

Abbey is a 2½-year-old European American female, the second of three children. Her mother and father represented her at the initial assessment, when they told me that she had made statements to them that seemed to allude to a sexual abuse incident. Her parents had been married for 11 years at the time of the initial assessment. Abbey's father worked at the local steel production factory and her mother was a registered nurse. The marriage between Abbey's parents was very stable and healthy. Abbey's elder sibling was a 5-year-old sister, and her younger brother was 8 months old at this time. There was no history of mental illness in either her mother or father's side of the family.

Abbey had been a full-term baby, and there were no immediate complications with her birth. When she was 1 year old, she'd had a bladder infection and reflux. Her symptoms were severe enough that she needed surgery, which occurred 7 months before she started showing symptoms of trauma. She began waking up at night moaning and crying. Her mother thought that her symptoms were the result of her surgery. Abbey was also experiencing severe nightmares, but those remitted a month after they had started. A month later, Abbey began creating spontaneous drawings of ghosts on which she would make puncture marks to show her mother where the "*owies*" were. She stated to her mother that a "bad guy" did it. She further indicated to her mother that the bad guy killed her, and that he killed her bottom. The next day Abbey identified the bad guy by name: her uncle, her mother's brother-in-law. Abbey picked him out of a number of pictures as the man who "gave me my *owie* on my bottom." Her nightmares returned after her initial disclosure. She further disclosed that the "bad guy" put his fingers on her eyes. Following this disclosure, her symptoms included (1) clinging to her mother, (2) mild separation anxiety, (3) free-floating fear, (4) marked anxiety, (5) avoidance of people, (6) mild aggressive behavior toward family members, (7) age-regressed behavior (especially verbalizations), (8) spitting on people, and (9) a fearful, reactive behavior toward the nurse examining her at the local child advocacy center ("Please don't hurt me!").

Based on the information I had received from the mother, Abbey's behavior began to make a lot of sense to me. The nightmares served as a signal of repressed material. She was experiencing behavioral deterioration with her avoidance of people, her aggression toward family members, spitting on people, and regressed behavior. These behaviors were attempts to disengage with the intrusive nature of the memories and the feelings that accompanied those memories. Her aggression could be viewed as compensatory behavior in which she was attempting to reempower herself from a victim complex. Spitting on people was her way of demeaning them, to show that she was superior to them—again, another response to the victim complex. Her clinging to her mother and separation anxiety were clearly symptoms consistent with an event that had overwhelmed her, from which she had generalized (cognition) that she was not safe in the world unless she was next to her mother. Her age regression was an attempt to return to a time before the intrusive event, when she was safe. Her fears and anxiety were consistent with the nature of the event that was perpetrated against her, and constituted an emotional decompensation. All of her symptoms were attempts to disengage from the reality of her experience, assuage the powerful feelings that came with the budding complex and intrusive memories, and to restore a temporary state of equilibrium. None of her symptoms led her toward engagement, and therefore true healing was not possible at that point.

I treated Abbey for 34 sessions. We began therapy the next week, and she spent little time acclimating to me and the room. She displayed a natural gift for symbolic play. Her first demonstrative working theme in play therapy occurred in the third session. For 20 minutes she sat on the table and cut pieces of paper, which she handed to me. The mood in the room at the time of her cutting the paper was somber and tense. As she continued to hand me pieces of paper, I hypothesized that she was showing me what happened to her as a result of her abuse. She felt cut up, broken into pieces, and as I received each piece of paper, I told her that I understood what she was doing and that I would take great care of the pieces of paper she was handing to me. She remained silent during this part of the therapy session.

As she was cutting the paper and handing me pieces of her broken self, she suddenly looked up and identified a plastic black bear on one of my shelves. This bear is rather menacing looking, with red eyes and a lowered head with its teeth exposed. She gasped and indicated to me that it was scary to her. She jumped down from the table and started to walk over to the bear, but stopped and gasped again. She then confronted the object onto which she projected her predator, stating, "I'm going to get your sword and kill him." She retrieved the bear from the shelf and placed it near me. She then retrieved the sword and handed it to me and instructed me to "kill him." I took the sword and began striking the bear repeatedly until she told me to stop. She then walked over to the bear and kicked it across the room, then jumped up and down on it, indicating that the bear was dead. This engagement was powerful for Abbey, and served to strengthen her ego for the work that was yet to come. In my countertransference I wanted this experience to indicate the end of her treatment, but her psyche had other work to do. I needed to contain my enthusiasm for the "end" of the bear's terror.

The next session Abbey enacted more of the same behavior as in the previous session, but her intensity toward the black bear was less powerful. She ended her session by cutting paper again. I gave her the 5-min-

ute warning indicating that our session was nearly over and I noticed that she had a tear in her eye. I noted this to her and she asked me, "I do?" I told her that I saw her tear and I was wondering if she was crying. She then disclosed to me that her uncle Rob "hurt my bottom." It was the confirmation that her parents needed to move forward to clearly identify who had abused their precious child. After I had the opportunity to tell the parents about the disclosure in the session, they informed the authorities and Abbey's abuser was taken into custody.

Two sessions later, Abbey introduced another play theme that was about protection. She retrieved a box of plastic blocks that can come apart on one side and join with other blocks. She had discovered how they worked when exploring earlier. She then began bringing over small, docile, and harmless animal figures to the table and she got back onto the table and began placing these animals into the blocks. She indicated to me that the animals were safe in there and that the mean bear could not hurt them in there. I hypothesized that Abbey still did not feel safe and that she needed to fortify her environment for herself and others. I responded to her with "Those animals sure must feel safe now that the black bear can't get to them." She instructed me verbally by stating that there were still more animals on the shelf that wouldn't fit into the blocks. I responded that she "wanted to make sure that all of the animals were safe," to which she replied "yes."

Her play continued to evolve over time, moving from one theme to another—each one connected to the complex created from her abuse. It became apparent that Abbey would need to "circumambulate" her complex in order to find the right way or order to resolve her complex. Jung defined this term to mean a circular movement that marked a sacred precinct around a central point. Jung (1968, para. 186, 188) came to see circumambulation as the containment of the ego in the broader and deeper dimension of the self. The Self archetype finds new and meaningful ways of engaging complexes stored in the unconscious. This dynamic is common for many of the children with whom we work, as they rarely land on the one and only true way to resolve complex material the first time they engage in a play theme. Often as therapists we witness a child engage in a play theme that seems like it should resolve the complex material, only to find that the child's symptoms have not subsided but may even have worsened. This process of healing is made possible as the Self becomes the dominant psychological force directing the child's play. Using the wheel motif introduced by Jung, it is possible to think of a child in the play therapy room as the hub of the wheel, and the outer circle of the wheel representing the ability of the Self to contain the ego in a healing capacity. The spokes would represent the different means by which the Self introduces healing themes to the ego. Simply because true healing and transformation do not occur immediately after a healing theme is introduced does not mean that the Self has directed the ego incorrectly. When different themes appear, it is safe to conclude that each theme represents different aspects of healing for the ego. It is the JAPT therapist's job to understand the different healing aspects of the different themes for the child's ego. No attempt is made to redirect the child's behavior to another theme. Our mission here is one of understanding the healing aspects of each theme on the child's ego.

Abbey presented several sessions later with a theme of marked regression. She physically played on the floor for most of the session. This physical change to her play level indicated to me that there was a clear age and time regression taking place. I hypothesized that she wanted to return to another time in her life before her abuse—a time when she was safe from harm. That session ended with a theme of being rescued. I was directed to rescue her from "bad guys." It was the first introduction of a rescue theme, and she directed it toward

herself. The combination of being in a regressed state and being rescued indicated clearly to me that she wanted to be rescued before the abuse occurred; she wanted to spare herself from the imminent abuse. I responded to her play with the following soft hypothesis: "Sometimes it feels good to go back to when we felt good. I understand why you want to go back there." She made eye contact with me and did not say anything. She then asked me to hold her for the remaining minutes we had left in the play therapy room. I obliged; then she asked me to sing to her, as if she were going to sleep. I once again obliged. When our time was up, she bounced to her feet and ran smiling to the door, opened it and ran down the hallway back to her mother in the lobby.

Several sessions later she began some serious and powerful water play. She sank different objects in the water, brought them back to the surface, allowed the water to drip off of them, and then allowed each object to float a while before repeating this play theme. Given that water is a powerful symbol for the unconscious, I hypothesized that she was bringing up material from the unconscious and making it conscious. My comments to her were about her play at this time, without interpretation, as that would have been too much for her to handle emotionally and psychologically. She then took a large ball and placed it in the water. The ball was too big to immerse in the water, but it was evident that she was going to continue her play theme of pushing things into the water and having them emerge. She pushed the ball down into the water and a good deal of water spilled onto the floor. This indicated to me that the unconscious material she needed to bring forward was going to get "messy." I told her that I understood why she needed to push the large ball into the water and why the water had made a mess. I also reflected to her that, "Sometimes when big things go into the water, they make a mess." She laughed a nervous laugh and conveyed some mild fear that she might be in trouble for making a mess. I assured her that it was nothing that couldn't be cleaned up and that she was in *no* way in trouble. She felt relieved and with that message delivered to her unconscious—that there was no mess that couldn't be handled in the play therapy room—we made room for more unconscious material to come forward. Full conscious and unconscious trust was now established in Abbey, and she spent the next four to five sessions making messes that were all contained with great ease.

The next move forward in her healing occurred when she introduced two new symbols of archetypal predation: an alligator and a snake. (The alligator, because it is both a water and land animal, represents predation on both a conscious and unconscious level. It also carries the bulk of unconscious energy. The snake has an obvious phallic quality to predation.) At this time in her therapy her ego had inflated sufficiently to directly confront the presence of these two powerful symbols of predation, and the sexual predation from the snake. She demonstrated fear of the animals at first, gasping and stepping back from them. She then found her courage and anger, saying, "I am going to get them and kill them." She then attacked them and threw them on the floor in front of me. I witnessed her courage and power and amplified the fact that she had killed the predators by verbalizing, "You are so brave and so powerful to kill those very dangerous animals." She then picked them up and handed them to me and, in my countertransference rage that was resonating with Abbey's, I threw them across the room and they banged off the door. I must admit that most of that energy came from me, and that it felt *wonderful*! We laughed together and celebrated their deaths.

It occurred to me at this point that the bear figure she previously had me kill, and that represented her uncle Rob, was someone she did not want to hurt or kill. It was the *evil and darkness of abuse*, represented by the snake and alligator, which needed to be killed. This distinction created a dilemma

in her work: How could she resolve the abuse perpetrated against her by her uncle without also hurting *him*? I have to admit to not being smart enough to imagine how to resolve this dilemma for Abbey. Luckily, Abbey's Self was directing the play therapy process.

Several sessions continued with themes of bad guys coming into the room. Little by little, the intensity of Abbey's emotions diminished. She began "playing" with different objects of predation and disempowering them so that they couldn't hurt her anymore. She placed them in spots from which they could not escape, from which they could not find their way back, and from where they could not do any harm. She exercised power over them and thereby depotentiated *their* evil powers. Then, halfway through a session, Abbey introduced a teddy bear into her play. She held it, nurtured it, loved it, and had me hold it for some time, infusing a strong nurturing theme into the field. In the same session, she took the black bear that had borne the burden of her abuse, brought him to me and told me, "This guy is nice." This behavior foreshadowed a powerful direction in which she would head to complete her healing. I responded to her on all three levels by stating, "He used to be bad, but now he is nice, and that feels good." She hugged the black bear and had me do the same.

At this time Abbey's symptoms began to diminish drastically. Her nightmares had disappeared, she had not engaged in age-regressed behavior for several weeks, she was experiencing hardly any anxiety, she was separating from her mother without any incident, and she was not clingy with her. She had, however, developed some anger toward her mother, expressed via noncompliant and limit-testing behavior. Abbey's mother understood that she had failed to protect her daughter, but there was more depth to Abbey's behavior than that, so I told her parents that it was probably a good idea to keep Abbey in treatment for a few more weeks. Also at this time, her uncle had confessed to abusing Abbey and was placed in jail, without Abbey having to be interviewed or testify in court.

In the next session Abbey's play presented a failed rescue theme again. She had selected two giraffes of different sizes (to represent herself and her mother). She got out the bucket of water that I have in the room for children to wash their hands, if needed. She selected another animal (a horse) and dropped it into the bucket. She told the mother giraffe to go get the horse out of the water. The big giraffe repeatedly tried, unsuccessfully, to extract the horse from the water. This enactment represented the failure of her mother to both protect her *and* rescue her. I understood the first part of this play sequence as a natural part of her abuse—that her mother had failed to protect her—but I did not fully understand the latter part about the failure to rescue her until later. Given the nature of Abbey's emotion, which expressed repeated disappointment in the mother's failure to rescue the little giraffe and the horse, I verbalized, "It sure feels sad when that one can't rescue that one in the water." She clarified the emotion for me and indicated that it made her "mad!" I told her that I understood.

The next few sessions were filled with a mixture of themes: nurturing, bad guys being contained, ensuring the safety of small animals within the play therapy room, and playing cooperatively. It is common for children to repeat and review their work, and this was the impression I got from Abbey's play behavior at this time. A small shift also occurred in that her play was becoming less symbolic and more "real," meaning that she was beginning to play more with the dollhouse, with people figures from the house, and with real-life toys. At the end of one of these sessions, she played out a healing theme with me as she took on the role of the doctor. She had me lie on the floor as she "healed" me from myriad illnesses that I was instructed to have. This "healer" role could not have been more powerful for her, and it was after this session that her

symptoms disappeared completely. Even her anger toward her mother disappeared, and she acted like her old self prior to the abuse.

Her parents wanted to stop her therapy sessions at this point, but they also had gained a lot of trust in me, so when I told them that I believed there was something left that she had not fully resolved, they agreed to leave her in therapy for another few sessions, and we would monitor her symptoms carefully over that time. The next session I had with Abbey proved to be one that definitely crystallized her healing.

This session held a compilation of all of the themes she had previously presented. Abbey began by playing in the dollhouse. She selected mother and father figures, who were in bed, and she indicated that she, Abbey, was also going to go to bed shortly. She then introduced another child figure that was sleeping, but the figure representing her (Abbey) was not sleeping because she had "something wrong with her eyes." The Abbey-figure falls down, but she tells me that she is okay, and then she goes to sleep. This process represented Abbey's struggle with unconscious material. She knew that she had to confront something dangerous, but she was afraid to do so. The Abbey-figure then wakes up and states "I forgot to brush my teeth." Now the door to consciousness is opened to her. She remains on the couch watching a movie. The father figure is now awakened, and he falls down. The Abbey-figure exclaims "Ouchy" in response to the father-figure's fall. She tells me that the dad is feeling sick, so she puts him to bed. She drags the bed out from the house and places it in a very prominent position in front of the house. She "fixes" Dad and then puts him to bed. The mother-figure is sick as well, and she stays in bed. My dominant soft hypothesis about this sequence is that Abbey understands the systemic wounding of the family due to her abuse.

Next Abbey retrieves a large, sturdy rhinoceros from the shelf of animals. She lets me know, however, that this is a horse. (The horse is a female symbol, representing the great mother that carries humans in the womb and later is the support of their inner lives.) She then takes the doctor kit, but soon shifts from this theme to engage with the black bear. This time she experiences ego deintegration, engaging the bear directly. She leaves it on the shelf but tells me that the black bear is there and that the animals are afraid. She begins to hide the small animals in the doctor bag—which represents healing, not hiding. This symbolic change from protection to healing is significant and powerful. She shifts back to the healing place she wants to create. She retrieves the plastic blocks and, in the middle of the floor where we are playing, she creates a "quarternity"—a block in the middle, with one block extending from each side of the middle block. This is a powerful symbol of wholeness. (Jung [1958, p. 167] wrote about this fourfold aspect of wholeness as forming the logical basis for any judgment, including the four functions of sensation, thinking, feeling, and intuition.)

Next the Abbey-figure has the "horse" carry the mother to the top of the quarternity, where she is given a shot to heal her. The mother is taken back to bed, and the father is now brought to the healing place by the "horse." Abbey then hands the healer role to me, to heal her father. I begin to replicate what she just did, but she tells me that I am not doing it right, and she grabs the shot away from me and heals her father. The "horse" then transports the father back to bed. The child-figure who was watching TV (Abbey) now comes down from her upstairs room and tells her mother, "Mommy, I feel sick." The mother replies, "Go back to bed and leave us alone." Abbey acts out profound sadness. This was the other part of her anger with her mother. The Abbey-figure is now transported to the hospital by the "horse," where Abbey gives her a shot in the heart to heal her. She dismisses the "horse," as the need to engage with this theme has run its course. She begins exploring and looking through the toys again.

Abbey finds a necklace that she wants to wear. (This is a symbol of office, station, and dignity, and a binding to that office.) She takes it to the water and washes it to purify it. She puts it on again and examines it closely, then takes the healed little girl back to her bed. Abbey returns to me at this point and places the necklace around my neck. She recognizes me as a healer as well.

Abbey washes the necklace again, retrieves a boat, and places the necklace in the water. (The boat represents adventure, fecundity, and fertility; it also rests on the axis between consciousness and unconsciousness.) She places the necklace in the boat and sets it adrift in the water. Now she takes the necklace from the boat and floats it on the water. Here she experiences what I see as a symbolic transformation from Abbey, the abused little girl, to Abbey, the Holy Priestess. She walks over and grabs the black bear off of the shelf, showing no signs of deintegration, and brings it over to the water, where she washes it clean. In a very real ceremonial manner, she baptizes the bear, dries it off, and presents it to me, telling me that it has changed, and that it is now "nice and clean." She further tells me, "He likes you," and "He wants us both." She then places the Abbey-figure, which was lying on the quarternity, in her own bed in the dollhouse and places the bear on the sacred place of healing. She gives the bear a series of shots. This play theme is accompanied by a reverent silence as a very deep and powerful process unfolds.

Breaking from this play theme altogether, Abbey now grabs a flashlight from the shelf. (It is one of those flashlights that has three different lenses so that it can shine three different colors.) She is putting a new light on things; she is seeing things more clearly. The radiance symbolizes new life from the divinity of her inner healer. (Light was the first element created; it has the power of dispelling the forces of darkness, of evil.)

Abbey plays with the light for a period of time and then tells me that it is making her dizzy. She falls into my lap for nurturing and celebration. She ends the session with 5 minutes remaining, telling me that she is "done." Abbey knew the moment that she had arrived at her truest and most meaningful integration and transformation.

Conclusion

As demonstrated by this case, it is the brilliance of every child's unconscious that makes sense of both conscious and unconscious material. Abbey had to endow and inflate herself to the level of the Holy Priestess to heal her abuser. It was not in her nature to kill and destroy. She needed to transform her abuser to achieve psychological balance and peace. Abbey, and only Abbey, knew the way out of the dilemma of both hating and loving her uncle. Only Abbey's unconscious knew where her true transformation and healing could take place. Her healing came from her unconscious, and there was no other force that could have restored her to a place of balance and peace in her life.

It is by understanding and respecting the internal world of children that the JAPT therapist is able to facilitate true healing and transformation. It is understanding the world of symbol and how archetypal material is manifested through the use of symbol in play that allows the JAPT therapist to fully join children in their healing process. It is the willingness of the JAPT therapist to courageously confront his or her own unresolved, unconscious issues that allows him or her to willingly move into highly charged unconscious material, emotionally and psychologically, and act as the interpreter, the witness, and the container. The JAPT therapist's understanding of his or her own issues allows him or her to use countertransference as an effective tool in the play therapy session. Understanding the dynamics of compensation and confirmation allows the JAPT therapist to more fully comprehend and make sense of the individual therapeutic process of each child. It is the absolute belief of JAPT therapists that the inner healer exists in every child. This belief promotes patience in the therapeutic process, allows the therapist to be a true champion of individual freedom for every child, and creates the *temenos* that allows each child to find his or her own way to healing and psychological wholeness.

REFERENCES

Boszormenyi-Nagy, I., & Ulrich, D. (1981). Contextual family therapy. In A. Gurman & D. Kniskern (Eds.), *Handbook of family therapy* (pp. 200–238). New York: Brunner/Mazel.

Campbell, J. (1949). *A hero with a thousand faces.* New York: Pantheon Books.

Jung, C. G. (1954). *Collected works of C. G. Jung: Vol. 17. The development of personality* (H. Read, M. Fordham, G. Adler, & W. McGuire, Eds.; R. F. C. Hull, Trans.). London: Routledge & Keagan Paul.

Jung, C. G. (1958). *Collected works of C. G. Jung: Vol. 11. Psychology and religion: West and east.* Princeton, NJ: Princeton University Press.

Jung, C. G. (1968). *Collected works of C. G. Jung: Vol. 12. Psychology and alchemy.* Princeton, NJ: Princeton University Press.

Jung, C. G. (1971). *Psychological types: Collected works, Vol. 6.* Princeton, NJ: Princeton University Press.

Landreth, G. (2002). *Play therapy: The art of the relationship* (2nd ed.). New York: Brunner-Routledge.

Peery, C. (2003). Jungian analytical play therapy. In C. Schaefer (Ed.), *Foundations of play therapy* (3rd ed., pp. 14–54). Hoboken, NJ: Wiley.

CHAPTER 23

Child Maltreatment

SAFETY-BASED CLINICAL STRATEGIES FOR PLAY THERAPISTS

Janine Shelby
Lauren E. Maltby

Treating children when they are currently unsafe is like trying to treat PTSD in the midst of a hurricane.
—DAVID PELCOVITZ (1999)

When childhood maltreatment is alleged, suspected, or substantiated, children are often referred to therapy. Unfortunately for many of these youth, maltreatment episodes recur despite their mental health service involvement. So, many mental health services are delivered in the shadow of the predominant—but undisclosed or unsubstantiated—child safety concern. Although several trauma-based therapies have been empirically validated for youth with past, substantiated traumatic events, little clinical consensus and even less research has emerged to guide therapists when ambiguous allegations or investigation findings, or when subthreshold concerns of child maltreatment, are present (e.g., soft indicators of child maltreatment that do not rise to the level of suspected child abuse). Complex role dualities emerge as therapists in these cases strive to provide psychotherapeutic interventions, address safety concerns, and simultaneously uphold the important divide between clinical and investigative work.

Ongoing Child Maltreatment and Mental Health Services

Few studies have examined how commonly youth experience maltreatment while they are concurrently involved in mental health services. Research from the child welfare field suggests that maltreatment is a frequent occurrence among youth concurrently receiving child protective services (CPS) interventions. In the National Survey of Children's Exposure to Violence (NatSCEV) annual report on childhood victimization in a nationally representative sample of more than 4,500 children (U.S. Department of Justice, 2009), more than half (i.e., 60.6%) of the sample had experienced or witnessed victimization in the past year. More directly related to those currently receiving psychotherapy, child maltreatment is known to occur at disproportionately high levels in clinical populations, and 14.5% of maltreated children enrolled in family preservation services within the past 5 years were subject to at least one additional substantiated occurrence of maltreatment, according to the most recent Child Maltreatment report of the U.S. Department of Health and Human Services (USDHHS, 2011). Because these statistics reflect only the rate of *reported and detected* maltreatment, population-based child maltreatment surveys yield estimates as much as 70 times higher than the rates cited in reports based on identified maltreatment (Agans et al., 2005). Furthermore, the majority of abuse or neglect reports made to CPS agencies are not substantiated (i.e., 58.9% of all referrals nationally were closed as "unsubstantiated" in 2011; USDHHS, 2012). Although some proportion of these cases are investigated and accurately closed, clinical anecdotes abound about cases in which child maltreatment persisted despite criminal or child welfare investigations. Thus, trauma recurrence during the course of therapy is not rare and may, in fact, be common among play and other child-focused therapists likely to treat youth with trauma histories and symptoms. In these cases, play therapists' clinical repertoires must also include safety-focused interventions.

Existing Trauma Treatments

A good deal of empirical and clinical attention has been devoted to treatment for youth with identified, past traumatic incidents. However, most of these treatments were developed for use in cases with substantiated traumatic incidents and without ongoing child maltreatment concerns. Trauma-focused cognitive-behavioral therapy (TF-CBT; Cohen, Mannarino, & Deblinger,

2006) has been soundly demonstrated to be effective in reducing trauma-related symptoms. Yet, the manual's safety-related module falls at the end of the protocol and—though it can be used at other points during the treatment when crises arise—the module primarily targets future rather than current safety enhancement issues. In fact, when ongoing maltreatment issues surface during the treatment, TF-CBT is typically delayed, not offered, or delivered in a modified manner (e.g., excluding the exposure) to reduce the risk of iatrogenic effect on an endangered child.

Another research-based treatment for victims of identified child physical abuse and their caregivers, alternatives for families CBT (AF-CBT; Kolko, Herschell, Baumann, & Shaver, 2009), targets both historical child physical abuse and current child abuse concerns. Early during the course of treatment, AF-CBT therapists develop a family safety plan and deliver an intervention designed to reduce the level of force the caregivers use with their children. In addition, therapists monitor the use of parental disciplinary practices on a weekly basis via different types of paper-and-pencil assessment sheets. Although this treatment incorporates ongoing safety concerns, it was developed to treat families for whom there are identified or substantiated incidents of physical abuse. When allegations are ambiguous, denied by caregivers, or there are only soft indicators of abuse, the treatment is typically delayed, not offered, or delivered using only portions of the full treatment package. In addition to these and other trauma-focused therapies, CBT and play therapy blended approaches have been proposed for use with traumatized children (Cavett & Drewes, 2012; Goodyear-Brown, 2012; Shelby & Berk, 2008), and several specific child-safety-focused intervention techniques have been described (e.g., Goodyear-Brown, 2012; Kenney-Noziska, 2008; see also Green, Crenshaw, & Kolos, 2010, for a description of issues related to preverbal trauma).

Play therapies have a long tradition of widespread use and provide developmentally sensitive methods in which youth can process their experiences via play. Particularly for young children, those with constraints on their verbal capacity, or in cases of ambiguous allegations, child-led play therapies provide a vehicle through which youth can reenact, process, and reveal their experiences, perceptions, and emotions. However, empirical examination of traditional play therapies and play-based interventions has been modest relative to the rapidly accumulating research for CBTs and other trauma treatments. Furthermore, play-based approaches provide an opportunity for themes and disclosures of maltreatment to emerge but do not directly target maltreatment. As a result, there is a need for safety-focused, developmentally sensitive intervention programs for cases involving ongoing maltreatment or the presence of maltreatment indicators, as well as for cases involving ambiguous allegations.

Fortunately, several leading authors in the field have suggested specific domains and content areas to guide safety-based clinical assessments (see Friedrich, 2002; Gil & Cavanagh-Johnson, 1993; Hewitt, 2012; Van Eys & Truss, 2012). These authors remind clinicians to use a multifaceted, individually tailored approach that includes multimodal, multisource methods to assess children and families (e.g., clinical observation, standardized and projective measures, clinical interviews with youth and families, historical data review, and information from CPS involvement), as well as a focus on developmental history, cultural factors, a general mental health assessment, and a trauma-specific interview that elicits an account of the child's experiences, exposure, and risk level. Research identifying factors associated with child maltreatment, though beyond the scope of this chapter, also provides guidance for clinical assessments (see Kolko & Swenson, 2002). Given the importance of this area, it is surprising that interventions targeting the identification and re-

duction of child maltreatment are not more pronounced in the existing treatments for childhood trauma. In this chapter, we seek to promote further discussion in this area, particularly given the critical importance of identifying maltreatment as quickly and accurately as possible.

A Safety-Enhancing Program for Cases of Probable Maltreatment

In the safety-based package of assessment and interventions that we propose, there are five intervention domains. First, the therapist engages in a thorough assessment based on existing data, relevant history, environment, and clinical interviews. Second, barriers to communication are explored and addressed, if necessary. The third level of clinical attention involves interventions focused on family patterns, boundary enhancement, and/or protective caregiver capacity. Therapists begin with the domain that is most beneficial to the child and follow these interventions with the other two areas, as indicated. The therapist progresses to the fourth level of intervention by monitoring the family's behaviors and interactions each week. At the fifth level of intervention, the child may also receive individual play therapy, sandtray interventions, or other forms of child psychotherapy. Figure 23.1 illustrates these levels of interventions. (Please note that all case material has been deidentified and clinical vignettes represent a composite of multiple families or children rather than any single child in order to protect confidentiality.)

Module I: Assessment

In the following material we briefly describe various types of assessment, including historical data gathering, home visits, and standardized assessment measures. Because families are more likely to divulge information after they have developed a strong therapeutic relationship with their

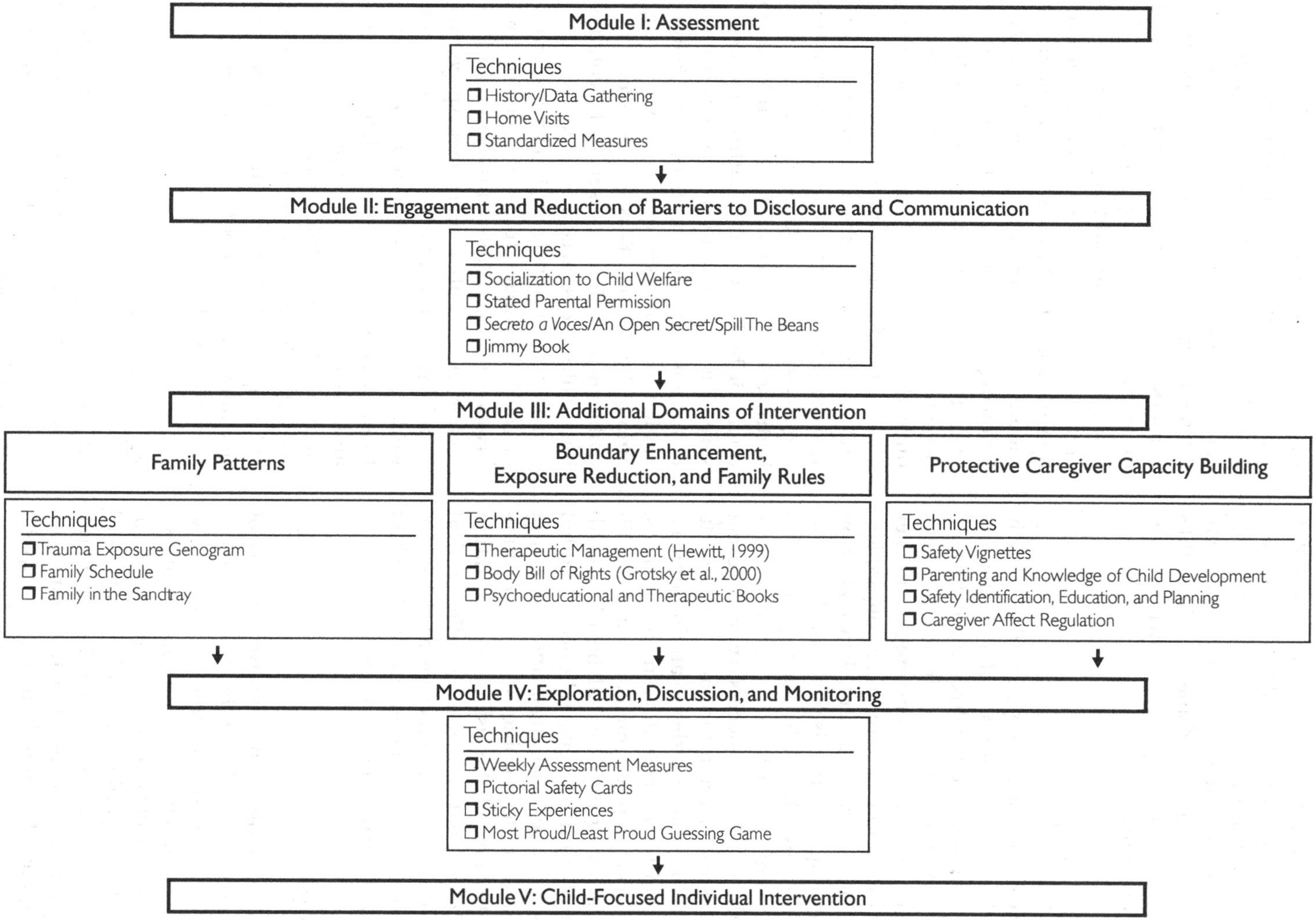

Module I: Assessment

Techniques
- History/Data Gathering
- Home Visits
- Standardized Measures

Module II: Engagement and Reduction of Barriers to Disclosure and Communication

Techniques
- Socialization to Child Welfare
- Stated Parental Permission
- Secreto o Voces/An Open Secret/Spill The Beans
- Jimmy Book

Module III: Additional Domains of Intervention

Family Patterns

Techniques
- Trauma Exposure Genogram
- Family Schedule
- Family in the Sandtray

Boundary Enhancement, Exposure Reduction, and Family Rules

Techniques
- Therapeutic Management (Hewitt, 1999)
- Body Bill of Rights (Grotsky et al., 2000)
- Psychoeducational and Therapeutic Books

Protective Caregiver Capacity Building

Techniques
- Safety Vignettes
- Parenting and Knowledge of Child Development
- Safety Identification, Education, and Planning
- Caregiver Affect Regulation

Module IV: Exploration, Discussion, and Monitoring

Techniques
- Weekly Assessment Measures
- Pictorial Safety Cards
- Sticky Experiences
- Most Proud/Least Proud Guessing Game

Module V: Child-Focused Individual Intervention

FIGURE 23.1. Safety enhancement for children with maltreatment indicators.

clinicians, as well as because of the possibility of new episodes of child maltreatment or trauma exposure at additional points during the treatment, it is important to engage in periodic reassessment of the child's history, trauma exposure, environment, and symptoms.

Historical Data

The caregiver of a young child is usually the primary adult source of information. In cases of suspected maltreatment, it is unwise to rely as heavily on a single caregiver's perspective as the therapist might in other clinical situations. Therefore, a comprehensive review of records and data collection from multiple sources is particularly important in cases where child safety concerns are present. Describing these procedures as both routine and necessary, we present consents to release information at the outset of treatment in order to attain information from CPS, law enforcement agencies, pediatricians, prior mental health facilities, the caregiver's mental health providers, probation officers, schools, extended family members, siblings, and child care providers, unless doing so is contraindicated because of the risk of stigmatization or other related concerns. A fuller clinical portrait of the child emerges as the therapist obtains information about the child from a range of vantage points.

Home Visits

A basic but often informative method of safety assessment is the home visit, which provides a basis for understanding the child's symptoms in a naturalistic context. As with consents to release information, the visit is described as both routine and necessary to understand the child and family's needs and to develop the best treatment plan. If family members express reluctance to schedule home visits, the therapist explores their understanding of the rationale for the visits, past experiences with professionals or others who have intervened or conducted past home visits, and any concerns (e.g., fear of scrutiny, discovery of immigration status, embarrassment related to living conditions). Persistent resistance to home visits in the context of an otherwise strong rapport with the therapist warrants additional exploration and may be suggestive of a safety concern. Specific aspects of assessment in the home should include, but are not limited to, the following: (1) safety-related considerations (e.g., general safety conditions in the home, persons living in the home, access to weaponry, the presence of dangerous elements, and exposure to community violence, crime, and public substance use); (2) privacy- and boundary-related considerations (e.g., co-sleeping arrangements, access to bedrooms, presence of doors and locks on doors of bedrooms and bathrooms, exposure to adult sexuality and sexual content from pornography or media for mature audiences); (3) food and substances (e.g., amount and type of—as well as access to—edible nutritive food, presence of alcohol or illicit substances, access to medications or poisonous substances); (4) characteristics of the living space (e.g., presence of toys, display of photographs of the child and the child's art, number of rooms, space free from distractions and conducive to homework completion, cleanliness, protection from overexposure to weather elements and insects/animals, and opportunities to monitor children while caregivers perform typical daily activities, such as cooking and cleaning); and (5) areas that children are not allowed to access (e.g., medicine cabinets, rooms, closets, or drawers).

Standardized Measures

Although psychological assessment is typically the domain of psychologists, other mental health practitioners can make use of the many commercially available, standardized instruments when working with high-risk families. The UCLA PTSD Reaction Index (both child and parent versions) contains items that assess cumulative trauma exposure (i.e., surviving different types of traumatic events). The instrument is useful as a means of assessing information that family members may not spontaneously reveal, and may also increase some family members' comfort level in revealing their histories because of the standardized, matter-of-fact questionnaire format. The UCLA PTSD Reaction Index is available from the National Center for Child Traumatic Stress (*www.nctsn.org*). Additional measures that help identify potential maltreatment risk include indices of parental stress (e.g., Parenting Stress Index; Abidin, 1995), parenting practices (e.g., Child Abuse Potential Inventory; Milner, 1986), and high-risk sexual behavior in young children (e.g., Child Sexual Behavior Inventory; Friedrich, 1997). All three of these measures are commercially available through Psychological Assessment Resources (PAR).

Module II: Engagement and Reduction of Barriers to Disclosure and Communication

The therapeutic relationship is often cited as an overarching factor in the success of mental health treatments. With caregivers who may be reluctant to disclose the full extent of their children's exposure to maltreatment, engagement is an indispensable element of family-based intervention. Because the therapeutic relationship is central to most psychotherapeutic approaches, clinicians have usually worked diligently to hew this skill. Yet, working in the context of ambiguous child maltreatment concerns presents unique challenges for clinicians, who must create and maintain empathic connections to both children and their caregivers.

Increasing Engagement

Therapists who work in child maltreatment settings often have unsettling experiences if caregivers respond with apathy, scrutiny, or overly negative biases toward the children for whom therapists also feel a sense of loyalty. At times, therapists may find caregivers' behaviors incredulous and experience a sense of overwhelm, anger, sadness, disgust, or fear. In these circumstances, it can be challenging to maintain positive regard for the caregiver, who may be functioning as best as he or she can at that moment, but whose behaviors are nonetheless psychologically or physically injurious to the child. It can be cognitively taxing for therapists to flip between embracing the parental perspective, empathizing with the child, and simultaneously developing strategies for exploration, assessment, and intervention. To enhance their ability to maintain empathic connections to these caregivers, some therapists remind themselves that the caregivers were once children whose hardships during their own childhoods may be linked to their current parental responses. Other therapists identify and connect with a particular aspect of the caregiver (e.g., a strength, parenting goal, or vulnerability). Yet, other therapists visualize how the family members would function if they were to embrace positive growth, and view the caregiver's reactions as a transient step along a clear path toward more adaptive caregiver behaviors. Whatever the strategy, it is helpful for therapists to remain hopeful, supportive, and resourceful when intervening with caregivers who may be extremely sensitive to disapproval, invalidation, or rejection. When engaging in this work, therapists are reminded to rely heavily on the support of supervisors and colleagues to prevent fatigue or burnout.

Reducing Communication Barriers

Family members' past experiences, family and cultural values, and fears about the consequences of disclosure may negatively impact open communication. Several techniques to address these issues are presented in the following sections.

SOCIALIZATION TO CHILD WELFARE SYSTEMS

Both children and caregivers may have anxiety, misinformation, or misconceptions related to the child welfare system. Some have had prior experiences that either promote or discourage the use of the child welfare system to enhance familial safety. For example, children may remain silent because of fear that they will be "taken away" from their parents if they reveal family information. Exploration of the family's prior child welfare experiences is critical, but it is also helpful to provide accurate or corrective information about child welfare processes and roles—or at least how the system is intended to work for those who have had unduly negative experiences. In some cases, the corrective information (e.g., CPS goals usually involve helping families stay together safely; most CPS dispositions do not involve detainment) allows family members to feel more at ease when discussing safety-related issues.

STATED PARENTAL PERMISSION

Many children receive mixed messages from their caregivers about whether or not it is acceptable to speak openly to the therapist. We recommend meeting with caregivers during the initial phase of treatment to discuss both adults' and children's comfort level with the child discussing feelings and experiences with the therapist. We explore and normalize parental reservations about their own and their children's disclosure, and affirm our desire to create a sense of acceptance and support. We describe our goals as helping family members develop trust in our motives, but more so, in their own ability to speak bravely about their realities. We stress how parental encouragement of open communication is related to safe and competent parenting as well as to children's current and future self-protective capacities; that is, as caregivers encourage youth to speak about safety concerns, the children are more likely to value their own

safety, verbalize inappropriate acts that might befall them outside their homes, and use self-protective strategies in their current and future relationships. When the caregiver can encourage open disclosure of information, conjoint child–parent sessions can be held and parents are asked to reassure the child that it is all right to tell the therapist anything, even if it has been a secret in the past. Parents are also asked to tell their child in the presence of the therapist that the child *should* tell the therapist if anything unsafe, uncomfortable, or frightening happens or has happened. Next, the therapist informs the family that he or she will be checking in about these things on a weekly basis, to give them the chance to practice open discussion and disclosure of safety-related incidents that occur between sessions.

SECRETO A VOCES AND "SPILL THE BEANS"

Proverbs or idioms about communication appear across ethnic and cultural groups, and they can create a familiar, culturally relevant base from which to address communication barriers. For example, in the *secreto a voces* (a "secret" that is already widely known) intervention, we demonstrate how a clown pops out of a jack-in-the-box toy. Then the lid is closed, the caregiver is asked to hold the box, and the child is asked to stand near the caregiver, without touching the jack-in-the-box. Everyone is asked to listen, and the caregiver is asked to begin cranking the handle slowly. The therapist asks the caregiver to pause long enough for the therapist to describe how everyone knows that there is something inside, even if it is not being discussed aloud. The therapist might further suggest that, at any moment, something might pop out and, as anticipation grows, the therapists can assess whether family members feel tense, excited, or relaxed. The therapist can then normalize the emotions that families often feel when waiting for something to "pop" out. As anticipation of the ejecting clown rises, the therapist can comment on the changes in affect. When the clown finally ejects, the release of tension becomes a natural point of discussion. The therapist can emphasize the changes in affect, how everyone knew what was inside even though it had not yet sprung forward, and that it was inevitably going to emerge at some point. They might also discuss how *talking* about something hidden is much easier than remaining silent about it. Afterward, the therapist relates this activity to family secrets and encourages family members to describe their *open secrets*.

In a similar intervention based on the *spilling the beans* proverb, family members are asked to try to remain silent as they carry large bags of beans from one side of the therapy room to the other. Because the bags have holes through which the beans inevitably spill, it is difficult for family members to remain silent. Family members usually find these interventions enjoyable, and the concept of open discourse provides an important foundation for future communication, self-protection, and safety-based therapeutic work.

JIMMY BOOK

For youngsters who find it difficult to speak about intrafamilial or other life experiences, I (Shelby) proposed using individually designed therapeutic booklets to facilitate discussions. In the Jimmy Book (Shelby, 2000), a drawing of a boy's face appears on the first page. A real shoelace is inserted into the page such that it is tied in a bow over the mouth of Jimmy, the boy in the drawing. Typically, young patients untie the string immediately to unseal Jimmy's mouth. The activity both enhances the child's level of intrigue and serves as a handy metaphor for the subsequent discussion. On the next page, the story reads, "Something happened but Jimmy doesn't want to talk about it. . . ." On an additional page, the child might draw what would happen if Jimmy talked about "it." This inter-

vention suggests that something has happened, and although it is not recommended for use with all children, it can be a useful tool when clinical judgment indicates sufficient reason to refer to an unidentified, negative event.

Module III: Family Patterns, Boundary Enhancement, and Protective Caregiver Capacity Building

After conducting the assessment, engaging the family in treatment, and reducing explicit barriers to disclosure/communication, the third level of intervention involves prioritizing each family's unique needs. Three broad domains (i.e., family patterns, boundaries, and caregiver capacity) are described in the following material as possible points of intervention, but clinicians and families collaborate to identify the most salient, initial area of focus, and other domains are targeted sequentially thereafter.

Family Patterns

Identification of family patterns (i.e., specific parental behaviors across time and multigenerational victimization experiences) can be particularly helpful in developing rapport, enhancing caregiver insight, and noting parental strengths.

TRAUMA EXPOSURE GENOGRAM

Similar to the technique commonly used in family therapy, trauma therapists can use genograms to assess intergenerational familial safety themes during collateral caregiver sessions. In this technique, the caregiver describes current and past generations of family members, and the therapist draws a genogram to depict intrafamilial relationships. Then the therapist inquires about relatively benign areas for each member (e.g., occupation, educational level, medical issues) before exploring family histories of mental disorders, substance abuse, intrafamilial conflicts, domestic violence, use of harsh disciplinary methods, criminal histories, victimization experiences, and perpetration histories. After the information is provided, the therapist and caregiver discuss intergenerational themes or patterns. In families with multiple victimization experiences, the use of different-colored highlighters to differentially shade the genogram symbols representing family members who had/have either victimization or perpetration histories can be a poignant means of visualizing the patterns of intergenerational violence and other forms of child maltreatment on the trauma genogram.

We also ask for information related to familial history involving noteworthy efforts to change situations for the positive. In this way, we can often point out that, despite family themes of intergenerational child abuse or domestic violence, the caregiver has heroically—and often uniquely—sought to end a tragic cycle for the family. Acknowledgment of caregivers' efforts is a powerful way to build rapport, reframe the purpose of therapy, and develop a safety-based goal.   Even if families do not endorse any familial experiences in the domains we assess, it is helpful to collect intergenerational family information as we assess various aspects of family functioning, and when we repeat the genogram during a later stage of treatment, additional information sometimes emerges. As an additional benefit, the trauma genogram technique provides a mechanism for identifying influential family members so that the therapist can determine their level of support for the child's psychotherapy involvement.

FAMILY SCHEDULE

Some caregivers may not recall, deem important, or spontaneously describe aspects of the child's life that pose safety concerns. For example, caregivers may want to present themselves in a positive light or may be limited in their ability to identify potentially dangerous situations. Identifying the components of a child's 24-hour schedule for each day of a typical week allows for parents to provide information that might not otherwise surface (e.g., mealtime, bathing and hygiene practices, adult supervision, exposure to other children or adults, and quality and amount of sleep). For example:

The father of two boys, ages 5 and 7, reported that the children's aunt (i.e., his adult sister) watched the children after school until he returned from work in the late evening. During a genogram activity, the father denied that anyone in his family had experienced or perpetrated child abuse, and he described his sister as a nurturing and appropriate disciplinarian. However, during the weekly safety check-in, the 5-year-old boy appeared to be anxious and sometimes cried. On one occasion he said, "I don't want to get hit again," but when his statement was reflected, he immediately denied that he had been hit and begged to change the subject. During the family schedule activity, we learned that Gordito, the father's sister's father-in-law, sometimes ate dinner with the boys during the afternoons they were at their aunt's house. The 5-year-old boy ultimately disclosed that Gordito hit and threatened him several times when the aunt took her afternoon walks with the dog. Gordito had not been included in the father's genogram because he was related only by marriage, and the father had forgotten that this relative by marriage was present with his children unsupervised. The father later revealed that his sister's husband acknowledged that Gordito had physically abused him when he was a child.

FAMILY IN THE SAND

Because objects can be hidden and discovered, sandtray techniques can be a particularly fruitful medium for exploring secrecy and undisclosed experiences. Here we describe specific sandtray techniques, and refer the reader to the substantial sandtray therapy literature for a more thorough description of the methods in common use. In this applied technique, children are asked to select an object that reminds them of a secret. They are then instructed to hide the object in the sand while the therapist looks away so as not to see the placement of the object. Next, the therapist begins to search for the item as the therapist describes his or her role to the child (e.g., "I help children talk or play about anything they want, and, if there are secrets, I help uncover them"; "I want you to know that I want to help if hidden things need to come out, but you are the one who knows where things are hidden"; or "If you help me find the secret thing, we can uncover it more quickly"). Children are then asked if they would give the therapist clues that would help him or her to locate the object. As children work together with therapists to uncover the hidden object, a sense of mutual collaboration develops, but children also learn that therapists are neither all-knowing nor oblivious to whatever lies hidden in the sand. Because we do not know which children hold dangerous secrets, sometimes we use this intervention with children whose secrets are benign and age-appropriate. Irrespective of their circumstances, children usually enjoy the activity and benefit from the collaborative rapport it generates. If therapists have cause to use a more suggestive intervention, children can be asked to create vignettes in the sandtray that show what is hidden in their families (e.g., any secrets they keep, secrets their caregivers or other adults keep, or emotions that are buried). On the other side of the sandtray or in a different sandtray scene, children can then depict how life would change if the secrets were revealed. For example:

Ariana, a 9-year-old girl, was introduced to the sandtray after showing multiple indicators of undisclosed abuse. When the therapist explored safety concerns, Ariana often responded suggestively, saying "I'm not allowed to talk about that," or "Only my mom can answer that question." Ariana often referenced "family secrets." During her first sandtray scene, Ariana hid objects in the sand

for the therapist to find. When the therapist began looking for the hidden objects, Ariana appeared nervous. The therapist normalized her response by saying that sometimes children feel nervous about the hidden thing being found. When invited, Ariana initially decided not to provide clues to help the therapist in her search for the hidden objects, but after some time elapsed, she began to provide hints as to their location. When the therapist reflected that Ariana had now decided to work with her to uncover the hidden things, Ariana said that she had decided she wanted the therapist to find what was hidden. The therapist eventually found the objects, and Ariana asked to repeat the activity multiple times during the session. The therapist noted that the hidden objects were difficult to find until Ariana helped her find them. In later sessions, this experience was used as a reference point to help Ariana understand her role in facilitating open communication and disclosure by collaborating with the therapist and other protective adults, who could not know the family's hidden secrets without Ariana's help.

Boundary Enhancement, Exposure Reduction, and Family Privacy Rules

Working with families to create or enhance physical and emotional boundaries, recognize unsafe or inappropriate environments, and develop effective family rules helps bolster safety related to both past and future traumatic incidents and exposure.

THERAPEUTIC MANAGEMENT/ SAFETY CONTRACT

Hewitt (1999) proposes a useful intervention in which family members separately create a list of appropriate and inappropriate interactions (e.g., types of touching, privacy arrangements, and exposure to adult content). The therapist then compiles and synthesizes the items on the list to form a final family safety contract. The caregivers then read the list to the child and specify that no one, not even they themselves, are allowed to engage in the prohibited activities. The contract is further strengthened by the caregivers' naming of trusted adults to whom the child should speak if anyone violates the safety contract. The therapist uses this contract as a basis for family safety monitoring in subsequent sessions.

BODY BILL OF RIGHTS

Grotsky, Camerer, and Damiano (2000) propose a technique in which the youth composes a bill of rights related to his or her own body. This activity, for older elementary school-age children or adolescents who may be familiar with the historical Bill of Rights, adds a more sophisticated element to psychoeducation and bodily integrity discussions by introducing the principle that not only do their own families need to abide by family safety contracts, but *all* children's bodies are deserving of protection and safety. In the intervention, youth create a "Body Bill of Rights" loosely based on the Bill of Rights contained in the U.S. Constitution. For example, in their bill of rights, children identify the rights that their bodies have to be fed, nurtured, housed, touched kindly, touched appropriately, and to be free from intentional or negligent injury.

PSYCHOEDUCATIONAL AND THERAPEUTIC BOOKS

Numerous developmentally appropriate bibliotherapy materials exist to facilitate caregiver–child discussions of bodily boundaries, sexual or physical abuse, and puberty. Therapists are encouraged to use these commercially available materials, author their own booklets, or work with youth in therapy to develop their own body "manuals" (e.g., youth can write questions on blank pages of a booklet, caregivers and therapists collaborate on the responses, and caregivers then read the booklet to their children).

Protective Caregiver Capacity Building

Some caregivers have underdeveloped abilities to detect threats to their own or their children's safety, and need assistance in learning to set developmentally appropriate expectations for children's behavior, communicate consistent safety-related messages (i.e., by consistency in both words and actions), and regulate their own affective responses. Using vignettes—rather than the family's own history—to enhance caregiver safety-related capacity often increases caregivers' comfort level and accelerates their ability to learn safety-based skills.

SAFETY VIGNETTES

Caregivers who have fundamental difficulty identifying threats to their children's safety and well-being are likely to be impaired in their ability to report these hazards during therapy sessions. To help develop caregivers' capacity in this area, we often begin by discussing fictionalized vignettes, rather than the caregivers' own situations. This use of fiction reduces the likelihood of caregiver defensive reactions. In the vignettes we present scenarios in which fictionalized caregivers face dilemmas about their children's safety or exposure to violence. We then ask parents to rate the children's level of safety on a 1–10 scale. Based on caregiver responses, we provide individualized psychoeducation about safety hazards, threats, and safe parenting practices. For example, in one vignette, a mother reveals that she and her children are now safe from exposure to domestic violence because her formerly abusive spouse has tearfully apologized, sent her flowers, and "won't drink for the next 30 days." Another example of a written vignette is as follows:

A single, hardworking mother of three young children works two jobs to be able to provide for her family. She was recently informed that her child care provider will be closed for a 2-week vacation. The mother has no family members who are able to care for the children, and she is unable to find anyone to watch her children for her. She fears that missing another day of work will result in the loss of her jobs. The neighbor offered to watch her children, and he has always been nice to them. She heard from someone that he had been accused of molesting the children of another family who lived in the apartment building last year. How safe is it to use him as a child care provider for 2 weeks?

When parents master the safety vignette tasks by demonstrating the ability to detect threats to children's welfare, we then introduce vignettes that involve dilemmas the specific caregiver might face. We often find that caregivers are then able to apply these newly developed skills to reevaluate their own safety-related parenting choices.

PARENTING AND KNOWLEDGE OF CHILD DEVELOPMENT

In the prevention of child abuse, parental knowledge of typical child development and successful use of child behavior management techniques are primary protective factors. Information on child development can help caregivers adjust unrealistic and unhelpful expectations of their children; learn parenting techniques based on these new, adjusted expectations; develop new strategies for managing their children's behaviors; and engage in more positive interactions with their children. The reader is referred to treatments such as Parent–Child Interaction Therapy (Chaffin et al., 2004) that have been shown to reduce child physical abuse recidivism.

SAFETY IDENTIFICATION, EDUCATION, AND PLANNING

In this intervention, caregivers are asked to identify a time in their childhoods—or in adulthood if caregivers have difficulty identifying a safe childhood experience—when they felt completely safe. Caregivers are then encouraged to describe this experience in terms of what, specifically, led to the feeling of safety (e.g., who was present, what was said or done, how the situation was handled, and so forth). The therapist elicits as much detail as possible and notes any specific actions or verbalizations described by the caregiver about his or her remembered experience of safety. Therapists can then use components of the caregiver's own experience to identify and discuss the specific elements that led to a sense of safety, protection, and comfort (e.g., the content of what was said, tone of voice, nonverbal communications, immediacy and effectiveness of any actions taken, level of verbal reassurance). The therapist discusses how a caregiver's words and actions can be either consistent or inconsistent, and how children respond to caregivers in each scenario, as described in Figure 23.2.

Following the description of this concept, the therapist may role-play demonstrations of each of these four primary scenarios: (1) Caregiver speaks and acts consistently to promote the child's safety; (2) caregiver speaks and acts inconsistently (e.g., saying reassuring things but not doing much to promote safety; taking safety-enhancing steps but not providing reassuring explanations to the child); or (3) caregiver neither speaks nor acts in safety-enhancing ways. When the parent demonstrates an understanding of the concept, the parent is then asked to describe what he or she has said and done to communicate safety-promoting messages to the child. Using a blank version of Figure 23.2, the parent is asked to note where his or her behaviors and statements would fall, and then to evaluate and identify additional actions that could be taken to either verbalize or enact safety-promoting messages to the child.

CAREGIVER AFFECT REGULATION SKILL

Because affective dysregulation can pose significant impediments to parents' ability

	Action Taken	Incomplete Action Taken	Action Not Taken
Talk (caregiver makes safety-enhancing statements)	Strong safety-enhancing message conveyed; child likely to feel supported ☺	Inconsistent message conveyed; child likely to feel confused and unsupported 😐	Message conveyed that safety is not a priority; child likely to feel unsupported, betrayed, and confused by inconsistency between words and actions ☹
Mixed Statements	Ambiguous message comveyed; child may not feel gratified by caregiver action ☺	Ambiguous message conveyed; child likely to feel confused 😐	Message conveyed that safety is not a priority; child likely to feel unsupported and betrayed by inconsistency between words and actions ☹
Talk (caregiver does not make safety-enhancing statements)	Partial safety-enhancing message may be conveyed; child may not feel gratified by caregiver action without accompanying verbal reassurance and description ☺	Ambiguous message conveyed; child likely to feel confused 😐	Message conveyed that child is undeserving of protection and safety; child likely to feel abandoned, unsupported, fearful, and angry ☹

FIGURE 23.2. Speaking and Doing Safety Chart.

to respond adaptively to their children, therapeutic activities designed to enhance distress tolerance and affect regulation skills, particularly pertaining to parenting issues, can be critically important adjunctive components of safety-based work. Addressing these or other caregiver mental health or substance use issues often includes not only a collateral caregiver focus on skill building but also linkage to, and close contact with, the caregiver's therapy provider.

Module IV: Ongoing Exploration, Discussion, and Monitoring of Child Safety

Many families acknowledge past and ongoing safety concerns after work is completed in the preceding domains, and ongoing monitoring solidifies the gains made in

these areas. Many youth in these families may be in a position to now benefit from trauma-focused or other forms of treatment. Even in cases without disclosures of maltreatment incidents, these monitoring strategies can be used to conduct weekly assessments of safety and intrafamilial interactions until maltreatment concerns have subsided, continuing, if necessary, while families are engaged in subsequent psychotherapeutic intervention modalities (e.g., TF-CBT or play therapy).

Weekly Assessment Measures

Administering weekly paper-and-pencil questionnaires or conducting verbal assessments of exposure to trauma, discipline, or other identified safety issues is a standard component of safety-based treatment (Gil & Cavanagh-Johnson, 1993; Kolko et al., 2009). By consistently assessing safety issues each week, therapists not only track familial progress or treatment needs, they also model the importance of safety.

Pictorial Safety Cards

As an alternative to paper-and-pencil questionnaires to monitor safety issues, we developed a set of picture cards that depict various parental and familial behaviors (e.g., completed homework, read a book to child, or played with child), including child maltreatment behaviors and potentially dangerous activities (e.g., domestic violence, lack of privacy during toileting or bathing, sexual abuse, physical abuse, access to weapons, substance abuse by caregivers). The pictures are accompanied by developmentally appropriate descriptions (e.g., "The grown-ups hit each other"). Pictorial representations of each situation are used, with the exception of sexual and aggressive content, which is implied rather than graphically depicted. Because the cards show pictures of the assessment items, younger children can participate in the monitoring task without parental assistance. When used in family sessions, each family member receives his or her own deck of picture cards and as each card is described by the therapist, the family members place the picture cards in one of three boxes labeled *Yes, No,* or *I Don't Know* to indicate whether or not the event occurred during the past week. Each family member silently reveals family experiences without other family members knowing which cards are being placed in which boxes. When the family is finished, the therapist reviews the cards privately and then discusses themes or issues (e.g., the lack of agreement or consistency across family members or themes across multiple weeks). The therapist inquires about endorsed items carefully to be sure that family members understand precisely which behaviors the children are

endorsing. Traditional Q-sort cards without the pictures can be used if older children and teenagers prefer them. This method provides both a strategic form of information gathering and some protection for family members who may not feel comfortable disclosing aloud. Both the content provided by the participants during the activity and the family members' responses to the intervention (e.g., willingness to disclose, level of direction seeking about whether or not to endorse events, discrepancies between family members' reports, intrafamilial reactions when endorsements or disclosures occur) provide valuable information. For additional information on how to use the pictorial safety cards, please contact me (Maltby).

Sticky Experiences

To add variety to the weekly safety monitoring intervention tools, Post-its can be placed on a wall for youth to pull off if the event occurred during the prior week (e.g., "Someone in the family had an argument"; "Someone yelled"; "Someone hit"; "Someone played with me"; "Someone read to me"). Though the intervention is designed to monitor safety, it is also important to assess positive familial interactions and to give youth the opportunity to notice positive experiences with their caregivers. The therapist can note the frequency of positive and negative experiences each week, the themes, and the ratio of positive-to-negative intrafamilial events. When caregivers are asked to complete the same task, their recollections can be contrasted with their children's and addressed either directly or indirectly by the therapist.

Very Proud/Not-So-Proud Guessing Game

In this assessment activity, both children and caregivers are asked to list, draw, act out, or use figurines to depict one of their own behaviors during the past week about which they are the proudest. Family members then indicate behaviors for which each family member should feel pride. Next, family members indicate behaviors about which they feel the least proud. This time, family members write or draw the incident without verbalizing it. Each family member then begins a new description or drawing to identify the behaviors the others might have chosen as their least proud moments. When family members share all of their least proud moments with each other, they are encouraged to apologize if necessary and to create a plan for how to handle similar situations in the future. This intervention not only assists the therapist in monitoring safety, but also increases comfort levels with direct communication and provides a natural format for coping and problem-solving activities.

Module V: Child-Focused Individual Intervention/Play Therapy

Many play therapy approaches have been articulated in play therapy's long history and wide literature, including those detailed throughout this volume. No matter which play therapy approach is used, the themes derived from children's play narratives can be invaluable in discerning their perceptions, feelings, and experiences. In safety-focused play therapy, themes related to problem solving, open communication, safety (i.e., the playroom, toys, sense of emotional safety, and physical safety), protection, and one's ability to influence difficulties or challenges in a positive manner are all highlighted and emphasized.

For example, the boy who builds a bridge with blocks might be told that he figured out how to solve the truck's problem of getting over the river. When a girl voices her baby-doll's cries, the therapist might say that the baby is using her voice to let us know that she needs or dislikes something. The therapist might further explain, "I want to understand, I can understand best when the baby uses her voice to let

me know." For a child who tries multiple approaches to opening a container of play dough, the therapist might highlight that sometimes it takes a lot of attempts before the thing that needs to come out can come out. In this way the therapist not only uses the reflection technique familiar to most play therapists, but more specifically emphasizes the core actions related to safety (e.g., problem solving, open communication, and repeated efforts). In many safety-based play therapy sessions, the child can be asked toward the end of the session what the characters or situations need to be safer or to make things better. Many children use this prompt to reveal or play out resolutions to the play scenarios they created. The therapist can then exercise clinical judgment as to whether or not these resolutions can be linked to the real-world issues the child perceives. Even if children say that nothing can be done to make the situation better, the therapist can use the opportunity to instill hope by speaking directly to the characters, reminding them that the therapist will not forget about them, and saying that the therapist and the child will return again next week, trying again to make a better/safer/happier world. These play therapy interventions facilitate the development of the warm, emotionally responsive therapeutic relationship that is central to all client–therapist bonds, but the interventions go one step further by decreasing barriers to disclosure and promoting safety-related values.

Conclusion

Despite the magnitude of their work, many child-focused therapists do not yet have best-practice parameters to guide their safety-focused interventions. This chapter is written to enhance the visibility of safety-based clinical interventions, to contribute to an underrepresented body of literature, and to propose specific safety-focused assessment and treatment strategies. For clinicians who work in the shadow of child maltreatment concerns, the development of an evidence-based, safety-focused treatment protocol would be invaluable. Until such a treatment emerges, we offer this discussion as support and guidance to the many therapists who seek to intervene both inside and outside the play therapy room to address child maltreatment concerns in as comprehensive a manner as possible.

REFERENCES

Abidin, R. R. (1995). *Parenting stress index: Professional manual* (3rd ed.). Odessa, FL: Psychological Assessment Resources.

Agans, R., Bangdiwala, S. I., Chang, J. J., Hunter, W. M., Runyan, D. K., & Theodore, A. D. (2005). Epidemiological features of the physical and sexual maltreatment of children in the Carolinas. *Pediatrics, 115*(3), e331–337.

Cavett, A. M., & Drewes, A. A. (2012). Play applications and trauma-specific components. In J. A. Cohen & A. P. Mannarino (Eds.), *Trauma-focused CBT for children and adolescents: Treatment applications* (pp. 124–148). New York: Guilford Press.

Chaffin, M., Silovsky, J. F., Funderburk, B., Valle, L., Brestan, E. V., Balachova, T., et al. (2004). Parent–Child Interaction Therapy with physically abusive parents: Efficacy for reducing future abuse reports. *Journal of Consulting and Clinical Psychology, 72*, 500–510.

Cohen, J. A., Mannarino, A. P., & Deblinger, E. (2006). *Treating trauma and traumatic grief in children and adolescents.* New York: Guilford Press.

Friedrich, W. N. (1997). *Child Sexual Behavior Inventory: Professional manual.* Odessa, FL: Psychological Assessment Resources.

Friedrich, W. N. (2002). *Psychological assessment of sexually abused children and their families.* Thousand Oaks, CA: Sage.

Gil, E., & Cavanagh-Johnson, T. (1993). *Sexualized children: Assessment and treatment of sexualized children and children who molest.* Ann Arbor, MI: Launch Press.

Goodyear-Brown, P. (2012). Flexibly sequential

play therapy (FSPT) with sexually victimized children. In P. Goodyear-Brown (Ed.), *Handbook of child sexual abuse: Identification, assessment, and treatment* (pp. 297–319). Hoboken, NJ: Wiley.

Green, E. J., Crenshaw, D. A., & Kolos, A. C. (2010). Counseling children with preverbal trauma. *International Journal of Play Therapy, 19*, 95–105.

Grotsky, L., Camerer, C., & Damiano, L. (2000). *Group work with sexually abused children.* Thousand Oaks, CA: Sage.

Hewitt, S. (1999). *Assessing allegations of sexual abuse in preschool children: Understanding small voices.* Thousand Oaks, CA: Sage.

Hewitt, S. (2012). Developmentally sensitive assessment methods in child sexual abuse cases. In P. Goodyear-Brown (Ed.), *Handbook of child sexual abuse: Identification, assessment, and treatment* (pp. 121–142). Hoboken, NJ: Wiley.

Kenney-Noziska, S. (2008). *Techniques–techniques–techniques: Play-based activities for children, adolescents, and families.* Concord, MA: Infinity.

Kolko, D. J., Herschell, A. D., Baumann, B. L., & Shaver, M. E. (2009). *Alternatives for families: Cognitive-behavioral therapy for child physical abuse–session guide* (Version 2.4). Pittsburgh, PA: University of Pittsburgh School of Medicine.

Kolko, D. J., & Swenson, C. C. (2002). *Assessing and treating physically abused children and their families: A cognitive-behavioral approach.* Thousand Oaks, CA: Sage.

Milner, J. (1986). *The Child Abuse Potential Inventory: Manual.* Dekalb, IL: Psytec.

Pelcovitz, D. (1999). *Child witnesses to domestic violence.* Presentation sponsored by Four Winds Hospital, Astor Home for Children, and Ulster County Mental Health, Kingston, NY.

Shelby, J. S. (2000). Brief play therapy with traumatized children: A developmental perspective. In H. G. Kaduson & C. E. Schaefer (Eds.), *Short-term play therapy for children* (pp. 169–243). New York: Guilford Press.

Shelby, J. S., & Berk, M. J. (2008). CBT, play therapy, and pedagogy: An argument for synthesis. In A. A. Drewes (Ed.), *Effectively blending play therapy and cognitive behavioral therapy: A convergent approach* (pp. 17–40). New York: Wiley.

U.S. Department of Health and Human Services, Administration for Children and Families, Administration on Children, Youth and Families, Children's Bureau. (2011). Child maltreatment 2011. Retrieved from *www.acf. hhs.gov/sites/default/files/cb/cm11.pdf.*

U.S. Department of Health and Human Services, Administration for Children and Families, Administration on Children, Youth and Families, Children's Bureau. (2012). Child maltreatment 2012. Retrieved from *www.acf. hhs.gov/programs/cb/research-data-technology/ statistics-research/child-maltreatment.*

U.S. Department of Justice, Office of Juvenile Justice and Delinquency Prevention. (2009). Children's exposure to violence: A comprehensive national survey (Juvenile Justice Bulletin October 2009). Retrieved from *www. ncjrs.gov/pdffiles1/ojjdp/227744.pdf.*

Van Eys, P., & Truss, A. (2012). Comprehensive and therapeutic assessment of child sexual abuse: A bridge to treatment. In P. Goodyear-Brown (Ed.), *Handbook of child sexual abuse: Identification, assessment, and treatment* (pp. 143–170). Hoboken, NJ: Wiley.

CHAPTER 24

Reunifying Families after Critical Separations

AN INTEGRATIVE PLAY THERAPY APPROACH TO BUILDING AND STRENGTHENING FAMILY TIES

Eliana Gil

Many families have crises that lead to critical separations in which children are placed under the custody of the state, typically when child protective services (CPS) concludes that one or more children have been, or are, at risk of child maltreatment of many kinds. The national statistics confirm that child neglect is still the most reported form of child abuse (U.S. Department of Health and Social Services, *www.acf.hhs.gov/programs/cb/resource/child-maltreatment-2011*) and represents one of the greatest risks for children whose families have serious stressors such as poverty, homelessness, drug abuse, family violence, parental physical illness or compromised parental functioning, and/or limited parental capacities to provide safe and nurturing environments in which children can thrive. In addition, some families elicit protective intervention due to physical or sexual abuse; lack of supervision, protection, and/or guidance; or other family issues such as drug abuse, homelessness, or do-

mestic violence (which also place children at risk of emotional and social difficulties; Kitzmann, Gaylord, Holt, & Kenny, 2003). Some children are viewed as more high risk or vulnerable than others, including children with developmental disabilities, sexual nonconformity, or other variables—factors that can put them at risk for abuse by nonfamily members (e.g., children who are bullied in person or via the Internet).

The Child Welfare League (*www.cwla.org/advocacy/statefactsheets/statefactsheet05.htm*) estimates that over 500,000 children are in foster care at any given time. Foster care was created to provide temporary care to vulnerable youngsters while their parents are given an array of services designed to optimize their caretaking capacities, address acute problems, and provide corrective action to restore safety. And yet the very system designed to protect children has been well documented to be a system with serious structural problems: Children are sometimes kept in foster care too long, with multiple placements, an array of social workers, and documentation of negative outcomes for the children. In addition, the fact that children don't always achieve stability in foster care, and a small percentage of them may even be abused or neglected in foster care, may contribute to difficulties in their behavior, their adjustment, and their parents' ability to maintain positive family changes.

Reuniting children in out-of-home care with their families is a mandate of the Adoption Assistance and Welfare Act of 1980, and family preservation has become a primary goal of child welfare (Jones, 1998). However, sometimes returning children to their parents is seen as the goal or conclusion of a separation, without careful consideration given to the tremendous challenge of bringing fractured families back together, and facilitating repairs, after each family member has been impacted by the separation and his or her experiences in foster care and/or in developing new family compositions. Premature reunification and failure to correct the family problems that caused state intervention in the first place can contribute to higher rates of reentry into the foster care system (Terling, 1999). Efforts have been undertaken to determine factors that can prevent children's reentry into foster care; Terling (1999), for example, emphasizes that service delivery is one of the factors under consideration.

Few mental health professionals have received specialized training to assist families in a reunification process and there are woefully few structured models developed beyond identification of criteria for moving toward reunification. Not surprisingly, clinicians therefore have mixed feelings about working with these cases (Gil & Roizner-Hayes, 1996; Roizner-Hayes, 1994). Yet few other family transitions are subject to such inherently painful ruptures and reunions. Play therapists are often called upon to work with child/family issues, and they are in a unique position to provide the necessary child-sensitive guidance to family

members. At the same time, play therapists may be intimidated or reluctant to accept these cases because they often include a multidisciplinary approach. However, play therapy is inviting and helpful to all families, particularly those who may present with feelings of shame and guilt.

Sibling Incest

Despite the fact that sibling sexual abuse is underreported and clouded in secrecy, my agency receives frequent calls for help in cases of sibling incest as well as sibling physical abuse. In fact, there are estimates that only 2% of sibling abuse is ever reported (Baker, 2002). Although several authors have focused attention on this issue, it continues to harm countless children and exert a traumatic impact that is similar to adult-inflicted child abuse (Caffaro & Conn-Caffaro, 1998; Wiehe, 1997).

It becomes clear in cases of sibling incest that the approach must be systemic and multimodal (Sheinberg, True, & Fraenkel, 1994), as well as capable of providing family members with individualized, parallel attention. For example, children who are victimized by siblings need parents to believe them, support and nurture them, and provide immediate and clearly identifiable evidence of their ability to provide safety and supervision. Adolescents who are the abusers (and usually referred to as "adolescent sex offenders") also need parental support as well as firm limit setting. In addition, they need to know that their behaviors are of grave concern and that they will need to participate fully in their specialized adolescent sex offender therapy process. Both siblings require specialized services by professionals who understand the complexity of sibling incest and the necessity for more active case management and clinical direction. Finally, because the family system changes at the point that disclosures of sibling incest are made, the subsequent loss of trust, sense of betrayal, and feelings of fear, sadness, and worry must be addressed on an individual and a family level, and hope must be conveyed.

My experience and the literature indicate that sibling incest creates an intense and serious family crisis and must be approached carefully and with certainty. The family has to negotiate a wide range of thoughts and feelings, and sound clinical guidance and clarity by the therapist is imperative. When parents attempt to deal with sibling incest "on their own," they may make informal efforts to separate their children for protection. When their efforts fail, they may seek help that often includes reporting to authorities and mandatory, formal removal of one child (even to relative placements). Thus, it is not unusual for cases of sibling incest to include brief or longer-term separations followed by the goal of reunification.

Parallel Treatment Processes

As mentioned, the children in sibling sexual abuse cases go through a parallel treatment process, with an eye toward meaningful therapeutic dialogues after both have had a chance to process the positive and negative aspects of their past relationship. Adolescent sex offenders are a large, heterogeneous group of children and youth who present with unique treatment needs (Ryan, Hunter, & Murrie, 2012). They don't all abuse for exactly the same reason, and their psychological, emotional, and social skills vary in addition to their family compositions and living environments. There is no "typical" adolescent sex offender, although the literature cites the characteristics of emotional immaturity, low self-esteem, social difficulties, and impulsivity in most of these youth, with aggression cited as also present in some (Barbaree & Marshall, 2006).

The impact of sexual trauma on children has been well documented as contributing to difficulties in physical, emotional, and behavioral regulation, as well as social interactions and attachment (Anda et al., 2006; Chiccheti & Toth, 1995; Cloitre et al., 2009; Cook et al., 2005), but these responses are mediated by many factors, including the presence of threats, force, or coercion; whether penetration occurred; the chronicity and intensity of the abuse; and what can best be described as signs of resilience or stress resistance. Having said that, some sexually abused children have been abused by people who cajole, entertain, or nurture them in order to gain their acceptance and compliance. Thus some young children view the abuse as a playful game and do not experience it as traumatic. It is important to conduct careful assessments to determine how to best help family members.

A Careful Model of Reunification

Over the years of working with sibling incest cases as well as sibling physical abuse cases, it has become very apparent that the best results occur when following a blueprint of reunification services. Although this blueprint is flexible and may need tweaking for individual family needs, it is a course that is charted, one that seems to help clinicians provide steady and careful assistance to families. This blueprint includes specialized, parallel services; clear and ongoing communication among treatment providers; individual and family interventions; and clinical confidence in navigating and guiding complex therapeutic issues.

An Integrative Approach to Reunification

Most contemporary treatment services of abused children include an identified theoretical anchoring, and they give attention to the growing research and evidence-based approaches (Ludy-Dobson & Perry, 2010; Osofsky, 2013). The "prescriptive" approach is gaining popularity because it acknowledges that no single therapy model will fit all clients (Goodyear-Brown, 2009). Clinicians using this approach consider the identifying problem, seek guidance from the research about what effective models are indicated, and then choose the evidence-based strategy that has the greatest likelihood of facilitating positive treatment outcomes. In the field of child sexual abuse, the current treatment of choice for victims is trauma-focused cognitive-behavioral therapy (TF-CBT; Cohen, Mannarino, & Deblinger, 2006); for adolescent sex offenders there are several models that also rely on CBT to achieve goals (Kahn, 2011).

The treatment model I describe in this chapter incorporates CBT with other expressive and systemic approaches. Such an integrative methodology increases the potential for engaging children and their families, for making therapy accessible and less threatening, and for encouraging a holistic approach that attends to cognitive and behavioral changes. In addition, children learn about themselves, the impact they have on others, and how their families have been changed by behaviors that have occurred—all of which facilitates in shifting their perspective. Family members are encouraged to understand how their behaviors will be altered, how their family roles will change, and how their future will be crafted to include preventive efforts so that the abuse does not recur. This is a realistic trauma-informed model of hope, resiliency, and respect in which therapists convey the relevance of their personal and collective investment in positive change. A collaborative, multidisciplinary approach is also applied to optimize family change.

Play Therapy: A Pivotal Strategy

In a previous publication (Gil, 2012) I articulated a treatment approach called *trauma-focused integrated play therapy* (TF-IPT), which evolved within the context of my clinical work over the last three decades. During this time, I prioritized the usefulness of play therapy in addressing victim issues. In particular, I paid special attention to clinical identification and encouragement of posttraumatic play, as well as the integration of directive and nondirective play therapy (as utilized by trained play therapists) and the use of playful therapeutic strategies within a structured, phase-based model of treatment, anchored in trauma theory. With particular attention to Herman's (1997) phases of treatment (establishment of trust and safety, processing of traumatic material, and affiliation with others), TF-IPT became an integrative approach designed to be user-friendly and respectful of client coping strategies. Importantly, this model also allows for client growth and development, as informed by Perry and Szalavitz's 2007 book as well as information on Dr. Perry's website (*www.childtraumaacademy.org*) and his neurosequential model of therapy, which suggests that therapists design the delivery of their interventions in a manner consistent with clients' brain development, specifically attending to parts of the brain that require stimulation first, and avoiding strategies that might override the individual's capacity to be helped. Since the hierarchical structure of the brain is such that the cerebral cortex is the last to develop fully, it appears pertinent and necessary to prepare the child to take part in varied therapeutic tasks that engage multiple functions of the brain.

As mentioned earlier, the experience of safety determines whether traumatized children can move on to the important work of directly processing their trauma. Since relational safety has been compromised in most complex trauma cases, clinicians are well advised to invest time in allowing the child to acclimate to a relationship that does not include relational threat. Acknowledging that children have defensive strategies that were learned in order to cope with overwhelming events and served to protect or help them in some important ways, this approach meets them where they are, and offers them different ways to engage and participate in the therapy process gradually, giving them the time they need to develop a sense of safety and trust in the therapy setting and in the clinician.

An integrative approach makes use of both child-centered play therapy (CCPT; well recognized for its positive treatment outcomes; Bratton, Ray, & Rhine, 2005) at the outset of treatment as well as directed, playful, expressive techniques designed to afford ample opportunities for self-expression, self-directed gradual exposure, and eventual assimilation of traumatic material (Gil, 2011). I believe that inviting children to utilize the *safe-enough distance* provided by play therapy often allows them to move at their own pace and gain genuine feelings of power and mastery; it also increases the possibility that they will participate in treatment in a more meaningful way. In this model, therapists are patient, allow children to find their own healing capacities, encourage self-expression beyond verbal therapy, and maintain a positive relationship with parents, coaching and supporting them to provide the most optimal recovery environment for their children. In addition, therapists also approach client resistance cautiously, gradually introducing more directive approaches to children who remain avoidant of traumatic memories, and who may develop symptoms that continue to signal that traumatic material needs resolution or closure.

There is a new respect for the engaging power of play, and many proponents of TF-CBT have paid special attention to the complementary value of play when delivering their model (Cohen, Mannarino, & Deblinger, 2012). However, important differences occur based on which theoretical approach takes the lead: There is a great difference between viewing play as a mechanism for advancing other goals, thinking of play or toys as a way to "break the ice," and, in contrast, utilizing play as the mechanism of change that has curative factors of its own.

One of the distinguishing features of TF-IPT is the use of play therapy to process traumatic experiences, not only as a way to engage children sufficiently to advance the goal of cognitive and verbal processing. That is not to say that cognitive-behavioral work is overlooked in this model; in fact, cognitive-behavioral methodology is highly valued when children are receptive to talk therapy, when they can engage in insight-oriented therapies, and when they are capable of meaningful cognitive reevaluations of their experiences. What this model offers children and their families (in individual and family formats) are fully valued alternative ways of working with difficult traumatic experiences, including active participation in play therapy and other expressive arts.

Clinical Case Example

The S. family consists of parents, Louise and Shane, both in their early 40s; their first-born son, Tom, 14; their 13-year-old daughter, Candice; and their "surprise child," Harry, 8 years old. Louise told me that she discovered the abuse by walking into her daughter's room to drop off folded clothes. She found Tom and Candice under the covers and Tom had his shirt off and his pants undone. She struggled to understand what was going on, but could not help but notice that Candice had a "faraway look in her eyes," staring at the wall. Louise discussed this incident with Candice's teacher who was legally mandated to report suspected sexual abuse to CPS. However, when Louise said that she was in the house when the abuse occurred and that Tom was not in a caretaking position, CPS did not open the case for investigation. The social worker did, however, encourage Louise to seek therapeutic services for her children, which Louise did reluctantly but with the understanding that something felt disquieting to her. Eventually, after Candice disclosed the full extent of the abuse, the case was again reported, this time to police who pursued the case in Juvenile Court and mandated Tom's participation in sex offender therapy.

Louise and Shane

Louise felt an array of upsetting and polarized feelings that are not unusual for mothers in cases of sibling incest. She was furious and disgusted by what her son had done, while at the same time she felt protective of him, finding it hard to imagine that he could end up in a juvenile detention facility. Sometimes she found herself minimizing what her son had done, hoping that it was less extensive than she thought, or that perhaps it was part of normal childhood sexuality and experimentation. Sadly, she eventually returned to an understanding that what had occurred was not normal, had affected her daughter greatly, and there was no turning away from her son's underlying problems. She talked about the guilt that overwhelmed her rational thoughts and her constant need to think about the past and what signs she had missed. She had not come up with much, except perhaps Shane's work-related absences being a factor and the fact that she might have relied on her son a little too much over the years. I reassured her that her feelings were normal in the context of what she had learned and that many parents feel precisely the same way as she. However, I also cautioned her from trying to latch on to single explanations because those would be hard to find. She did insist, however, that she would have known if her son had been exposed to sexual abuse in the past and had eliminated that from the range of possibility.

Shane felt less guilty and conflicted and kept questioning whether or not his wife was exaggerating the potential impact of what had occurred. He reported that when he was young, maybe 12 or so, his 17-year-old babysitter had introduced him to sexual activity. He claimed that he felt "lucky" to have had this experience, and he remembered going to school and telling all his friends—who couldn't get enough details.

Shane seemed to minimize Candice's experience and saw her as "dramatic" and "spoiled." It was clear that he had more positive feelings about both his boys and either did not understand or relate to his only daughter, or had never invested the time and energy to develop a strong bond with her. This differential treatment was noticeable in the first session that he attended. It was also apparent that Shane and Louise had become distant with each other and lacked healthy modes of communication. At the first joint meeting with them, the parents seemed to be discussing the issues for the first time and often seemed surprised at each other's reactions.

After meeting the parents, it was clear that they were struggling with the news of their son sexually abusing their daughter; that their ability or willingness to problem-solve and communicate was limited; and that they might not see each other as a source of emotional support. In addition, Shane's schedule seemed literally impossible in terms of establishing any kind of regular therapy for them. He conveyed the message that he wanted *us* to "fix this situation" as quickly as *we* could.

Tom

Tom was a charismatic 14-year-old youngster with an easy way of communicating candidly and openly. Initially, he denied the extent of the abuse, but he did not deny "mutual sex play" with his sister. He rejected the idea of abuse because he felt he had not forced her at any time and "if she had said for me to stop, I would have." Tom declared with conviction that his sister seemed to "like experimenting" with him as much as he did with her. He admitted to touching, oral sex, and inserting his fingers in her. He shied away from saying how long this had gone on or how many times it had occurred. (We later found out from Candice that it had started over a year ago and had happened maybe twice a week since it started.)

One of the most interesting aspects of this case was that Tom was so forthcoming about the sexual abuse of his sister, albeit not the chronicity. In some ways, his initial bravado seemed to reflect many thinking errors: It was not forced contact, it was experimental and fun, his sister liked it, and she had never said no. In other words, his initial perception was one of mutuality and thus the notion that he was abusive was minimized and dismissed. His father had told him to tell the truth, and he did so without apology. His presentation was somewhat atypical in his willingness to admit to his sexual behaviors with his sister, more typical in how he depicted them and in his reluctance to disclose fully the chronicity and extent of his behaviors. Over the course of his treatment he became more able to admit fully the extent and compulsive nature of his sexual activities with his sister, as well as his involvement in watching pornography almost daily, and videotaping himself performing oral sex on his sister and sharing the tape with some of his friends at school.

Candice

Candice, 13 years old, was more reticent to speak to me about what had happened with her brother, and it took a good 3 months before she felt comfortable enough to confide the specifics of her abuse. She seemed very worried that she had caused trouble for everyone in the family and that her mother was so upset and crying all the time. She also got very quiet when discussing her father and how he wanted her to "get over it" quickly so they could move on with their lives. Candice seemed sad and somewhat detached early in treatment. Not uncommon in children who have been abused chronically, she had a faraway look at times, and seemed uncomfortable with having a voice, or visibility, in her family. She asserted that she felt safe in her family, that her mother was not allowing Tom to be alone with her, and that Tom's new therapist had met with the family and spoken openly about the fact that Tom was "on notice," and was not allowed to scare, threaten, or otherwise in-

timidate his sister. Candice felt comfortable that Tom would not disobey his dad or he would be "in big trouble." She would not specify further what "big trouble" meant in her family. Candice was especially grateful that she did not have to live with Tom: He had moved to his grandparents' home (who had become foster parents).

Harry

Harry was a sweet younger brother and was close to his sister. He was very involved in school, got good grades, and did lots of after-school activities. He seemed unaware of what had happened between his siblings and informing him became a topic of great discussion in therapy. The parents seemed reluctant to say anything to him initially, but after several questions about where his siblings were during therapy appointments, the parents agreed to give him some basic information, do some prevention training, and increase his understanding of the family's challenges. Often nonabused children can be kept in the dark longer than needed and are confused by their awareness of the unexplained stress the family is undergoing. They also need to be included in order to restore family health. Harry participated in many of the family therapy sessions.

Criteria for Reunification

Although social service agencies are gravely concerned with the need to identify factors that could decrease the reentry of children into the foster care system once they have been reunified, few models exist for reunification services. Generally speaking, the following issues are considered relevant in our reunification model:

1. Completion of specialized services for adolescent sex offenders (which usually involve individual, group, and family therapy) and treatment recommendations specific to investment in therapy.
2. Adherence to probation requirements

in cases when adolescents are adjudicated and asked to meet specific probation conditions.

3. Completion of victim-specific services for child victims of sexual abuse.

4. Sibling sessions in which the offender provides a credible and genuine apology based on new understanding of the impact of the abuse on the victim(s); accountability sessions in which offenders hold themselves accountable for their behaviors.

5. Family therapy designed to identify and correct underlying family dynamics that might have contributed to starting or maintaining the problem behaviors in the home; to ensure parents' cooperation and supervision; to create new patterns, roles, and methods of interacting in safe and appropriate manners.

Generally speaking, treatment (delivered both individually and in family therapy formats) falls into three broad categories: (1) acknowledgment and breaking through denial; (2) trauma-focused exploration of family dynamics that contribute to abuse; and (3) restructuring family dynamics with a focus on strengthening emotional connections, clarifying safety, decreasing secrecy, and building healthy coping strategies. As mentioned earlier, victim–victimizer work occurs in parallel fashion and eventually incorporates sibling sessions followed by family therapy. Even so, the first category is designed to encourage all family members to decrease all forms of denial without minimizing, rationalizing, or justifying abuse. Trepper and Barrett (1989) delineated several ways in which denial could occur: denial of facts, of details, of impact, and of culpability (Trepper & Barrett, 1989). These issues are addressed directly during this initial phase of intervention.

During the second phase of treatment, family dynamics that might have contributed to the emergence of sexual abuse in the family are explored. During this time, it is important for everyone to be cognizant that exploring family dynamics does not mean minimizing the perpetrator's responsibility or shifting of responsibility away from the person who has been abused. This simply means that other factors can come into play and must be acknowledged and addressed sufficiently to prevent recurrence of abuse.

Lastly, the third phase of treatment, restructuring family dynamics, addresses the family's future, with obvious attention to how each family member has shifted his or her perceptions when it comes to reestablishing family relationships and family dynamics. These stages are sequential and any one of them might take more time than another. The first phase, breaking denial, can sometimes be tough to negotiate; however, the second and third phases of treatment will not proceed well without a full investment in acknowledging the problems that have occurred.

Incorporating Play Therapy

Play has unique qualities that allow us to invite a fuller, often less guarded participation in the work of reunification. Families participating in reunification come to therapy with varying levels of hesitancy, ambivalence, pain, confusion, fear, anticipatory anxiety, pessimism, and optimism about their futures.

It is very important to engage families in treatment by being genuinely interested in their difficulties and in finding specific and concrete ways of helping them. From my point of view, play therapy and other expressive arts techniques may help families communicate more easily and deeply, may encourage them to view therapy as playful and nonthreatening, and may give everyone alternative ways of communicating with each other and expressing their substantive concerns. In my experience, play therapy is engaging, immediately helpful, and disarming to clients. It allows us, as therapists, to invite a different kind of emotional connectedness and it promotes and advances important goals in treating sibling sexual abuse. I describe three play therapy interventions that might be helpful in each of the three phases of treatment outlined above. I selected these interventions because they are used in the family therapy phase of treatment, they facilitate positive treatment outcomes in many cases of reunification, and they can be amended for other types of underlying issues.

Puzzle Pieces to Chronicle Proximity and Distance

One way that I have encouraged families to work through this early processing of different experiences is to take a piece of poster board and cut it in half, not with a straight line, but with jagged edges or curves that would fit together like a puzzle. I ask the separated family members to take collage pictures and fill in their halves or portions with images, drawings, words, or anything that communicates what their experience has been living away from their families. I ask them to do this in separate rooms or on different sides of the table. The first step is to name the images that they have included. I coach all of them to simply understand that time has passed, they have

been separated, and each of them has had different experiences. If parents are inappropriate (i.e., use this exercise as a way to instill guilt or shame), I will stop the session, meet with parents alone to encourage them to soften their delivery and put their children's needs ahead of theirs, and allow them to vent all they want with me, not with their children who now need guidance to address the separation.

In later sessions, we make strips of red and brown construction paper: The red strips represent *roadblocks* or obstacles that remain in the way of family members getting closer to each other and achieving an easier reunification; the brown strips represent *building blocks* or specific ways that family members identify positive actions they can take to draw closer to each other. These roadblocks and building blocks are reviewed weekly until the family begins to feel that the building blocks are beginning to outnumber the roadblocks.

As Figure 24.1 illustrates, Shane, Louise, Candice, and Harry filled in the right side of the poster board with images of picnics, camp, friendship, and other symbols that were placed by Candice and likely related to the abuse: a sign that said *danger*, a pic-

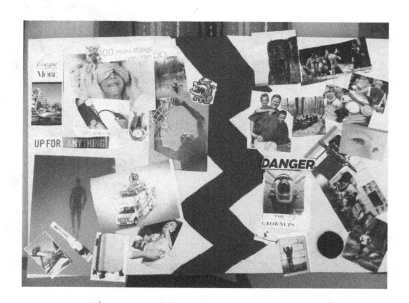

FIGURE 24.1. Acknowledging the rupture.

ture of a child backed up to a wall, a person falling off a cliff. At this particular reunification session, I invited Tom to come with his grandparents, as they were part of the solution to this family's crisis and had also made serious adjustments to provide ongoing care and supervision of Tom, in spite of being older and more conservative in their ways. Tom's grandparents had had a crash course in sexual abuse, trauma, porn, and sexting. Initially reluctant to learn details, they were now fully on board with treatment and cared deeply for their first-born grandson. Tom respected them and reciprocated their affection, but insisted it was "too quiet" in their house and he was eager to return home.

On the left side of the poster, you see grandparents' words (*up for anything, watch this, 100 more things you can do, escape more*) and collage pictures showing some of the changes that had occurred. Grandfather placed the picture of the RV with the car and motorcycle on the top, tied down with rope. "This is pretty much how it's felt," he said. "We haven't been able to travel as we did before." When he noticed Tom's sad look, he touched his hand and said, "but we've gotten used to having him around." Tom added a basketball hoop, a canoe, a suitcase (saying, "I can't wait to get home and get all my stuff back"), the blood pressure machine, and the man with paddles of a defibrillator on his chest. Tom stated that he often worried about his grandparents and hoped nothing bad happened to them "on his watch." His parents felt good to see their son taking some caring responsibility for his grandparents. Once this project was complete, I asked family members to take a look at what they'd made together, make comments or observations (several of which are included), and talk about associations that they had made during the project and share them with each other, including asking questions.

As Figure 24.2 illustrates, the family focused on documenting building blocks that would draw them closer as well as the obstacles that keep them from drawing closer and addressing their problems. The obstacles include secrecy, lack of communication, isolation (from each other), and feelings of insecurity and low self-esteem. Conversely,

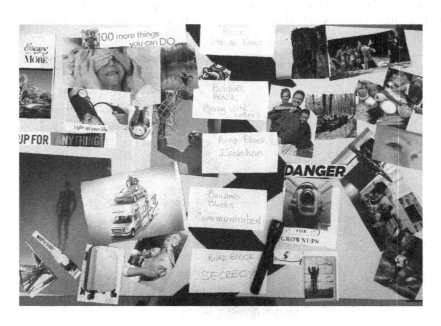

FIGURE 24.2. Building repairs, setting foundations.

the bridges with building blocks include the cell phone (communication), laughter, spending time together, Dad being home more of the time, plus visibility (the flashlight). It was clear that family members had recognized that they were often going in different directions, didn't talk with each other, spent a lot of time alone, and were not feeling good about themselves or their resources.

Acknowledging the Goal of Reunion

The puzzle-piece exercise is used throughout therapy to gauge each person's perception of the progress that is being made toward reunification. The first task that family members are asked to do is to show, using two (or more) portions of the poster board, how close or far they think they are from accomplishing the goal of reunification. I have seen parents bring the opposite puzzle pieces very close together, whereas their children join the pieces at one point on the bottom and make the separation very wide at the top (see Figures 24.3 and 24.4).

These perceptions are documented and often reflect the family's ambivalence about the reunification process that inherently includes losses and challenges for everyone. In this case, although Tom was eager to get home, he also recognized that being around his sister elicited strong and difficult emotions that he did not feel quite ready to confront. Tom's ability to express his ambivalence about coming home as well as his admission of needing more help with his emotions was a very good sign of his progress in treatment.

Another useful benefit of this exercise is that it makes the abstract concrete. Giving the separation and reunification experiences a concrete form (in the poster board and what the family includes as roadblocks and building blocks) allows family members (1) to communicate more safely through image or metaphor, (2) to "see" what they are doing and how they are doing it, and (3) to reflect on their experiences. One of the most pivotal contributions of using play and expressive arts is the possibility these modalities offer to reflect on what

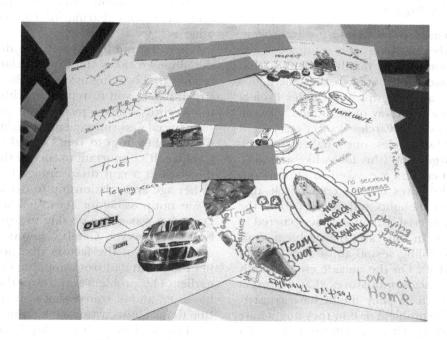

FIGURE 24.3. Concrete representation of the separation.

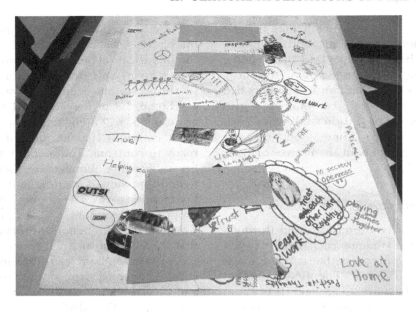

FIGURE 24.4. Concrete representation of closeness/distance.

the unconscious mind has brought forward through symbol and/or through conscious reflection.

The Circles Project

When denial in all its forms is broken, the family moves on to a trauma-focused exploration of the family dynamics that might have contributed to the emergence of sexual abuse. Using the Circles Project might be a good way of introducing the salient issues. The Circles Project consists of drawing two circles, one smaller circle inside a larger one (this looks like a donut). Family members are asked to choose and place miniatures in the center circle that show their thoughts and feelings about the problem or crisis situation that occurred in their lives. In this case, the problem situation was sibling sexual abuse (not the discovery of it). On the outside circle, family members place miniatures that represent how they think they might have contributed to the problem or how they might have kept it going. This is a delicate process for child victims and must be clearly explained. Given that this is the second phase of treat-

ment, child victims might have understood that they made a contribution by keeping the abuse secret. This fact does not place blame on the child but simply explains that children have many limitations that prevent them from sharing information with others.

When the family is given the directive, the clinician takes the lead to clarify the request that is being made: "In the outside circle, I want you to represent with miniatures, words, collage pictures, or drawings your initial and subsequent thoughts, reactions, and feelings to Tom's sexual abuse of Candice. It's important to specify that Candice was at a real disadvantage here, due to her age and relationship to her brother. It was not possible for her to tell Mom and Dad what was going on due to fear of her brother. However, Candice knows that secrecy is one of the factors that prevented her mom and dad from stopping the abuse earlier. The problem was Tom's threats to his sister, and of course that's his contribution to the abuse lasting a long time. I say to the family, "I ask that you dig deeply, look carefully at yourself and your family dynamics, and see what you now see or understand that you didn't see or understand when the abuse was going on." Family members are also asked to include representations of what has helped them, who has been of help, and what (or who) provided them with guidance, support, encouragement, and so forth. This is a very active exploration of family members' insights into their own functioning and how sexual abuse came to emerge and be addressed in their family.

As Figure 24.5 shows, the abuse was described in very specific terms: clouds, lightning, fire, freedom (represented by the girl raising her arms), and a clown removing a mask. The things on the outer circle that had helped were therapy and therapists, church, connecting more on an emotional level, Dad staying home more, doing fewer outside activities, and spending more time with each other. Candice also included her best friend (whom she confided in), as well as her new boyfriend, and Tom included the miniature of the clown taking off his mask (which he had used in many other projects). When the family shared about the objects they had chosen, Candice talked about feeling "hit by lightning, in that lightning was always scary, always came out of nowhere, and was physically painful." This session was the first where Candice began to discuss the emotional *and* physical hurt that Tom had caused her. Her mother and father put their arms around her, literally

and figuratively, offering her support and encouragement for beginning to speak directly to her brother about her perceptions of the abuse. This project is the conduit for reflection and verbal communication, as well as recognition of what thoughts and feelings were at play in the past and need to be managed differently in the future.

Family Aquarium

The family aquarium project is undertaken in the third phase. All family members are asked to draw a picture of a fish, "any fish at all." This project usually takes two or three sessions, but the first is always dedicated to drawing, cutting out, and decorating the fish. Family members are offered glue, glitter, puffy balls, feathers, markers, and crayons. Their task is done individually yet family dynamics are on display.

Shane and Tom drew their chairs closer and seemed to be making jokes about what they were drawing, somehow excluding the family. I waited to see how Louise would handle this situation, and given that we were further along in family therapy, I expected her to take action instead of simply feeling rejected and then isolating herself. I looked at her briefly as she was watching Shane and Tom from the other end of the table, and she suddenly took her chair, moved it between them, and said, "I want

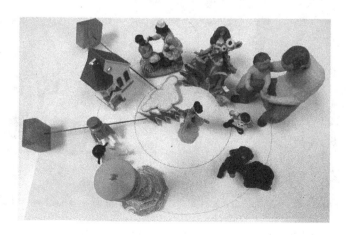

FIGURE 24.5. A solution-focused activity: acknowledging the problem and how it was addressed.

some of the fun!" Tom took the cue immediately and moved closer to his brother to see what Harry was working on. Dad then asked Candice to come to the other side of him and she willingly moved, with a smile on her face. I commented that it looked like the family had taken action to change one of the dynamics we had discussed in other sessions, and I complimented Louise on taking the risk of pulling her chair up, Shane for being receptive and inviting Candice to join them, and Tom for taking the cue and then redirecting his attention to his brother. The family completed their fish drawing/ decorating project with a few laughs and comments about "artistic endeavors."

In the second session, the family is invited to use a poster board as an "aquarium," in which their fish will reside together. Their first directive is this: "As a family, decide together what kind of an aquarium it's going to be . . . decide ahead of time the environment that the fish will share." This directive is open-ended and encourages clients to use projective skills to identify and express what seems important, necessary, and critical for their fish to survive and even thrive.

In addition, another relevant directive is where the fish are going to be placed (eventually glued down) in relation to each other in this environment. Needless to say, this project raised many important issues regarding boundaries, family roles, negotiation of space and privacy, perceptions of danger and safety, etc.

This family made a strong emotional investment in this project, one of the last joint projects that we did in concluding family therapy. The aquarium project became a metaphor for their future and the many ways they felt they had addressed and resolved their crisis, as well as the permanent changes that were implied, and the ongoing need for clarity, safety, openness, and boundaries to be maintained.

The final product was informative for all, and each family member was very proud of what he or she had accomplished and the many therapeutic dialogues that had occurred as they all reflected on their family environment.

As Figure 24.6 shows, an enclosure went up spontaneously around Tom's fish (lower left quadrant), something that even Tom

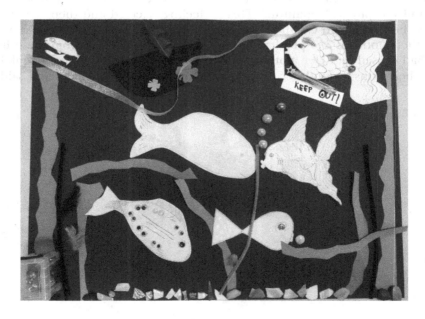

FIGURE 24.6. The type of aquarium where fish coexist.

contributed to, although they never fully agreed on who had started it. In addition, Tom had placed about 6 pairs of eyes on the body of his fish, and he talked about how he both wanted and hated people checking on him. He talked about how he felt he had betrayed everyone's trust and he had to earn it back. At the same time, he seemed aware that external controls would be in place for him for quite a time to come.

Candice was able to put little bells on the door to Tom's container, noting that it would be hard for her to have him live at home again, and that she would want him to have "bells on his door," so that everyone knew when he was coming in and out. The parents also talked about how they had moved Tom away from her sister's room into an attic that created an artificial but very concrete barrier to his sneaking into her room. In addition, Candice had requested a new bed, and her mother took the opportunity to redecorate her room completely, something Candice relished. This room would be "off limits" to her brother, and she had asked that he not be allowed to go in it and that she have a lock and key so that she could keep it private. Mother had acquiesced to this request but also kept a spare key for emergencies.

Father had initially placed himself in a peripheral position in the aquarium, suggesting the distance that he had maintained in the past. Everyone noticed and complained and asked him to join them. The final picture reflects the hope that Mother and Father would be working more closely together and that Dad would stop working out of the home so much. Harry had drawn a small sailboat, to show that people come and go from the aquarium, but the final project does not include the sailboat heading away without a passenger. Rather, Harry chose to put that in his notebook to take home with him (another example of his wanting his dad closer). It took Dad a little while to dismiss his guilt in favor of understanding and accepting what an important part of the family he was to everyone.

When the family reflected on their aquarium project, Tom burst into tears and hugged his mother. He had already had sibling sessions with Candice and had read a prepared statement to her. She had listened attentively and then read her prepared statement to him. Both children had worked diligently to make clear statements to each other, to listen, and to respond. Tom talked about what he had learned about why he abused his sister, how he had manipulated her to be silent, and how he had minimized and justified what he was doing. Candice talked about how the abuse had "taken over her childhood" and had left her feeling dirty and "weak." She said that at first she was mostly afraid that he would hurt her again, especially for telling Mom about the abuse, but later she started feeling stronger and knew that she would not let him hurt her again. Tom and Candice had met in joint sessions with their own therapists first, and then met with their parents so that they could hear what each felt important to say. In addition, Tom had prepared a heartfelt apology to his parents for all the trouble he had caused, for betraying their trust, and for hurting his sister. Candice expressed her anger at her dad for not being around, for not paying as much attention to her as to the boys, and for being mean to her mother at times, teaching Tom that it was okay for boys to be mean to girls. These family therapy sessions raised many strong feelings from everyone, and the family was making real headway addressing the underlying family issues that contributed to the abuse.

During the aquarium project, Tom seemed very moved and blurted out some things to his sister while crying: "I'm sorry for what I did, I feel horrible about it now. I was wrong and I've learned that, and you don't have to believe me right now, but I promise I won't touch you badly ever again, I promise. I want to be just your regular brother from here on out and I know that I can be good now." This spontaneous communication seemed genuine and Candice listened, stating quietly, "That's good you know what you did was wrong." She also said quietly, "I don't trust you yet, and you have to earn that from me and everybody." We worked together on the metaphors that emerged during the aquarium project for about six more sessions and at the end of that time, they framed the aquarium and placed it in a central place in their home as a reminder of the crisis and how it was being overcome.

Conclusion

Parents and their children can be separated for an array of reasons, some voluntary, some not. In cases of parental abuse and neglect, CPS may remove children into foster care when children are at risk of harm from their caretakers. In cases of sibling incest, CPS is called initially and they may refer the case to juvenile justice agencies, which become involved with adolescents who are committing criminal behaviors, such as sexual abuse or physical assaults. There are no standardized responses and depending on a number of factors, cases of sibling sexual abuse can be dismissed with or without legal consequences. In some cases, children are referred for treatment alone, and in other cases parents are encouraged to obtain help if they choose to do so. Consequently, there is little guidance for parents about what to do in situations involving sibling sexual abuse.

When legal or protective services are involved, children may be placed in foster care or relative placements. During family separations, the family is asked to comply with a number of requirements before their children are allowed to return to their homes. One of those requirements is reunification treatment, although few clinical models and resources exist to guide this treatment.

In this chapter, a reunification model is proposed that utilizes an integrative therapy approach that incorporates a variety of theoretical perspectives and models, including a systemic or contextual perspective, CBT, and expressive therapies such as art and play therapy. In addition, the reunification model is delivered in individual, conjoint, and family therapy sessions and has three general phases of treatment: acknowledgment and breaking through denial; trauma-focused exploration of family dynamics that contribute to abuse; and restructuring family dynamics with a focus on strengthening emotional connections, clarifying family roles, parental provision of safety and protection, decreasing secrecy, and building healthy coping and communication strategies.

Over the years of working with sibling incest cases, including those involving physical abuse, it has become very apparent that best results occur when following a structured model or blueprint which remains flexible throughout. This blueprint includes specialized, parallel services for victims and victimizers; clear and ongoing communication among treatment providers; individual and family interventions; and clinical confidence in navigating and guiding complex therapeutic issues. The goals of reunification services are clearly outlined at the outset of therapy and are advanced through integrative therapy models designed to engage and invite families to fully participate in the therapeutic process, decreasing their hesitancies and resistances toward treatment. A combination of directive and nondirective expressive therapy techniques seem most appropriate and yield optimal results.

REFERENCES

Anda, R. F., Felitti, V. J., Brenner, J. D., Walker, J. D., Whitfield, C., Perry, B. D., et al. (2006). The enduring effects of abuse and related adverse experiences in childhood: A convergence of evidence from neurobiology and epidemiology. *European Archives of Psychiatry and Clinical Neuroscience, 256,* 174–186.

Baker, L. (2002). *Protecting your child from sexual predators.* New York: St. Martin's Press.

Barbaree, H. E., & Marshall, W. L. (Eds.). (2006). *The juvenile sex offender* (2nd ed.). New York: Guilford Press.

Bratton, S. C., Ray, D., & Rhine, T. (2005). The efficacy of play therapy with children: A meta-analytic review of treatment outcomes. *Professional Psychology: Research and Practice, 36*(4), 376–390.

Caffaro, J. V., & Conn-Caffaro, A. (1998). *Sibling abuse trauma: Assessment and intervention strategies for children, families, and adults.* New York: Haworth Press.

Cichetti, D., & Toth, S. L. (1995). A developmental psychopathology perspective on child abuse and neglect. *Journal of the American Academy of Child and Adolescent Psychiatry, 34*(5), 542–565.

Cloitre, M., Stolbach, B. C., Herman, J. L., van der Kolk, B., Pynoos, R., Wang, J., et al. (2009). A developmental approach to complex PTSD: Childhood and adult cumulative trauma as predictors of symptom complexity. *Journal of Traumatic Stress, 22*(5), 399–408.

Cohen, J. A., Mannarino, A. P., & Deblinger, E. (2006). *Treating trauma and traumatic grief in children and adolescents.* New York: Guilford Press.

Cohen, J. A., Mannarino, A. P., & Deblinger, E. (2012). *Trauma-focused CBT for children and adolescents: Treatment applications.* New York: Guilford Press.

Cook, A., Spinazzola, J., Ford, J. D., Lanktree, C., Blaustein, M., Cloitre, M., et al. (2005). Complex trauma in children and adolescents. *Psychiatric Annals, 35*, 390–398.

Gil, E. (2011). *Helping abused and traumatized children: Integrating directive and nondirective approaches.* New York: Guilford Press.

Gil, E. (2012). Trauma-focused integrated play therapy. In P. Goodyear-Brown (Ed.), *Handbook of child sexual abuse: Identification, assessment, and treatment* (pp. 251–279). New York: Wiley.

Gil, E., & Roizner-Hayes, M. (1996). Assessing family readiness for reunification. In E. Gil (Ed.), *Systemic treatment of families who abuse.* San Francisco: Jossey-Bass.

Goodyear-Brown, P. (2009). *Play therapy with traumatized children: A prescriptive approach.* New York: Wiley.

Herman, J. L. (1997). *Trauma and recovery: The aftermath of violence-from domestic abuse to political terror.* New York: Basic Books.

Jones, L. (1998). The social and family correlates of successful reunification of children in foster care. *Children and Youth Services Review, 20*(4), 305–323.

Kahn, T. J. (2011). *PATHWAYS: A guided workbook for youth beginning treatment* (4th ed.). Brandon VT: Safer Society Press.

Kitzmann, K. M., Gaylord, N. K., Holt, A. R., & Kenny, E. D. (2003). Child witness to domestic violence: A meta-analysis review. *Journal of Consulting and Clinical Psychology, 71*, 339–352.

Ludy-Dobson, C. R., & Perry, B. (2010). The role of healthy relational interactions in buffering the impact of childhood trauma. In E. Gil (Ed.), *Working with children to heal interpersonal trauma: The power of play* (pp. 27–43). New York: Guilford Press.

Osofsky, J. (Ed.). (2013). *Clinical work with traumatized children.* New York: Guilford Press.

Perry, B. D., & Szalavitz, M. (2007). *The boy who was raised as a dog: And other stories from a child psychiatrist's notebook–What traumatized children can teach us about loss, love, and healing.* New York: Basic Books.

Roizner-Hayes, M. (1994). *Therapists' attitudes towards the reunification of incestuous families after treatment.* Unpublished doctoral dissertation, Boston University.

Ryan, E. P., Hunter, J. A., & Murrie, D. (2012). *Juvenile sex offenders: A guide to evaluation and treatment for mental health professionals.* New York: Oxford University Press.

Sheinberg, M., True, F., & Fraenkel, P. (1994). Treating the sexually abused child: A recursive multimodal approach. *Family Process, 33*(3), 263–276.

Terling, T. (1999). The efficacy of family reunification practices: Reentry rates and correlates of reentry for abused and neglected children reunited with their families. *Child Abuse and Neglect, 23*(12), 1359–1370.

Trepper, T., & Barrett, M. J. (1989). *Systemic treatment of incest: A therapeutic handbook.* New York: Brunner/Mazel.

Wiehe, V. (1997). *Sibling abuse: Hidden physical, emotional, and sexual trauma* (2nd ed.). Thousand Oaks, CA: Sage.

CHAPTER 25

Play-Based Disaster and Crisis Intervention

ROLES OF PLAY THERAPISTS IN PROMOTING RECOVERY

Anne L. Stewart
Lennis G. Echterling
Claudio Mochi

The 4-year-old dancer struck an elegant pose, her arms outstretched above her tiny frame, as if she were still wearing the bangles that previously adorned her wrists. With the older children and adults singing and clapping their encouragement, she began to dance with a grace and poise that belied her age. Just weeks earlier, the tsunami had wreaked havoc on her beloved Sri Lanka, destroying entire communities, killing thousands of people, and leaving countless survivors without their homes, livelihoods, and loved ones. Now, on the site of her devastated village, the child performed a traditional dance to welcome the arrival of play therapists who were members of an international disaster recovery team. Later, the therapists invited the children to engage in play-based activities designed to enhance their ability to focus, regulate their emotions, and adaptively cope with the countless challenges they would face in the midst of the annihilation left in the wake of the tsunami. However, at this moment, the play therapists were bearing witness to this inspiring welcoming ritual that they recognized as reflecting the deep, abiding bonds of attachment among these villagers.

The child no longer possessed the bangles she had used in her dancing before the tsunami, but her manner was so entrancing that everyone there could almost hear the musical chiming of her bracelets. As vital members of the disaster recovery team, the play therapists brought none of the materials necessary for rebuilding the physical infrastructure of this village. Instead, they welcomed and graciously accepted the child's dance, noted how the community members took such obvious delight in the child, and appreciated how wholeheartedly the community had helped create and enter her imagined reality. In other words, the villagers honored a creative experience that facilitated their recovery of their most important and fundamental infrastructure of all: the supportive, interwoven, and interdependent web of human attachments that characterized their resilient community.

Research and Theory

In the wake of a devastating natural disaster or in the aftermath of the horrific violence of a war, play may seem to many to be a frivolous, trivial, and inconsequential activity. However, as play therapists, we recognize its power as a dynamic, life-affirming process that can be intrinsically fulfilling, thoroughly absorbing, and ultimately rewarding, especially in times of crisis. In fact, play is an essential component of the recovery process. Many children use play to act out their traumatic experiences, but they also can demonstrate their resilience in their play. The U.N. High Commission on Refugees commissioned a study of the physical and psychological well-being of children displaced from their homes in Syria. The resulting report, *The Future of Syria: Refugee Children in Crisis* (UNHCR), includes a discussion of the importance of play and describes play-based programs in place to help children mitigate the disruptive impact of displacement and violence (UNHCR, 2013). Many nongovernmental organizations (NGOs) are now promoting sport and play as innovative recovery strategies in postdisaster and postconflict situations (Kunz, 2009). By participating in all forms of play, including games and sports, children and families engage in the process of re-creation by strengthening their ties of attachment, regulating their emotions, enhancing their self-esteem, and reinvigorating themselves.

By creating specialized play-based interventions, play therapists can normalize reactions, invite children and families to try out new coping strategies, modify cognitive distortions, increase self-soothing, enrich relationships, enhance social support, and offer a sense of hope (Echterling & Stewart, in press; National Child Traumatic Stress Network, 2013). Play provides opportunities to respond to novel situations, practice newly developed behaviors, and engage in creative problem solving (Pellegrini, Dupuis, & Smith, 2007; Smith, 2010). Because it is universal, individuals can engage in play to connect quickly with those from other cultures. Play therapists are especially adept at creating a safe haven that can serve as a refuge for children and families who

are coping with catastrophic events (Dugan, Snow, & Crowe, 2010).

In this chapter we describe the contributions play therapists can offer in crisis and disaster intervention programs. We begin by highlighting the research on the psychological impact of disasters and providing a conceptual framework that integrates the concept of resilience and attachment theory. Next, we discuss the challenges that confront play therapists in crisis and disaster interventions. We then provide an overview of the roles that they can fulfill as vital members of disaster response teams. Finally, we conclude this chapter by offering practical, play-based techniques that play therapists can use in any of the roles they may serve in disaster intervention—consultant, trainer, supervisor, or therapist—under circumstances that are dramatically different from the usual play therapy office. Readers may be surprised to find that they can adapt these play therapy activities to creatively address needs during virtually any phase of the disaster recovery process.

Negative Consequences of Disasters and Toxic Environments

By 2050, the violence, devastation, and chaos of wars, social conflicts, and natural disasters will have directly affected at least 2 billion individuals throughout the world (Ronan & Johnston, 2005). Researchers have documented that, in addition to the physical, environmental, and economic consequences, these catastrophic events can have a psychological impact (Gulliver, Zimering, Carpenter, Giardina, & Farrar, 2014). Disasters threaten to upset children's emotional well-being and disrupt their developmental trajectories by inflicting pervasive trauma, wrecking infrastructures, undermining regular social interactions, and sabotaging families' support networks (Catani, Jacob, Schauer, Kohila, & Neuner, 2008). In addition to documenting the impact of these disastrous events, researchers have gathered disturbing evidence of the corrosive effects of ongoing biologically and psychologically toxic conditions on children's well-being. Furthermore, children's emotional, mental, and behavioral disorders are interconnected and stem largely from a set of common conditions, including the harmful impact of poverty (National Research Council & Institute of Medicine, 2009; Yoshikawa, Aber, & Beardslee, 2012).

Unfortunately, our practice and research endeavors continue to treat children's problems as if they were isolated and not related to each other, to the detriment of their overall mental and physical health. Based on these findings, Biglan, Flay, Embry, and Sandler (2012) argued that our intervention efforts should create *nurturing environments*. They described nurturing environments as ones that promote healthy development by reducing threats from toxic events, encouraging prosocial behaviors (including self-regulation), and fostering mindful reflection. The emphasis on working to establish nurturing physical and psychological environments is especially relevant for play therapists who conduct their work in community, school, and health care settings. The framework illustrates the crucial role for play therapists in fostering collaborative help-giving efforts across a variety of disciplines, agencies, and conditions, particularly during crisis conditions.

Resilience

We live in a time of highly publicized crises and catastrophes during which the news media bombard the public with countless narratives portraying survivors as pitiable victims. Occasionally, one or two individuals are spotlighted as inspiring heroes who overcome extraordinary obstacles. However, in contrast to these misleading portrayals, the vast majority of disaster survivors are neither helpless nor superhuman. Instead, the research has documented that they are typical individuals doing their best to adapt to abnormal circumstances—in

other words, most children and families are resilient (Prince-Embury & Saklosfske, 2013).

In physics, *resilience* refers to the extent that a material can endure strain and return to its original shape. Recently, ecologists, political scientists, and economists have found productive ways to apply the concept of resilience to disasters. For example, environmental scientists and engineers are collaborating to design resilient coastlines that can withstand the impact of hurricanes. Personal resilience is a core concept of the emerging positive psychology movement (Cohrs, Christie, White, & Das, 2013), and social scientists now have expanded the concept of personal resilience to that of social resilience to reflect the posttraumatic recovery of communities as they transform and adapt (Keck & Sakdapolrak, 2013). In the wake of a disaster, communities vary greatly in their ability to recover and reinitiate normal social functioning. In some cases, entire societies are so profoundly affected that they disintegrate and are lost to humanity. In other cases, not only do they quickly attain some semblance of normal functioning, but also they eventually grow and thrive (Norris, Sherrieb, & Pfefferbaum, 2011).

Resilience has provided an exciting conceptual framework for providing play-based disaster intervention services. Instead of concentrating on only identifying the psychological casualties of catastrophes, play therapists can offer interventions that promote resilience and avoid pathologizing the reactions of survivors. Moreover, Calhoun and Tedeschi (2006) have proposed the concept of posttraumatic growth (PTG) to reflect the profound and positive changes that most trauma survivors demonstrate later in their lives. These benefits include more confidence, enhanced relationships, deeper compassion, and greater maturity. Fundamentally, resilience is the process through which disaster victims become survivors who can then go on to thrive in their lives.

Attachment Theory

Why should play therapists be concerned about the quality of a child's attachment in times of disaster? How can promoting more secure attachments enhance our disaster intervention work? One compelling reason to use the attachment perspective is that catastrophes threaten children's relationships with parents, teachers, and peers. In addition, many children's posttraumatic symptoms reflect basic difficulties in their regulation of behavior, thoughts, and feelings. Disturbances in the felt security of relationships and disruptions in regulation are central concerns addressed in attachment-based interventions.

Attachment theory provides a holistic framework through which to understand resilience. Atwool (2006) stated:

> Attachment theory adds weight to resilience theory by clearly outlining the significance of relationships as the key to all aspects of resilience—culture, community, relationships and individual. Integrating attachment theory and the concept of resilience clarifies the adaptive nature of behavior and refines our understanding of the types of relationship experiences necessary to promote positive adaptation. (p. 327)

The secure pattern of relationship development is the attachment pattern most associated with resilience (Grossmann, Grossmann, & Waters, 2006). Children with secure attachments are better at social problem solving, are more successful academically, have fewer behavior problems, are at lower risk for psychiatric problems, and are more likely to be law-abiding citizens (e.g., Sroufe, 2005; Sroufe, Egeland, Carlson, & Collins, 2005). In fact, the brain of a securely attached child continues to develop an increasingly sophisticated structure of neural connections and subroutines that results in enhanced social competence (Schore, 2001). Therefore, overall goals of an attachment-based play therapist is to reorder and organize the child's internal experiences through attuned and responsive interactions, so that the child's automatic feelings and behavior become more resilient.

A review of the resilience and attachment research identified four factors that promote successful resolution of crises and disasters (Echterling & Stewart, in press). These four pathways to recovery include receiving social support, making meaning, managing emotions, and learning coping strategies. Later in this chapter we offer examples of play-based disaster intervention techniques that promote dimensions of resilience and attachment and provide opportunities for children and families to connect with and explore both their natural and relational worlds.

Play Therapists as Disaster Interveners

In recent years mental health professionals have gained the well-earned acceptance and respect as integral members of crisis and disaster response teams throughout the world. In particular, the professional training, experiences, and techniques of play therapists make them uniquely qualified to serve as resources in disaster recovery programs, especially for the children and families who are survivors of such catastrophic events (Jordan, Perryman, & Anderson, 2013).

Play-based disaster interventions encompass a wide range of services, including assessment, consultation, training, supervision, and program evaluation, in addition to any rapid, brief, and direct assistance to survivors (Echterling, Presbury, & McKee, 2005), as well as intensive therapies designed to facilitate successful problem resolution (Steele & Kuban, 2013).

Challenges of Crisis and Disaster Intervention

In your typical practice as a play therapist, you probably offer your services at appointed times in a well-equipped private office that reinforces a sense of safety and security for your clients. You also probably have immediate access to therapeutic tools that may not be easily transported. Toys, figures, puppets, and children's books are often within hand's reach to help you encourage a child's emotional expression and personal growth. Diplomas, certificates, and textbooks—the artifacts that speak to your legitimacy as a mental health service provider—may cover the walls, reassuring clients of your professional expertise. In your play therapy practice, you also ordinarily conduct a parent intake, consult with other professionals, complete a comprehensive assessment, develop a treatment plan, and establish therapeutic goals before you fully engage in play therapy.

In contrast, your crisis interventions with the survivors of large-scale conflicts, wars, and natural disasters are likely to be unscheduled and take place any time during the day or night. You may be working in a nontraditional setting, such as the gymnasium in a devastated town, the corner of an emergency shelter, or a tent in a refugee camp. Without an appointment schedule, your encounters with survivors may last a couple of minutes or go on for several hours. Although the appearance of your usual practice may contrast dramatically with your practice in the face of crises and disasters, there is one common element connecting these situations—you. In every therapeutic encounter, whether taking place in your familiar office or a debris field, your most important and reliable play therapy tool is *yourself* (Echterling & Stewart, in press). Across a broad range of circumstances, you will connect in attuned and supportive ways to demonstrate your ability to make a positive difference for survivors and colleagues.

First, Know Thyself

Given the fact that you are your most important tool, before you explore deployment possibilities as the member of a disaster response team, you must engage in a process of honest self-reflection and assessment to determine your readiness to offer effective interventions following a catastrophic event (Echterling & Stewart, in press). In this regard, the American Psychological Association has offered guidelines based on the recommendations of the Inter-Agency Standing Committee (IASC; 2007), the primary group that facilitates decision making in response to complex emergencies and natural disasters.

First, you must be willing to be deployed under an appropriate sponsoring organization. Self-deployed interveners, or "lone wolves," run the risk of sabotaging the coordinated efforts of those disaster response teams who are responsible for providing services. Furthermore, your deployment will necessarily use some of the resources that are already critically limited, so being a part of an official disaster recovery organization will ensure that food, clothing, and shelter will be available as much as possible to those with the greatest needs.

A second fundamental guideline for you to follow is to be properly trained in disaster mental health practices, fully prepared to endure the inevitable hardships, ready to tolerate the confusion inherent in the chaos of disaster sites, and willing to follow the policies of your sponsoring organization. You may be an excellent play therapist with traumatized children and families in traditional therapeutic settings. That said, it may not be a good match for you to work under chaotic, primitive, or hazardous conditions. Consult with your colleagues and refer to your discipline's professional practice standards and code of ethics to inform your decision making in this regard. In particular, you must take care to not compromise the interests of your current play therapy clients, undermine the mission of your practice, create undue burdens on your colleagues who may be covering for you, or sacrifice the well-being of your family and friends.

Third, you must examine your motivations to engage in disaster intervention. Are you working out your own unresolved issues from previous catastrophic events that you have personally endured? Certainly your own crisis and disaster experiences can provide you with an empathic bridge to the suffering of survivors, but you may also find yourself overidentifying with their pain and opening up old wounds of your own. Are you hoping to be the valiant rescuer of passive and pathetic victims? If so, then you are not only likely to be ineffective, but you may actually do more harm than good. These first three guidelines underscore a simple and important fact: Every member of the disaster response team should represent an added value to the recovery process.

A final important guideline is that you must ensure that your interventions will respect and celebrate the local languages, cultures, and customs. Your training in multicultural issues and your experience working with diverse client populations can help to some extent in this regard. However, it may be especially challenging when you find yourself immersed in a different country in which not only the climate, but also the dominant culture, is radically unlike your own. Being a stranger in a strange land, particularly in the wake of a disaster, can be disorienting and confusing. Nevertheless, as a play therapist, you have been thoroughly trained to embrace the stance of not knowing, which is an essential therapeutic quality. Stepping down from that expert pedestal to learn from survivors about their hopes, dreams, needs, and values will guide you throughout your disaster work, from designing meaningful interventions to selecting culturally appropriate animal puppets, relying on traditional crafts, and using suitable rituals. For example, in preparing play-based disaster interventions following a tsunami, it was learned that monkeys in Sri Lanka are not considered to be silly animals, as they are in most Western societies. Instead, monkeys are respected as wise creatures, and turned out to be excellent characters for dispensing sage advice about coping strategies.

The Good News

After you have fully addressed these difficult considerations, the good news is that if you are ready, willing, and able to provide interventions under the "ground zero" circumstances of a disaster, you can make an enormous contribution to the resilience of children and families who have endured catastrophic events. One of the most robust and consistent findings in child development—as well as disaster, trauma, and crisis research—is the positive influence of a significant relationship in helping a child to recover, avoid negative outcomes, and even thrive later in life (Stewart & Echterling, 2014). Your therapeutic presence means that you may be creating one of those transformative experiences, significant interactions, and healing relationships. The purpose of crisis intervention is not to achieve a cure. Instead, it is to promote resilience by supporting the innate potential for hope and resolve that all children and families possess. Because you intervene at such a crucial turning point in a child's life and a family's history, a seemingly small intervention can make a profound difference for years to come.

Roles of Play Therapists on Disaster Response Teams

Well-prepared play therapists have vital roles to perform in optimizing the ability of children, families, organizations (e.g., schools and mental health agencies), and communities to prosper and thrive after catastrophic events. By using your clinical expertise, encouraging healthy parent–child interactions, following recommended practices, and designing culturally sensitive interventions, you can assist stakeholders, community leaders, first responders, teachers, faith-based organizations, neighborhoods, and parents in the rebuilding process by offering training and consultation. In some circumstances, you may deliver direct services as a response team member or as a model for local interveners, who observe, assess, and adapt potentially helpful intervention methods.

As a member of a disaster response team, you must follow protocols and fulfill certain roles, but you also must be flexible while you are engaging in play-based interventions involving children, families, and entire communities (Baggerly & Exum, 2008). This is a dialectical and dynamic process in which you are both intentional and spontaneous. Just as you do in your play therapy practice, you need to vary your interventions in disaster work according to the specific situations. Nevertheless, you also follow fundamental principles: You provide survivors with the support of a nurturing environment, opportunities for meaning making, practice in managing emotions, and resources for coping. In the next section we describe the different roles a play therapist may fulfill as a member of a disaster response team.

Because your goal is to facilitate a successful and sustained disaster recovery, your roles will vary according to the current needs and circumstances of survivors. For example, at the initial impact of a disaster, you may *provide psychological first aid* (National Child Traumatic Stress Network, 2013), in which you engage in the evidence-informed strategy of reaching out with compassion, giving social support, and creating a nurturing environment. At this point of the recovery process, you are primarily concerned with ensuring the safety and security of the survivors, providing physical and emotional comfort, offering a calm and caring presence, engaging in reassuring conversation, and limiting their exposure to distressing stimuli.

Another role you may be fulfilling early in the aftermath of the disaster is that of *needs assessor* or *program evaluator*. Effective community-wide programs require accurate assessment information on the impact of the catastrophe not only on the local environment, economy, and physical infrastructure, but also on the psychological well-being of the community residents. Your expertise in child development, interviewing skills, insight into system dynamics, and case conceptualization abilities are valuable resources in gathering meaningful data regarding the psychological impact of the disaster on children, youth, and families. Just as it is the case in your play therapy practice, your interventions in disasters should be based on accurate assessments of the needs of the clients and should include methods of evaluating your therapeutic effectiveness. Research has shown (e.g., Pearson & Mitroff, 1993; Reyes & Jacobs, 2006; Wickrama & Wickrama, 2011) that programs which are not attuned to the culture, the needs of the survivors, or the assets of the community can produce unintended but seriously damaging consequences.

Other important roles that you may perform, especially if you are deployed to a foreign country, are those of *consultant, trainer,* and *supervisor.* Performing these roles in a disaster response team can have a "pyramid effect." By collaborating and sharing your expertise with a number of indigenous helpers, each of whom can offer direct services to many more survivors, your knowledge can be adapted for the culture and circumstances in the most beneficial and widespread form. Because they are members of the local community, the indigenous providers are likely to be much more effective and to remain there throughout the recovery process.

While you are offering these "indirect services," you need to keep in mind that in any community reeling from a catastrophe, all its members are survivors. They may not have been at the epicenter of the disaster or have lost any loved ones, but everyone has been profoundly affected, perhaps even vicariously traumatized, by the disaster. Therefore, whenever you work with indigenous consultees, trainees, and supervisees, always assume that you are also intervening with disaster survivors. Your demonstrations, experiential learning activities, feedback, and discussions may not only enhance their knowledge and skills, but also promote their own personal resilience. They may leave these encounters with a profound appreciation for the power of play-based interventions. Ultimately, as a result of collaborating with local community resources and equipping indigenous workers with play therapy skills, your work can be not only more effective, but also self-sustaining. Of course, your effectiveness as a consultant, trainer, or supervisor is enhanced when you can accompany indigenous helpers in their fieldwork, model the skills they are learning, observe their performance, and give them practical and immediate feedback.

Strategies and Techniques

All catastrophic events share certain commonalities: overwhelming devastation, disorienting chaos, and pervasive suffering. Nevertheless, they vary tremendously in their causes, circumstances, processes, and effects. The precipitating causes may be climate, geology, war, human greed, nationalism, religious ideology, accidents, or ethnic violence. The circumstances may include historical trauma, poverty, marginalization, geography, available resources, and culture. The process may have been sudden, haphazard, or predictable. The impact may have affected entire communities, including such infrastructures as transportation, power, and communication, whereas other infrastructures may be virtually unaffected. Because of this multilevel diversity, all interventions must necessarily be improvisational.

In this section, we describe a sampling of techniques that you can use in any of the roles you may be performing in the wake of a disaster; we believe that these approaches are also relevant to your regular therapeutic work with everyday crises. The techniques require minimal materials and can be implemented in virtually any setting, however primitive the conditions. The activities can take any form of creative expression—playing, drawing, singing, sculpting, dancing, storytelling, and making music. You can find descriptions of many other play-based activities for disaster survivors in Echterling and Stewart (in press) and from the National Child Traumatic Stress Network—Terrorism and Disaster Branch (2005). Although you will not have the luxury of a well-stocked play therapy room when you do disaster work, you can create a portable tote bag of toys and other materials for play-based interventions (Landreth, 2012). In this chapter we introduce a new resource for promoting survivors' well-being: the great outdoors.

With special attention to maintaining physical safety or exposure to harsh scenes, you may be able to explore the outdoors or collect items from nature for use in your activities. This intentional connection with nature, particularly when a natural disaster has occurred, is an untapped resource for play therapists. Research findings indicate that exposure to, or interaction with nature enhances creativity, attention and focus, and an overall sense of well-being (Louv, 2011; Wells & Evans, 2003). Disengagement from nature has been associated with increased levels of anxiety, depression, and higher incidences of attention-deficit disorder (ADD) and attention-deficit/hyperactivity disorder (ADHD) (Taylor & Kuo, 2006). In a study of school-age children, Wells and Evans (2003) found that the presence of nearby nature bolsters a child's resilience against stress and adversity, particularly among those children who experience a high level of stress. We strongly encourage play therapists to explore ways to strategically incorporate outdoor experiences with their clients as part of their interventions and to select natural items for use in the playroom. Therapists can help promote a playful and relationship-based reconnection to nature for survivors of natural and human-induced disasters.

Basic Principles

Before describing specific play-based techniques, we want to mention some basic principles of effective disaster intervention. First, you should always intervene with LUV—listen, understand, and validate—the essential ingredient of any therapeutic encounter (Echterling et al., 2005). When you offer LUV, you are actively *listening* to the child's verbal and nonverbal messages, communicating your empathic *understanding* of the child's thoughts and feelings, and *validating* unconditionally the child's innate worth. When children and families do not experience LUV, your play-based interventions, however elegant, can seem to be only manipulative ploys or meaningless stunts. By offering your LUVing presence, you create a safe haven, a psychological refuge, and a nurturing environment in troubled times.

Another basic principle of disaster intervention is to recognize and value the resilience of children and families—to presume that they are survivors, not pathetic and passive victims. In the midst of the physical devastation and emotional turmoil, disaster survivors also have undiscovered strengths, overlooked talents, and unnoticed resources. As children and families begin to experience their own sense of empowerment, recognize their untapped capabilities, and reconnect to sources of sustenance and nurturance, they build the psychological scaffolding for disaster recovery.

Social Support

The purpose of these interventions is to help children and families connect with one another to find support, comfort, and nurturance as they embark on the journey of recovery.

Pebble Pictures

Invite the family or small group of children to take a walk outside (through a park,

their backyard, along a river, or along a neighboring street) and find a pebble that is interesting to each of them. Once found, these unique pebbles can be painted with any image or phrase that is meaningful to the pebble holder. After the pebbles have been painted, ask the family members to describe what they found special about their pebble and what influenced the design they created.

You can comment on the similarities and differences in the collection. The pebbles are similar to the complexity of a family system or group, and each pebble is unique. Some pebbles may have bumps or sharp edges and others may be smooth and worn. Each pebble has had unique experiences that shaped it into its exclusive form, and when these pebbles (and family or group members) come together, they create a strong foundation upon which to rebuild and thrive. As an alternative, the pebbles would not be painted and family members could simply comment on how the pebble's shape, color, and other characteristics reflect their own strengths and values.

Group Puppet Play

Due to the helpful influence of routines, group puppet play can be a regular activity for children (or a family) to play, focusing on different topics chosen by the therapist or children. A variety of puppets or figures are needed for the activity. Children can also draw the animal or character they wish on paper and fasten it to a stick. The therapist poses a situation or theme—such as "a big storm is coming" or "an important lesson I learned"—and each child selects a puppet (or figure) to use. When the puppet/character selection is done, the children are invited to imagine they are all gathered in a safe place. Each puppet character is asked to tell about his experience and perspectives, including who and what helped then and now, and what advice the character has for the other characters in the play (adjust according to the children's age and topic).

An example demonstrates the power of this technique. After a devastating earthquake, the surviving children had repeatedly conducted puppet shows and were making good progress in their recovery. However, some of the young children continued to be fearful when strong winds blew, a common occurrence in the area. It was decided to involve the children in a play about "What I do when the strong winds blow." The children chose their puppets. After a moment of silence, a little girl of 7, acting as a horse, proudly said that she would run fast when the winds blew strong, and in this way, she could escape any danger.

Another young boy said, "I'm a very fast monkey. I find safe places to hide because earthquakes come with the wind."

Suddenly, a boy with his puppet bear announced, "A friend told me that the wind and earthquake do not go together."

The play therapist interjected, "I agree with the bear! The grown-ups are here to help you stay safe when the wind is loud and fast. Wind does not make an earthquake."

The play therapist then asked the bear, "So what could we all do when the wind is blowing very strong?"

The child with the bear puppet said, "We will be brave. If we are afraid, we can go to our family. We will tell each other that the wind is wind and not an earthquake." The other puppets agreed with him and cheered the bear for his idea.

The play therapist shared the children's play with other leaders and family members. The bear's advice was then linked with additional exercises (e.g., deep breathing) to help children regulate their hyperaroused symptoms. As in this case, an underlying and often overlooked assumption of these techniques is that children are also resources in times of crisis. Providing children with the opportunity to make a positive difference during troubled times can promote their own sense of resilience.

Meaning Making

Meaning-making activities offer children and families opportunities to give form to raw experiences, gain some sense of cognitive mastery, and make important discoveries about their strengths and resources.

Creating a Safe and Secure Place

Invite children or family members to close their eyes, relax, and think of a time in an outdoor place when they felt safe and secure. Ask them to recall their surroundings—the sights, sounds, and smells—and reminisce about who was with them, what they experienced, and how they felt. Invite them to gather items to build a small, safe place that creates those same feelings of security that they experienced in their imagination. Ask them, children or family members, to then choose an item to represent themselves and place it in the safe place (sometimes they have already done this in their creation). Children and family members share stories about the safe places in nature they recalled and how they might be used to help them survive this crisis.

You can collect items and have them on hand for survivors to use, or you can incorporate a walk together or invite them to collect items from nature and bring to the next meeting. Familiar items collected to build safe and secure place constructions include seeds, plants, stones, leaves, shells, sticks, moss, flowers, grasses, and bark.

Collecting items in nature following a natural disaster may help establish a sense of normalcy and hope. You may wish to intentionally go on a walk to look for signs of hope in nature. Technology can be used productively in this activity. Perhaps you carry a photo (paper or on your phone) of a place that provides comfort, peace, or solace for you. A few weeks after Hurricane Katrina, along the saltwater-saturated coast, we were inspired to take this photo of a bright green sprig of fresh growth in the midst of acres of decay (Figure 25.1).

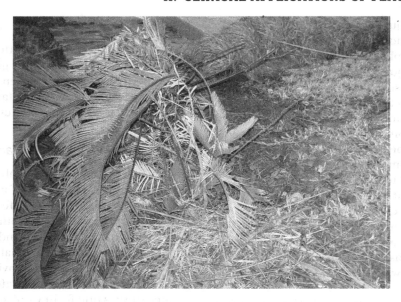

FIGURE 25.1. Sign of hope.

Nurtured by Nature

Over time, the following activities integrating items from nature can help children to transform their crisis experiences into survival stories. In each instance, the children share their creation with you, their family, or others in a group, creating a more coherent narrative of their own experience and bearing witness to the resilience of others.

And Then . . . !

The children or family members are seated in a circle with the collected natural materials in one bag. You begin the story by establishing the people, place, and plot. Use phrasing that distances the story from the current surroundings and time. For example, you might say, "It was a chilly day in a land far away and the brave villagers were just waking up," or "Long ago, the Brio family decided to spend the day together in a magical and fun forest." When you pause, a child or family member then pulls an item out of the bag and uses it to "fill in the blank." For example, your story might start this way, "One day, just as the sun was going down, some friends were walking in the meadow. One friend's name was _____!" A child who pulled out a stick could volunteer, "Stick!" or "Woody!" The story continues with you incorporating the child's comments directly. For example, "Woody turned to his friends with his eyes opened wide with surprise. They could not believe what they saw walking across the meadow. It was an ever so small _____!" Adjust the complexity, content, amount of structure, and twists and turns in the story to match the children's therapeutic goals, verbal ability, and familiarity with the activity. Using a variety of sensory, movement, thinking, and feeling prompts, always include a problem (attainable) or challenge. It is useful to include more than one failed attempt before a resolution to the dilemma is achieved. When the story has an end, it can be recapped and recited together, with everyone pitching in to put the details of the narrative in the correct order. There are often amusing mistakes and reauthoring as the tale is retold. (Thanks to Janet Stewart for sharing this collective storytelling activity.)

Word of Hope on Stone

Help children select a stone and then draw a symbol or write the name of who or what helps them feel safe, hopeful, happy, peaceful, etc., in times of crisis.

Circle of Strength

Children make a circle in the sand or dirt and put in items from nature that help them know they are stronger, confident, have friends, etc. Of course, you can complete this activity with other meaningful items and use a circle of string or a circle drawn on paper.

Then, Now, Next

Children or families select natural objects that represent them before the disaster, at this moment, and in the future. They tell why they chose the particular items and create a story about their journey. You may comment on shared struggles, accomplishments, or destinations.

We believe that using materials from the natural world offers a creative and in-spirational alternative to more traditional objects. We hope you will consider trying some of these variations to meet the needs and goals of survivors, while monitoring the "on-the-ground" conditions of physical and psychological safety.

Regulating Emotions

The Volcano Speaks

This activity was introduced to us by David Crenshaw and combines several therapeutic tasks, including problem identification, labeling of emotions, and verbal mediation with problem solving in an engaging metaphor. The activity begins with asking children to think of an event that made them angry (or other intense emotion). Next, they choose a symbol (e.g., volcano, dragon, storm) to depict their anger and draw it. You then introduce verbal mediation by telling the children to pretend the symbol can talk and give words to the anger it feels—what would it be saying? Interview and expand the ideas in metaphor. Figure 25.2 was drawn by a 10-year-old girl, who proclaimed that the volcano said, "Burn it down! Every-

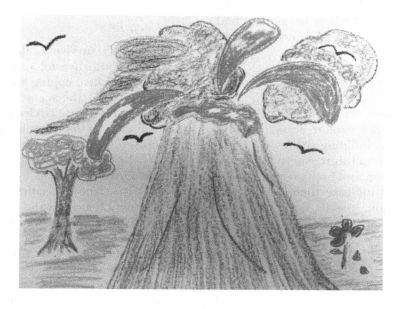

FIGURE 25.2. The volcano speaks.

thing is destroyed!" Collaboratively identify alternatives that could prevent the strong angry feelings, thoughts, or behaviors from occurring by asking, "What could it do to stay calmer?" and "What might other people do that would be helpful?" The girl who drew this picture decided that the volcano would say, "Don't come near me right now! Stay away!" Once the activity is conducted with a particular emotion, names for different levels of intensity could be introduced. In this example, emotions such as frustration, irritation, or rage could be examined in addition to anger. The activity also provides playful openings to explore other intense or unwelcome feelings, such as grief or sadness, along with corresponding vocabulary and coping strategies.

Name (and Count) That Feeling!

Read a book together and make a note of each emotion the characters could be feeling. Write the feeling on a card and put it in a basket. Children can name, sort, and count up the feelings they identified at the end (can even graph them). Great books to use include *Dumbo* and *Alexander and the Terrible, Horrible, No Good, Very Bad Day*. Discuss with the children when they had similar feelings and crises and how they dealt with the strong emotions.

Coping Strategies

These play-based activities can help children and families explore ways to begin the process of rebuilding their lives. Once they begin to see a future, survivors gain a sense of direction and hope, become more motivated, and increase their momentum toward resolution.

A Banner Day

Keep in mind that even though children and their families have not recovered from the disaster, they have successfully survived it. You can invite children and families to explore the achievements that they have already accomplished by creating a banner with a slogan announcing those achievements. By drawing attention to these instances, you can assist survivors in discovering unknown strengths, appreciating unrecognized resources, and achieving a sense of hope.

Worry Bully

Talk with survivors about what a worry is and have them identity a specific worry. Depending on the purpose of the activity, you can suggest that the children identify a worry related to the crisis. Ask them to draw this as a "worry bully," as something that is pushing them around and causing them trouble (externalizing the worry). Together, you and the survivors can generate ways to make the worry bully give up, disappear, and stop causing trouble. Lastly, ask the survivors to draw a picture of the worry bully defeated and discuss ways to use the strategies generated in everyday situations. The picture can be used as a trigger for positive coping statements and behaviors (adapted from Huebner, 2005).

Hula Hoop Toss

In this activity survivors, along with you, can practice affective tolerance and regulation with positive coping statements and behaviors. To set the scene, lay out three Hula Hoops (or create circles with sticks or stones) at varying distances from the standing position (make a line on the floor or ground). In this fun and mildly challenging task, introduced to us by Scott Rivere, survivors are asked to predict in which ring they can toss a foam ball and to make an encouraging statement before and after their attempt. You can vary the challenge by moving the hoops or changing to different types of balls or objects (a rubber chicken or alien doll are great choices). The activity can be used as a metaphor to discuss goal setting and the process of achieving a goal.

Conclusion

When you reach out as a play therapist to crisis and disaster survivors, you are often on their turf—not in your safe and secure office—and your very first intervention is likely to be expressing your gratitude to them for welcoming you as a guest. You will also discover that crisis and disaster intervention can be gut-wrenching, painful, and even heartbreaking at times, but as a play therapist who engages in this work, you will also find tremendous fulfillment in your encounters with survivors whose courage, compassion, and hope will amaze you. You will have countless opportunities to bear witness to the resilience of these children and families. That lesson will continue to serve you well in your more traditional play therapy work. After all, in your daily practice you are a guest who is invited into the inner worlds of your clients. You may find yourself appreciating even more the gracious and welcoming hospitality of the children and families who have allowed you into their lives through play therapy. In an emergency, something new emerges. Don't be surprised if you emerge with a renewed and expanded sense of your own professional calling.

REFERENCES

Atwool, N. (2006). Attachment and resilience: Implications for children in care. *Child Care in Practice, 12*(4), 315–330.

Baggerly, J., & Exum, H. A. (2008). Counseling children after natural disasters: Guidance for family therapists. *American Journal of Family Therapy, 36*, 79–93.

Biglan, A., Flay, B., Embry, D., & Sandler, I. (2012). The critical role of nurturing environments on promoting human well-being. *American Psychologist, 67*(4), 257–271.

Calhoun, L. G., & Tedeschi, R. G. (2006). *Handbook of posttraumatic growth: Research and practice*. Mahwah, NJ: Erlbaum.

Catani, C., Jacob, N., Schauer, E., Kohila, M., & Neuner, F. (2008). Family violence, war, and natural disasters: A study of the effect of extreme stress on children's mental health in Sri Lanka. *BMC Psychiatry, 8*(33), 1–10.

Cohrs, J. C., Christie, D. J., White, M. P., & Das, C. (2013). Contributions of positive psychology: Toward global well-being and resilience. *American Psychologist, 68*(7), 590–600.

Dugan, E., Snow, M., & Crowe, S. (2010). Working with children affected by Hurricane Katrina: Two case studies in play therapy. *Child and Adolescent Mental Health, 15*, 52–55.

Echterling, L. G., Presbury, J., & McKee, J. E. (2005). *Crisis intervention: Promoting resilience and resolution in troubled times*. Upper Saddle River, NJ: Merrill/Prentice Hall.

Echterling, L. G., & Stewart, A. L. (in press). Creative crisis intervention techniques with children and families. In C. A. Malchiodi (Ed.), *Creative interventions with traumatized children* (2nd ed.). New York: Guilford Press.

Gulliver, S. B., Zimering, R., Carpenter, G. S., Giardina, A., & Farrar, J. (2014). The psychological consequences of disaster. In P. Ouimette & J. P. Read (Eds.), *Trauma and substance abuse: Causes, consequences, and treatment of comorbid disorders* (2nd ed., pp. 125–141). Washington, DC: American Psychological Association.

Grossmann, K. E., Grossmann, K., & Waters, E. (2006). *Attachment from infancy to adulthood: The major longitudinal studies*. New York: Guilford Press.

Huebner, D. (2005). *What to do when you worry too much: A kid's guide to overcoming anxiety*. Washington, DC: APA Magination Press.

Inter-Agency Standing Committee (IASC). (2007). *IASC guidelines on mental health and psychosocial support in emergency settings*. Geneva: Author.

Jordan, B., Perryman, K., & Anderson, L. (2013). A case for child-centered play therapy with natural disaster and catastrophic event survivors. *International Journal of Play Therapy, 22*(4), 219–230.

Keck, M., & Sakdapolrak, P. (2013). What is social resilience?: Lessons learned and ways forward. *Erdkunde, 67*(1), 5–19.

Kunz, V. (2009). Sport as a post-disaster psychosocial intervention in Bam, Iran. *Sport in Society: Cultures, Commerce, Media, Politics, 12*(9), 1147–1157.

Landreth, G. (2012). *Play therapy: The art of relationship* (3rd ed.). New York: Routledge.

Louv, R. (2011). *The nature principle: Human restoration and the end of nature–deficit disorder.* Chapel Hill, NC: Algonquin Books.

National Child Traumatic Stress Network. (2013). *Psychological first aid: Field operations guide* (2nd ed.). Los Angeles: Author. Retrieved from *www.nctsn.org/content/psychological-first-aid.*

National Research Council & Institute of Medicine. (2009). *Preventing mental, emotional, and behavioral disorders among young people: Progress and possibilities* (M. E. O'Connell, T. Boat, & K. E. Warner, Eds.). Washington, DC: National Academies Press.

National Child Traumatic Stress Network—Terrorism and Disaster Branch. (2005). Tips for helping school-age children. Retrieved from *www.nctsnet.org/nctsn_assets/pdfs/pfa/TipsforHelpingSchool-AgeChildren.pdf.*

Norris, F. H., Sherrieb, K., & Pfefferbaum, B. (2011). Community resilience: Concepts, assessment, and implications for intervention. In S. M. Southwick, B. T. Litz, D. Charney, & M. J. Friedman (Eds.), *Resilience and mental health: Challenges across the lifespan* (pp. 149–161). Cambridge, UK: Cambridge University Press.

Pearson, C. M., & Mitroff, I. M. (1993). From crisis prone to crisis prepared: A framework for crisis management. *Academy of Mangagment Perspectives, 7*(1), 48–59.

Pellegrini, A. D., Dupuis, D., & Smith, P. K. (2007). Play in evolution and development. *Developmental Review, 27*(2), 261–276.

Prince-Embury, S., & Saklofske, D. H. (Eds.). (2013). *Resilience in children, adolescents, and adults: Translating research into practice.* New York: Springer.

Reyes, G., & Jacobs, G. (2006). *Handbook of international disaster psychology: Interventions with special needs populations.* Westport, CT: Praeger.

Ronan, K. R., & Johnston, D. M. (2005). *Promoting community resilience in disasters: The role for schools, youth, and families.* New York: Springer.

Schore, A. N. (2001). Effects of a secure attachment relationship on right brain development, affect regulation, and infant mental health. *Infant Mental Health Journal, 22*(1–2), 7–66.

Sroufe, L. A. (2005). Attachment and development: A prospective, longitudinal study from birth to adulthood. *Attachment and Human Development, 7*(4), 349–367.

Sroufe, L. A., Egeland, B., Carlson, E., & Collins, W. A. (2005). *Placing early attachment experiences in developmental context.* In K. E. Grossmann, K. Grossmann, & E. Waters (Eds.), *Attachment from infancy to adulthood: The major longitudinal studies* (pp. 48–70). New York: Guilford Press.

Smith, P. K. (2010). *Understanding children's worlds: Children and play.* Hoboken, NJ: Wiley-Blackwell.

Steele, W. & Kuban, C. (2013). *Working with grieving and traumatized children and adolescents.* Hoboken, NJ: Wiley.

Stewart, A. L., & Echterling, L. G. (2014). Therapeutic relationship. In C. Schaefer & A. Drewes (Eds.), *Therapeutic powers of play* (2nd ed., pp. 157–169). New York: Wiley.

Taylor, A., & Kuo, F. (2006). Is contact with nature important for healthy child development?: State of the evidence. In C. Spencer & M. Blades (Eds.), *Children and their environments: Learning, using and designing spaces* (pp. 124–140). Cambridge, UK: Cambridge University Press.

UNHRC. (2013). The future of Syria: Refugee children in crisis. Retrieved from *http://unhcr.org/FutureOfSyria/index.html.*

Wells, N. M. & Evans, G. W. (2003). Nearby nature: A buffer of life stress among rural children? *Environment and Behavior, 35*(3), 311–330.

Wickrama, K. A., & Wickrama, T. T. (2011). Perceived community participation in tsunami recovery efforts and the mental health of tsunami-affected mothers: Findings from a study in rural Sri Lanka. *International Journal of Social Psychiatry, 57,* 518–527.

Yoshikawa, H., Aber, L., & Beardslee, W. (2012). The effects of poverty on the mental, emotional, and behavioral health of children and youth. *American Psychologist, 67*(4), 272–284.

CHAPTER 26

Play Therapy with Military-Connected Children and Families

Jessica Anne Umhoefer
Mary Anne Peabody
Anne L. Stewart

As a result of their military affiliation, military-connected families face unique challenges and stressors, including multiple relocations, extended work hours, additional financial and caregiving burdens, and extended family separations often involving war-zone deployments. Data compiled from 2011 show that the Department of Defense consists of almost 2.3 million military personnel across active duty and reserve populations, and that 43.9% of these military personnel have one or more children (Department of Defense, 2012). This number does not take into account the additional children who are connected to the military through siblings or extended family members' involvement. Since September 11, 2001, nearly 2 million children in the United States have been affected by a military member's deployment (Flake, Davis, Johnson, & Middleton, 2009). Given the unique challenges and stressors that military-connected children face, it is important to understand how play therapy can be used to support these children through times of great stress.

This chapter provides a brief introduction to the many stressors with which military-connected children and families must cope, followed by an overview of how play therapy can be used with this unique population. The extended pathways to resilience model for military families (P2R-Military Families) is presented as a framework to promote resilience in children dealing with military-induced separations. Finally, clinical case examples are provided to illustrate how this model can be applied within a play therapy framework.

Description of Military-Connected Children and Families

In order to work with military-connected children and families, it is important to understand the challenges they face, as well as the differences they may experience. There are several different branches and types of military employment, each with its own culture and traditions. Overall, a hierarchical system characterizes the

U.S. military. One can voluntarily join the military either. as enlisted (i.e., typically high school diploma) or as an officer (i.e., minimum bachelor's degree). In addition, military members can choose the specific branch to join (e.g., Army, Navy, Air Force, Marines, Coast Guard), each of which offers different career tracks and specialized training, as well as whether they would like to make the military their full-time career or part-time employment (e.g., active duty, reserves, National Guard). Military members can then work their way up through different ranks based on their performance evaluations, which are determined by their superiors, and their continuing education and training.

Although military members encounter some stressors that are similar to civilian careers, unique aspects of the military lifestyle lend additional stressors that impact both the military members and their families. For example, similar to police officers and fire fighters, military employment can put one in harm's way and under extreme stress on a regular basis. General safety of the military member then becomes an ongoing concern for the family. In addition, in order to access different training and career opportunities, a military member is often required to move regularly and may have little say about the place of relocation or the timing. As a result, military-connected families often move across the country, or world, multiple times throughout a military career. These frequent relocations create additional burdens for the children and families, as they must create new social connections and support networks, not to mention switching schools every couple of years.

Military families also face a unique set of stressors as a result of the current military conflicts. Specifically, separation from a loved one due to a war-zone deployment can create challenges for military families and children that many civilian children do not face. Additionally, recent research has suggested that the unique experiences of the more recent cycle of war-zone deployments (i.e., Iraq, Afghanistan) can have a negative impact on the children of military personnel (Lowe, Adams, Browne, & Hinkle, 2012). For example, during deployment children from military families exhibit higher levels of emotional and behavioral problems (Chandra et al., 2010; Flake et al., 2009; Kelley et al., 2001; Morris & Age, 2009) and higher rates of symptoms related to depression and anxiety (Lester et al., 2010; Waliski, Bokony, Edlund, & Kirchner, 2012; Wickman, Greenburg, & Boren, 2010). Furthermore, there are higher rates of parental distress and higher reported difficulty for parents in supporting and connecting with children (Flake et al., 2009; Lowe et al., 2012).

Supporting Children and Families through Military-Induced Separations

In order to assist families through military-induced separations, it is important to understand the specific context and stressors that are at play, unique to each family. Military personnel and their families can have different experiences depending on their branch of service, their military rank, and whether they are on active duty, part of a reserve unit, or part of a National Guard unit. Although the global media tend to convey the impression that a soldier deploys with a large unit from the same military base, this is not always the case. Furthermore, families who are part of a National Guard or reserve unit, rather than an active duty unit, may have to cope with additional stressors, including living away from military bases and military support systems, and possible reductions in their family's income while deployed (Tollefson, 2008).

Although military deployments are the most researched and widely known type of family separation, military-connected children can face a variety of separations as a result of their family member's military career. In addition to deployment, military-connected families may be separated as a result of an unaccompanied tour in which a military member is assigned a change-of-duty station to a high-risk location such that their family is unable to move with them, as well as by a temporary duty assignment in which a military member is sent away for a short period of time to complete a specific short-term job or to access training. In addition to the type of separation, families can have different experiences depending on the branch and rank of the military member. For example, a Navy sailor on sea duty may be on a regular rotation whereby he or she is at sea for 6 months, then home for 6 months, over a period of several years. In addition, this cycle would not be considered a deployment, but would be part of their regular job duties and expectations. Regardless, this type of intermittent separation and reunion cycle would affect the military member and family. Knowing the type of separation can suggest the amount of time the family will be apart, as well as the amount of danger and/or stress the military member will be under while away.

Independent of the type of separation, a cycle of feelings and challenges, generally referred to as the *deployment cycle*, appears to play out. One such cycle, developed by Pincus, House, Christensen, and Adler (2001), includes five stages: predeployment, deployment, sustainment, redeployment, and postdeployment/reintegration. The predeployment stage begins when the military member is notified of the deployment and ends with his or her departure. The deployment stage consists of the entire length of time when the military member is away. During this period, the family may move into the sustainment stage, which begins once the family develops and engages in new routines in the military member's absence. Throughout the deployment there may be times of short-term reunions, when the deployed member returns for "rest and relaxation" breaks, which can cause the family to enter the redeployment stage. This stage can create anticipation of a re-

union; however, the military member is usually home only for a short duration, so it can cause the family to have to renegotiate the deployment cycle after the member leaves again, and upset the family schedule and routines. As a family moves toward reunion and the postdeployment/reintegration stage, in which the military member returns, the family must again create new routines and renegotiate roles. Researchers have also examined how children's emotions can vary across the deployment cycle (Flake et al., 2009).

Although the majority of the research has focused on identifying the negative outcomes of deployment on military members and their families, a growing literature base is pushing for the identification of the protective factors and positive outcomes of deployment for families. This approach calls for the use of a resilience model to guide research and intervention (Goldstein & Brooks, 2013). The co-director of the Resilience Research Centre, Dr. Michael Unger, describes resilience as follows:

> In the context of exposure to significant adversity, resilience is both the capacity of individuals to navigate their way to the psychological, social, cultural, and physical resources that sustain their well-being, and their capacity individually and collectively to negotiate for these resources to be provided in culturally meaningful ways. (Unger, n.d., para. 1)

During deployment children and families face added stress and are at significant risk for a number of negative emotional and behavioral effects. Finding ways to assist children and families to cope during deployment can help them remain resilient during this stressful time.

Military-Connected Children and Families and the Practice of Play Therapy

Military families often demonstrate incredible resilience in the face of many uncertainties, yet ongoing separations can create high levels of stress for even the healthiest of families. Children are extremely sensitive to the behaviors and emotions demonstrated by the significant adults in their lives, including parents, grandparents, teachers, and other adults. Therefore, interventions and therapeutic approaches that attend not only to the child, but to the relationships and emotional health of parents and caregivers in the child's life, are vital. With distinct challenges confronting children and their families at each phase of deployment (Horton, 2005), it is incumbent upon schools, military resource centers, and community clinicians to ensure that children who need additional support receive developmentally appropriate mental health interventions from culturally competent clinicians.

Culturally competent clinicians understand the worldview of others. Specifically, clinicians should take time to understand the uniqueness of the military culture, including the norms and beliefs of individual service members and their families. The unique culture of the military requires clinicians to be cognizant of their own values, biases, preconceived notions, and limitations through engagement in self-reflection and clinical supervision. Treatment is not about political agendas, but rather supporting children and families as they navigate roles, transitions, relationships, change, and resiliency. Adjusting to change is a reality in the lives of military families. Virtually all military families deal with constant change and transition, which is often accompanied by various levels of loss (Hall, 2008). Many families are faced with transitions and changes on such a consistent basis, that they may not even realize they have not grieved the previous transition before planning for the next (Hall, 2008). From a child's perspective, few life changes are as unwelcome as parental separation. Most children feel powerless over the decisions that military life brings, and they experience a range of feelings as they travel through the emotional stages of deployment. While children deal with the primary loss of their deployed parent, there are often secondary or intangible losses such as loss of routine, loss of a sense of safety, and loss of special time with their parent (Fiorini & Mullen, 2006).

When a military-connected child is in need of emotional support, play therapy may be the most developmentally appropriate intervention because it utilizes the natural language of play throughout the therapeutic process (Landreth, 2002). Because play therapy is tailored to children's developmental characteristics, it can enhance their wellness by providing supportive emotional scaffolding as they experience familial change and transitions (Pedro-Carroll & Jones, 2005; Vygotsky, 1978). By definition, play therapy is "the systematic use of a theoretical model to establish an interpersonal process wherein trained play therapists use the therapeutic powers of play to help clients prevent or resolve psychosocial difficulties and achieve optimal growth and development" (Association for Play Therapy, 2013, p. 2).

As such, a play therapist is purposeful and intentional in the selection of theoretical models, interventions, and specific techniques. Although play techniques are plentiful, techniques without a theoretical underpinning or guiding framework for how and when to use them in treatment do not constitute best practice. As Goodyear-Brown (2010) states, "It is easy to feel adrift in a sea of interventions" (p. xv). The integration of play therapy with the following P2R-Military Families is an example of the systematic use of a theoretical model that uses the therapeutic powers of play to help clients prevent or resolve the psychosocial difficulties associated with military deployment and to achieve optimal growth and development, specifically resilience. By merging play therapy and play-based interventions with this six-factor model of resilience, clinicians intentionally guide the selection of interventions that are especially relevant for deployment stages. Clinicians skillfully facilitate their own therapeutic responses designed to promote a child's sense of power or control, encourage expression of feelings, modify any cognitive distortions, teach coping skills, promote a sense of hope despite uncertainty, and recognize and enhance strengths and social support.

The P2R-Military Families

The P2R-Military Families was developed to include those dimensions, identified from the research literature, that are necessary to build resilience in military-connected children and families facing a deployment (Umhoefer, 2013). The six dimensions of the P2R-Military Families provide a framework to guide intervention, and can be adapted to meet the needs of each individual child and family. Figure 26.1 provides a visual representation of this model.

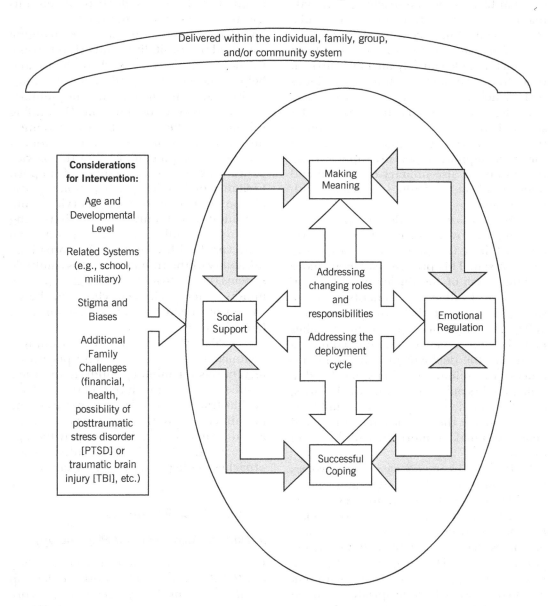

FIGURE 26.1. The extended pathways to resilience model for military families (P2R-Military Families).

The original pathways to resilience model (P2R; Echterling, Presbury, & McKee, 2005) was developed to support individuals who are facing crisis or times of extreme stress. The model has been applied in interventions to address populations as diverse as international landmine survivors and domestic school shooting survivors (Echterling & Stewart, 2010; Stewart et al., 2011). The four original factors include reaching out, making meaning, facilitating emotional regulation, and enabling successful coping.

Reaching out refers to the social support on which people can rely during a difficult time. In this context, reaching out includes seeking help during a crisis, as well as others reaching out to support the person under stress (Echterling et al., 2005). During a time of deployment, families can reach out for social support, especially support from those who are also military-connected and understand the difficulties associated with deployment.

Making meaning includes the process of creating a narrative of how the stress and crisis fit into the person's life story and sense of self. This process usually includes making sense of the difficulty or trauma, as well as finding the benefits and the strengths within it (Echterling & Stewart, 2008). Throughout deployment, families may develop a belief and understanding regarding the deployment and the importance of the military member's role. In addition, people's opinions around the families, as well as media reports about the military, may challenge the families' narratives and beliefs and make it more difficult for them to cope.

Facilitating *emotional regulation* involves helping families acknowledge and appropriately express the emotions they are experiencing (Echterling & Stewart, 2008). Families experience a variety of emotional outcomes that can vary throughout the deployment cycle. They may need additional support and opportunities that assist them in learning ways to appropriately express these emotions.

Finally, enabling *successful coping* includes helping the person begin to take action and use resources to address his or her situation (Echterling et al., 2005). Frequently, one goal of intervention is to teach appropriate coping skills and to assist families in utilizing available resources.

The P2R-Military Families model posits that extending the four dimensions of the original P2R to include two dimensions specific to military families (i.e., [1] acknowledging and addressing the changing roles and responsibilities and [2] addressing the deployment cycle) builds resilience and helps children and families move toward positive growth when facing the military-related stressor of deployment. Grounding this model is the idea that any intervention must take into consideration the factors of age and developmental level of the participants, other coexisting systems of support, hesitancy of families' participation because of the stigma of receiving services, and any additional family stressors impacting the families' ability to cope (e.g., financial concerns, health concerns). The broad applicability of the framework across multiple systems (i.e., individual, family, group, community) offers a clinician choice in the selection of interventions that best suit each family's needs.

The P2R-Military Families encourages a clinician to select purposeful playful interventions for military children and their families that align with the six dimensions. To illustrate this overlay, we first examine nondirective play therapy approaches, followed by integrative, directive play therapy approaches. Woven into the different approaches are hypothetical case examples.

Clinical Case Examples

Individual Child-Centered Play Therapy

During individual child-centered play therapy (CCPT), the clinician works to develop a safe relationship by creating the core conditions of the person-centered theory:

(1) empathy—entering the child's world and seeking to understand this frame or perception of the world; (2) unconditional positive regard—conveying acceptance and warmth to the child; and (3) congruence—interacting in a genuine and real manner (Rogers, 1951). The core conditions of the person-centered approach are considered the techniques, with the fundamental "technique" being the therapeutic relationship (Ray, 2009). Specific nonverbal and verbal skills guide the therapist's communication (Landreth, 2002; Ray, 2009).

A child-centered therapist working with military-connected children coping with deployment might include military-related play materials in the playroom, such as military figures or vehicles, extended family figures, a variety of playhouses, play telephones, or military dress-up clothes. These materials would be added to the variety of expressive materials available. Staying within the child-centered model, the child would choose whether to play with the toys or not. As in all play therapy, some children may find playing with toys or materials that are literal representations of the current stressors too threatening, and may instead choose toys that symbolically represent their stories or narratives, thereby providing the necessary distancing through metaphor.

Case 1

Susie (vignette not based on an actual case), a 6-year-old girl referred for play therapy, presented with significant behavioral challenges (i.e., oppositional and disruptive behavior) that had increased since her father's deployment. Mother reported that Susie and her father had a close relationship and that he was the main disciplinarian. Susie's grandmother had moved into the house to offer support; however, Susie's mother and grandmother had differing views on parenting and discipline. Simultaneously, Susie was starting a new school. Using the P2R-Military Families, several areas were explored in designing a treatment plan for Susie and her family.

CONSIDERATIONS FOR INTERVENTION

Prior to designing interventions, the clinician considered relevant background factors, including Susie's age and developmental level, coexisting systems of support, and additional family stressors. Given that Susie was 6 years old, individual play therapy and collateral work with Mom, Grandmother, and Susie's teacher was selected. Gaining awareness of additional family challenges for the mother and grandmother, including caregiving styles of behavior management, was critical in the assessment stage to help guide interventions.

REACHING OUT

One consideration within the P2R-Military Families was an exploration of the social supports available to the family. Given that the family had recently moved to the area, and that Susie would be starting a new school, it was important to help the family members connect with other families and resources in the area. Military-sponsored or community groups that help connect families were explored, as well as assessing if the mom was interested in faith-based groups or recreational activities. Taking time to match individual family interests with available resources helped ensure that the family would not only take the initial steps to attend and find support, but also continue involvement, thereby building a stronger social support network over time. Additional social support was also inherent in building the therapeutic relationship between the counselor, Susie, and her family.

MAKING MEANING

To assist Susie in making meaning of the deployment experience, a nondirective CCPT approach was selected. Providing therapeutic responses, along with the core conditions of CCPT, helped Susie express the emotional content underneath her externalized behavior. From a child-centered approach, the therapist looked for common themes in Susie's play over time. For example, military-connected children frequently reenact the experiences of moving and undergoing transitions during their play. Feelings of confusion, anger, and helplessness became evident as Susie used toys to express familial moves. Glimpses into Susie's play themes of power and control, change and transition, are shared below.

SUSIE: Let's play musical chairs!

THERAPIST: You've decided what you want to play.

SUSIE: I'm lining up all the dollhouse chairs and here . . . you move this doll when I sing.

THERAPIST: You know just how you want this to go.

SUSIE: (*Starts singing.*) Now move. Go, chair to chair, place to place! Move, move, move!

THERAPIST: You're in charge of the moves in here.

SUSIE: (*Stops singing.*) Ha! Ha! (*Takes chair away from the doll.*) You can't stay here. There, it's time to move again! Even if you really like this chair . . . pack up! (*in a marching tone*) You can't stay in that chair any more.

THERAPIST: You decide when to stay, when to pack up, and when it's time to move. You're the powerful decision maker.

Through such play, children assert their sense of control and power, even though in reality they have no control over when and where they will move. Being powerful in the playroom, facilitated by a trained clinician, allows children the experience of control and power, which internalizes into their sense of self. Sharing experiences through play also brings the feelings held inside, outside to be shared, thereby lessening the intensity of the emotion. Verbally reflecting an understanding of desires, feelings, and themes to children in the metaphor of their play helps to increase growth and awareness as part of making meaning. Providing facilitative responses along with the core conditions of CCPT helped Susie express a range of emotional content through the medium of her play.

FACILITATING EMOTIONAL REGULATION

The opportunity to release emotional content in an environment of safety and through the natural language of play is part of how young children learn emotional regulation. During Susie's individual play sessions, emotional regulation was often braided with meaning making. The nature of the therapist's responses that reflected feelings back to Susie provided her with "feeling words" that increased both Susie's self-awareness and her affective vocabulary. Reflections of feelings helped Susie feel listened to, and acknowledged her needs and wants, so that her need for negative attention-seeking behavior began to minimize. By its nature, CCPT provides the child with control and power to make choices and turns responsibility for decisions back to the child. These skills all promote self-regulation. Given that Susie's behavior was often externalized, consistent limit setting using the three-step ACT model (Landreth, 2002; Landreth & Bratton, 2006) was utilized during play sessions. This model utilizes the following sequence:

- A—acknowledge the child's feelings, wants, wishes or desires. "Susie, I know that you think throwing the ball at the ceiling light is fun."
- C—communicate the limit (clearly and briefly). "But the ceiling light isn't for being thrown at with the ball."
- T—target acceptable alternatives by providing one or more choices depending on the age of the child. "You can throw the ball at this wall or in the basket."

Consistent limit setting taught Susie self-control and responsibility for her own behavior by allowing her to experience the consequences for her choices and decisions. In an effort to ensure that this limit-setting model was generalized at home and school, the clinician held a psychoeducational session with the mother, grandmother, and Susie's new teacher. By bringing both home and school together to provide a united front in supporting Susie, the social support net continued to expand. During this session the limit-setting model was demonstrated, role-played, and written materials were shared. The child-centered skill of providing "choices as consequences" was taught as another skill in promoting self-regulation. For example: "Susie, when you choose to pick up your toys by the time Grammy returns from the store in about 10 minutes, you choose to have 20 minutes on the computer after dinner. When you choose not to pick up your toys before Grammy returns, you choose not to have computer time after dinner."

ENABLING SUCCESSFUL COPING

Although individual CCPT was selected for Susie initially, the therapist chose to teach some skills during family sessions in anticipation of forming a filial play therapy group with other parents in the near future. Filial therapy instructs parents on how to apply CCPT techniques and principles in their interactions with their children. Specifically, filial therapy trains parents to conduct special nondirective play sessions with their children, along with providing parental psychoeducation, so that parents can begin to understand their children's feelings and motivations through the themes in their play. Treatment begins as supervised play sessions under the direction of a trained therapist, and moves toward encouraging parents to use the skills learned at home. Chawla and Solinas-Saunders (2011) argue that filial therapy can be successfully used with military families to strengthen the parent–child bond and to reduce child stress and externalizing behaviors. In Susie's case, the therapist made the decision to conduct individual play therapy first, teaching several skills to Mom and Grandmother during family sessions, and to conduct filial group play therapy after an optimal number of military parents could be referred to form a group. Ideally, the filial group would occur after Dad returned from deployment, enabling him to join his wife in the group experience with other parents. This arrangement would extend social support, build upon his current relationship with Susie, and strengthen his ability to be an emotionally responsive parent.

ADDRESSING THE DEPLOYMENT CYCLE

Considering that the family was within the deployment part of the deployment cycle, it was important to help prepare family members for the father's return and reintegration. This preparation included informing the family of changes to expect as they neared reintegration, and discussing how to effectively communicate expectations with one another. Both individual play sessions and family sessions began to deal with Dad's return. As the conversations about her father's return became more prominent, Susie would include him in her drawings and dollhouse play more frequently. Susie was anticipating his return as a happy event and talked about activities she wanted to do as a family upon his return.

ADDRESSING CHANGING ROLES AND RESPONSIBILITIES

Given that family members were moving toward reintegration, it was especially important to prepare them for how roles would change once Susie's father returned home and attempted to reenter the family system. Just as the family had had to adjust their roles and responsibilities when Susie's father left for deployment, his return meant renegotiating those roles and responsibilities. Finding ways to incorporate Dad into "playtimes" was of critical importance and could best be achieved by using the relational power of play to reconnect Susie with her father after his absence.

Directive Approaches: Group/ Community-Based Interventions

Although the basic conditions of a relational child-centered approach influence the work of many child therapists, some therapists prefer a more directive approach. Other therapists use an integration of both nondirective and directive approaches as their preferred method (Drewes, 2009; Gil, 2003b), whereas still others find that using a prescriptive approach, which matches the best evidenced-based intervention to the presenting needs of the client, is ideal (Schaefer, 2003). Clearly, a range of interventions is needed for a comprehensive treatment plan that includes not only individual or group work with the child, but consultation with parents and schools across and between ecosystems (O'Connor & Ammen, 1997).

A frequently used directive play therapy approach to strengthen resiliency across multiple populations is cognitive-behavioral therapy (CBT). Paris, DeVoe, Ross, and Acker (2010) argue that CBT strategies such as cognitive processing, reframing, and relaxation can be used within the framework of a relationship-based intervention when a child experiences anxiety or distress related to a separation. Many play therapists have incorporated play-based interventions into the key components of CBT (Drewes, 2009; Goodyear-Brown, 2010; Knell, 1993; Knell & Dasari, 2009).

A promising group intervention that combines CBT and a psychoeducational approach and is specifically designed for military-connected children in grades K–6 is called *Same Sky Sharing*. Although Same Sky Sharing is in its developmental stage, its goals and focus match well with the P2R-Military Families model. Same Sky Shar-

ing uses play-based interventions across 8 weeks with groups of children experiencing parental deployments (Peabody & Johnson, 2009). Designed for use in schools, military support groups, or community programs, the psychoeducational curriculum focuses on fostering a supportive group environment, facilitating the expression of feelings, teaching coping skills, and identifying strengths in the child, his or her family, and other potential supports outside the family (Peabody & Johnson, 2009). Play-based activities include identifying current support systems and untapped resources, the use of artwork to identify self and family strengths, and a focus on how deployment has changed the family in positive ways. All activities are paced sequentially over time to be introduced as the group becomes more comfortable with sharing and being together. This second hypothetical case study provides an illustration of how the P2R-Military Families could be applied within a group and community intervention.

Case 2

Paul (vignette not based on an actual case), a 9-year-old boy referred for psychological services, presented with significant challenges (e.g., regressive behavior, developmentally inappropriate attachment to his mother, social and peer difficulties). His stepfather was recently deployed, and he was living with his mother. Contact with his biological father was infrequent and unpredictable. Paul initially refused to participate verbally in treatment; however he did engage through artwork, and his art often included themes of war, destruction, and fear.

CONSIDERATIONS FOR INTERVENTION

To start, the clinician considered relevant background factors, including age and developmental level, coexisting systems of support, and any additional family stressors. Through an assessment interview with the mother, it became apparent that both Paul and his mother had little social support. Their extended family was geographically distant, and their ability to help with everyday needs was extremely limited. At the start of treatment, neither Paul nor his mom were involved in any extracurricular activities and had become each other's sole companion. Paul was showing difficulty at school with peer conflicts and friendships. His increasing emotional outbursts were beginning to impact whether his peers wanted to play with him. His inability to regulate his emotions and behavior began to spill into his academic learning. His emotional dysregulation was impacting both his social and academic worlds.

REACHING OUT

Given Paul's social difficulties and lack of social connections, the clinician looked for both school-based group and community interventions. The clinician collaborated with Paul's school counselor to utilize the Same Sky Sharing curriculum for Paul and other children experiencing parental deployment. Simultaneously, the clinician worked on assessing Mom's personal interests and explored whether a woman's group, faith-based group, or school-related parent group might be a match for her. Given the availability of a community group starting for military families, the clinician offered this experience for both Mom and Paul.

MAKING MEANING
AND EMOTIONAL REGULATION

These two dimensions of the P2R-Military Families are addressed together in this case example, as each was closely intertwined with the other in the choice of play interventions. Children often communicate primary feeling states more potently through their art than through their words (Gil, 2003a; Malchiodi, 2008). Paul was no exception, as he expressed his initial feelings and

thoughts through the variety of art-related play interventions in the Same Sky Sharing curriculum. As he became more comfortable drawing and sharing, he wanted others to understand his story. It became clearer as he described his artwork that anxiety was his primary feeling state, although his inability to regulate the anxiety was characterized by agitated emotional outbursts. Paul, with the guidance of the group facilitators, began to express how anxious he felt about his stepfather's deployment, the changing roles that deployment brought for himself and his mother, the constant uncertainty of moving, and his sadness over the lack of close friends. During the fourth group, Paul asked his peers if other children had both a stepdad and a real dad.

PAUL: Do you have two dads?

MATT: No. Do you?

PAUL: I have a real dad that I never see and a stepdad, but now he's gone too . . . it stinks!

THERAPIST: It's really hard to not be able to see people you love as often as you want.

PAUL: I don't really remember my real dad anyway . . . but my stepdad . . . I miss him.

THERAPIST: You have different memories of them. Right now, you miss your stepdad.

MATT: You get to talk on the phone and Skype with your stepdad, right?

PAUL: Yeah . . . but I wish he was here in person . . . that's when it's the best.

THERAPIST: You like it best when he's here with you and your mom. Let's make a list of what helps you deal with the feelings of missing your stepdad—like a menu of coping ideas.

MATT: I have some things that work for me, Paul.

PAUL: Can I draw it out, like a real restaurant menu?

THERAPIST: Absolutely, you're so artistic! Both of your ideas can be part of this menu.

This exchange prompted the counselor to ask Paul's mom about her perceptions of Paul's feelings surrounding the inconsistent relationship with his biological father. Mom shared that the inconsistency was certainly difficult, but Paul rarely, if ever, talked with her about his biological dad. Mom also offered that she, admittedly, worked hard to avoid the subject with Paul, instead putting her energy into ensuring that communication with his stepdad was as consistent as possible.

Paul's artwork continued to be his preferred expressive medium in group and the primary vehicle for allowing difficult conversations to take place. Artwork gave him the opportunity to make sense of the changes and his current life situation in a language that was safe for him. With Paul's permission, several examples of his artwork were shared with his mom during their subsequent family sessions. With the guidance of the therapist, Paul's art from the structured group activities became the bridge and catalyst for Paul to teach his mom about his feelings and how he made meaning of their current deployment situation.

SUCCESSFUL COPING

Through both the group and community experiences, Paul was introduced to new coping skills. He particularly enjoyed the bubble blowing activity that taught the skill of deep breathing. He thought the bubbles were both fun and competitive, as he tried to change his breathing pattern to control the physiological aspects of coping through this activity. As the group facilitator spoke about emotions that cause anxiousness and how focused breathing can calm one down, Paul suggested he teach his mom this activity as a homework assignment.

As Paul's network of social peer support widened, he showed an interest in playing community baseball, as one of the boys in the community support group was playing on a team. As part of the mental prepara-

tion before each game, the coach used deep breathing and mental visualization, similar to some of the skills talked about in the group formats. When Paul shared with the coach that he already knew how to do these skills, the coach invited Paul to be the captain of the pregame mental warm-up. Paul was a bit hesitant at first, but with guidance from the coach, it wasn't long until Paul was leading the warm-up by himself and feeling empowered in front of his peers.

The clinician continued to work with Paul's mother around parenting issues to help her become more aware of her tendency to blur the roles of mother and friend. Mom began to recognize that she was sending confusing messages to Paul regarding peers, companionship, roles, and responsibilities. In support of Paul's play therapy treatment plan, the clinician guided Mom's exploration of parenting topics, issues, and practices, including the use of coping skills to reduce anxiety on a daily basis so that the skills became natural; good limit-setting practices; scheduling peer playdates for Paul; and ensuring frequent communication with the stepdad via Skype. The clinician also coached the mom in how to talk with Paul about the relationship with his biological father.

ADDRESSING THE DEPLOYMENT CYCLE

Paul and his mother had just recently entered the deployment segment of the deployment cycle. Within the deployment group, Paul and his peers could directly discuss the deployment cycle and the accompanying changes and feelings. In one session, Paul created figures out of clay representing his mom, his biological father, and his stepfather. He shared that he "was the man of the house now," a comment frequently reinforced by both parents. Paul also placed feeling cards with the words *happy* and *worried* next to his clay. Together, Paul and the clinician were able to share this with his mom in a family session. The clinician was able to help both Paul and his mom identify and address appropriate responsibilities during this time of changing roles.

ADDRESSING CHANGING ROLES AND RESPONSIBILITIES

Both group experiences addressed the changes in roles and responsibilities that accompany deployment. The community group helped support Paul's mother in understanding and meeting the demands of her new role as a "single parent" and connected her with resources that could support the two of them as they tried to create their "new normal." For Paul, becoming more involved in age-appropriate activities, having scheduled peer playdates, and helping the family focus on what a 9-year-old boy should be doing versus a mindset of being "the man of the house," all contributed to a lessening of his anxiety. Paul gained more positive peer experiences through age-appropriate social involvement. Additionally, during phone and Skype conversations his mom was able to explain to the stepdad about the need to use alternate language with Paul to encourage him to be a 9-year-old helper to her.

These case studies provide examples of how the P2R-Military Families model can be used to guide and select play therapy or play-based interventions when working with military-connected children and families. Although the model is not an intervention, in and of itself, it denotes those dimensions that are critical to cover in any intervention addressing families during a deployment. Using the model's six dimensions as a framework can help clinicians successfully assist families in coping with myriad deployment-related stressors and in remaining resilient throughout the deployment process. These case studies also illustrate the flexibility of the model in that it can be adapted to work with children of differing ages and developmental levels, and it can be applied within different intervention formats and settings (e.g., individual, group, family, and community).

Conclusion

Drewes (2009) suggests both "play in therapy" and "play as therapy" as having therapeutic potential. Whether it is through a specialized summer camp experience for military-connected children, structured family play therapy, a community-based psychoeducational group experience bringing together military children and their parents, or a parent participating in filial therapy where the skills of nondirective CCPT are taught, several treatment approaches and interventions exist. Play in therapy and play as therapy offer nonthreatening experiences for children to connect therapeutically through the medium of play.

This nonthreatening appeal is specifically important to military families, who currently find themselves in the early stages of a military cultural shift around counseling and mental health services. In the past, seeking mental health services was not encouraged and many felt that securing treatment would negatively impact future career promotions (Hall, 2008). The current military culture is taking encouraging steps to change the stigma associated with seeking mental health services. This type of cultural shift takes time. Fortunately, children are remarkably resilient, particularly when the adults surrounding them provide predictability, security, and safety. Our military families deserve effective strategies and services, such as play therapy, to help them build on family strengths, foster resilience, and thrive while in service to our nation.

REFERENCES

Association for Play Therapy. (2013). About play therapy: Overview. Retrieved from *www.a4pt. org/ps.playtherapy.cfm?ID=1158*.

Chandra, A., Lara-Cinisomo, S., Jaycox, L. H.,

Tanielian, T., Burns, R. M., Ruder, T., et al. (2010). Children on the homefront: The experience of children from military families. *Pediatrics, 125*, 13–22.

Chawla, N., & Solinas-Saunders, M. (2011). Supporting military parent and child adjustment to deployment and separations with filial therapy. *American Journal of Family Therapy, 39*, 179–192.

Department of Defense. (2012). 2011 demographics: Profile of the military community. *Military OneSource.* Retrieved from *www.militaryonesource.mil/12038/MOS/Reports/2011_Demographics_Report.pdf.*

Drewes, A. (2009). Preface. In A. A. Drewes (Ed.), *Blending play therapy with cognitive behavioral therapy: Evidenced-based and other effective treatments and techniques* (pp. xvii–xx). Hoboken, NJ: Wiley.

Echterling, L. G., Presbury, J., & McKee, J. E. (2005). *Crisis intervention: Promoting resilience and resolution in troubled times.* Upper Saddle River, NJ: Merrill/Prentice Hall.

Echterling, L. G., & Stewart. A. L. (2008). Creative crisis intervention techniques with children and families. In C. A. Malchiodi (Ed.), *Creative interventions with traumatized children* (pp. 189–210). New York: Guilford Press.

Echterling, L. G., & Stewart, A. L. (2010). Pathways to resilience at Virginia Tech. In J. Webber, D. D. Bass, & R. Yep (Eds.), *Terrorism, trauma and tragedies: A counselor's guide to preparing and responding* (3rd ed., pp. 83–88). Washington, DC: American Counseling Association.

Fiorini, J. J. & Mullen, J. A. (2006). *Counseling children and adolescents through grief and loss.* Champaign, IL: Research Press.

Flake, E. M., Davis, B. E., Johnson, P. L., & Middleton, L. S. (2009). The psychosocial effects of deployment on military children. *Journal of Developmental and Behavioral Pediatrics, 30*, 271–278.

Gil, E. (2003a). Art and play therapy with sexually abused children. In C. A. Malchiodi (Ed.), *Handbook of art therapy* (pp. 152–166.). New York: Guilford Press.

Gil, E. (2003b). Family play therapy: "The bear with short nails." In C. E. Schaefer (Ed.), *Foundations of play therapy* (pp. 192–218). Hoboken, NJ: Wiley.

Goldstein, S., & Brooks, R. B. (2013). Why study resilience? In S. Goldstein & R. B. Brooks (Eds.), *Handbook of resilience in children* (2nd ed., pp. 3–14). New York: Springer.

Goodyear-Brown, P. (2010). *Play therapy with traumatized children: A prescriptive approach.* Hoboken, NJ: Wiley.

Hall, L. K. (2008). *Counseling military families.* New York: Routledge.

Horton, D. (2005). Consultation with military children and schools: A proposed model. *Consulting Psychology Journal, 57*, 259–265.

Kelley, M. L., Hock, E., Smith, K. M., Jarvis, M. S., Bonney, J. F., & Gaffney, M. A. (2001). Internalizing and externalizing behavior of children with enlisted Navy mothers experiencing military-induced separation. *Journal of the American Academy of Child and Adolescent Psychiatry, 40*, 464–471.

Knell, S. M. (1993). *Cognitive-behavioral play therapy.* Northvale, NJ: Jason Aronson.

Knell, S. M., & Dasari, M. (2009). CBPT: Implementing and integrating CBPT into clinical practice. In A. A. Drewes (Ed.), *Blending play therapy with cognitive behavioral therapy: Evidenced-based and other effective treatments and techniques* (pp. 117–133). Hoboken, NJ: Wiley.

Landreth, G. L. (2002). *Play therapy: The art of the relationship.* New York: Brunner-Routledge.

Landreth, G. L. & Bratton, S. C. (2006). *Child parent relationship therapy (CRPT): A 10 session filial therapy model.* New York: Routledge.

Lester, P., Peterson, K., Reeves, J., Knauss, L., Glover, D., Mogil, C., et al. (2010). The long war and parental combat: Effects on military children and at-home spouses. *Journal of the American Academy of Child and Adolescent Psychiatry, 49*, 310–320.

Lowe, K. N., Adams, K. S., Browne, B. L., & Hinkle, K. T. (2012). Impact of military deployment on family relationships. *Journal of Family Studies, 18*, 17–27.

Malchiodi, C. A. (2008). *Creative interventions with traumatized children.* New York: Guilford Press.

Morris, A. S., & Age, T. R. (2009). Adjustment among youth in military families: The protective roles of effortful control and maternal social support. *Journal of Applied Developmental Psychology, 30*, 695–707.

O'Connor, K. J., & Ammen, S. (1997). *Play therapy: Treatment planning and interventions.* San Diego, CA: Academic Press.

Paris, R., DeVoe, E. R., Ross, A. M., & Acker, M. L. (2010). When a parent goes to war: Effects of parental deployment on very young children and implications for intervention. *American Journal of Orthopsychiatry, 80*, 610–618.

Peabody, M. A., & Johnson, D. B. (2009). *Same Sky Sharing: A curriculum for children in our military families.* Rochester, NY: Children's Institute.

Pedro-Carroll, J., & Jones, S. H. (2005). A preventive play intervention to foster children's resilience in the aftermath of divorce. In L. A. Reddy, T. M. Files-Hall, & C. E. Schaefer (Eds.), *Empirically based play interventions for children* (pp. 51–75). Washington, DC: American Psychological Association.

Pincus, S. H., House, R., Christensen, J., & Adler, L. E. (2001, Apr/June). The emotional cycle of deployment: A military family perspective. *U.S. Army Medical Department Journal*, pp. 15–23.

Ray, D. (2009). *Child-centered play therapy treatment manual.* Denton, TX: Child and Family Resource Clinic.

Rogers, C. (1951). *Client-centered therapy.* Boston: Houghton Mifflin.

Schaefer, C. E. (2003). Prescriptive play therapy. In C. E. Schaefer (Ed.), *Foundations of play therapy* (pp. 306–320). Hoboken, NJ: Wiley.

Stewart, A. (2013, April). *Supporting the children of military families through play therapy.* Paper presented at the Mid-Atlantic Play Therapy Training Institute, Alexandria, VA.

Stewart, A., Echterling, L., Macauley, C., Hamden, H., Neitzey, N., & Ghannam, G. (2011). Pathways to resilience workshop: Leadership and peer support. *Mine Action Information Journal, 15*, 3.

Tollefson, T. T. (2008). Supporting spouses during a military deployment. *Family and Community Health, 31*, 281–286.

Umhoefer, J. A. (2013). *Supporting military-connected children and families throughout deployment.* Unpublished doctoral dissertation, James Madison University, Harrisonburg, VA.

Unger, M. (n.d.). *What is resilience?* Resilience Research Center Homepage. Retrieved from *http://resilienceproject.org.*

Vygotsky, L. S. (1978). *Mind in society: The development of higher psychological processes.* Cambridge, MA: Harvard University Press.

Waliski, A., Bokony, P., Edlund, C. N., & Kirchner, J. (2012). Counselors called for service: Impact of parental deployment on preschool children. *Family Journal, 20*, 157–163.

Wickman, M., Greenburg, C., & Boren, D. (2010). The relationship of perception of invincibility, demographics, and risk behaviors in adolescents of military parents. *Journal of Pediatric Health Care, 24*, 25–33.

CHAPTER 27

Play Therapy with Children on the Autism Spectrum

Kevin B. Hull

Perhaps there is more understanding and beauty in life when the flaring sunlight is softened by the patterns of shadows. Perhaps there is more depth in a relationship that has weathered some storms. Experience that never disappoints or saddens or stirs up feeling is a bland experience with little challenge or variation of color. Perhaps it's when we experience confidence and faith and hope that we see materialize before our eyes this builds up within us a feeling of inner strength, courage, and security. We are all personalities that grow and develop as a result of our experiences, relationships, thoughts, and emotions. We are the sum total of all the parts that go into the making of a life.
—VIRGINIA M. AXLINE (1964, p. 215)

Robert, a 10-year-old boy, enters the play therapy room accompanied by his play therapist, Ellen. Robert is talking excitedly about a new Lego set he is carrying that he got for his birthday and is eager to show Ellen, who tells Robert that she wants to know all about it. Robert sets his new Lego creation in the center of the floor and Ellen joins him, sitting and watching as Robert shows all the parts of the Lego creation and the new mini-figures that came with the set. Ellen tries to ask Robert questions about the creation, but Robert talks so quickly and without any pauses that Ellen cannot complete a sentence. Robert makes no eye contact with Ellen and is so intensely focused on sharing the information about his Lego creation that he appears to not even notice when she sneezes.

Ellen scoots closer to Robert on the floor and faces him. She does not interrupt him and simply waits for him to notice her. After

a few moments, Robert looks at Ellen. He pauses from talking to adjust some pieces on his Lego creation. Ellen tells Robert that she likes his creation and is very happy that he brought it. She tells Robert that today they are going to play with Legos again and that his new set can be part of the play. Ellen and Robert play together using the Lego creation, and Ellen uses Lego mini-figures to help Robert talk about a bullying situation at school. Some of Robert's classmates have been making fun of him by taking his pencils and hiding them, which makes Robert very upset. Ellen uses the mini-figures to help Robert see the situation from different perspectives and to teach him skills in learning to deal with bullies.

Robert is diagnosed with autism spectrum disorder (ASD), formerly known as Asperger's syndrome. Although Robert is able to verbally communicate and his intelligence is in the normal to moderately high range, he struggles to form connections with peers and his only interest is Legos. Robert's parents brought him to play therapy at the urging of Robert's pediatrician and teacher, who were both concerned about the difficulties that Robert was having at school and home. Robert struggled to make friends and exhibited emotional "meltdowns" when things did not go his way, and his parents could not understand how such a bright boy struggled so much. Ellen has helped Robert's parents understand that although Robert is very bright, he, like many diagnosed with ASD, has difficulty understanding social cues, is easily emotionally overwhelmed, and has difficulty seeing situations from another person's perspective.

Perhaps the most helpful information that Ellen shared with Robert's parents was how his brain entered into a state of dysregulation when a threat was detected. For Robert, these threats or "triggers" are a crowded room, his father taking a driving route with which Robert is unfamiliar, or loud noises. These threats are different for each child and the reaction to the threat varies. The perceived threat triggers the sympathetic nervous system ("fight-or-flight" response), which leaves the child emotionally overwhelmed and results in tantrum-like behavior. Ellen helped Robert's parents understand that his rigid, repetitive behavior sequences were Robert's way of trying to self-soothe and that these behaviors help him feel safe. Ellen explained that play therapy was about giving Robert a warm, safe, and accepting space that would help him learn about himself and grow.

Over time, the play sessions were very helpful to Robert. Ellen incorporated Robert's love of Legos into the play therapy to teach him to deal with negative emotions, and helped him learn to see people and situations from a different perspective, which helped Robert to better adapt in social situations. Through the use of Lego mini-figures, Robert was able to see challenging social situations from a different perspective that helped him choose better behavior options. Robert also became more self-confident and began to try new things, and his emotional meltdowns lessened in intensity and frequency.

This case illustration provides a brief picture of a child diagnosed with ASD and how play therapy can help. Although Robert's behavior shares common elements that are found in all individuals diagnosed with ASD, it must be remembered that each child on the autism spectrum is unique and has his or her own "bundle" of challenges—but with those challenges also come many strengths and gifts. Children diagnosed with ASD are extraordinary, with many facets to their thinking and behavior; play therapy offers a rich and unique approach that is ideal in forming connections with these children and helping them learn and grow. This chapter provides an overview of research in this area and describes techniques that are helpful in understanding how play therapy can be used with children diagnosed with ASD, both in forming a therapeutic bond that provides a foundation for growth, and in guiding the child on a path of reflection, exploration, and a deeper sense of self-understanding.

Clinical Considerations

Is Play Therapy Effective with Children on the Autism Spectrum?

Play therapy is an effective therapeutic approach with children and adolescents (Bratton, Ray, Rhine, & Jones, 2005; Leblanc & Ritchie, 2001), and in recent years there has been an increase in studies that specifically demonstrate play therapy's effectiveness with children diagnosed with ASD. Various types of play therapy have been used with children with ASD for increasing social skills (LeGoff & Sherman, 2006; Tricomi & Gallo-Lopez, 2012); improving emotional control and decreasing negative emotions (Cashin, 2008; Greig & MacKay, 2005; Hull, 2009; Kenny & Winick, 2000); increasing verbal expression and overall adaptability (Lu, Peterson, LaCroix, & Rousseau, 2009; Solomon, Ono, Timmer, & Goodlin-Jones, 2008); helping ease the transition of the adoption process (Rubin, 2007); strengthening relational connections (Ray, Sullivan, & Carlson, 2012; Solomon et al., 2008); increasing coping skills in dealing with divorce and grief and loss (Hull, 2011); helping to enhance family relationships (Hull, 2011); creating a process of individuation and self-healing (Green, 2012); and teaching symbolic play that can generalize into the child's daily life, resulting in better coping skills and adaptability (Barton & Wolery, 2008; Herrera et al., 2008). Play therapy is also effective as a group therapy approach to help young people with ASD deal with the emotional and social issues that typically create immense challenges for them (Hull, 2013).

A number of books have been written in recent years about the application of play therapy for children and adolescents with ASD (Bromfield, 2010; Gallo-Lopez & Rubin, 2012; Hull, 2011). These works, like the one you are reading, are in response to the vast and increasing numbers of young people being diagnosed with ASD. What should be exciting for the reader to notice is that as awareness of ASD has grown in the medical and psychological fields, and as the numbers of those diagnosed have increased, the field of play therapy has responded by offering innovative and creative approaches that are as unique as the young people on the autism spectrum. As more is learned about ASD, the field of play therapy stands ready to continue to meet the psychological and emotional needs of children and adolescents diagnosed with ASD. It is imperative that current practitioners and future play therapists be prepared to work with this remarkable population.

The Play Therapist and ASD: Important Characteristics Needed for the Amazing Journey

The therapeutic alliance with a child or adolescent is one of the foundational elements of play therapy (Crenshaw & Mordock, 2005; Saunders, 2001), and from this bedrock emerges the trust and safety that are necessary for the young person's sense of freedom to explore and grow (Crenshaw & Mordock, 2005). However, building the therapeutic alliance with a child with ASD can be a daunting task. For example, one child with ASD may choose not to speak at all, whereas another child, like Robert, may talk incessantly. A child with ASD may be overwhelmed with the many choices of toys in the playroom, triggering feelings of being unsafe, and as a result the child may stay rooted to the couch and refuse to move. Another, stimulated by the roomful of toys, might bounce from toy to toy, energized by the sights and sounds of a new place and eager to explore. The play therapist choosing to work with children with ASD will never be able to predict how the child will respond upon entering the playroom or what form of play will be most useful for that child. However, if the therapist is open and willing to set aside preconceived notions and agendas, he or she will be able to create a space that is both wonderful and deeply meaningful. Obviously, there are many characteristics required of a play therapist in working with any child who has exceptional needs and abilities, but here I discuss three that are of utmost importance when working with children diagnosed with ASD.

The first characteristic is one that I call simply, "just be." To "just be" means that the therapist has abandoned an agenda, is not reactive or controlling, is not seeking to "change" or "fix" the child before him or her. To "just be" means that the therapist is curious and is simply in awe of the child, waiting patiently and without rushing the child, merely creating a space of acceptance and warmth that fosters exploration. Meeting new people and encountering new experiences are often anxiety-provoking for children diagnosed with ASD; however, with the therapist's attitude of unconditional acceptance and his or her ability to create a space of safety, the child's anxiety level will likely decrease and match the emotional climate of the environment of the playroom (Badenoch & Bogdan, 2012).

A second important characteristic is to be comfortable with silence. The play therapist working with this population must be prepared for the possibility that, at least early on, the child may not communicate verbally. During the initial phase of trust building, while the child becomes familiar with both the therapist and the playroom, allowing him or her to explore freely and interact with the space created is central to forming the therapeutic alliance. The beauty and freedom of using play therapy with these children is that for those who are nonverbal, the play experience provides a path to connection and healing.

Third and last, the therapist must bring his or her imagination to the process. A vivid and broad imagination is essential in working with children with ASD. The ideas of the child are limitless; the spectacular worlds and beastly fears that may be conjured up during the play sessions have no bounds. Certainly, interpretation and intervention have their place when working with children with ASD, and these are addressed later, but therapists must be able to resist the urge to make sense of something based on their interpretations of the world and instead surrender their imaginations to the world that the child is creating. For it is by entering the child's world that the therapist truly meets her; where the therapist truly sees him; and there, in that world, is where the truth of the child's experience is made known. Siegel (2010) echoes this phenomenon by reminding therapists that the way in which a client is viewed creates connections at a neural level that are made "real" in the form of the therapeutic relationship.

Play Therapy and ASD: Potential Challenges

The characteristics of ASD can create potential challenges in play therapy. One possible challenge arises in the area of forming a relationship and the therapeutic alliance.

Children with ASD often struggle in forming relationships with others due to deficits in joint attention, "mindblindness," also known as a deficit in theory of mind (ToM), and alexithymia. *Joint attention* refers to the combination of pointing, gaze monitoring, and showing signals (Baron-Cohen, 2008) that one uses to focus the attention of another toward an object of interest. *Mindblindness* is a term used to explain the incapacity of the person diagnosed with ASD to predict and comprehend the behavior of other people (Baron-Cohen, 1995; Hull, 2011). Another way of saying this is that the individual with ASD has a hard time understanding a situation from another person's perspective. *Alexithymia* is described as the difficulty in recognizing and understanding emotions in others and oneself, and in identifying/describing emotions using words (Fitzgerald & Bellgrove, 2006). A high number of individuals with ASD exhibit alexithymia, which creates problems in forming and sustaining relationships. Others, including the play therapist working hard to create connection with the child, may interpret his or her behavior as indicating an absence of feeling or lacking the capacity for empathy. However, although many individuals diagnosed with ASD demonstrate alexithymia, it should be remembered that this does not mean that they are incapable of exhibiting empathy (Bird et al., 2010). The play therapist working with children with ASD must be aware of the impact that joint attention deficits, mindblindness, and alexithymia have on their ability to form and sustain relationships, and must be patient in working to form the therapeutic alliance.

Another potential challenge is the restricted interest and unique characteristics of children with ASD. Play therapists who work with neurotypical children are used to children who, more often than not, have a wide interest in toys and engage in pretend play easily. Children diagnosed with ASD, in contrast, may like only one type of toy or game and completely refuse to join in anything other than what he or she likes. Many believe that children with ASD do not engage in "pretend play," and sadly this has led many to think that play therapy is not a viable treatment option. It is most helpful to remember that although the play of a child with ASD may appear "different" (Rubin, 2012, p. 31), it is *play* nonetheless. Play therapists must be flexible in their expectations, learn what the child's interests are, and then be willing to adapt the play process to those interests. It is recommended that the therapist meet with the parent or caregiver prior to meeting with the child to learn about the child's interests.

Although all children are unique, children with ASD can have very different preferences about things commonly found in the playroom, such as toys that other children have played with or the sandbox. For example, a child with ASD may be revolted by the sandbox, not wanting to get his or her hands dirty, no matter how much the therapist tries to explain that the sand is clean. Another child, very afraid of germs, may be repulsed at the thought of playing with toys that others have touched. In such instances it is important for the play therapist to remember that the child's behavior is related to feeling safe and the child's attempts to control his or her environment are an attempt to self-soothe. The message of unconditional positive regard sent by the therapist will be important to help the child with ASD feel comfortable and safe in the playroom.

What Type of Play Therapy Is Effective for Children with ASD?

The question of which play therapy approach is most effective when working with children with ASD is not easily answered. Certainly, there are many forms of play therapy, and many variations exist within those forms. To complicate matters further, each play therapist often adapts his or her individual play therapy approach based on the particular needs of the population he

or she serves. The characteristics of children with ASD requiring therapeutic intervention are vast and complicated. Similar to the concept that no two snowflakes are alike, the uniqueness of the child diagnosed with ASD and the variations of his or her struggles create a web of interlaced, delicate connections. These connections, representing a mixture of strengths and gifts, intertwine with underdeveloped skills and developmental challenges. Children with ASD who struggle to form and sustain relationships and who have difficulty communicating within relationships, represent a population that requires a treatment approach that is both broad enough to create connection so a bond of trust and safety is formed, yet precise enough so that individual problems can be addressed.

Nondirective play therapy, or client-centered play therapy (CCPT), is useful with children with ASD, especially in the early stages of helping them feel comfortable and safe in the playroom. Ray and colleagues (2012) state that CCPT is beneficial for use with children with ASD because it is relationship-based and serves as a model for building relationship and fostering communication. A second benefit of CCPT is that the therapist's full acceptance of the child fosters the child's sense of safety, which increases because he or she feels understood and his or her "motivation to interact with the external world increases" (Ray et al., 2012, p. 167). A third benefit of CCPT is the nonverbal approach; the child is not forced to communicate with the therapist. For children with ASD, this is a welcome change from most of the environments they encounter. Finally, CCPT is beneficial for use with children with ASD because the focus is on fostering a positive sense of self in them; the children are completely accepted for who they are and are not seen as needing to be "fixed" or changed (Ray et al., 2012, p. 166).

Directive play therapy also provides valuable tools for the play therapist working with children with ASD. Directive play therapy, also known as "prescriptive" play therapy (Schaefer, 2001), can be used to address specific challenges associated with ASD, such as understanding and overcoming negative emotions, decreasing mind-blindness, increasing social skills, decreasing negative behaviors, and strengthening family relationships (Hull, 2011). Based on the intricate challenges of ASD, as well as the vast array of unique characteristics of the children who live with those challenges on a daily basis, an integrative approach that utilizes both nondirective and directive techniques is best in treating children with ASD in play therapy. An integrative approach, also known as a client-focused theoretical approach (Kenny-Noziska, Schaefer, & Homeyer, 2012), is "a theoretical approach tailored to the individual needs of a client" (p. 249), and allows the play therapist to incorporate pieces of both approaches in a way that best serves the child with ASD. This tailor-made aspect of the therapy can be seen in the interactions of Robert and his play therapist Ellen, and is further demonstrated in the case example at the end of the chapter.

Play Therapy Techniques for Children with ASD

Sandtray

The use of the sandtray is an effective play therapy tool for children with ASD (Green, 2012; Hull, 2011; Richardson, 2012). Incorporating the sandtray in treatment is useful in helping the child develop a sense of self (Green, 2012), increase communication skills and relationship building (Richardson, 2012), increase spontaneous and imaginative play (Lu et al., 2009), increase his or her sense of self-worth (Hull, 2011), and deal with troubling negative emotions (Hull, 2011). Interacting with sand is a nonverbal experience in which the child can construct his or her own world. This autonomy to create and express freely in

the sandtray helps the child work through distressing emotions and achieve a sense of safety and relaxation (Richardson, 2012).

All that is needed to begin sandplay is a simple introduction. I never know how a child, whether neurotypical or diagnosed with ASD, is going to respond when seeing the sandtray for the first time. I wrote earlier how some children with ASD find the sandtray "icky" because they do not want to get their hands "dirty," or because of sensory issues, or simply because it is something "new" and their anxiety prevents them from engaging in the experience. Should the child reject the sandtray, I recommend allowing him or her to have that freedom in a nondirective manner. However, because sandplay is such a powerful tool in which internal conflicts and confusing emotions can be brought safely to the surface, the therapist should reintroduce it as the therapeutic alliance is strengthened.

Use of the sandtray has been adapted to many different theoretical orientations and approaches. The most important part of using the sandtray with children with ASD is to simply give them the freedom to create without judgment or direction; the therapist's role is that of an observer. The child's personal experience with the sandtray carries the therapeutic value, not the therapist's interpretation (Green, 2012). The child is provided with a selection of objects/miniatures to be used in the sandtray so that he or she can make a "sand world." The therapist can simply prompt the child to "make a world however you want it to be." I provide objects related to the child's specified interest for use in the sandtray, such as Legos or miniature horses. After the child creates his or her world, the therapist may ask about that world, such as what certain objects represent and what characters would say to one another, if they could speak.

Some children will not use objects in the sand at all; they may simply sculpt the sand or create patterns. A child with whom I worked asked for a sandtray with wet sand so that he could sculpt it. He created an island and made a sand "ball," which he used to represent himself, then made several other "balls" representing his family members and placed those "far, far away from *my* island." This simple picture was a representation of how he, being diagnosed with ASD, felt "different" and excluded from his neurotypical parents and siblings. This representation was powerful in helping this child create a picture that signified his feelings and thoughts related to his family. His simple sculptures paved the way for a more positive sense of self to emerge. This increased sense of self-worth was evidenced by increased social interaction with his family and his peers at school.

Puppets and Stuffed Animals

Children are often attached to stuffed animals and find them appealing, and many children enjoy engaging in therapeutic play using puppets. Puppets are a useful tool to use with children with ASD, specifically to help them articulate their fears and to increase their perspective-taking abilities (Bromfield, 1989; Hull, 2011). Stuffed animals can be used to help children describe their family members or their classmates from school. I have used stuffed animals and puppets to help children with ASD play out bullying situations and use the animals to tell the story of what happened. For instance, the child can be directed to select a stuffed animal that represents the bully and one that represents him- or herself. If the child seems at a loss, I may prompt with a statement such as "Show me what happened when the bully approached you" or "What did you say after he called you that name?" This technique can help children process emotional content, such as fear over a certain situation or sadness about a death or loss. Puppets and stuffed animals provide excellent tools for introducing the skill of perspective taking to younger children, by getting them to imagine what another person might be thinking or feeling.

Expressive Arts

Expressive arts are effective in helping children with ASD develop cognitively, socially, emotionally, and behaviorally (Gilroy, 2006) because they provide these children with a medium through which to integrate information. As Goucher (2012) so eloquently describes, working in expressive arts media "leads to increased ability to integrate and creatively express experiences, allowing an individual with autism the opportunity to begin to build a more fully realized self" (p. 301). A common finding among individuals with ASD is that they possess great strength in the area of visualization, yet struggle with verbalizing what the mind's eye sees. The use of the expressive arts provides the means with which they can exercise this strength and, at the same time, create new neural pathways as they bring to life an internal image and attempt to articulate what is within (Goucher, 2012). Expressive arts can be nondirective by simply providing a child with the space and tools to create, and can also be directive in nature, with the therapist prompting the child to draw or sculpt an object or scene. Children with ASD may benefit most from a combined approach, depending on their abilities and interests. Some children with ASD do not like art and may approach the activity with great hesitation, experiencing heightened anxiety sitting before a blank piece of paper with markers, crayons, and pencils lying about. In these situations, it is helpful to direct the child to draw something ("Make a person, any way you want to") or engage in the activity with him or her. I will sometimes draw for the child in order to get things moving, allowing him or her to come up with an image in the mind's eye while I create a rough sketch. This not only helps to get the child talking about internal images, but can prompt him or her to practice verbalizing what he or she sees. I used this technique to help a boy overcome his fear of monsters and masks (Hull, 2011). Although very hesitant at first, he eventually began drawing his own monsters as a result of watching me draw. We put silly hair and lipstick on the monsters, and some of them wore dresses and had suitcases attached to their heads. This activity helped him grasp the concept that monsters were not real, but could be created in the mind's eye—which created a real picture but not reality. This case is an example of how the use of expressive arts created a pathway to confidence and growth in overcoming fear where verbal engagement alone had failed to do so.

Legos, Lincoln Logs, Tinkertoys, and Other Building Materials

Building toys, such as Legos, Lincoln Logs, and Tinkertoys have been found to be useful in play therapy for increasing children's sense of self-worth and overcoming fears (Hull, 2011), increasing social skills and problem-solving abilities (LeGoff & Sherman, 2006; Owens, Granader, Humphrey, & Baron-Cohen, 2008), and creating a sense of structure and safety in the play process (Norton & Norton, 1997). Building toys such as Legos tend to interest young people with ASD "due to the fact that people with autism are particularly attracted to systems" (Owens et al., 2008, p. 1945). Playing with toys such as Lincoln Logs and Tinkertoys can help instill a sense of self-confidence and freedom in exploration as the child begins to build; the completed product is a representation of something that the child envisioned in the mind's eye and brought to life by his or her own hands. Children will often incorporate other toys with the building materials; for instance, using the building made of Lincoln Logs as a parking garage for toy cars, or pretending that the Tinkertoy creation is a robot that will defend the city made of Legos. I have used building toys to also help children with ASD learn impulse control and patience through the "one block at a time" notion that is a natural part of play with building toys.

Legos are unique building toys because they include mini-figures, small Lego "people," that come in both genders and a variety of uniforms and fields. Because they are miniature representations of people, the mini-figures can be used to act out social situations, explain family dynamics, and demonstrate perspective taking for children with ASD. This is done through simple questions such as "What do you think Luke is thinking when he finds out that Darth Vader is his father?" or "How might this character feel when his classmates ignore him?" I have found that using mini-figures help children with ASD verbalize thoughts and feelings about family members or classmates—something that is ordinarily hard for them to do. Lego bricks can be used to build representations of familiar places, such as the child's home or school, and provides the opportunity for the child to share her thoughts and feelings about such places.

Lego bricks and pieces come in thousands of various shapes, sizes, and colors and allow children to freely create any type of building, vehicle, spaceship, or device. This freedom helps provide a sense of structure and safety and instills a sense of self-worth as the child sees his or her creation in finished form. Legos and other building toys are also useful in group therapy settings for increasing children's social skills (Hull, 2011; LeGoff & Sherman, 2006).

Superheroes

Superheroes are a powerful tool to use in play therapy (Rubin, 2007) and can be particularly useful with children with ASD (Scanlon, 2007). Individuals of all ages identify with a superhero of some sort, and children with ASD often have a favorite superhero character that they love and with whom they identify. Due to the tendency of children with ASD to engage in solitary or parallel play, and because of the phenomenon of "echoplaylia," which is defined as the tendency to "mimic" various cartoons or movies the child has seen (Scanlon, 2007, p. 177), the use of superheroes with these remarkable children can be beneficial in important ways.

First, the superhero is a representation of power, but more importantly, superheroes use their power to overcome obstacles and adversity in an effort to fight evil and help others. The backstories of most superheroes contain themes of rejection, struggle, and overcoming negative emotions such as anger and fear. Many children diagnosed with ASD suffer with low self-worth and often feel weak and rejected, and identify with the superhero model's characteristics such as bravery, loyalty, and believing in oneself. No one cheered louder than I when a young boy named Harry Potter burst onto the world's stage, and child after child, with book in hand, found strength and comfort in this character who seemed so much like them ("He wears glasses just like me!"). Harry and his friends, as well as the enemies, came alive in the office as I helped to cultivate inner strength and a sense of value and worth through these amazing stories and characters.

Second, there is rich metaphorical material embedded in the stories of superheroes. The "enemies" in the stories provide valuable metaphors for bullies, obstacles, challenges, and negative emotions. The character attributes of the superhero as well as the various abilities and gadgets (e.g., Batman's "utility belt") provide symbols with which children can identify and incorporate into their way of thinking. The metaphor of Batman's utility belt was useful with a child with ASD who loved Batman and was experiencing bullying. We examined Batman's belt and then came up with "tools" for this young man: Getting to safety, physically standing in a firm stance (just like Batman!), using his strong verbal skills, and telling an adult were all part of an internal "utility belt" that the child could keep with him at all times. This extended metaphor helped to provide a sense of safety and increased this boy's

confidence in not just surviving the school day, but doing so with confidence—and his social interactions improved as a result. Superheroes also provide wonderful ways for children to deal with life's difficult transitions, such as divorce and adoption (Rubin, 2007), as well as improving emotional "literacy," the ability to "identify and express different emotions quickly and accurately" (Sayers, 2007, p. 91).

Video/Computer Games

Video/computer games have grown in use as a play therapy tool (Hull, 2009) and have specifically been used with children who have ASD to overcome fears, increase self-worth, and conquer bullying and social rejection (Hull, 2011). Many children with ASD are naturally interested in video/computer games and serve as their specified interest. Attwood (1998) notes that incorporating a child's specified interest into the therapy process often motivates the child to engage in the therapeutic process, which is important for children with ASD who may be wary of a new environment such as the playroom.

The first benefit of using video/computer games in play therapy is that the games can be used to build the therapeutic relationship by helping to establish a sense of safety and trust between therapist and client. Second, video/computer games can serve as an assessment tool by revealing how the child responds to failure, deals with frustration, and solves problems (if at all). For example, a child who continues to try at a game after failure and does so by learning from the failed attempts shows great resolve and problem-solving skills—valuable information that the therapist can use later in the therapy process. Third, video/computer games are valuable teaching tools for such areas as increasing frustration tolerance and impulse control, dealing with negative emotions such as anger and fear, learning to make good choices, and relying on others for help. Fourth, video/computer games are useful to help children overcome challenges such as bullying, a parent's divorce, or stressful life transitions. I often use the game Super Mario Bros., with all of the various villains and obstacles, with children who are being bullied as a way to view the situation from a safe distance through play and learn coping skills to overcome the challenging situation.

Video/computer games can be used in individual therapy sessions as well as group sessions and are effective ways to teach social skills such as turn taking, responding to joint attention cues, and offering encouragement to peers who are engaged in a task. Video/computer games are effective in strengthening family bonds between parents and caregivers of children with ASD by creating opportunities for the parent's greater understanding of the child through observing and joining in game play (Hull, 2012). These games are also useful in helping a child with ASD with the challenge of risk taking and trying something new. The characteristics of ASD discussed earlier cause the child to be very resistant about trying new food, engaging in different routines, and visiting new places. Trying a new video/computer game, or trying a new part of a game with which the child is unfamiliar, serves as a metaphor for the child to try something new in real life and grow. A consideration that must be addressed is that video/computer games can be isolating, especially for children on the autism spectrum. A solution to deal with this problem, should it arise, is to choose interactive games with a two-player option so that the therapist can join in the play.

The Play of Drama and Dance/Movement

Drama therapy allows children with ASD to express and explore emotions and learn to understand others through interacting with peers and modeling their behavior. This approach, which can be adjusted to the ability level of the child, helps with improving child's flexibility and improvisa-

tion in new or difficult situations (Tricomi & Gallo-Lopez, 2012). The ACT Method© uses a group format in a school setting and a number of drama-based techniques such as "dramatic play, improvisation, role play, theater games, puppet and mask work, the use of costumes and props, scripted readings, playwriting, movement, music, visual arts, and performance" (p. 278). Members meet weekly and at the end of the school year craft a public performance, which provides them with a sense of self-worth and an opportunity for validation from those observing the performance.

Dance/movement therapy has a rich history and has been found to be a helpful approach with children with ASD by helping to regulate their nervous systems, which are often over- or underactivated (Devereaux, 2012). Dance/movement therapists (DMTs) observe the child's movements, which are often stereotyped, repetitive, and restricted. Integrating these movements into larger patterns of motion through dance "provides a broader range of responses that children can use to communicate and cope with their environment" (Devereaux, 2012, p. 341). Gradually, as children's confidence grows, they can leave their isolated worlds and branch out to new environments, now more aware of themselves and others.

Play Therapy with Families

Filial therapy (FT) is "a theoretically integrative psychoeducational model of therapy in which parents serve as the primary change agents for their children" (VanFleet, 2012, p. 193). FT guides parents in nondirective play therapy techniques that result in deeper family relationships and provides the parents with greater understanding of their child's needs. FT is especially useful for families with children with ASD because it helps break down communication barriers, build better relationships between parents and child, and create better relationships between the child and his or her siblings (VanFleet, 2012).

The PLAY (Play and Language for Autistic Youngsters) Project is another play therapy approach that incorporates parents-as-professionals to help their child up the developmental ladder. Parents are trained in play techniques to better understand their children and help them overcome the developmental challenges that accompany ASD (Solomon, 2012).

DIRFloortime®, another play approach that puts the parent in a therapeutic role, is an "interdisciplinary framework that enables play clinicians, parents, and educators to construct a comprehensive assessment and intervention program based on the child's and family's unique developmental profile that addresses these core deficits" (Hess, 2012, p. 231). This effective approach uses play as a way to build relationship between parent and child, increase parental understanding of the child's needs, and foster the child's growth to the highest possible rung of the developmental ladder (Greenspan & Wieder, 1999; Hess, 2012).

Clinical Case Example

The following is a composite case example of a child diagnosed with ASD and how play therapy helped with his challenges. Jonathan, a 9-year-old boy, was referred for play therapy because he was overwhelmed by negative emotions, mainly anxiety. Like many children diagnosed with ASD, Jonathan's strengths included a vivid imagination, high intelligence, and a very caring heart. Jonathan struggled with emotional intensity, which created a roller coaster of feelings and thoughts, and the most devastating emotion for him was fear. When Jonathan became triggered by a fear, he would mentally obsess about it and play scenarios over and over in his mind, until he became mentally and emotionally exhausted. Jonathan's main fear was connected to "robbers who would break in his house and steal things." Jonathan's fears would usually "ramp up" in the evenings, after dark,

and he constantly checked the locks on the doors and windows of the house. Lately, his mother explained that his fear of robbers was also triggered when he was out in public, especially if Jonathan saw a police car parked in the grocery store parking lot or other public place. It is important to note that this fear was not related to a life event; neither Jonathan nor anyone he knew had ever been a victim of theft.

Jonathan was hesitant and cautious on his first visit to the playroom, but soon relaxed upon seeing the variety of toys, especially a Nintendo Entertainment System. He was very knowledgeable about old video game systems and was a "big fan" of Mario and Luigi from the game Super Mario Bros. Jonathan asked if we could play the game; he became very excited during game play and recited the history of the characters and how Mario and Luigi have evolved over the years. He paid particular attention to the villains of the game, such as the goombas, koopa troopas, and piranha plants, referring to them as "bad" guys because they try to stop Mario and Luigi from saving the princess. Each time Jonathan maneuvered his character through a patch of villains, he would release a sigh of relief and push the pause button on the game to gather his thoughts and refocus before he went on. This cautious way of playing the game was revealing, as it showed how Jonathan approached situations that he viewed as threatening.

In the next few visits Jonathan expanded his exploration of the playroom. Although he still wanted to play Super Mario Bros. for part of the time, it did not consume the whole session. During the second session, while playing Super Mario Bros., Jonathan brought up the topic of "robbers" and his fear of them. He did so at a point in the game in which his character had to fight the "boss" at the end of one of the levels, and it worried him to think of "failing" and having the boss "beat" him. While the game was stopped, he told me all about what robbers do and how they terrify him.

"That's why it feels so good to beat the bad guys in Mario Bros.," he said. He and I both agreed that a game like "Beat the Robbers" would be a great idea for a video game. The player could be a police character and work together with other law enforcement personnel to capture the robbers and put them in jail. I gave Jonathan a legal pad and asked him to sketch out the game on the paper; he included storyboards and various elements of what the game would look like.

Jonathan liked to invent things and often brought sketches or models of the various ideas that he had come up with earlier in the week. One unique aspect of Jonathan's play was that he liked to take elements from various videogames, TV shows, etc., and combine them to form a game that was his distinct invention, and he also liked to act them out or use objects, such as Legos to bring them to life. Suddenly, he sprang into action and asked me to help him: He wanted to construct a city. We set to work using Legos and wooden building blocks for buildings that we positioned on the floor. Next, we gathered various cars: a "getaway" car for the robbers and police cruisers and emergency vehicles for the police and fire department. Jonathan chose a small golden figurine, which we called an "idol," and placed it at the top of one of the buildings the robbers would attempt to steal. Once the scene was ready, Jonathan began to play out the scenario of the robbers taking the idol and the police successfully apprehending the offenders.

Jonathan played this scenario out over four sessions and insisted that I join him in play. At times, I would be in charge of the robbers' vehicle, and sometimes I was Jonathan's "assistant" in helping catch the robbers. Other toys and figures were used from time to time, such as Batman and Mario and Luigi figures made of Legos. He liked it when I talked in an Italian accent and pretended to be Mario and Luigi. I incorporated them into the story as two brothers who were once afraid of robbers but who had realized that there was a force

of "good," such as police officers and concerned, watchful citizens, that helped keep the robbers away. Later in the play sequences, Jonathan liked it when I spoke in a gruff voice pretending to be the robbers. I said things like, "We have no chance against the police force"; "We're not as smart as the good guys"; and "Crime never pays—we always get caught!" He would laugh and remark, "Those guys sure are dumb. They get caught every time!"

Over the course of five to seven sessions, Jonathan's fear of robbers completely disappeared. His play shifted from cautious and fear-based, to confident and intentional. He showed humor when talking about robbers instead of closing his eyes and cowering, and he was able to verbalize his insight about knowing that law enforcement existed to protect people like him, something that he was unable to grasp before coming to play therapy. Jonathan's mother reported that he no longer checked the doors at night and that he was relaxed and no longer showed any signs of mental or emotional distress once it became dark. She shared that one day, in front of their church, a woman's purse was snatched, and Jonathan watched as the police came and conducted their investigation. She said that he was able to show genuine concern for the woman, and instead of becoming emotionally overwhelmed, he was able to go home and play after commenting that he hoped the police caught the person who committed the crime. His mother stated that just a few months prior, an event such as that would have traumatized him.

Conclusion

Play therapy has many dimensions and possible applications and is an effective therapeutic approach to use with children with ASD. This fascinating therapeutic medium, complete with many unique tools and techniques, assists those brave clinicians who help children, parents, medical professionals, and educators face the developmental dragon of ASD. Play therapy not only helps these children reach key developmental milestones, but also provides a vehicle for communication and understanding, and more importantly, creates fertile ground for the development of the child's self.

REFERENCES

Attwood, T. (1998). *Asperger's syndrome: A guide for parents and professionals.* London: Jessica Kingsley.

Axline, V. M. (1964). *Dibs: In search of self—personality development in play therapy.* New York: Ballantine Books.

Badenoch, B., & Bogdan, N. (2012). Safety and connection: The neurobiology of play. In L. Gallo-Lopez & L. C. Rubin (Eds.), *Play-based interventions for children and adolescents with autism spectrum disorders* (pp. 3–18). New York: Routledge/Taylor & Francis.

Baron-Cohen, S. (1995). *Mindblindness: An essay on autism and theory of mind.* Cambridge, MA: MIT Press.

Baron-Cohen, S. (2008). *Autism and Asperger syndrome: The facts.* Oxford, UK: Oxford University Press.

Barton, E. E., & Wolery, M. (2008). Teaching pretend play to children with disabilities: A review of the literature. *Topics in Early Childhood Special Education, 28*(2), 109–125.

Bird, G., Silani, G., Brindley, R., White, S., Frith, U., & Singer, T. (2010). Empathic brain responses in insula are modulated by levels of alexithymia but not autism. *Brain, 133*(5), 1515–1525.

Bratton, S. C., Ray D., Rhine T., & Jones, L. (2005). The efficacy of play therapy with children: A meta-analytic review of outcomes. *Professional Psychology: Research and Practice, 36*(4), 376–390.

Bromfield, R. (1989). Psychodynamic play therapy with a high-functioning autistic child. *Psychoanalytic Psychology, 6*(4), 439–453.

Bromfield, R. (2010). *Doing therapy with children and adolescents with Asperger syndrome.* Hoboken, NJ: Wiley.

Cashin, A. (2008). Narrative therapy: A psychotherapeutic approach in the treatment of adolescents with Asperger's disorder. *Journal of Child and Adolescent Psychiatric Nursing, 21,* 48–56.

Crenshaw, D., & Mordock, J. (2005). *Understanding and treating the aggression of children: Fawns in gorilla suits.* Lanham, MD: Aronson.

Devereaux, C. (2012). Moving into relationships: Dance/movement therapy with children with autism. In L. Gallo-Lopez & L. C. Rubin (Eds.), *Play-based interventions for children and adolescents with autism spectrum disorders* (pp. 333–351). New York: Routledge/Taylor & Francis.

Fitzgerald, M., & Bellgrove, M. A. (2006). The overlap between alexithymia and Asperger's syndrome. *Journal of Autism and Developmental Disorders, 36*(4), 573–576.

Gallo-Lopez, L., & Rubin, L. C. (Eds.). (2012). *Play-based interventions for children and adolescents with autism spectrum disorders.* New York: Routledge/Taylor & Francis.

Gilroy, A. (2006). *Art therapy: Research and evidence-based practice.* London: Sage.

Goucher, C. (2012). Art therapy: Connecting and communicating. In L. Gallo-Lopez & L. C. Rubin (Eds.), *Play-based interventions for children and adolescents with autism spectrum disorders* (pp. 295–315). New York: Routledge/Taylor & Francis.

Green, E. (2012). The Narcissus myth, resplendent reflections, and self-healing: A Jungian perspective on counseling a child with Asperger's syndrome. In L. Gallo-Lopez & L. C. Rubin (Eds.), *Play-based interventions for children and adolescents with autism spectrum disorders* (pp. 177–192). New York: Routledge/Taylor & Francis.

Greenspan, S. I., & Wieder, S. (1999). A functional developmental approach to autism spectrum disorders. *Journal of the Association for Persons with Severe Handicaps, 24*(3), 147–161.

Greig, A., & Mackey, T. (2005). Asperger's syndrome and cognitive behaviour therapy: New applications for educational psychologists. *Educational and Child Psychology, 22,* 4–15.

Herrera, G., Alcantud, F., Jordan, R., Blanquer, A., Labajo, G., & De Pablo, C. (2008). Development of symbolic play through the use of virtual reality tools in children with autism spectrum disorders. *Autism, 12*(2), 143–157.

Hess, E. (2012). DIR/Floortime: A developmental/relational play therapy approach for treating children impacted by autism. In L. Gallo-Lopez & L. C. Rubin (Eds.), *Play-based interventions for children and adolescents with autism spectrum disorders* (pp. 231–248). New York: Routledge/Taylor & Francis.

Hull, K. (2009). Computer/video games as a play therapy tool in reducing emotional disturbances in children. *Dissertation Abstracts International: Section B: Sciences and Engineering, 70*(12-B), 2010, 7854.

Hull, K. (2011). *Play therapy and Asperger's syndrome: Helping children and adolescents grow, connect, and heal through the art of play.* Lanham, MD: Aronson.

Hull, K. (2012). *Bridge building: Creating connection and relationship between parents of children/adolescents on the autism spectrum.* Lynchburg, VA: Liberty University Press.

Hull, K. (2013). *Group therapy techniques with children, adolescents, and adults on the autism spectrum: Growth and connection for all ages.* Lanham, MD: Aronson.

Kenny, M. C., & Winick, C. B. (2000). An integrative approach to play therapy with an autistic girl. *International Journal of Play Therapy, 9*(1), 11–33.

Kenny-Noziska, S. G., Schaefer, C. E., & Homeyer, L. E. (2012). Beyond directive or nondirective: Moving the conversation forward. *International Journal of Play Therapy, 21*(4), 244–252.

Leblanc, M., & Ritchie, M. (2001). A meta-analysis of play therapy outcomes. *Counselling Psychology Quarterly 14*(2), 149–163.

LeGoff, D. B., & Sherman, M. (2006). Long-term outcome of social skills intervention based on interactive Lego play. *Autism, 10*(4), 317–329.

Lu, L., Peterson, F., LaCroix, L., & Rousseau, C. (2010). Stimulating creative play in children with autism through sand play. *Arts in Psychotherapy, 37*(1), 56–64.

Norton, C. C., & Norton, B. E. (1997). *Reaching children through play therapy: An experiential approach.* Denver, CO: Pendleton Clay.

Owens, G., Granader, Y., Humphrey, A., & Baron-Cohen, S. (2008). Lego® therapy and the social use of language program: An evaluation of two social skills interventions for children with high-functioning autism and Asperger's syndrome. *Journal of Autism and Developmental Disorders, 38*, 1944–1957.

Ray, D. C., Sullivan, J. M., & Carlson, S. E. (2012). Relational intervention: Child-centered play therapy with children on the autism spectrum. In L. Gallo-Lopez & L. C. Rubin (Eds.), *Play-based interventions for children and adolescents with autism spectrum disorders* (pp. 159–175). New York: Routledge/Taylor & Francis.

Richardson, J. F. (2012). The world of the sand tray and the child on the autism spectrum. In L. Gallo-Lopez & L. C. Rubin (Eds.), *Play-based interventions for children and adolescents with autism spectrum disorders* (pp. 209–227). New York: Routledge/Taylor & Francis.

Rubin, L. C. (2007). "Luke, I am your father!" A clinical application of the *Star Wars* adoption narrative. In L. C. Rubin (Ed.), *Using superheroes in counseling and play therapy* (pp. 213–224). New York: Springer.

Rubin, L. C. (2012). Playing on the autism spectrum. In L. Gallo-Lopez & L. C. Rubin (Eds.), *Play-based interventions for children and adolescents with autism spectrum disorders* (pp. 19–35). New York: Routledge/Taylor & Francis.

Saunders, S. M. (2001). Pretreatment correlates of the therapeutic bond. *Journal of Clinical Psychology, 57*(12), 1339–1352.

Sayers, J. M. (2007). The Incredible Hulk and emotional literacy. In L. C. Rubin (Ed.), *Using superheroes in counseling and play therapy* (pp. 89–101). New York: Springer.

Scanlon, P. (2007). Superheroes are super friends: Developing social skills and emotional reciprocity with autism spectrum clients. In L. C. Rubin (Ed.), *Using superheroes in counseling and play therapy* (pp. 213–224). New York: Springer.

Schaefer, C. E. (2001). Prescriptive play therapy. *International Journal of Play Therapy, 10*(2), 57–73.

Siegel, D. J. (2010). *The mindful therapist.* New York: Norton.

Solomon, M., Ono, M., Timmer, S., & Goodlin-Jones, B. (2008). The effectiveness of parent–child interaction therapy for families of children on the autism spectrum. *Journal of Autism and Developmental Disorders, 38*, 1767–1776.

Solomon, R. (2012). The PLAY project: A train-the-trainer model of early intervention for children with autism spectrum disorders. In

L. Gallo-Lopez & L. C. Rubin (Eds.), *Play-based interventions for children and adolescents with autism spectrum disorders* (pp. 249–269). New York: Routledge/Taylor & Francis.

Tricomi, L. P., & Gallo-Lopez, L. (2012). The ACT project: Enhancing social competence through drama therapy and performance. In L. Gallo-Lopez & L. C. Rubin (Eds.), *Play-based interventions for children and adolescents with autism spectrum disorders* (pp. 271–291). New York: Routledge/Taylor & Francis.

VanFleet, R. (2012). Communication and connection: Filial therapy with families of children with ASD. In L. Gallo-Lopez & L. C. Rubin (Eds.), *Play-based interventions for children and adolescents with autism spectrum disorders* (pp. 193–208). New York: Routledge/Taylor & Francis.

CHAPTER 28

Play Therapy with Children with Attention-Deficit/Hyperactivity Disorder

Heidi Gerard Kaduson

Attention-deficit/hyperactivity disorder (ADHD) is one of the most commonly diagnosed neurobehavioral disorders in children. Controversy surrounding ADHD, as well as our understanding of the disorder, continues to evolve. Although ADHD was once characterized primarily in terms of overactive and inattentive behavior, and later by marked impulsivity, it is now described by deficits in executive function (Barkley, 2012) and motivation (Sonuga-Barke, 2005). Challenges with activity level, attention, and impulsivity are viewed as behavioral manifestations of problems in the capacity for self-regulation and corresponding deficits in planning and successfully completing goal-directed activities.

ADHD is one of the most prevalent mental disorders diagnosed in children, affecting about 3–5% of children globally (Frank-Briggs, 2013). A study by the Centers for Disease Control and Prevention (2011) reported that approximately 11% of U.S. children ages 4–17 years (6.4 million) have received a medical diagnosis of ADHD. This constitutes an increase from 7.8% in 2003,

and has raised concerns about the overdiagnosis and overmedication of children by some (Schwarz & Cohen, 2013). Although psychostimulants continue to be the most dominant treatment implemented, the use of medication for ADHD actually decreased from 15% of visits (to the pediatrician or psychiatrist) in 2003 to 6% in 2010, and the management of ADHD in the community has shifted away from pediatricians to psychiatrists. It is important for play therapists to reach out and communicate with the other professionals, such as psychiatrists, physicians, psychologists, teachers, and occupational therapists, working with the child and family.

Most of research conducted on treatment effectiveness has examined the impact of medication, behavioral therapy, or cognitive-behavioral therapy for ADHD, and some professionals have questioned whether play therapy could be an effective intervention for the disorder. Over the last 20 years, the efficacy of play therapy with children with ADHD has been reported clinically and empirically, and play therapy is increasingly recognized as a helpful tool to use for this population (Barzegary & Zamini, 2011; Bratton et al., 2013; Kaduson, 1993; Ray, Schottelkorb, & Tsai, 2007). The therapeutic powers of play, such as problem solving, self-regulation, and direct and indirect teaching (Schaefer, 2014), can help children with ADHD identify and communicate their problems through play and participate more fully in treatment. A vital aspect of using play therapy is that the child is *actively engaged, practicing, and developing needed skills* in treatment. Play therapy treatment for children with ADHD focuses on remediation of skill deficits and also allows children to work through any related psychological issues, such as anxiety and poor self-esteem. The play therapist facilitates this psychological work by keeping the child focused on his or her own play, simultaneously working on important issues and skills, without distraction. Another vital aspect of successful intervention is parent education and consultation. This collaborative effort permits more therapeutic engagement to occur directly with the child.

The fifth edition of the American Psychiatric Association's (2013) *Diagnostic and Statistical Manual of Mental Disorders* (DSM-5) provides a consistent set of criteria to use to confer a diagnosis of ADHD. Evidence of inattentive or hyperactive–impulsive symptoms must occur before age 12, be present across two or more settings (e.g., at home, school, recreational setting), and interfere with functioning or development. The symptoms of inattention may include trouble maintaining attention when engaged in tasks or play activities, often failing to finish schoolwork, difficulty organizing tasks, or being easily distracted. Hyperactivity and impulsivity symptoms can be displayed in the form of frequent fidgeting, inappropriate running about, talking excessively, and trouble waiting for a turn. There is no definitive test with which to diagnose ADHD, and many other problems (e.g., anxiety, trauma, depression, certain forms of learning disabilities) have similar symptoms, so play therapists should work in close collaboration with other professionals and the family to make sure that the diagnosis and treatment are appropriate.

As can be seen, the constellation of symptoms that make up ADHD is quite varied and the presentation can change over time, making it one of the most complex disorders with which to work. Based on the nature of the symptoms, three types of ADHD can be diagnosed applying the DSM-5 criteria: combined presentation, predominantly inattentive presentation, and predominantly hyperactive–impulsive presentation. The symptoms of ADHD affect children's interactions in all areas of their environment and result in an inability to meet situational demands in an age-appropriate way (Imeraj et al., 2013). Children with ADHD typically experience difficulty with home, school, and community behavior, including peer interaction, academic achievement, and general adjustment. Their behavior is frequently enigmatic to their parents and teachers. Their uneven, unpredictable behavior creates additional stress and leads to the erroneous belief that these problems are solely problems of motivation and desire rather than physically based disabilities.

ADHD symptoms can cause significant and pervasive impairment in children's day-to-day interaction with the environment. The adults in their lives primarily determine, create, and maintain the familial, social, and academic demands placed on the children (Goldstein, 2002). However, when a child enters school for 6 hours a day, the adult interventions from home cannot work, and the teachers do not always understand the manifestations of the disorder. When that confusion occurs, the focus of concern can become the "bad behavior" that a child exhibits, rather than an understanding of the symptoms of ADHD as a disorder. Children with ADHD can begin to feel different, without knowing why and without understanding how to cope adaptively. Furthermore, ADHD appears to significantly and negatively impact the child's emerging personality and cognitive skills, resulting in negative feedback in various areas (Barkley, 2012). Children with ADHD do not understand the impact it has on their own functioning. They are brought to treatment by their parents, who have either been told by the school or by other family members to get help, and the children generally have no choice in this matter.

Although there are many different modes of treatment, play therapy works directly with children to help remediate the skill deficits while also increasing their self-esteem and self-confidence. In addition, play therapy allows the therapeutic powers of play to assist in healing psychological difficulties in the context of a caring relationship. Children who experience years of negative feedback, negative reinforcement, and an inability to meet the reasonable demands of family, friends, and teachers because of such skill deficits will certainly be affected. Play therapists must be aware not only of the core symptoms of this disorder, but also of the significant secondary impact they have on both the child and family members (Barkley, 2012; Kaduson, 2000). Play therapy gives children a safe place where they are accepted as they are and it allows them the freedom to learn coping mechanisms and to feel the self-confidence they need.

To facilitate the healing of children, parents must be trained in how to understand and manage their children's behavior and how to be the advocate they need. A multimodal approach also includes education of the parents regarding the facts about the diagnosis and treatment of ADHD. Parent training is conducted on a weekly basis, incorporating medication referrals (when indicated), classroom interventions, teacher consultation, social skills training, and individual play therapy to help the children understand the characteristics of the disorder as well as to learn adaptive coping and satisfying play skills. In a study of on-task behavior by children with ADHD and non-ADHD children, it was found that the

children with ADHD were significantly less attentive only during tasks that required high self-regulation, information processing, and motivational demands, and developed similarly in the music and art classes (Imeraj et al., 2013). This difficulty with on-task behavior would also impact children's play skills and impair the emotional and therapeutic value of play for processing psychological difficulties.

While parents may need guidance with respect to being advocates for their children, it should be noted that not all parents will be able to function in this role. The play therapist will need to try to educate them about their children's particular needs and help them understand the value of parental input.

Clinical Application

In all the years I have worked with this population, the most rewarding part is to see a child succeed and feel productive as he or she begins to cope with the disorder and starts the healing process. Since these children rarely get the typical positive responses from others, allowing them to be in an environment where they are free to be who they are, without judgment, will begin the process of healing that other children can experience perhaps without therapy.

Play therapy for children with ADHD involves a combination of theories and techniques. Cognitive-behavioral therapy and behavioral therapy have been successful for many children who have ADHD (Antshel, Faraone, & Gordon, 2012; Curtis, Chapman, Dempsey, & Mire, 2013; Miranda, 2000), and it is from this approach that some of the applications are derived. Cognitive-behavioral play therapy (CBPT; Knell & Dasari, 2009) focuses on children's ability to learn more adaptive coping skills. Play therapy allows children to learn how to cope by *doing* rather than being told to behave in a certain way or reading about a desired behavior. Children with ADHD are about one-third behind their age-mates in social and emotional growth (Barkley, 2013). With appropriate modifications, play therapy can be used into the teenage years for children who continue to find it easier to express and relate through play (Kaduson, 2006).

To begin the treatment, the play therapist must do a complete intake with the parents only. This is crucial to make sure that the therapist is aware of cultural differences, family dynamics, prior treatment, and biological factors that could impact treatment (e.g., parents having ADHD and perhaps finding compliance with the child's therapy schedule difficult). The Child and Family Interview Questionnaire (Kaduson, 2006) can be used to help the therapist gather all necessary information.

The next step is one I have found important for my treatment approach. I inform the parents that the child's willingness is an integral part of treatment, so if the child doesn't want to come back after his or her intake, then I recommend that a referral should be made to another therapist. This simple information lets the parents know that you respect their desire to help, but that they must respect their child's input about this undertaking as well. I believe it is my obligation to make the child want to come back during the intake; there are so many obstacles for children with ADHD, and the play therapist must remain a totally safe place for this child to understand, learn, explore, and heal. Of course, each therapist must devise his or her own approach.

During the next session, the child intake, the play therapist must try to be different from a teacher, parent, or other authority figure. The play therapist is a guide to help children with ADHD work through their play—the language of all children. It is very difficult for children with ADHD to maintain focus in a thematic form of play without the play therapist assisting with the focus and tracking of the play. The inability to stay focused and distractibility cause children with ADHD to have great trouble

working through problems and/or finding solutions on their own. In addition, children with ADHD have experienced an excessive amount of discipline and criticism from adults. As a result, many children don't feel that they are capable of much and can give up when faced with even small challenges.

The intake with the child should not be challenging at all and is very structured to assess auditory processing and attention spans, fine motor skills, anxiety, and hyperactivity. The therapist must maintain a lighthearted and welcoming demeanor so that the child feels comfortable in the setting. I typically assess the child's capabilities with the use of a family drawing and the game Guess Who, by Milton Bradley. This game can be used to informally assess auditory processing, attention span, and communication abilities (I recommend that the play therapist not win and that the game be played at least three times so that initial anxiety can pass). At the end of this game, the play therapist brings a self-control-type game into play (e.g., Rebound by Mattel). Once again I recommend that the therapist not win so that several games can be played to see if the child exhibits self-control in a game format. These are quick games so that the child will not get bored or feel challenged. Each activity helps in assessing the level of planning ability and self-control (executive functioning) the child exhibits in this setting. By the end of the child intake, the play therapist likely will know whether or not the child wants to come back, and in most cases, he or she will want to return.

Weekly sessions are structured to provide the parents a focused 10-minute education/ training session specifically created for their child. This is a time to teach; all other comments or information should be sent by voicemail or e-mail so that the 10 minutes can be solution focused. Research shows that incorporating parent training, especially for preschoolers, is the treatment of choice for children with ADHD (Charach et al., 2013). Including parents also ensures the best possible opportunities for generalization of treatment. Weekly child sessions include a structured, directive portion and a more child-centered time. Within the structured portion of the child session, the child is given the opportunity to release anger and verbalize feelings through strategies created by the therapist. In the child-centered portion of the sessions, the child is able to use the playroom to play out difficulties in his or her emotional life. The play therapist also uses play techniques to teach self-control and increase attention span.

The play therapist should have a general idea of how each play session will be structured, and at the same time, the therapist must be able to keep the therapy child-centered. Whether the therapist is nondirective or directive, the goals set for increasing attention span and self-control and releasing frustrations are all part of the therapeutic powers of play and the appropriate play therapy for children with ADHD. In addition, whenever the child initiates play, the play therapist must be ready to help the child continue the play as he or she works through the problem at hand to gain mastery or management of whatever comes to the surface.

Strategies and Techniques

The ability to integrate techniques and strategies, while keeping the focus on *child-centered* play therapy, is a skill that many play therapists already have once the relationship is established. Agendas are not scripted for each session, but to help children with ADHD manage their difficulties the play therapist must be ready to put into play some techniques to help in this process while keeping the fun and enjoyment of learning.

The following techniques are used to assist children with ADHD stay with their play so that they can work out emotional difficulties. The main difficulties for most children with ADHD are short attention span, impulsivity, and hyperactivity, as well as some disruptive behavior or anger. Directive play therapy interventions can be integrated into each session for short periods of time, then transitioned into a more nondirective format, if needed/desired.

Beat the Clock (to Increase Attention Span)

Materials

30 poker chips
Coloring page (or create original)
Stopwatch
Crayons

Beat the Clock is a simple technique that can be done during the session to increase the child's attention span. The play therapist introduces the activity as a game that will be played, and announces that a prize may be won at the end of it. At first, the play therapist draws a simplistic flower or design with large spaces for the child to color in while being timed. The therapist plays the first round of the game to determine the child's baseline attention span. The child is given 10 poker chips and the drawing to color. Most children will be very impulsive with this task, so offer this instruction: "You must keep your eyes on your work the entire time without looking up or stopping. If you do that, then at the end of the timing, you will receive 10 more chips. You need a total of 25 chips to pick a prize." Any questions are answered before the game begins. (Expect the child to not fully understand how the game works even though he or she said otherwise.) Remember that children with ADHD have difficulty with rule-governed behavior, so nothing will be said about the misinterpretation if it is shown, other than to laugh it off and repeat how to do it. After the first round of perhaps 30 seconds, the next round will take the same amount of time. It is very important to help the child stay in the game by, for example, praising the child for having good concentration, strong focus, etc. When and if the child looks up once, the play therapist takes away one chip, and then returns to the praising.

In a three-trial game, the child could lose some chips, but the success depends on whether or not he or she understands what to do, exhibits what is expected, and shows pleasure when he or she succeeds. The therapist might say to the child that the timing is for 30 seconds, but if there are too many distractions, it is best for the therapist to say, "You made it" (even if the time has not been fully met). Then give the next 10 chips, and begin the next round. The training is done every week for short periods of time, increasing the time limit by either seconds or minutes depending on the child's ability. To train in a new skill in a way that ensures more success over time, one must be sure to train within the child's "zone of proximal development" (Vygotsky, 1978). After the child has acquired 25 or more chips (three rounds), then he or she can pick a prize from the play therapist's treasure box.

Strategic Board Game Play (to Decrease Impulsivity)

Materials

Trouble (Milton Bradley) or Sorry (Hasbro) board game

Strategic board games have been shown to decrease hyperactivity and increase self-control in a group format (Kaduson, 1993). Many children are familiar with typical board games, such as Trouble (Milton Bradley) or Sorry (Hasbro). Use of a game such as Trouble can help the therapist decrease the child's impulsivity. Board games, by definition, require waiting for one's turn, staying focused on the game, and thinking before making a move. The therapist has to be familiar with all games that are used so that he or she can win or lose at will. If the game were only a chance game, it would not be beneficial as a therapeutic medium. To facilitate this type of play, the therapist introduces the game, and the child picks the color he or she wants to be. The therapist

should not decide on the color, and if the child responds with something indecisive, the play therapist must tell the child that he or she has to pick one. Then the therapist can either talk about the rules of the game when it is his or her turn or read the rules at the beginning of the game. The purpose of using familiar board games is to avoid the rule reading, if possible. Because auditory processing difficulties have been highly correlated with children with ADHD (Lucker, 2007), the therapist must remain attuned to how the child receives the information by observing his or her play behavior during the game. To allow for the training of self-control, the therapist will only comment on each of her or his own turns, speaking aloud about each move he or she is making. This verbalizing allows the child to see and hear how to strategize without feeling threatened or pressured. In most cases, the child will begin to model waiting his or her turn, looking around at all pieces before moving, and ultimately increasing self-control. After this game is mastered, then other strategic games can be played with skill only so that the child's self-control can be exhibited and praised consistently.

Rebound (to Develop More Advanced Self-Control)

Materials

Rebound (Mattel)

The game Rebound is very useful in helping the child develop more advanced self-control because it involves sliding ball bearing pieces on a plastic board game, so that they bounce off two rubber bands, and then land in the target zone. At first, this game can be very challenging, and once again, the play therapist must be able to play the game to win or lose at will. I believe that losing a game will negatively impact the treatment strategy for the child. The best strategy is to try to keep the score even, going up one point at a time and down a point to desensitize the child's fear of losing. Playing Rebound can be done for as long as the child is interested in the game, and the more winning experiences he or she gets, the more the child will want to continue just for the fun of it. For this reason, it is a good idea to have the child practice before joining in the play. During the practice time, the therapist will praise the child's self-control when it is exhibited, and minimize the negativity of sliding it too hard and off the board. Examples of statements such as "That was a lot of self-control," "I think you lost some of that self-control," "Good thinking about that one" and "Wow—too fast—missed that target" can be used to allow the child to become aware of what self-control feels like.

Slow Motion Game (to Decrease Hyperactivity)

Materials

Box of actions (created by the therapist)
Stopwatch

The Slow Motion game (Kaduson, 2001) allows the child to become aware of the difference between moving in slow motion speed and moving at hyperactive speed. Whether it is played in a group or individual treatment, this is a game that most children enjoy because the play therapist has to do it also. A stopwatch is given to the child who is shown how to use it. The watch is set for 60 seconds. There is a box of actions to pick from (e.g., shoot basketball, turn page in book, brush teeth). Then the therapist picks a card and does the acting first, thereby modeling how slow motion looks, as well as being silly and talking aloud about how hard it is to do. A sound machine or metronome can be used if needed to set the slow pace of the action. Since children with hyperactivity are not hyperactive all the time, they do not focus on the difference between fast and slow actions. But most of the attention they get will generally be negative, when they are more hyperactive ("Sit still," "Slow down," "Stop tapping,"

etc.). After the first action is completed, the play therapist takes the stopwatch and the child picks from the box of actions. If the slow motion is too difficult for the child to do, the therapist can say that the time is up (before the actual 60 seconds passes) so that the child does not feel that he or she can't do it.

Splat Eggs (to Release Anger/Anxiety)

Materials

Splat Eggs (Oriental Trading Company) (rubberized eggs with water and rubber yolks inside; wet paper towels or balls of clay can be substituted for the Splat Eggs)
Whiteboard
9"–11" latex balloons
Paper towels

Probably the most popular technique for children with ADHD is Splat Eggs. The play therapist takes one egg and the child gets one egg. The therapist illustrates how to play the game by throwing the egg at the white board while saying something that the therapist dislikes, and then removing the egg from the whiteboard for the next turn. The play therapist must not throw the egg too hard because it will put pressure on the child; this initial demonstration is simply to show the child how the game is played. When it is the child's turn, he or she first makes the anger statement and then throws the egg. If it misses the board, then the play therapist can say, "Wow, you must really dislike that one because now you have to throw it again until it lands on the whiteboard." If when throwing, the egg breaks (which seems to be the ultimate goal of all the children), then it is celebrated by either throwing the rubber skin into a "Mad Holding Box" (a cardboard box that is filled with other children's eggs if they don't want to throw them on the ceiling, to keep the anger at the office and not take it home with him) or up to the ceiling tiles, where it will stick for some time.

When the egg splat is broken, the water comes out, and the yolk will stay in or it can be removed. Using the yolk creates the "shaky balloon," which can be discussed as a representation of hyperactivity. The child pushes the yolk into the balloon with the assistance of the play therapist, and then he or she pumps up the balloon and ties it off. This technique is so popular that sometimes it is the focus of the entire session. The release of anger and/or anxiety is immediately felt. If there is time after the egg throwing (which would be the last training intervention), the therapist can shift to a nondirective phase where the child leads the therapist into play and the therapist can reflect or enhance verbalization of the feelings, while following the lead of the child until the end of the session.

Because many children with ADHD have great difficulty anticipating and planning for transitions, 5-minute warnings are given. The use of a visual timer, in addition to the statements, can be very helpful. Setting limits is part of therapy, for without limits there is no therapy. Follow-through must be maintained to keep the playroom a special, safe place to work through any difficulties.

Clinical Case Example

Joey, age 10, was referred for treatment by his school counselor due to disruptive behavior, including impulsive responses to peers and teachers, excessive moving during class, and being very easily distracted. The parents, Mr. and Mrs. K., were concerned about whether Joey was learning in school and if the teacher was capable of "handling a boy like him."

The initial intake with Mr. and Mrs. K. revealed a biological predisposition for anxiety and ADHD. Mr. K. admitted that he was just like Joey, but he knew how to follow the rules. Mrs. K. reported that she had always been a "worrier." and it seemed that this recommendation to get treatment

for Joey was exacerbating her symptoms. Both parents were having difficulty managing Joey's behavior at home. When asked what discipline they use, and if it works, they both agreed that nothing seemed to work. Using an example from the parents' own complaints, I illustrated how ADHD can interfere in the family's interactions.

The behavior the parents agreed was problematic was Joey's inability to comply with everyday rules, for example, coming to the dinner table the first time he was called. I empathized and went on to describe how children with ADHD are not likely to comply with the first requests because of possible difficulties such as auditory processing disorder, short attention span, slow cognitive processing, or simply overfocus on enjoyable tasks. As we discussed how the scene typically played out, it became evident that the parents usually called to Joey from the kitchen, when Joey was in the family room playing videogames. The parent's quickly acknowledged the challenge they were facing by shouting to an occupied child in another room. In addition, because the parents did not expect Joey to comply, they called to him over and over again with different statements about coming to dinner. I noted that it may be oppositional behavior, but many times it seemed like ADHD itself was interfering with Joey's ability to comply. Joey's parents also admitted that they sometimes threatened to take away toys and cancel TV programs, which they do not really want to do. Mr. and Mrs. K. said that they often did not follow through with their threats after Joey got upset. As a result, the dinnertime scene involved frustrated parents sitting with an angry or crying child, who was still not at the dinner table.

I continued to dialogue with the parents and found that when Joey did respond before the requests escalated, the parents typically said nothing or just thanked him for coming to dinner. As we examined this problematic scenario, I pointed out to the parents how negative attention was significantly more prominent than positive attention and how ADHD symptoms seemed to be ruling the household. We identified a few strategies to try, such as directly approaching Joey, saying his name while touching his shoulder, making eye contact, and giving him 5-, 3-, and 1-minute "alerts" for dinnertime. We also discussed the possibility of using humor (one parent feigning extreme hunger) or having a walking race to the dinner table.

The intake with Joey followed 3 days later. He came into the waiting room with his mother; I greeted him and asked him to come see the playroom. Joey came very willingly, and as we entered, I told him that this is a special playroom and he can do almost anything he wants in it, but he must *never clean up*. Puzzled by my odd request, he asked why. I said that it was my decision to allow the mess making and that I would do the cleanup. Joey was agreeable. I asked Joey to then sit down at the table with me and draw a picture of a person with a body, and not a stick figure. He was compliant, but the picture was done without any care. The house and tree were done the same way, without details. Then I asked if he would draw a picture of his family; he could use stick figures if he wanted to, and so he did. Dad was first, and he was very tall (although not in reality), followed by Mom, who was standing apart from Dad and close to Joey. Then Joey added his dog Snowflake to the picture right next to him. I reflected what he was drawing and encouraged him to continue.

When it was done I then asked Joey if he knew how to play Guess Who? He said he did, and we began the game. He chose to be blue and he asked me to go first. That could have been due to misunderstanding of how to play or to his desire to show what he believed to be socially appropriate behavior. I began and asked if his person was a girl. He said no and I put down the five girls that were on the board. He decided to ask me if mine was a girl, and I said no. He then seemed excited, which made me realize that he was going to put down all

the boys and leave only the girls up. Before he began to do it, I said, "Remember, I do not have a girl here. I only have a boy." That seemed to assist him in doing the proper deletion. When we finished the first game, I had him win by guessing whom I had and pretending it was the one he said. That allowed for the self-confidence and we played two more games.

Throughout all the games, Joey's confusion over which people to eliminate was consistent, and could be a red flag for auditory processing difficulties. We followed Guess Who? with a few games of Nok Hockey (Carrom Company) because he plays it at camp and told me he is the top player of the camp. I was able to set up his shots to make success happen, and I could see that although he had a low level of self-control, it existed. When we finished three games of Nok Hockey, he was the winner. It was clear to me that he was having a good time, and I asked him what he wanted to play with now. He chose to take out the racing pull-back cars and said he wanted to have a race with me with them. I certainly could not control this competition, so I said that I wasn't sure how to play with them. He was more than willing to show me, and this was how the racing was played—he would show me how the car is supposed to go, and I would try to make it go the same way but would fail in order to follow his lead. I gave the 5-minute warning, and he dropped the cars and took out some of the army men with vehicles. I reflected his play and his interest in many different things at the same time, but he stayed with the army men until the end. When the intake was over, I walked him back to the waiting room and asked Mrs. K to make another appointment, so she knew all went well.

Joey's treatment started the next week when he came in with his mother. I said that I was going to talk to Mom for about 10 minutes, and I set up Joey in the playroom and showed him the office where I would be talking to Mom. I knew from our initial session that he had enough self-control not to just pull out all the toys. Mom reported some success with getting Joey to come to the dinner table. Importantly, she indicated that it did not seem like such a hardship and that she and her husband were actually having some fun creating innovative ways to let Joey know dinnertime was approaching. I explained I wanted her and her husband to work on the Good Behavior Book, maintaining a record of Joey's good behavior observed in detail (Kaduson, 2000). I gave her a tablet in which to record the good behavior, along with an instruction sheet to show Dad. I focused on how easy it was to remember only the bad items and forget all about the expected behaviors that Joey does without reinforcement at all. Overdosing the positive was needed.

I then went into the playroom with Joey and told him that Mom was bragging about all the good stuff that he does, and I'd asked her to keep a record of it. He didn't comment at all but asked what we could play with. I told him that first we had a game to play called "Beat the Clock." and I explained that a prize would be given at the end of it. He took the 10 chips and began to color the picture, sloppily but consistently, and was able to focus for 1 minute before he began to look around. Using that 1-minute focus as the baseline, I gave him 10 more chips. He was excited that he would earn the prize. In the second round, with 1-minute timing, he was distracted twice toward the end, so that two chips were removed. However, when I was complimenting him on his focus and attention to the drawing, he was smiling. By the third trial, Joey's attention was less focused because he was getting bored with doing the coloring and clearly ready for something else. He did make it to the end of the third trial, and he was rewarded with the poker chips first, and then the treasure box was shown so he could pick the prize he wanted.

Due to Joey's difficulty with attending for a 3-minute segment of the session, I introduced the Splat Eggs game. When he saw me demonstrate the Splat Eggs, he was

thrilled and couldn't wait to go. The first item I used was "homework," and he had no problem saying what he hated. Since we were meeting during the school year, and the school had referred him, it seemed very appropriate to use. He went next and he said he hated "tests," and then he threw an egg onto the whiteboard, saw it flatten and return to shape, and was thrilled to do it again. I was not involved in turn taking and he was totally engaged in the expression of his feelings of anger. He said he hated when his friends were mean to him; hated when he had to write an essay or book report; hated when he is blamed for something he didn't do; hated when the teacher asked him to read in class; hated when his parents told him what to do over and over again; hated school; and hated getting up early to go to school. When he said the last one, the egg exploded and the water went all over the floor, which was very funny, and I made sure that he understood that it was supposed to happen and not that he did something wrong. It was clear to me that he was concerned when it broke initially, even with the earlier instructions about what would happen when an egg breaks. I asked if he wanted to put it on the ceiling or in a Mad Box. He chose the ceiling and then asked me for another egg. This intervention lasted the rest of the session, and Joey actually looked less tense when we stopped for the day. I told him that he was great fun to be with, and he said "Thanks."

The next session was split the same as the first, and Mom's Good Behavior Book was reviewed to make sure it was done in only a positive format. She said she found it difficult to write the good things he does when he can't even get out of bed in the morning. I reframed it for her that he does go to school every day, so he succeeds in getting out of bed. I asked her if she could continue making entries in the Good Behavior Book, and she said she would. I then introduced to her the next parenting lesson of spending 10 minutes a day with Joey doing whatever he wanted, without direction, question, or evaluation. Since he liked to shoot hoops, I gave her an illustration of how to engage in the activity and only to focus on him.

When I joined Joey in the playroom, he asked where the eggs were. I said we were going to do the Beat the Clock game first and maybe then we could do one more thing that is fun before the eggs. He was compliant because he wanted the prize from the Beat the Clock game. He did much better this week, with an increased attention time of 1 minute and 30 seconds. It seemed that when he knew the limits of the game, he was able to stay focused more and exhibited much more self-control. He lost only one chip and picked his prize.

This session I introduced the game Rebound. He hadn't played it before, so I told him that since I had played it, it was only right for him to have practice time. When he slid the first ball bearing, it did not reach the target, and I reflected that happens to many people. Then on his second try, it went too fast, which I also reflected as normal when one first begins the game. He began to show more self-control his 10th attempt, and I complimented his ability to control his speed, and how easy it seemed for him to learn something fun, etc. He then asked me to join, and we played five sets. He won the first four and I won the last. He seemed fine with the loss, although he had told me he wins almost all the games he plays.

Now the eggs were brought out again. Without hesitation, Joey was ready to let out what he hates. I was not a participant in the game; however, I reinforced the clever throws he made, the strength of his throwing, and the weird flying egg. During this second session, he was already telling me more about what he hated. He listed fewer things that he hated this time (having been so thorough in our first session), but this time explained a lot of them, especially about other kids being mean to him. I reflected his feelings, and he began to express more and more regarding school in general: hating to sit all day; hating to redo work he'd already done; hating when he

forgot to hand in something he'd already completed. He was opening up very quickly about how vulnerable he felt with regard to school-based problems. I reflected his frustration and disappointment.

After he had broken two eggs, I asked him what else he wanted to play. He went back to the army men and now was able to increase his play, which allowed for the reflection of his feelings through this metaphor. He had one small, injured army man who would never give up the fight, but needed a lot of help to get to the computers so that he could control the way the army attacked the evil others. Adding sound effects during this play enhanced his involvement in it as well, and even after the 5-minute warning, he stayed in the play.

Sessions continued for approximately 3 months (12 sessions), with the parent training lesson being specifically addressed each week, and Joey had time to set up his army play during the time I spoke to his mother. He began to work through the feelings of being different that no one had really communicated to him, and he was able to increase his attention span in the Beat the Clock game up to 5 minutes for three trials. That was enough time for him to complete homework, so he began to feel more successful. Each week that followed, to the end of the treatment, he expressed a few hates with the Splat Eggs. Joey's self-control on the Rebound game became so good that he asked if we could make a DVD of it so that he could prove to his dad that he has self-control. He was very proud of himself and he was clearly feeling the more positive parenting that his parents were doing. Joey was able to express his anger in a more appropriate way at home, but at school, he still kept it in. He did, however, exhibit more self-control and less hyperactivity in the classroom.

In the last session, Joey and I reviewed all of his successes since we had started. He was more involved in sports now, so the timing of termination was actually facilitated by having a very scheduled day with practices. He wanted to throw one more egg at the end of this session. He started to say what he hated was not to come here anymore, and I intervened and told him that he was doing great, but if he needed to come back, the door was always open. That seemed to help him transition.

Conclusion

The basic premise is that children with ADHD need to feel successful because they rarely encounter success due to their impulsivity and/or inattentiveness. The play therapist's work with children with ADHD is valuable because it facilitates experiences of success for the child, and helps guide the parents through parent training sessions tailored to their child. Once the initial symptoms of the child are minimized in the playroom, then the child can use the therapeutic powers of play to work through underlying psychological issues that any typical child might do in play therapy. Children with ADHD are on the same continuum as typical children, and although the typical behaviors they exhibit are more intense, more frequent, and may last longer, they too need the play to help them succeed and work through and with the difficulties they experience. Play therapy gives children with ADHD the ability and freedom to feel successful in their own lives.

REFERENCES

American Psychiatric Association. (2013). *Diagnostic and statistical manual of mental disorders* (5th ed.). Washington, DC: Author.

Antshel, K. M., Faraone, S. V., & Gordon, M. (2012). Cognitive behavioral treatment outcomes in adolescent ADHD. *Journal of Lifelong Learning in Psychiatry, X*(3), 334–345.

Barkley, R. A. (2012). *Executive functions: What they are, how they work, and why they evolved.* New York: Guilford Press.

Barkley, R. A. (2013). *Taking charge of ADHD: The complete authoritative guide for parents.* New York: Guilford Press.

Barzegary, L., & Zamini, S. (2011). The effect of play therapy on children with ADHD. *Procedia–Social and Behavioral Sciences, 30,* 2216–2218.

Bratton, S., Ceballos, P., Sheely-Moore, A., Meany-Walen, K., Pronchenko, Y., & Jones, L. (2013). Head Start early mental health intervention: Effects of child-centered play therapy on disruptive behaviors. *International Journal of Play Therapy, 22*(1), 28–42.

Centers for Disease Control and Prevention. (2011). Attention-deficit/hyperactivity disorder: Data and statistics. Retrieved from *www.cdc.gov/ncbddd/adhd/diagnosis.html.*

Charach A., Dashti, B., Carson, P., Booker, L., Lim, C. G., Lillie, E., et al. (2013). Attention deficit hyperactivity disorder: Effectiveness of treatment in at-risk preschoolers—long-term effectiveness in all ages; and variability in prevalence, diagnosis and treatment. *Academic Pediatrics, 12*(2), 110–116.

Curtis, D. F., Chapman, S., Dempsey, J., & Mire, S. (2013). Classroom changes in ADHD symptoms following clinic based behavior therapy. *Journal of Clinical Psychology in Medical Settings, 20*(1), 114–122.

Frank-Briggs, A. I. (2013). Attention deficit hyperactivity disorder (ADHD). *Journal of Pediatric Neurology, 9,* 291–298.

Goldstein, S. (2002). *Understanding, diagnosing, and treating ADHD through the lifespan.* Plantation, FL: Specialty Press.

Imeraj, L., Antrop, I., Sonuga-Barke, E., Deboutte, D., Deschepper, E., Bal, S., et al. (2013). The impact of instructional context on classroom on task-behavior. *Journal of School Psychology, 51,* 487–498.

Kaduson, H. G. (1993). Self-control game interventions for attention-deficit hyperactivity disorder. *Dissertation Abstracts International, 54*(3-A), 868.

Kaduson, H. G. (2000). Structured short-term play therapy for children with attention-deficit hyperactivity disorder. In H. G. Kaduson & C. E. Schaefer (Eds.), *Short-term play therapy for children* (pp. 105–143). New York: Guilford Press.

Kaduson, H. G. (2001). The slow-motion game. In H. G. Kaduson & C. E. Schaefer (Eds.), *101 more favorite play therapy techniques* (pp. 199–202). Northvale, NJ: Aronson.

Kaduson, H. G. (2006). Short-term play therapy for children with attention-deficit/hyperactivity disorder. In H. G. Kaduson & C. E. Schaefer (Eds.), *Short-term play therapy for children* (2nd ed., pp. 101–142). New York: Guilford Press.

Knell, S. M., & Dasari, M. (2009). CBPT: Implementing and integrating CBPT into clinical practice. In A. Drewes (Eds.), *Blending play therapy with cognitive behavioral therapy: Evidence-based and other effective treatments and techniques* (pp. 321–352). New York: Wiley.

Lucker, J. R. (2007). History of auditory processing disorders in children. In D. Geffner & D. Ross-Swain (Eds.), *Auditory processing disorders: Assessment, management and treatment* (pp. 3–24). San Diego, CA: Plural.

Miranda, A. (2000). Efficacy of cognitive-behavioral therapy in the treatment of children with ADHD, with and without aggressiveness. *Psychology in the Schools, 37*(2), 169–181.

Ray, D., Schottelkorb, A., & Tsai, M. (2007). Play therapy with children exhibiting symptoms of attention deficit hyperactivity disorder. *International Journal of Play Therapy, 16*(2), 95–111.

Schaefer, C. E. (2014). *The therapeutic powers of play*. Northvale, NJ: Aronson.

Schwarz, A., & Cohen, S. (2013). ADHD seen in 11% of U.S. children as diagnoses rise. *New York Times*. Retrieved from *www.nytimes.com/2013/04/01/health/more-diagnoses-of-hyperactivity-causing-concern.html?_r=0*.

Sonuga-Barke, E. J. S. (2005). Causal models of attention-deficit/hyperactivity disorder: From common simple deficits to multiple developmental pathways. *Biological Psychiatry, 57*, 1231–1238.

Vygotsky, L. S. (1978). *Mind and society: The development of higher psychological processes*. Cambridge, MA: Harvard University Press.

CHAPTER 29

Filial Therapy for Children with Anxiety Disorders

Louise F. Guerney

This chapter describes the rationale for the application of filial therapy (FT) with children with anxiety disorders. How FT can be used to help these children and its method of application is in contrast to cognitive-behavioral therapy (CBT), which appears to be the most commonly used therapeutic approach for this type of disorder. The goal is to suggest that FT has a legitimate place in psychological interventions for these kinds of problems in children under the age of 13. The major difference between the methods is that CBT is directed toward overt behavioral manifestations of the anxiety, whereas FT directs efforts toward the internal psychological life of the child (see the chapter on FT in O'Connor & Braverman, 1997, which expands on the rationale for FT, and in this volume as well). FT uses the child-centered play therapy (CCPT) approach, which has been used for 60 years by professional therapists. FT differs only in that nonprofessional therapists, primarily parents, serve as the change agents.

Child-Centered Play Therapy

The CCPT approach encourages the child to play in any way he or she chooses. The therapist addresses the accompanying feelings by accepting them and empathizing with the child in understanding these feelings. There is no direct effort to help the child control or suppress feelings. The assumption is that the child brings up the issues that need to be dealt with and resolves them through the play. For example, a child who is afraid of going to school might set up role plays that represent her anxieties about performance and anticipated criticism. She might become very angry with others involved in the "school" until she reaches a point where she feels that she is not a victim of their powers. Following that shift, she might move on to becoming the teacher who is helpful to children and is fun to be with. The child has reduced the fear by playing out a class situation that is frightening and moved on to a class situation in which she is very functional, frequently taking the role of the "good teacher." In these symbolic ways the child works out anxieties and their mastery as opposed to talking about them in a conscious way and using deliberate strategies for controlling anxiety directly, as in CBT. The play therapy process described in this chapter follows the same course when conducted by parents or other nonprofessionals.

CBT with Anxious Children

CBT is frequently recommended for dealing with anxieties, fears, and behaviors rooted in anxiety, such as inappropriate displays of temper. CBT therapists believe dealing directly with the maladaptive behaviors is preferred, with the goal of helping the child control them by some cognitive means (e.g., telling himself that he is starting to feel anxious, to be followed by a strategy to control that anxiety; Wood & McLoud, 2008).

CBT practitioners make a case (Wood & McLoud, 2008) for employing parents to implement homework in some of their programs. FT is based exclusively on the use of parents and/or paraprofessionals to provide CCPT to these children. Thus common elements are present in the application of both CBT and FT, despite their very different theoretical orientations. Empirical evidence exists for the reduction of anxiety and in reaching therapeutic goals in both CBT and CCPT.

There will be no effort in this chapter to compare the respective value of CBT to CCPT. Both the methods clearly have a place in a child/family therapist's armamentarium. There is no need, as I see it, to feel locked into a single approach. The in-

tent is to broaden the choices for clinicians so they can best assist children troubled by anxiety disorders.

Anxiety

Before considering the treatment of anxiety in children, it is important to describe this family of disorders and their incidence and effects on children.

Anxiety takes many forms, ranging from low-level feelings of discomfort, unease in anticipating an expected situation, to panic attacks at the extreme or complete withdrawal from the anticipated dread. Symptoms can be quite notable, including somatic reactions such as vomiting, as well as striking out in an attempt to extricate oneself from the dreaded situation. Anxiety can even take the form of externalizing behaviors such as anger and aggression. In this form anxiety is often treated only as an acting-out behavior. The anxiety component is so hidden that it may not be addressed appropriately. However, two diagnoses can be made: an externalizing label, and one of internalizing fear and anxiety. The anxious child may harbor one or more anxieties under the surface, which become apparent only when the child is faced with the actual stressors responsible for them. For example, a child with an imagined fear of his community being struck by a tornado becomes anxious every time a dark sky and wind appear. The fact that the tornado does not occur does not allay his fears. Stressors that activate the anxieties can be limitless— from very innocuous to extreme responses to obviously fearful situations. For example, a mildly autistic infant became extremely anxious at the sight of a towel fastened onto a refrigerator door.

Because removal of the stressor offers great relief, children will spend considerable energy trying to get rid of or avoid their particular stressor. Such behaviors are what generally bring their anxiety problems to the attention of adults. For example, the child fearful of tornados refuses to leave his room and stays hidden under his blanket until convinced that all threat is gone. At this level, adults would recognize the incapacitation created by this anxiety. Depending on how frequently such behavior occurred, psychological help might be sought. Some families are more casual and accepting of these deviations than others. There's an old story of two families whose children began to play with matches. One family took the child to a psychiatrist and the other hid the gasoline.

Children will often cover up or disguise their anxieties in social situations, such as in the classroom, so they are not detected by teachers, counselors, or peers.

A secondary anxiety can develop in an effort to hide the initial anxiety. For example, a child may fear that he will be picked on because he's not good at hitting a ball. He then fears going to the playground where the ballgames are played. This type of avoidance could be viewed as a positive coping mechanism, but if used repeatedly, can narrow the child's choices so that he becomes avoidant of many activities of his age group.

Performance anxiety is probably one of the most pervasive anxieties in both children and adults. As long as it remains tied to few unimportant demands (e.g., making public speeches) it will not be crippling. Crippling anxiety develops when the anxiety state is associated with a wide range of stimuli and impairs functioning. These broader anxieties are difficult to treat because of the number of situations that they encompass.

One in eight children under the age of 13 is diagnosed with anxiety (Anxiety and Depression Association of America, 2013). Furthermore, "A large, national survey of adolescent mental health reported that about 8 percent of teens ages 13–18 have an anxiety disorder, with symptoms commonly emerging *around age 6*" (National Institute of Mental Health, 2013, emphasis added).

Specific fears such as fear of the dark, particular animals, crowds, or clowns are more readily remedied. Simple avoidant strategies such as providing nightlights and keeping away from the feared objects are handled in the course of ordinary living. When anxiety cannot be handled by these kinds of straightforward strategies, clinical intervention may be necessary. A simple traumatic experience such as a dog running up to a toddler can generalize into a fear of the street where the dog appeared or to any barking sound from any source. What began as an uncomplicated stressor can be ruminated upon to a point where the child becomes anxious in any area where a dog could appear or once appeared. Children can develop stomachaches and other somatic symptoms, inability to sleep, as well as fear of school. When the anxiety interferes with the demands of the child's life (e.g., school), action is required. Unfortunately, common-sense solutions on the part of parents (and some professionals) can make matters worse. Coaxing a child to pat a dog that she is terrified of while assuring her that the dog won't hurt her can result in greater fear. The accompanying anxieties cannot be driven away by the successful accomplishment of touching the dog. These anxious feelings are stronger than the success of patting the dog.

Commonly, younger children experience anxieties and fears at stages of normal development. Most frequent is separation anxiety in relation to the mother or major caregiver. Typically these anxieties do not develop into anxiety disorders because children are learning to regulate their feelings and extend their interest beyond the family members upon whom they are totally dependent. Separation anxiety that appears in school-age children—SAD (separation anxiety disorder)—has estimated prevalent rates of around 4% (Briggs-Gowan, Horwitz, Schwab-Stone, Leventhal, & Leaf, 2000). To receive a diagnosis of SAD, the symptoms must be present for 4 or more weeks.

A further complication in treating anxiety is the frequent contributions of parents and other adults who experience anxieties of their own and express those to their children, consciously or unconsciously, in such a way as to reinforce children's anxieties. For example, the fear of a child who is very frightened of new or more mature situations is inadvertently reinforced by the mother who protects the child from these situations in order to reduce her anxieties. The mother explains that she provides this assistance to allay her own anxieties about her child's fears.

Parental Contributions to Anxiety

Mental health professionals have long believed that parental behavior is a major component in the generation and perpetuation of anxiety disorders in children. Although temperament undoubtedly plays a role in having a predisposition to anxiety, some researchers have been able to demonstrate that parental attitudes and involvement with their children are salient factors in the development or absence of anxiety. Parpal and Maccabee (1985) were able to demonstrate that very young children whose mothers were less intrusive in their children's free play were able to manage themselves better in the play situation and be more compliant than the children of the more intrusive mothers. Wood (2006) cites Carlson and Harwood (2003): "Parents who act intrusively tend to take over tasks that children are (or could be) doing independently and impose an immature level of functioning on their children" (p. 43). The intrusiveness of the parent's behavior would be perceived differently depending on the age and stage of the child's development. What might be helpful for a toddler would be major interference for a 5-year-old, for example. Parental intrusiveness can take a variety of forms including helping older children with dressing, displaying

excessive affection, and using vocabulary that is below the child's age level (Wood & Mcloud, 2008).

Treatment of Anxiety

Current treatment of childhood as well as adult anxiety includes medications such as Prozac, Zoloft, and Xanax. Although commonly prescribed, questions remain about the appropriateness of the use of such medications for children because most studies on the efficacy and safety of these kinds of medications have been conducted primarily with adults (Alavi & Calleja, 2012; Loewit-Phillips & Goldbas, 2013; McCabe, 2009; Wolfe, 2005). Many practitioners believe that these medications can provide a bridge until more appropriate coping skills are attained. CBT as the nonmedical, psychological approach is probably the most commonly recommended treatment (AADA NIMH).

CCPT therapists and filial therapists teaching CCPT to parents are quite certain that anxiety in children can be significantly reduced through nondirective play therapy. There is considerable evidence that CCPT is successful with internalizing as well as externalizing problems in children (Bratton, Ray, Rhine, & Jones, 2005; Guerney & Stover, 1971; see Ray, Chapter 32, this volume).

CBT advocates cite that following treatment, 50% of children participating in CBT no longer reached the criterion of anxiety (Wood & McCloud, 2008). If the criteria that CBT therapists use to determine the success rate of CBT with anxious children were to be applied to FT, I believe that the success of FT would equal or exceed that attained through CBT.

Family Involvement in Treatment

The value of including family members in the treatment along with the target child is apparent in CBT programs as well as in filial programs. In play therapy the meta-analysis revealed that using parents as play therapists resulted in a higher effect size than when therapists provided the play therapy (CCPT) (effect size = 1.15 vs. 0.80) (Bratton et al., 2005). Family-based CBT programs report a 70% positive response (Wood & McCloud, 2008).

FT is a variation of CCPT. The unique feature of FT is that parents or other care-givers are the providers of the play therapy to children. Using nonprofessionals as play therapists requires careful training and close supervision by professional therapists during the entire process. In addition to conducting the play sessions, parents receive a great deal of attention to their feelings about their role as therapists, their concerns about parenting, and their relationship with their children. Thus, both parents and children are the recipients of emotional and social support. In a wait-list control study, Sywulak (1978) reported that parents who had completed only the training phase of FT before starting FT play sessions reported positive changes in their perceptions of their children. The changes were significantly greater than those of the wait-list control parents. This finding suggests that the training alone has therapeutic effects.

Transfer and Generalization Stage

There are advantages to parents and other caregivers serving as change agents. Development of rapport between play therapist and child moves more rapidly when a known figure rather than an unknown play therapist is offering the therapy. Generalization and transfer are more likely to occur when the positive changes in the adult–child relationship established in the play session are carried to home life. Although filial sessions are held and observed in the therapist's office when needed, home play sessions are generally relied upon to attain full therapeutic effects. Current technology permits parents to record their home sessions, and those videos are observed and supervised by the therapist. Giving parents the therapeutic role makes them genuine partners in helping the child and appears to facilitate change. A change in the child's behavior leads to positive changes in parental behavior—a finding that has been demonstrated over the years (e.g., Bratton, 2005; Guerney & Stover, 1971; Landreth & Bratton, 2006).

When sufficient progress in play sessions has been attained, the focus shifts to the transfer and generalization of these appropriate skills to real-life situations. Therapists spend sufficient time in this phase to be certain that the parents' application of these is appropriate.

For example, CCPT sessions have a clear structure and limits that are consistently enforced. Parents who have trouble exerting sufficient control of their children gain from being taught the clarity and consistency of limit setting. Parents who have problems understanding their children's feelings gain from the empathic skills that are taught, the backbone of the child-centered approach. These changes in relating to their children, learned in play sessions, frequently lead to parents' initiating the same changes at home.

During play sessions, parents have an opportunity to see their children responding differently than they typically see them outside the play session. With a tighter structure and clear limits, children who don't cooperate outside the play session reveal that they are capable of greater compliance. This shift allows parents to observe potential of which they were not aware in their children. Similarly, children perceive their parents in a more positive light. Recognizing that in the play session their parents are more understanding, flexible, predictable and consistent, children often say that they like their parents better in the play session.

Role of the Therapist

The role of the FT therapist is multifaceted. Equal in importance to teaching the skills of CCPT to parents (or parent substitutes) is the therapist's responsibility to be sensitive and responsive to parents' feelings and attitudes toward their learning and execution of the play therapist role. As a co-developer of FT (Guerney & Guerney, 1987), I believe that a major power of this method to bring about change is this use of empathy with the parents in addition to teaching them the skills of play sessions and the transfer of skills to the home. Our rationale initially for including this important component was that parents do not have a chance to express themselves and be understood when they are serving as play therapists. Play sessions are child-centered, with the playing adult focused entirely on the child's feelings and activities. It was evident to us that the parents would do a far better job of carrying out responsibilities of the CCPT therapist if they had ample opportunity to deal with their own feelings about their roles as play therapists and as parents in the home setting (see the exchange between a therapist and a parent later in this chapter). This component enables parents to face some of their negative feelings and to recognize how these are expressed in counterproductive ways. In the microcosm of the play session, parents gain insights that did not seem to be available to them when operating in the complexity of the larger environment.

In learning to conduct appropriate play sessions, parents tend to struggle with the same issues that they also struggle with outside of the play session. In providing feedback, the FT therapist is careful to be understanding and constructive with any comments. The example below illustrates parenting control issues in the parent–child relationship. If a parent struggles to accept the child's feelings and cannot refrain from criticizing or directing the child, the play therapist deals with these feelings in a ther-apeutic way, providing a great deal of empathy to enable the parent to gain insight into what makes it hard to follow the therapeutic role. For example, say a mother finds that she cannot stop telling her child that certain things he does are not correct. This kind of behavior is totally out of bounds for a CCPT play therapist, as the parent has been taught. When a parent cannot follow the prescribed behaviors of the play therapist role, his or her feelings are considered to be getting in the way and are dealt with empathically. The following brief example illustrates such a situation.

A parent has a problem responding to her child's feelings in the play sessions. She feels that in real life she is also more concerned with getting the child to comply and accomplish what the child should be doing. Realizing that the mother's feelings are the dominant issue here, the therapist focuses on those. The filial therapist firmly believes that unresolved feelings of the parents will serve as a barrier not only to mastering their role as play therapists but to their relationships with their children.

PARENT: Well, I'm not doing too badly in the play sessions, but I still find myself wanting to see that he does things correctly when he plays.

THERAPIST: You'd like to say less about how he plays. You feel that is not the best thing for him as well as it is not following the rules of conducting the play session.

PARENT: Yes, I guess I'm thinking that if he doesn't do things the right way in the play session, it will carry over to real life and he will think he can get away with sloppy performances, even in school. How does he know the difference between real life and playing?

THERAPIST: Just seems to make sense to you that the way he is allowed to act in the play session will be transferred to other places where that kind of behavior is not appropriate.

PARENT: Well, sure! If he doesn't get corrected, how will he know better? Isn't that the way it is?

THERAPIST: It just seems that that kind of transfer would happen.

PARENT: Yes!

THERAPIST: It may seem to be different than what would be the case with some other kinds of learning, but years of this type of play therapy have demonstrated that children, even young ones, quickly recognize the difference between the special play therapy circumstances and conditions in real life. It is very interesting to me how children will change games around in the playroom to win but in real life grasp that that is not the way games are played. And even more interesting to me is evidence that children play more honestly at the end of a course of play sessions when they are feeling confident in themselves. They no longer need to manipulate outcomes to feel that they are competent. They know they can win and lose depending on circumstances, that outcomes are not a reflection of their "goodness."

PARENT: It's pretty hard to see how that could happen, but I guess we'll just have to see. My friend down the block had great success with this method, and so I know it can work. What you're saying seems right, but I am a "doubting Thomas."

THERAPIST: You're willing to give it a try, and I think that's great. I feel confident that you will find that Billy will follow the pattern we know is typical. I think it is wonderful that you are trying so hard to help your son.

After such a short exchange with the parent, the therapist would return to the business at hand and the play session. Having an opportunity to experience empathy for her feelings, the parent would generally become attentive to the topic being covered in the play session supervision and be more receptive to the skills training work. The combination of the processing of feelings and the didactic teaching component led the early filial developers to label FT as both dynamic and didactic (Addronico, Guerney, Fiddler, & Guerney, 1967). We still believe that this blending of training with a processing of feelings permits parents to achieve a high level of performance in the play sessions and to make significant progress in relating to their children (e.g., Eardly, 1978; Guerney & Stover, 1971).

Clinical Case Example

Sam is a 10-year-old Caucasian boy from a well-to-do family that resides in an upper-middle-class community. The parents are very involved with him, although his father has less time and his executive position requires him to travel often. Sam has an older sister, 13 years old, who appears to be free of any psychological difficulties. Sam was a very shy preschooler and had trouble staying in the preschool without distress. As a consequence his mother frequently came in to see what she could do to support him. The very competent teacher recommended that the mother come less often to stay with Sam, but his mother continued to come frequently. Although Sam did not always welcome her, things smoothed out while she was there until it was time for her to leave. Sam would go off and play by himself after she left.

Although Sam's current academic achievement is acceptable, he gets upset in class when he cannot get things right or if he has to write on the board where others can see him. When Sam indicates that he is worried about what he has to do at school, his mother frequently comes in to work with his class and to unobtrusively observe Sam, thus indirectly reassuring him. When Sam is particularly anxious and stressed, he develops a very noticeable eye tic. Sam has one good friend with whom he plays after school; otherwise he does not play much with other children. Sam cannot sleep at night without his parents coming up to reassure him of safety a number of times. Sometimes his mother stays with him until he is soundly asleep. Sam was given the DSM-5 diagnosis of adjustment disorder with anxiety (DSM-5).

Sam's mother is overinvolved in his life. Although she would prefer that he be more independent, she appears to accept his need for her constant presence. Sam's father thinks Sam should not require this kind of companionship at 10 years of age. This causes tension in the marital relationship. Sam is difficult to manage at home, as he frequently makes excessive demands. His parents are always uncertain about how much they should go along with these demands and are often uncomfortable doing so.

When Sam is frustrated with his own shortcomings or those of others, he becomes aggressive. He may grab his mother's shirt and yank on it very hard and has been known to throw things at her and hit her in these frustrating moments. His mother feels helpless and cries at these times. She cannot understand why Sam is so angry with her.

The parents brought him to a private practice clinic because they felt that he was too fearful and aggressive and that these issues might lead to an inability to perform to his potential, both academically and socially. Sam's parents had come to the clinic with an expectation that a behavioral program would be offered, having heard about such programs from other parents. They were surprised and somewhat disappointed when the therapist described the filial approach. It did not seem as relevant as a behavior modification program would be.

Sam's parents accepted the recommendation but remained unconvinced that it was the best approach. Their trust in the therapist appeared to outweigh their doubts, however. The therapist convinced them that because Sam's problems affected the whole family, a family approach might be more

fruitful. They also had doubts about the idea of playing as opposed to a more direct behavioral strategy. The therapist was able to explain the value of play therapy to children with fears, anxieties, and dependence issues. She stressed that through play, children are able to explore the feelings that are getting in the way of their successful functioning. They can be relied on to focus on the feelings that are behind their psychological problems. In turn, they play out these problems in ways that are therapeutic for them.

Training

Both parents were trained in three 60-minute sessions that involved practicing all the kinds of statements a play therapist would make. The therapist used a number of role plays to increase the parents' skill level. Following the usual training protocol, the therapist added a special emphasis on empathy and limit setting, which seemed to be the neediest areas for them.

The mother conducted the 30-minute sessions for 2 consecutive weeks. The third week the father played, and in the following weeks the parents conducted the play session on an alternating basis. Had circumstances been favorable, both parents could have had a play session each week. With the exception of both parents' desire to praise and Sam's fearfulness about undertaking play on his own, the sessions went very well. After three sessions Sam improved in his attitude toward school and was more willing to volunteer and not as fearful of performing in the classroom. To everybody's surprise and delight, Sam suggested that his mother not remain after she had joined his classroom.

Play Sessions

In his play sessions Sam beat up the Bop Bag vigorously. At any pause, Mom hastened to point out to Sam that there were more constructive things to play with, that she would be happy to play a game with him. When Sam would spontaneously move on to more constructive play, both parents would be more responsive and reinforcing than to the aggressive play, thus providing nonprescribed differential feedback. In feedback Sam's mother realized that she was more anxious when Sam was being aggressive (such anxiety is not uncommon in parents conducting FT sessions). Early sessions were extremely aggressive, but later sessions were more restrained as Sam developed better control of his aggressive feelings. As his aggression was reduced, Sam occasionally invited his parents to join him in shooting games. On one occasion he handcuffed his mother, saying, "Wherever I go, you're coming with me." The therapist saw this behavior as a step forward in the play therapy, toward that of nurturance/attachment, where the focus is on being cared for and caring for others. Other nurturing themes appeared at this point in Sam's therapy, generally connected with rescuing people from various kinds of accidents. At the final mastery stage Sam showed his skill in demonstrating control over the Bop Bag by targeting specific places as opposed to enacting gross aggression. It was clear that his control over his emotions had advanced as well as his motor skills.

Sam played for a total of 14 sessions: six with his father, eight with his mother. The teacher continues to report positive gains in Sam's classroom behavior and schoolyard interactions. At this point it's been recommended to the parents that they continue at least having "special times" at home with Sam to maintain the gains he has made in FT.

Following one of the mother's early play sessions, when she was still struggling with trying to allow her son to move at his own pace, the mother and the therapist had the exchange noted below to work through the mother's anxieties about his not performing. When Sam seemed afraid to try some of the new toys in the playroom, his mother began to tell him that he *should* play with them because they would be fun and he would learn new things. Sam's continued hesitation led to the mother's admonishments; for example, at one point she urged, "You need to try new things and you can make up your mind to do it." (Such parent statements are inappropriate in CCPT because "the child leads the way and the therapist follows" [Axline, 1969, p. 47]). The therapist talked to the mother following this play session:

THERAPIST: Mrs. K., it is really hard for you to allow Sam to go at his own pace. He seems to be hesitant when you feel he should be getting involved in things. It's hard for you not to say something. Remember, the child leads the way, and we, the therapists, follow.

PARENT: I thought if he would just start playing with some of those things, then he would learn how to use them and he could realize that he is more capable than he thinks he is.

THERAPIST: It's very important to you that Sam take advantage of every opportunity. You don't want him to miss out.

PARENT: Yes, he won't try anything. He just wants to stand around and let other kids do stuff while he does nothing. What will happen to him?

THERAPIST: Seems to you if you could just kind of give him a little push, he might be willing to attempt some new and ultimately rewarding activities.

PARENT: Yes, I really believe that if he would just try, he would find it's much easier than he thought it would be and he would do a lot more than he thinks he can. He's always so afraid of new situations. He plays with the same things he did when he was 5. What's gonna happen to him?

THERAPIST: You can't help but worry about his future. That's why you'd like to see him be different now.

PARENT: Yes, that's why we're here—to help him not be so shy and afraid.

THERAPIST: You really want to see some change in Sam that would make you feel more hopeful about him.

PARENT: Yes, I haven't seen much happening in the play sessions yet. Do you think that he will really change with this kind of therapy?

THERAPIST: So far you haven't seen much to make you feel that things will change. You'd like to know that this method will get you and Sam to where you think it's important for you to go.

[After the therapist addresses the parent's feelings, she provides some information.]

THERAPIST: Sam has had three play sessions and if you recall, we talked about 10 sessions minimum being sort of average for seeing any meaningful change. Since Sam seems to enjoy this special kind of time with you, there seems to be no reason to think that further sessions will not lead to some observable gains. If, after about 10 sessions, nothing seems to be moving forward, we would try to help you find another approach that might be more productive. Let's wait and see how it develops. I think that you are doing a good job. You do need to work on your strong need to try to motivate Sam to do certain things in the play session that he isn't inclined to do. This kind of direction goes against the principles of these play sessions. One of the strengths of this therapeutic play is that the children move at their own rate to undertake what they wish to attempt at that time. Next time, try to make it your goal to give no direction or hints to Sam about what to do. We will talk about it next time. I am thinking that in a few more sessions Sam will be realizing that he is not going to be criticized if he makes any mistakes and will dare to undertake more challenging things; that

would mean that his self-confidence is increasing. We'll talk about how things are going after your next session.

Parent Involvement

In FT the parents are taught the methods of creating these special child-led play sessions. In CBT parents are frequently involved as well by supervising their children's exercises and assisting with appropriate labeling.

In summary, the contrast between CBT and CCPT, as conducted by therapists or parents, is primarily the directive versus nondirective approach to symptom reduction. CBT practitioners often have trouble believing that nondirective approaches to symptom reduction can be effective. The major difference between the nondirective and directive approaches is that directive approaches focus on the anxious behaviors per se, and try to reduce them through therapeutic measures, whereas the nondirective approach does not direct the therapy toward the anxious behaviors but rather to the underlying feelings that "create" the symptoms of anxiety.

CBT is very straightforward and makes instant sense to professionals and consumers alike; therefore it has more instant appeal than CCPT. It is difficult for the public to see that a child playing, concretely or abstractly, can actually work on his or her psychological problems and resolve them through the play itself. Helping people trust the process is probably the biggest challenge to filial therapists when training parents.

REFERENCES

Addronico, M., Guerney, B., Fiddler, J., & Guerney, L. (1967). The combination of didactic and dynamic elements in filial therapy. *International Journal of Group Psychotherapy, 27,* 10–17.

Alavi, Z., & Calleja, N. G. (2012). Understanding the use of psychotropic medications in the child welfare system: Causes and consequences and proposed solutions. *Child Welfare, 91*(2), 77–94.

Anxiety and Depression Association of America. (2013, October 1). Facts and statistics. Retrieved from *www.adaa.org/about-adaa/press-room/facts-statistics*.

Axline, V. (1969). *Play therapy*. New York: Ballantine Books.

Bratton, S., Ray, D., Rhine, T., & Jones, L. (2005). The efficacy of play therapy with children: A meta-analytic review of the outcome research. *Professional Psychology: Research and Practice, 36*, 375–390.

Briggs-Gowen, M. J., Horwitz, S. M., Schwab-Stone, M. E., Leventhal, J. M., & Leaf, P. J. (2000). Mental health in pediatric settings: Distribution of disorders and factors related service use. *Journal of the American Academy of Child and Adolescent Psychiatry, 39*, 841–849.

Carlson, V. J., & Harwood, R. L. (2003). Alternate pathways to competence: Culture and early attachment relationship. In S. M. Johnson & V. E. Whiffen (Eds.), *Attachment processes in couple and family therapy* (pp. 85–99). New York: Guilford Press.

Eardley, D. (1978). *An initial investigation of a didactic version of filial therapy dealing with self-concept increase and problematic behavior decrease*. Unpublished doctoral dissertation, Pennsylvania State University, State College.

Guerney, L. F., & Guerney, B. G. (1987). Integrating child and family therapy. *Psychotherapy, 24*(35), 609–614.

Guerney, B. G., & Stover, L. (1971). *Filial therapy: Final report on NIMH Grant 1826401*. (Available from NIRE/IDEALS, 12500 Blake Road, Silver Spring, MD 20904)

Landreth, G., & Bratton, S. (2006). *Child parent relationship therapy (CPRT): A 10 session filial therapy model*. New York: Routledge.

Loewit-Phillips, P. M., & Goldbas, A. (2013). Psychotropic medications for the nation's youngest children. *International Journal of Childbirth Education, 28*(1), 32–37.

McCabe, P. C. (2009). The use of antidepressant medications in early childhood: Prevalence, efficacy and risk. *Journal of Early Childhood and Infant Psychology, 5*, 13–36.

National Institute of Mental Health. (2013, October 1). Anxiety disorders in children and adolescents (Fact Sheet). Retrieved from *www.nimh.nih.gov/health/publications/anxiety-disorders-in-children-and-adolescents/index.shtml*.

O'Connor, K. J., & Braverman, L. D. (1997). *Play therapy theory and practice: A comparative presentation*. New York: Wiley.

Parpal, M., & Maccoby, E. E. (1985). Maternal responsiveness and subsequent: Child compliance. *Child Development, 56*, 1326–1334.

Sywulak, A. E. (1979). The effect of filial therapy on parental acceptance and child adjustment. *Dissertation Abstracts International, 38*(12), 6180B.

Wolfe, S. M. (2005). *Worst pills: Best pills*. New York: Gallery Books.

Wood, J. J. (2006). Parental intrusiveness and children's separation anxiety in a clinical sample. *Child Psychiatry and Human Development, 37*, 73–87.

Wood, J. J., & Mcleod, B. D. (2008). *Child anxiety disorders: A family-based treatment manual for practitioners*. New York: Norton.

CHAPTER 30

Play Therapy with Adolescents

Brijin Johnson Gardner

Ode to Emerging Adolescents: Teen To-Do List

Grow up!
Get rid of these zits
Figure out who I am?
Get them to add unlimited texting to my plan
Figure out a way to change my clothes in PE without anyone seeing my junk
Make my parents proud of me, maybe?
Figure out who I want to be . . . wtf
Make friends/fit in . . . who is gonna like me?!
Decide what I want to do when I grow up . . . now? Seriously?
Figure out if I like girls OR boys . . . then what?!
Download that friggin' awesome video of Katy Perry
Post a made-up status on my Facebook account
Decide what I believe in
Pierce my nose
Make out or have sex, maybe?
Be okay with who I am

"Ode to Emerging Adolescents" is an amalgam of developmental tasks and paraphrased reflections teen clients have offered up along the way—a crazy mix of enormous life endeavors that can predict future outcomes for a teen fused with daily desires, needs, hopes, and questions. Much like the to-do list above, a teen's focus can fluctuate from simple to savvy in moments, making it a confusing experience for everyone involved. Consequently, while teens are wondering about all those "to dos," they are sorting through many complicated and abstract developmental tasks, meeting them with occasional success and frequent frustration. If adolescence were a ride at an amusement park, it might be named *Daunting Developmental Destinations*—a title that honors the big, scary, exciting, confusing, hellacious, hilarious, exhilarating experience that is all wrapped up into the almost 15-year life stage.

The goal of this chapter is to help the clinician gain a more robust understanding of adolescence overall and the developmental tasks related to becoming an adult. I consider the impact of attachment and identity development in terms of the relevant theories, as well as how those theories apply to clinical issues when treating teenagers. To illustrate the use of play therapy with adolescent clients struggling with identity issues, play therapy techniques and examples of their use are described.

There is significant research and information about adolescence that provide sequence and a semidefined roadmap of what one could expect to happen along the way (Blanc & Bruce, 2013; Ehrlich, Dykas, & Cassidy, 2012; Highland & Tercyak, 2014; Raudino, Fergusson, & Horwood, 2013; Romeo, 2013; Sentse & Laird, 2010; Van Doorn, Branje, & Meeus, 2011). However, when you are "in it" (adolescence), it's hard to read the map, see the signs, and navigate effectively. It is vital that clinicians working with adolescent clients find ways to be a useful companion on their journeys, shoring up their strengths and interests, demonstrating attunement and genuine care. Adolescents are inherently suspect of adults and advice, particularly if it comes in the form of a therapist they are likely being obliged to see. When we focus on the relationship and find ways to show up differently than other adults in their life—by being attentive, attuned, accepting, genuine, playful, and present—then there is more room for teens to safely explore themselves, their history, as well as experimenting with their future. Adolescents are increasingly being called upon to learn how to become adults without the support necessary to accomplish this task. Many times their parents and caregivers are in the same position of not knowing what they need to do to equip and support their adolescent. The hope throughout treatment is to traverse the daunting terrain alongside them on their trek toward self-discovery and adulthood.

Adolescent Development

The main developmental adolescent tasks that are identified consistently throughout adolescent research and literature (American Academy of Child and Adolescent Psy-

chiatry, 2011; Kroger, 2007; Patel, Flisher, Hetrick, & McGorry, 2007) can be categorized into three fundamental goals:

1. Autonomy—separation from parents or caregiver figures.
2. Individuation—explore roles and interests and create a more defined identity and sense of self.
3. Belonging—develop or reattach to the adult world and establish relationships.

It is the hope that teens negotiate and find resolution to each of these aims as they move into adulthood. The developmental tasks are a framework to help conceptualize what essentially needs to happen in order for an adolescent to develop into a mentally healthy, functioning, relational, and contributing adult. By understanding these key tasks, we can better assist teens and their parents to understand where they are on the adolescent roadmap, normalizing and validating their experience through a developmental lens.

Adolescence is a remarkable period of life, sandwiched between childhood and adulthood; it is a critical point in the lifespan that is characterized by a tremendous pace in growth and change that is second only to that of infancy. From the biological processes such as the onset of puberty to developing cognitive abilities such as abstract thought, it is a long and confusing journey for adolescents and adults alike. This stage of life brings to the surface many insecurities and challenges that can have enduring effects. Many of the negative behaviors exhibited during adolescence are related to individuals' struggles to navigate these developmental tasks. The duration and defining characteristics of these tasks vary across time, cultures, and socioeconomic situations. No teenager moves through and completes each stage in order, and regardless of resolution, development continues, proving to be a complex and frustrating endurance task for both the teen and the caregiver.

The biological determinants of adolescence and puberty are largely universal, with marked physical changes in both males and females. The time frame of puberty to young adulthood involves substantial changes in body functions and structure, including hormones, skeletal structure, overall body growth, and brain structure. These exceptional and furious changes take place only during one other period of life: from conception to birth.

Coinciding with the physical and sexual transitions that happen during puberty, a parallel process of social, emotional, and cognitive development is occurring. Teens begin to seek out and acquire skills necessary to connect in the adult world, exploring relationships and roles. When providing treatment, it is important to gauge where the teen fits on the continuum of physical, cognitive, and social–emotional adolescent development. Many times teens present physically at their chronological age, but due to life experiences and other factors, their cognitive or social–emotional development is at a much lower developmental stage. As we look over the three stages of adolescence, bear in mind that teenagers naturally vary from the descriptions provided. However, the information is considered to be what is within the range of normal adolescent development. Many times parents need help understanding the time span and range of adolescent growth that starts around age 10 and ends at age 25 (American Academy of Child and Adolescent Psychiatry, 2011).

Early Adolescence

An "explosion of awkward!" That was how a 13-year-old girl described in a session how she was feeling about the changes in her body and moods now that she was "officially a teenager." She was definitely on to something. This initial adolescent stage spans from age 9 to 13 years old; physically, development has begun. Girls experience the onset of menstruation, breast growth, and hip development, and boys have physical growth in testicles and penis, along with a deepening of the voice and other hormonal changes. Both genders experience physical growth in height and weight and begin to experience sexual interest in others. During this period, physical changes can become a large part of self-concept and identity formation, as adolescents evaluate self and others on their physical acceptability. Many early adolescents have an increased need for privacy, both physically and emotionally, as they tend to feel self-conscious about their bodies and the changes that are happening to them.

Cognitively, early adolescents, occasionally referred to as "tweens," have an increased capacity for abstract thought, moral thinking, and begin to have intellectual interests. However, they are still very "black-and-white" thinkers, especially in how they process information and relate to others. They also begin to make their first attempts at independence, separating from their parents or caregivers physically and emotionally. They are heavily focused on the present, with their developing self-concept and identity being wrapped up in a usually intense need and desire to fit in with peers—to be accepted by, or belong to, a group.

In the social–emotional domain, early adolescents are moody, encounter increased conflict with their parents, and begin to test rules and limits in relationships. When experiencing stress or other intense emotions, many tweens regress and use developmentally younger coping skills, such as throwing temper tantrums to express their feelings. Their behaviors are not based on thoughtful reflection, but on the presenting circumstances and the emotions they are experiencing.

Middle Adolescence

From the age of 14 to 18 years puberty runs its course and the physical changes are complete; it would seem that we could pack up this stage of life and put it all behind us. However, the engine of adolescence is just getting started! Cognitive abilities continue to stretch, increasing the ability to set goals, consider moral reasoning, and begin to think about the meaning of life as well as whom they are becoming as a person. This middle stage of adolescence is a highly self-absorbed time when the teen is focused on self-concept, the need for acceptance by peers, and the continuing need to adjust to their "new" bodies and abilities. The distance and tension between parents and teens increase at this time, as the fight for independence is mingled with the need for dependence and some coregulation by the parent. Parents are no longer at the center of the child's existence, and neither are their beliefs or opinions as teens begin to question values and beliefs. This is a push–pull time of separation and a need for closeness within the parent–child dyad—a time when the teen is no longer a child, but still miles away from being an adult. Although many teens will test limits and present some rebellious behaviors, they are able to maintain the difference between right and wrong and are behaviorally more capable to control impulses and thoughts.

It is primarily during midadolescence when teens begin to struggle with developing a unique identity by trying out various roles, experimenting with different characteristics and qualities, and then experiencing the diverse outcomes and consequences associated with those roles or traits. Additionally, by trying on these different roles and identities, adolescents are trying to figure out how they want to be perceived by others. The experimentation allows teens to experience outcomes that arise from, for example, dying their hair purple, propelling themselves into athletics, wearing all-black clothing, or just doing whatever they can to set themselves apart from adult culture. This proves to be a time-consuming and laborious process, which may be one of the many reasons the span of adolescence is so long!

Late Adolescence

Late adolescence: Just when you wish it were over, there are a few miles left to go! Neuroscience demonstrates that the brain matures from the back to front, starting with the brainstem, moving to the middle regions, and finally ending at the frontal lobes that are responsible for, among many things, executive decision making. So, a person is not working with a fully developed brain until age 25. Although one would think that the life stage of adolescence is over when a person hits the magic 2-0, it is not the case. Our culture places a good deal of attention on the physical development of adolescents and does little to represent the other pieces of the young person, such as social–emotional and cognitive development. A developed brain with the enhanced ability for complex thought, paired with the ability to engage in reciprocal and healthy relationships with other people, are major components of functioning as a successful adult. This is the final stage of prepping for entering the adult world, with attempts to finalize vocational aims and determine a sense of personal identity. Psychologically, during late adolescence, there is less need for peer approval and a definite sense of independence from parents.

Adolescent Development and Theory

Erikson's psychosocial theory (1968) remains significant to conceptualizing developmental stages and is widely used in the study of adolescent development. The fifth of Erikson's eight stages and the primary task of adolescence is creating an identity versus experiencing role confusion. During this stage, adolescents seek resolution between the extremes of childhood and becoming an adult, attempting to answer and integrate information about who they are while forming a sense of self and shaping a coherent narrative. During this critical stage of development adolescents experiment with different possible roles to find ones that seem to fit. When adolescents are able to integrate their answers to the "Who am I?" and "Who do I wanna be?" questions, their personal narratives take shape and set the foundation of their ongoing identity development as young adults.

The path to becoming a unique individual is an unmarked road for many adolescents; however, there are certain conflicts and changes that are universal and can be anticipated as they unfold. How do adolescents know who they are? What criteria do they use to define themselves? Who can safely join them in their journey? Throughout the process of identity formation, the adolescent is sorting through situations, historical information, and other important life assignments such as determining vocation, sexual identity, and personal values. This process represents the viewpoint that adolescent development is the product of the interplay between genetic makeup, personal experiences, and family upbringing. Making sense of these areas solidifies into a foundational understanding of who they are and who they will become. By discovering the person they are, they are more equipped to assert and assimilate themselves into adult society. In the book *Disconnected: Parenting Teens in a MySpace© World*, Clark and Clark (2007) define the process of adolescence as

> developmentally the process where we travel from a world where we do not have to think about who we are or what we do (childhood) toward a destination where we must have the confidence that we can not only survive but also thrive in the multiple relationships and expectations of adult society. . . . [Adolescence is] the overall task of moving out of childhood and preparing to engage in mainstream society as a peer with other adults. (p. 49)

Considering this definition, how many adolescent clients are prepared to cross the bridge of "becoming" an adult? How many adolescent clients possess the skills to navigate relationships, understand nuances of interactions, and possess the language and cognitive ability to enter into the adult world, let alone in successful ways? The path toward becoming a unique individual begins long before the onset of puberty; rather, it begins prenatally. In Erikson's first psychosocial stage, which occurs throughout the first year of life, a child encounters the basic existential issue of trust versus mistrust. When children experience responsive and warm care, they gain trust in their primary caregivers and adults in general and learn that the world can be a good and dependable place (Main, Kaplan, & Cassidy, 1989). However, if children's initial experiences in the world are filled with severe or harsh interactions, or they do not receive care that is responsive to their needs, they learn to mistrust their caregivers and ultimately other grown-ups who will enter their lives (Flaherty & Sadler, 2011).

Early emotional life is primarily physical; we learn about the world by the way we are held and cared for. Bonding, separating, feelings, needs, and their fulfillment are all first experienced through the body. The quality of a child's early emotional existence is determined by the primary caregiver's responsiveness: how, when, and why a baby is picked up, put down, held close, or pushed away. For better or for worse, what is learned and experienced during that early time frame forms the template of children's subsequent emotional lives, their perceptions of self and others, and their sense of identity. Considerable research has reported the important link between early attachment patterns of infant–parent dyads and later social and emotional adjustment, including problem solving, coping styles, identity development, self-image, and the presence or absence of depression and other mental health concerns (Conners, 2011; Kroger, 2007; Patel et al., 2007).

This link between early attachment and adolescent development emphasizes the need for clinicians to explore the attachment histories of their clients and families, particularly when working with teens struggling with identity development. Children receive their first understanding of the world and "self" through their primary caregiver's actions and responses. Clinicians can gain valuable insight into the narrative of the emerging adolescent by examining, observing, and learning about the parent–child dyad. As humans, we crave connection and a "home base," a person to go to with our feelings and fears, from whom we receive unconditional acceptance. Attachment theory highlights the necessity of a secure base for infants and young children, so that they can safely go off and explore the world around them, in turn learning about themselves and creating a sense of self or identity. Bowlby (1988) confirmed that individuals who have secure attachment relationships experience more positive mental health, compared to individuals who have an insecure attachment with primary caregivers. This kind of finding suggests that secure attachments contribute to healthy identity development and bolster an adolescent's ability to safely navigate separation and individuation from caregivers: a milestone in identity formation.

Play Therapy with Adolescents

In the book *Play Therapy with Adolescents* (Gallo-Lopez & Schaefer, 2005), the authors explore reasons and research that validate why play therapy is a viable and effective treatment for many adolescents struggling with developmental issues. For example:

- Playful interactions and environments can invite, validate, and normalize regressive inclinations an adolescent may experience.
- Using expressive and playful techniques allows the adolescent to safely have a foot in both worlds: childhood and adulthood.

- The control belongs to the adolescents; they decide how to engage and to what degree to participate in their own therapeutic process.
- Offering expressive, kinesthetic, and visually interesting props or toys kindles the desire and need to be expressive and to demonstrate and explore identity.
- The nondirective approach neutralizes the battle over what to reveal and what to keep hidden.
- A casual, playful approach counteracts fear and exposure to painful thoughts and feelings.
- The combination of symbolic and expressive play with verbal dialogue provides the capacity for healing and resolution of developmental issues.

Most adolescent clients come into therapy by force, not by choice. When behaviors and concerns get "big" enough to affect the parent–child relationship, that is when the adolescent shows up on therapy's doorstep. Although treatment of the dyad is paramount, it is essential for the clinician to establish a trusting and genuine relationship with the teen. This implies that the therapist is the teen's therapist, first and foremost. Upon referral, the adolescent should be included in the intake with the parents. Initially, I dialogue with parents, sharing that my first goal is to establish rapport with their child and that this can be achievable only if the teen is assured that his or her feelings, experiences, and information are safe. Conversations about confidentiality are essential to let the parent and teen know that "what is said in the room, stays in the room" and to let the teen know that the only time information will be shared outside the session with the parent is if the teen is in danger of hurting him- or herself or someone else or if he or she has been hurt or threatened by someone.

Safety cannot be achieved by having the parent ask at the end of the session, in front of the teen, "What did you talk about?" Communication with the parent is important; however, conversations in front of the teen can put the therapeutic relationship at risk. Upon intake, I encourage parents to e-mail me prior to, or after, a session with their questions or concerns. Every six to eight sessions I offer a parent session or consultation, providing updates on treatment, answering questions they may have, and gathering their thoughts and feelings about how the process is going. Another way to increase the parents' involvement in their child's treatment is to provide them with some "assignments" to complete while we are in session (see Figures 30.1 and 30.2). This is a way for them to become more engaged in the process, as well as providing valuable information to them about the treatment process and providing the therapist with a better understanding of their thoughts, feelings, worries, and perceptions of their teen.

Treatment

Adolescents frequently have difficulty expressing and communicating their thoughts and feelings; play therapy and expressive techniques can empower and support the message that needs to be communicated. The necessary work on identity development can be assisted through various play therapy techniques that allow for distance,

metaphor, and self-reflection. One caution to the developing therapist is that of placing too much value and focus on the use of props and techniques. Although much value and information can be derived through play therapy techniques, what is truly healing is found in the therapeutic relationship.

In life, teens retreat to places where adults are not welcome. They seek safety in relational places with other peers (directly or via technology), frequently escaping the high pressures of adolescence, including the pressures of adult expectations. As therapists, we need to sit on the steps of their world and learn from them, letting them guide us to a world that we can only understand with their assistance.

Knowing what is important to adolescents and discovering their interests are key components of establishing a therapeutic relationship, as well as learning about their developing identity. You don't need to be a detective, nor will they be responsive to that approach. Listen with your eyes! Every session, kids bring us clues on how to connect with them, from their coiffure to their Converse sneakers. In the search for belonging and identity teens also crave uniqueness; individuals' style and clothing are frequently used as ways to demonstrate "who" they are. Slowly seeing and observing the unique parts and pieces that make

---

The following information will help me better understand your wishes, wants, and worries concerning your teen, as well as allow you to share experiences from your adolescence. Please complete the following sentences:

1. One wish I have for my teen is . . .
2. One thing I wonder about my teen's life is . . .
3. One thing I think my teen really likes is . . .
4. One worry I have about my teen's social life/friends/social media is . . .
5. One thing I want for my teen is . . .
6. When I was a teen, I worried most about . . .
7. When I was a teen, I remember wanting to be . . .
8. When I was a teen, the most important person/people in my life were . . .
9. The most important person in my teen's life is . . .

FIGURE 30.1. Parent/caregiver "wish/want/worry" worksheet.

Please complete the following sentences:

1. Things in our [parent–teen] relationship will feel better when my teen . . .
2. I will know things are getting better when this happens . . .
3. There was a time when things were better between me and my child; that was when . . .
4. My favorite age/time to parent my child was when he or she was . . .
5. When we are done with therapy, I know things will be better because . . .
6. I will feel better when my teen . . .

FIGURE 30.2. Parent/caregiver "better when" worksheet.

up the adolescent client serve as baby steps toward attunement. Therapists need to recognize that many of our clients have never had the experience of truly being "seen" by another person, especially by an adult. This is an event that can be extraordinarily gratifying and excruciatingly painful all at once. The therapist honors the adolescent's pace to receive this experience and to tentatively accept the foreign feelings of being understood and valued.

Techniques

Mostly Me

This is a structured and simple game I created that allows the therapist to gain insight into the client's life experiences, what the client relates to, and his or her perceptions of self and the world around them.

- *When to play it*: Assessment stage.
- *Who plays*: This can be played with an individual client and therapist or led by the therapist with a parent–child dyad.
- *Supplies*: Ready-made list.
- *Goals*
  o Engagement.
  o Allow for appropriate disclosure between teen and therapist.
  o Provide a playful interaction to build rapport and learn about the client.
  o Gain insight into teen's sense of self through identifying and explaining his or her choice.

I introduce the game by saying the following: "I am going to say two words. Each of us will pick and say out loud the word we are mostly like, like the most, or identify with. There are no wrong answers, so say the first thing that pops in your head. After we say which word we've picked, we each will give a quick reason why we made that selection—no more than a 20-second explanation. We don't get to ask questions, we just listen to what the other person says. There may be some pairs of words that you don't like, but choose one anyway and then explain why you don't like it during the 20 seconds." A working list of word pairs is included in Figure 30.3.

This is a simple game that I frequently have parent–teen dyads play early on; it allows for safe disclosure, a place to claim what one believes and feels, and there is no wrong answer. It can provide the clinician with information about how the parent and teen interact in a noninvasive way. Throughout the course of playing this game with many teens, I have discovered that many parts of a teen's life experience, interests, historical information, relationships, beliefs, and perceptions are revealed.

While the game is played, the therapist is structuring the activity by prompting the word pairs, keeping the time for the brief explanations, and guiding the parent or teen back to the game if either starts to debate the other's choices. There are several observations that can be made when this is played by the parent–teen dyad. For

☐ Blue / Yellow

☐ Hamburger / Hot Dog

☐ Fireworks Display / Sparkler

☐ Sneakers / Flip Flops

☐ Grapes / Bananas

☐ Family / Friends

☐ Taylor Swift / Justin Bieber

☐ Thunder / Lightning

☐ McDonald's / Taco Bell

☐ Toes / Fingers

☐ Hike / Bike

☐ Mom / Dad

☐ Skateboard / Scooter

☐ Fruits / Veggies

☐ Exhaust Pipe / Engine

☐ Athlete / Observer

☐ Sister / Brother

☐ Bulldozer / Dump truck

☐ Coffee / 5-Hour Energy

☐ Outside / Inside

☐ Text / Talk

FIGURE 30.3. "Mostly me" working list of word pairs.

instance, does the parent correct the teen for his or her choice or invalidate the teen's response (e.g., "No, you never go outside! How can that be your answer?")? Are there certain word pairs for which both parent and teen give the same answer but for different reasons? Does the parent accept the answers given by the teen, and vice versa? This game can also provide an opportunity for the parent and child to learn about each other as well as determine commonalities.

Wonderful Junk

- *When to play*: Assessment and termination stages.
- *Supplies:* A small box of "wonderful junk" (Figure 30.4) containing no more than 30

small items that cover a broad representation. I do not use sandtray miniatures for this box; rather I have a small collection of items, buttons, and objects no larger than an inch. The collection can fit easily in a 4″ × 5″ plastic container.

- *Goals*
  - Provide teen with control to share portions of his or her history.
  - Gain historical information and client's perspective on his or her experiences.
  - Provide opportunity for narrative to coalesce and progress.

This technique is an engaging assessment that requires few materials; the small number and size of miniatures used can reduce anxiety that a large selection of miniatures can create. I introduce a small box of "wonderful junk" and invite the teen to look through the items and pick out a few items that show parts of his or her life "up

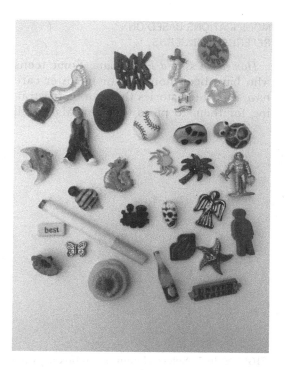

FIGURE 30.4. Box of "wonderful junk."

to now." The teen selects as many or as few items as he or she wants and sets them out in an order (see Figure 30.5). Sometimes kids need to use two or three items clustered together to help represent a certain time in their life; there are no restrictions, and teens are encouraged to use whatever they need. Once the items are selected, invite the teen to walk through the choices, telling a bit about each one. This undersized technique provides a concise and visual story that is a catalyst for teens to discern and integrate their personal narratives as well as explore their identity within the context of their historical experience. For teens who have had traumatic life events, this activity provides a safe way to represent the experience while staying in the present moment, a safe distance from the event and in a safe environment where they can reflect on their feelings and the visual representation of the experience. The following sections offer modifications for teens with specific referral concerns.

MODIFICATIONS BASED ON REFERRAL CONCERNS

Homelessness and Foster Care. Some teens who have been homeless or in foster care have disjointed stories that can be frustrating for them to piece together. Many will

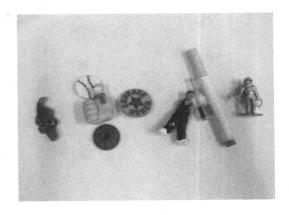

FIGURE 30.5. Selected items from box of "wonderful junk," placed in order.

struggle with the initial goal of representing all their experiences in one timeline. If that is the case, I invite them to pick items to represent each of the homes/families/shelters in which they have lived, acknowledging that each experience can be unique and impactful.

Adoption. Teens who have been adopted and are struggling with reconciling their experience can be invited to make a timeline of their life before the adoption (or what they think or believe their life before was like) and another timeline to show their life after the adoption. If the teen was adopted at a later stage in life, he or she can focus the timeline on the experience of being adopted. Teens who were adopted during infancy and do not recall their biological parents frequently wrestle with issues of abandonment. I have used this technique to help them explore the story they have created in their minds to understand why they were given up for adoption. Many times there is little information around why the child was adopted. Nevertheless, many children will create a narrative to make sense of that "why"; this technique allows them to create a concrete representation of what they believe to be true.

Sexual Abuse. For teens who have been sexually abused, this technique can be used to show how they felt or experienced their life before the abuse, as well as showing a timeline for when the abuse was happening.

In my practice, Wonderful Junk has helped teens explore and begin to comprehend the cumulative effect of their life experiences, both negative and positive. It can be a springboard to igniting their ability to reflect on the pain of the past or present while seeing the promise and possibility in their future, providing a visual timeline that helps them express their feelings and perceptions about experiences without having to use words. Sandtray items are a possibility to use with this technique; however, I have found that the smallness of the buttons and other objects provides a sense of psychological safety. Clients have reflected that using the tiny objects "gave [their] brain a smaller [and more manageable] picture." Many teens also indicate that the smaller items help them see things as "not as big or bad" as they are depicted in their head.

Teen-O-Gram

- *When to play*: Working stage.
- *Supplies*: I use the box of wonderful junk (see Figures 30.4 and 30.5) or Jenni-Jane Personality Buttons (Figure 30.6).
- *Goals*
  - Provide tools for the client to explore different facets of his or her personality.
  - Explore how the client views traits and characteristics of self and others.
  - Determine connection of others as they relate to the teen's relationships.
  - Explore interplay of social supports and family connections in the client's life.
  - Gain a representation of the client's perspective on his or her identity, including with whom and how he or she identifies with others.

Adolescents' social worlds expand tremendously as they grow, exposing them to many different types of individuals and experiences. Teens have dynamic private lives, about which the caregivers and adults in their lives know little. Teen-O-Gram (Figure 30.7) is one play therapy technique I have created that has helped teens to see a concrete depiction of their relationships, their self-labels, and the various pieces of their forming identity. Although adolescent cognitive processes are increasingly savvy, the use of labels returns to an earlier age when children have developed their *categorical self* (Oswalt, 2013), which is a concrete way of viewing themselves in "this or that" labels that are used to explain children's self-concept in very observable terms. I have found that moving teens out of the frontal lobes of verbal defenses into concrete and visual representations allows for a truer expression of self.

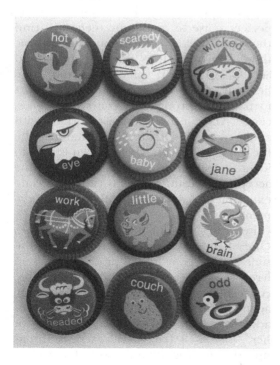

FIGURE 30.6. Jenni-Jane Personality Buttons.

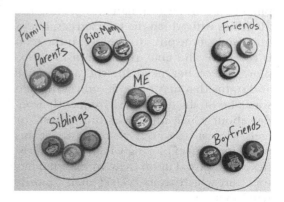

FIGURE 30.7. Teen-O-Gram.

To begin, I introduce the idea of how their world is growing and changing, compared to when they were younger when they dealt with just home, school, day care, and maybe an activity or two. On a large piece of paper, we draw a circle in the center that represents them and then section off the paper using lines or circles to represent parts of their life, including relationships and activities. Most teens identify their main groups as friends, boy/girlfriend, sports/activities, school, and their families (divorced, adopted, or other types of family transitions are denoted by separate circles or as directed by the teen). Either the teen or I write the label or group name within a section. The teen is invited to pick objects or buttons to represent the significant people who make up the various groups. After the items are selected and placed, I invite the adolescent to share something about each grouping and his or her thoughts or reasons behind the selection; this invitation typically evokes stories and involve histories revealing insight into the teen's understanding of others.

The therapist can follow up this technique by wondering about what influences affect the client's selection of labels or objects, including the external factors that shape all of our thoughts, including social media, peer interactions, group affiliations, and personality traits. The therapist then turns the conversation inward, to the teen's perspective on the labels he or she applied to his or her own name, exploring the identities with which the teen agrees, bucks up against, or aspires to achieve. If the teen is receptive and able, the therapist can explore his or her need for the acceptance and status that may be achieved via the personas he or she assumes. I frequently wonder about which identity is the "truest" or feels "closest" to who teens really are at this point in time, exploring which characteristics are imposed upon them by external factors and which traits reflect their "mostly true" identity.

Conclusion

"Some changes happen deep down inside of you. And the truth is, only you know about them. Maybe that's the way it's supposed to be" (Blume, 1981). This quote resonates with the adolescent experience. Throughout life, our external and emotional experiences amalgamate internally, shaping and shifting who we are becoming, frequently without recognition by the world and others around us. However slight, significant, or curious the difference of the change may be, it impacts the individual we become, no matter our age.

I recall reading books by Judy Blume throughout junior high school, late at night with my door closed, pretty sure it wasn't something I wanted my mom to catch me reading or ask me questions about. Looking back, these books, and many others, became my safe companion throughout my own daunting adolescent journey. Although the books were written years before my teens, the pains, hopes, problems, and needs expressed by the characters made perfect sense to me. Some teens will find their trustworthy companion in the music they listen to, others through sports and activities; however, some teens and families will reach out for additional support to navigate through the course of adolescence. And for any therapist working with adolescents, this is the task at hand: to be the "someone" with whom a teen is able to identify, feel safe with, experience genuine acceptance from, and who can appreciate experimental deviations—all without judgment.

Learning occurs through experience. One of the ways we develop into "responsible adults" is by lots of practice being an irresponsible, experimental, demanding, confusing, silly, hateful, frustrating teenager. And this is the developmental job of adolescence, and when a teen does his or her "job" well (i.e., totally screws things up), the therapeutic hope would be to create and integrate an experience that cultivates understanding and acceptance of self. So, prepare the teen, parent, and yourself for the wrong turns, twists, and metaphorical speeding tickets that will accompany the adolescent journey, knowing that what we experience along the way is incorporated into the formation of our identity, at any age.

And, a final verse to the Adolescent Ode:

Screw things up—royally!
Hang on tight
Learn/grow from my screw-ups with the help
    of some trusted adults
Cool . . . I think I just found ME!

REFERENCES

American Academy of Child and Adolescent Psychiatry. (2011). Normal adolescent development: Parts I and II. Facts for families. Retrieved April 13, 2013, from *www.aacap.org*.

Blanc, A. K., & Bruce, J. (2013). Commentary: Explicit attention to age and gender disparities is key to understanding adolescent experiences and outcomes. *Journal of Research on Adolescence, 23*(1), 191–192.

Blume, J. (1981). *Tiger eyes.* New York: Dell.

Bowlby, J. (1988). *A secure base: Parent–child attachment and healthy human development.* New York: Basic Books.

Clark, C., & Clark, D. (2007). *Disconnected: Parenting teens in a MySpace® world.* Grand Rapids, MI: Baker Books.

Conners, M. E. (2011). Attachment theory: A "secure base" for psychotherapy integration. *Journal of Psychotherapy Integration, 21,* 348–362.

Ehrlich, K. B., Dykas, M. J., & Cassidy, J. (2012). Tipping points in adolescent adjustment: Predicting social functioning from adolescents' conflict with parents and friends. *Journal of Family Psychology, 26*(5), 776–783.

Erikson, E. H. (1968). *Identity: Youth and crisis.* New York: Norton.

Flaherty, S. C., & Sadler, L. S. (2011). A review of attachment theory in the context of adolescent parenting. *Journal of Pediatric Health Care, 25,* 114–121.

Gallo-Lopez, L., & Schaefer, C. E. (Eds.). (2005). *Play therapy with adolescents.* New York: Aronson.

Highland, K. B., & Tercyak, K. P. (2014). What twin studies of adolescent behavior can teach us about shared environmental and genetic risk. *Journal of Adolescent Health, 54*(1), 1–2.

Kroger, J. (2007). *Identity development: Adolescence through adulthood* (2nd ed.) Thousand Oaks, CA: Sage.

Main, M., Kaplan, N., & Cassidy, J. (1989). Security in infancy, childhood and adulthood: A move to the level of representation. In I. Bretherton & E. Waters (Eds.), *Growing points in attachment theory and research. Monographs of the Society for Research in Child Development, 50,* 66–106.

Oswalt, A. (2013). Early childhood emotional and social development: Identity and self-esteem. Retrieved April 28, 2013, from *www.sevencounties.org*.

Patel, V., Flisher, A., Hetrick, S., & McGorry, P. (2007). Mental health of young people: A global public-health challenge. *Lancet, 369,* 1302–1313.

Raudino, A., Fergusson, D. M., & Horwood, L. J. (2013). The quality of parent/child relationships in adolescence is associated with poor adult psychosocial adjustment. *Journal of Adolescence 36*(2), 331–340.

Romeo, R. D. (2013). The teenage brain: The stress response and the adolescent brain. *Current Directions in Psychological Science, 22*(2), 140–145.

Samuolis, J., Layburn, K., & Schiaffino, M. (2001). Identity development and attachment to parents in college students. *Journal of Youth and Adolescence, 30,* 373–384.

Sentse, M., & Laird, R. D. (2010). Parent–child relationships and dyadic friendships as predictors of behavior problems in early adolescence. *Journal of Clinical Child and Adolescent Psychology, 39,* 873–884.

Van Doorn, M. D., Branje, S. J. T., & Meeus, W. H. J. (2011). Developmental changes in conflict resolution styles in parent–adolescent relationships: A four-wave longitudinal study. *Journal of Youth and Adolescence, 40,* 97–107.

CHAPTER 31

Play Therapy Interventions for Adults

Diane Frey

What do most Nobel Laureates, innovative entrepreneurs, artists, and performers, well-adjusted children, happy couples and families, and the most successfully adapted mammals have in common? They play enthusiastically throughout their lives.

—Stuart Brown (2008)

Somehow between childhood and adulthood play becomes outdated. More and more of adults' time and energy are spent on work. For adults play is often associated with idleness, laziness, or pointlessness. Recently, with children being overscheduled, trained, and prepared for college in elementary school, play is being viewed as dispensable for children as well, with some school districts eliminating physical education or recess. However, as Elkind (2007) stated, "Play is not a luxury, but rather a crucial dynamic of healthy, physical, intellectual, and social, emotional development at all age levels. Play, love, and work are operative throughout the human life cycle" (p. 4). Philosophers from Plato to the present time have observed that people are most human when they play.

> It is proposed that the theories of the function of play, especially those emphasizing mastery of the environment, mastery of painful experiences, and pleasure in function, should be uniformly extended to include play activity throughout the life of the individual and not limited to childhood or special categories of adults. (Adatto, 1964, p. 839)

Sutton-Smith (1997) posited that "a play theory of any comprehensiveness must grasp this strange companionship of the very young and the very old, the first waiting to begin and the second to finish" (p. 48).

There is a reciprocal relationship between play and learning. A play competence spiral develops in which learning leads to more sophisticated play, and play results in mastery that leads to more learning, which leads to more play, and so forth. This play competence spiral helps children reach an adult level in the cognitive, affective, and behavioral domains. Play can be viewed as an apprenticeship for adult life. In addition, the learnings a person develops through childhood play are those that are useful in his or her culture. It is through play that an individual becomes acculturated into society. Those adults who did not play much in childhood have little apprenticeship for adult life. They often lack the skills for coping with negation, rejection, cooperation, and competition that are learned in childhood play. The result is often that these individuals do not feel integrated into society.

Clinical Application

There is a large repository of research data from neurophysiology, developmental and cognitive psychology, animal play behavior, and evolutionary and molecular biology supporting the value of play in adult lives (Brown & Vaughn, 2009). Play optimizes learning, enhances relationships, improves health and well-being, potentiates novelty, and revitalizes us. Einstein (1964) stated that "play seems to be the essential feature in productive thought—before there is any connection with logical construction in work or other kinds of signs which can be communicated to others" (p. 171). Thus, playing with ideas was essential before Einstein began to think more completely. A review of the literature shows a number of lifelong benefits of play, including:

- *Play bonds people to each other.* Through play individuals develop empathy, compassion, trust, and intimacy.
- *Play fosters creativity, flexibility, and learning.* Play helps individuals to adapt and solve problems and arouses creativity and curiosity.
- *Play is an antidote to loneliness, isolation, anxiety, and depression.* Through play endorphins are released. Play offers distraction from pain, fear, and other burdens.
- *Play teaches perseverance.* The reinforcement from learning or mastering a new game teaches the value of perseverance. This trait is necessary for a healthy adulthood. Perseverance and violence are rarely found together.
- *Play results in happiness.* There is a joy in play. Play can preserve and nourish the human heart.
- *Play enhances relationships.* Playing together brings joy, vitality, and resilience to relationships. Play can heal resentments, disagreements, and hurts.
- *Play helps to develop and increase our social skills.* Through the give-and-take of play, social skills are learned.
- *Play teaches cooperation.* Play may be an

antidote to violence. Those who avoid or have never learned to play may develop fears, rage, and obsessive worry.

Adults and Play Therapy

In general, play enhances well-being in adults, and play *therapy* offers many opportunities for personal growth and healing for adults (Bludworth, 2014; Schaefer, 2011). The themes of adult play cluster around the major issues of this age group: depression, stress, anxiety, loss, and issues about aging. Developing a psychohistorical viewpoint of life is one of the developmental tasks of maturing adults and, in struggling to master this task, many concerns are manifested. Through play therapy adult clients can develop insight, reduce stress, improve communication, and gain more self-affirmation. The following model for processing sessions with adults in play therapy involves six steps (Frey & Carlock, 1991):

- Step 1. *Introduction.* The therapist discusses the rationale for the technique with clients.
- Step 2. *Participation.* Clients respond to the guidance of the therapist but should be allowed to decline if the material proves to be too threatening.
- Step 3. *Articulation.* Clients share reactions and observations about what happened.
- Step 4. *Processing.* Clients are asked to discuss patterns or dynamics they became aware of during the technique.
- Step 5. *Reflection.* Clients are asked to think about hypotheses and/or generalizations that can be inferred from the process.
- Step 6. *Application.* Clients begin to realize the relevance of the technique to their everyday life and generalize the learning(s).

By utilizing this process, the themes and insights developed from play therapy become more relevant for adults. The use of this process is illustrated in case examples provided later in the chapter.

Adults with certain psychological dynamics and from certain populations are especially well suited for play therapy. Adults who come to traditional talk therapy with a great deal of resistance are one example. Such clients may be mandated into treatment by the court and/or persuaded into therapy by others. Clients could also have resistance that comes from within. An adult, for example, who refuses to talk to the therapist or is very evasive will usually draw or play a board game. The client doesn't view the technique as a way of cooperating with the therapist. However, it is nonetheless enlightening for the play therapist. Older clients threatened by traditional approaches to therapy may respond to music, art, and other play therapy approaches, and most adults who are verbally challenged can often draw their feelings. This approach is especially effective with adults who have developmental disabilities or have been diagnosed with autism.

Adults who are in denial can also benefit from play therapy. An adult who denies an alcoholism problem will usually reveal something about it when engaging in play therapy techniques such as drawing, sandtray, or board games, but may not admit to the presenting problem directly through traditional talk therapy. In addition, emotionally constricted adults who live predominantly in the cognitive domain and have lost touch with their affective side and their own playfulness will benefit from play therapy. Many adults function well enough in the work world but have little opportunity to express their creativity. For these clients life has become work. With no play in their lives, life can become boring and/or depressing. As such, these clients frequently lose touch with their own creative aspects, which then open up in the world of play. Stressed and overworked adults may engage in play therapy for stress relief and to develop new coping skills.

Adults who are psychologically unaware of what is troubling them or the etiology of their difficulties obviously cannot verbalize as much to the play therapist. For example, if a client was raised in a dysfunctional, alcoholic family, he or she might not realize the impact of that history on his or her current functioning, but such concerns could be manifested in the sandtray.

Clients who are customarily able to discuss concerns but who are inhibited about expressing feelings on certain topics can benefit from play therapy. An adult who is inhibited about discussing intimacy and sexual issues can find it easier to discuss this topic through the use of a board game. When adults who are normally verbal reach a point in therapy where they feel vulnerable and less able to verbally process what is happening, play therapy can be helpful. Clients who are usually verbal can sometimes reach a plateau. The concern related to this plateau usually emerges through play therapy.

Lastly, it is important to remember that even play therapists can feel overwhelmed and/or stressed as they are busy helping others, and as a result, lose sight of their playful side. If a play therapist cannot play, his or her clients will find it difficult to play. While play therapists monitor the process of clients' play, they also need to be spontaneous and playful themselves.

Contraindications for the Use of Play Therapy with Adults

Adults for whom playfulness is threatening are not good candidates for this approach. Often these adults have a history of psychological damage in play or close relationships. The adult may have felt seduced by play as a child, only to be betrayed. Other clients may have experienced incest introduced as a "game." Some clients can use play as a defense. Play can serve to mask hostility, and some clients become playful to avoid dealing with anger or resentment.

Other adult clients use play to seduce or disarm the therapist. Such dynamics slow the progress of therapy.

Some adults use play as a way to control and manipulate the therapy environment and the therapist from the larger treatment goal. For example, an adult client might insist on playing chess with the therapist long after the value of this technique has ceased. Some adults become addicted to play, as is evident in many Internet games adults play incessantly while totally ignoring their family. Play therapy should be used cautiously with such clients who have allowed a form a play to become addictive.

Some might contend that many of these client types could benefit from play therapy to help them overcome the issues they have associated with play. Seductiveness, defensiveness, manipulation, inhibitions, and addiction can also be helped through play therapy. However, it is generally considered desirable to begin with traditional talk therapy with such clients, and then gradually introduce play therapy when clients have a readiness for it. In general, however, great caution is needed when working with these clients in play therapy.

Play therapists need to monitor the impact of play therapy with adults. Failure to identify these dynamics and/or engage in a client's pseudoplayfulness can result in collusion. It is necessary to monitor the degree to which play techniques are therapist-initiated, client-initiated, or conjointly initiated. The play therapist's keen awareness of these dynamics is extremely important for the successful use of play therapy with adults.

Play therapy can help adults develop a positive association with the affective domain. Through play therapy, feelings are not seen as so threatening. When adults develop a positive association with the affective domain, profound insight can develop. Such adults can then develop the capacity for tenderness, affection, and humor, which they have never experienced, through the use of game play, fantasy, and artwork.

Strategies and Techniques

A variety of play therapy techniques are commercially available for adults. In addition, the therapist and/or the client can create many play therapy techniques. Spontaneous, creative interventions often are very productive.

Card games are a modality very suitable for adults. The Ungame card game (family version; Zakich, 1983) helps family members learn how to communicate more effectively. The author of the game recalled that the first time her family played the game, she learned more about them in 20 minutes than she had in 12 years. The card game comes with two decks, one more lighthearted, whereas the other elicits more in-depth responses. Examples of these cards are: "What is likely to cause you to 'blow' up?", "Who do you think is the most loving member of your family?", and "You may ask any player one question or comment on any subject you choose." The game is noncompetitive and encourages active listening and self-disclosure about family concerns.

Play therapists can obtain blank playing cards and design a game for unique adult problems. Or a traditional deck of cards can be used and developed for therapeutic uses. One such example is a nonverbal card game intended to improve communication by focusing on the nonverbal domain. Each type of face card is assigned a feeling of the therapist's choice: for example, ace = love, king = joy, jack = anger. Each player is dealt six cards. When the playing begins there is no talking. The player decides which feeling card he or she is going to act out nonverbally and places it face down on the table. After observing, the other player(s) assesses what feeling is being portrayed. If the observing player has that card(s) in his or her hand, he or she places it face up on the table. If there is a successful match, all cards are discarded. If there is not a match, all players retrieve their cards. Playing continues with each player taking a turn until a player discards all cards. That player is the winner. The player has learned how to give and receive accurate nonverbal messages.

Toys can also be used with adults in play therapy: thumballs, stuffed animals, fortune cookies, and objects introduced to the client. Thumballs (Answers in Motion, 1990) are produced in different sizes with different feelings printed on the ball. The therapist tosses the ball to the client. The client catches the ball, looks under his or her thumb, and reads what it says. It could say "excited," "angry," "sad." The client tells about a time he or she felt like this feeling. The technique increases the person's ability to identify and express feelings.

Stuffed animals are sometimes held by clients for support and nonverbal caring. It is common for adults in play therapy to pick up toys that are present for children and use them therapeutically. A 66-year-old client who was grieving the loss of her husband and attending a hospice grief group reported that another group member had handed her a teddy bear as a source of comfort in a group session. This was so helpful to the client that she brought her own teddy bear to individual adult play therapy sessions.

Fortune cookies can also be used in play therapy with adults. The message inside should be relevant to the adult's dynamics. Examples of such fortune cookie messages include "Whether you think you can or you think you can't, you're right," or "Look forward to the butterfly instead of stepping on the caterpillar." After reading the message and discussing the relevancy to the client, the client is invited to eat the cookie. This technique can be used in an individual or group adult play therapy format.

Another play therapy technique for adults is board games. Much can be learned from the process of playing board games. The therapist can learn how the client problem-solves, how he or she reacts to success and failure, and how the client deals with conflict. Some adults argue about the rules of the game, manipulate the play therapist, succumb to defeat long before it is neces-

sary, blatantly or covertly cheat, and/or worry a lot about winning.

One board game used in adult play therapy is An Enchanted Evening (Games Partnership, 1989; available for purchase online). The goal of this game for two people is to increase self-disclosure and sharing about sexual intimacy. The cards can elicit positive and supportive statements and suggest gentle touching. One card states, "If you saw your partner at a dinner party, what might first attract you?" Another card instructs, "How much feeling can you put into a kiss contest that has just begun? You are a contestant. Give your partner the winning kiss." The game content assists couples in dialoging about their sexuality and intimacy. This is an excellent game to assist partners and couples in expressing their desires about an intimate topic, which is often difficult to articulate more directly in traditional talk therapy. It is also a gender-neutral game, thus facilitating the discussion of this topic among gay and lesbian couples.

The Chronic Care Challenges (Enasco, 1994) is a board game for adults who are caregivers of their parents or in a health center. The game focuses on the concerns of people who are helping others who have Alzheimer's, other forms of dementia, arthritis, asthma, chronic pain, diabetes, or experience elder abuse. Each of these separate topics has a set of cards associated with it. One general game board allows the therapist to insert whatever cards are appropriate for a client in individual or group play therapy.

Self-Esteem Bingo (Frey & Carlock, 1991) is a board game for adults designed to increase awareness of the characteristics of those with high self-esteem and to facilitate the acquisition of these qualities. Twenty-five techniques known to foster high self-esteem are placed on a bingo card. Players try to obtain bingo by finding individuals who engage in these self-esteem-enhancing activities. This game is a fun way to learn how to improve self-esteem.

These board games are just a representative sample of the many different board games available for adults in play therapy. Chess and checkers have also been used in a therapeutic fashion with adults. Other board games for adults in therapy focus on such topics as gender bias, midlife crisis, and communication skills. The American Association for Retired Persons (AARP; 1990) developed a board game for retired individuals entitled Limbo, a game designed to assist adults in transition to retired life.

Expressive arts activities can also be used with adults in play therapy. The art can be structured or unstructured. In more structured approaches the client is asked to draw a specific event or respond to a specific stimulus. The *Anti-Coloring Book for Adults Only* (Striker, 1983) is a good resource to help clients develop insight, creativity, and imagination. A graphic stimulus is placed on each page, and the client is asked to respond to the content by drawing whatever comes to mind. Examples of the various pages include content such as "What do you think your id looks like?", "What would you like to tell your spouse that you never had the courage to say?", "When you are old, what will your fondest memory be?", "What would you like to tell a shrink?", and "If you could go back to the womb for a while, who or what would you take with you?" A series of six anti-coloring books, also by Striker, for ages 6 and up, is also available. The therapist can choose appropriate content from numerous stimulus pages.

Interactive games can also be used with adults in play therapy. One such game often used as a warm-up technique for adults in group play therapy uses a Koosh ball or any other type of ball. Participants sit in a circle, and one at a time each person tosses the ball to another while stating his or her own name. When all have finished, phase two progresses. In this phase each person tosses the ball and states the name of the person to whom he or she is throwing the ball. Phase three involves each person tossing the ball while stating the recipient's name and telling the recipient one thing about the thrower. Next, each person tosses the ball to another while telling about a feeling he or she has. Lastly, the participant tosses the ball and can ask the recipient a question. Play continues until everyone has had a turn in each phase. This is a playful way of getting to know group members.

A game called Three Changes (Frey & Fitzharris, 1999b) helps clients become more aware of others, perceive others accurately, and realize the value of a social support system. This activity is suitable for adult group therapy. Two teams are formed: Team A and Team B. Teams form parallel lines, with the two teams facing each other. Each person on Team A has a partner on Team B. Participants are given a short period of time to observe their partner. Then Team A faces away from Team B while each person on Team B makes three changes to his or her appearance. Participants then face each other again, and Team A members try to guess what three changes their partners on Team B made. Following this, Team A members make three changes while Team B is turned away from them. Team B members then try to determine what changes have been made. This continues for two or three rounds. Participants usually start to comment about how few choices they have to make changes on themselves. Eventually the group realizes they can borrow from each other. Discussion can ensue about the value of a social support system.

Another interactive game that can be used for adults in play therapy is a scavenger hunt. Clients, for example, could be sent on a scavenger hunt to find six different ways to effectively manage stressors, enhance their self-esteem, or cope with difficult people. Clients would then observe and/or interview others about these topics. The topics can be changed to fit the needs of specific clients.

Drama and guided imagery can also be used with adults in play therapy. A guided imagery suggested by Dayton (1991) involves asking the client to imagine having everything he or she wants very much in life. The client is then asked to participate in life as if this desire were reality. After the client has fulfilled this desire in his or her mind, the client is asked to return to full consciousness and process the experience.

An imagery technique that has been used with adults and children in play therapy is Rosebush Identification (Stevens, 1991). In this experience the client is guided through an imagery in which he or she imagines a rosebush, its identity, lifestyle, environment, and feelings. When completed, the client is asked to draw the rosebush. Discussing the rosebush as a metaphor for self-processes completes the activity.

Dayton (1991) uses another imagery, Taking Care of the Child Within, in which the client is asked to see an image of him- or herself as a child. The client is then asked to imagine that the child self needs something from the adult client, something the client is able to give. The client then actually stands and puts the child self in his or her chair and gives the child self what has been requested. The client nurtures the child self and lets the child self know that he or she will return. When the client is ready, he or she returns her attention to the room and processes the experience. This is a powerful way to reparent the inner child. Dayton states that she learned this technique from Zekra Moreno, the doyenne of psychodrama.

Role playing can also be used in play therapy with adults and can help adults practice problem solving, rehearse behaviors, develop empathy, and reenact or reconstruct events. An example of rehearsing a particular behavior might involve the client practicing how to express anger prosocially toward her sister, while the therapist plays the role of sister. A client can develop empathy by playing the role of a significant other while the therapist plays the role of the client. Simulation games for adults would also be examples of the use of role playing.

Puppets can also be used in adult and family play therapy. In family play therapy each member is asked to choose a puppet and create a play. The therapist then processes with the family the symbolic meaning of the play as it relates to their family dynamics. Adults have also used a Freud puppet (Myrstad, 1988) to help them express feelings.

Sandtray therapy gives adults the opportunity to reveal symbolically thoughts, feelings, and behaviors that may be too difficult to express verbally (Garrett, 2013). Sandtray play shows clients unconscious material that could be influencing their lives. Carl Jung reported playing in the sand alone on a Swiss lakeshore, experiencing catharsis and developing new, creative ideas. He said, "Often the hands know how to solve a riddle with which the intellect has wrestled in vain" (Jung, 1981, p. 13). A following case example illustrates the value and uses of sandtray play with adults.

Violet Oaklander (1978) stated that "one of the most predictable ways to make oneself attractive to a child is to show them a few magic tricks" (p. 174). This applies to adult clients also. Even the most resistant client will usually respond positively to magic. It is helpful for therapists to collect magic tricks that have therapeutic metaphors embedded in them. One such trick often used with adult clients who feel "stuck" in life is called Drink the Water. In this trick the therapist holds a glass of water and asks the client to push down on his or her arm to prevent him or her from drinking the water. The therapist informs the client that he or she can drink the water in spite of the client holding down his or her arm. The therapist then switches the glass to the other hand and drinks the water. A discussion can ensue about how one can really feel "stuck" in life and think change is impossible when, through therapy, other avenues are often opened to clients.

Movie therapy can also be used with adults. "Movies have become the dominant art form in our culture; and like other art forms, movies reflect both the deep inner suffering, and the unlimited capacity for joy that make up our humanness" (Kristberg, 1980, quoted in Solomon, 1995, p. 9). In video play therapy clients are assigned a movie to watch between sessions. When they return they can role-play various characters, draw scenarios as they would like them to have been portrayed, reenact scenes in the sandtray, and/or use puppetry to act out relevant scenes. If a picture is worth 1,000 words, a movie can be worth a trillion words. Many people have not had anyone in their lives to listen to them and/or give them life messages. One unique feature of movies is that clients can hear and see life messages whenever they want and as many times as they want. Two resources helpful to therapists are the *Motion Picture Prescription* (Solomon, 1995) and *Rent Two Films and Let's Talk in the Morning* (Hesley & Hensley, 2001). These resources guide therapists in what movies to assign for various dynamics. Guidelines are also provided for processing the movies.

Bibliotherapy—using books to help the client in therapy—is also a helpful technique for adults in play therapy. The therapist could recommend a self-help book or a book in which the main character is similar to the client. The content of the book can be processed according to the guidelines for using bibliotherapy, as in traditional therapy, but can also be used in play therapy by adding sociodrama, role playing, art, and/or sandtray. Listings of appropriate books for various psychological concerns are available on the Internet (*www.tipperarylibraries.ie,   www.kilkennylibrary.ie, http://psychologicalselfhelp.org*).

Occasionally adults will jokingly comment about materials they see child clients holding while they are coming to or leaving therapy. A comment might be "Maybe I'll play with clay today," or "I can draw pictures too." Such comments can often be clues that the adult wants to enter the world of play. Looking for these opportunities can be rewarding for both therapist and client.

Clinical Case Examples

Glasser (2001) stated that when people are having fun, when they play and engage, they are learning, and that learning provides the health and growth necessary to become a fully functioning person. Without play, people are not really experiencing life. Play is necessary throughout all developmental stages of life. Anaïs Nin (1977) highlights why play therapy is such a necessary and useful modality for adult clients, stating, "We do not grow absolutely, chronologically. We grow sometimes in one direction, and not in another, unevenly. We grow partially. We are relative. We are mature in one realm, childish in another."

The asynchronicity of human development lends itself well to play therapy. In traditional therapy it is often assumed that the client is at the same level with regard to cognition, affect, and behavior. Through play therapy the specific areas of unevenness in development are revealed for each client. The following case studies are examples of what both Glasser and Nin stated.

Case 1

Joan was a 24-year-old single female who presented in therapy with severe depression. She stated that she had to force herself to get up in the morning and go to work. The therapist inquired about the client's satisfaction in various aspects of her life. She reported that she liked her job and had friends, a supportive family, and a boyfriend she liked. It did not appear that she was trying to be evasive or resistant, since she reported that she was desperate for help. The therapist then inquired about a family history of depression, and the client reported no such family history. The therapist inquired about angry feelings, which Joan might be internalizing. She denied any awareness of such feelings.

At this point the therapist decided to switch to play therapy since the client was unable to identify any source of her depression. The client was asked to respond to a page from the *Anti-Coloring Book* (Striker, 1983). The stimulus at the bottom of the page asks clients to draw anyone they would really like to call on the phone. Joan drew

three babies and said she would give anything if she could communicate with these
babies. It was discovered through further
discussion that slightly over a year ago she
had delivered triplets. About 2 months
after the births, one baby died, 2 weeks
later another baby died, and shortly thereafter the other baby died. Further exploration revealed that she had been dating a
man she loved very much and expected to
marry him. She became pregnant, and he
disappeared from her life. She was unable
to locate him anywhere. Her parents were
very supportive and indicated that they
would help her as much as possible. When
it was discovered she was carrying triplets,
her parents suggested that she move in with
them, which she did. Since she was a print
model for a local department store, she lost
her job temporarily. During a short period
of time she lost the love of her life, her lifestyle, her job, her independence, and her
three babies.

It was curious to the therapist why Joan
did not mention these losses when discussing her depression. Joan responded that
her parents and she agreed that the best
way to deal with all this loss in a short period of time was to close the door on that
chapter in their lives and never discuss it
again. Joan had so repressed these events
that she did not even think to mention
them in therapy. It was obvious to the therapist that this was the cause of her depression. Anniversary syndrome was also very
evident.

Joan's case is an excellent example of one
category of adults for whom play therapy is
effective—those clients who are psychologically unaware of what is troubling them. If
the client is unaware of the source of the
problem, it is difficult to discuss the issue
in traditional talk therapy. In this case play
therapy was used for diagnosis and insight
development, and it also helped Joan to
increase her verbalization skills about this
issue.

In addition to using the *Anti-Coloring
Book* (Striker, 1983) for diagnostic pur-

poses, Joan was also asked to participate in
the Grief Game (Kingsley, 1996). The game
is designed for children, adolescents, and
families experiencing grief. Through playing this game several times, Joan developed
insight into her grief. Sociodrama and fantasy play therapy were also used with Joan,
as was music. In one session Celine Dion's
song "My Heart Will Go On" was played.
Joan drew pictures of the babies and a symbol for how she will remember them. Since
no actual funeral services were conducted,
Joan played out the burial of the babies in
the sandtray. When therapy was completed,
Joan reported her amazement about how
effective play therapy had been for her, for
it had helped her to develop the necessary
coping skills to deal with her concerns.

Case 2

"If two wrongs don't make a right, what
do two rights make?" These were the first
words out of the mouth of a 42-year-old
client named Jim. He answered the question by saying "an airplane," referring to
the Wright brothers. Living in Ohio, he
was keenly involved with Ohio history and
culture. The therapist soon realized that
Jim's way of dealing with stress was through
humor. An attorney who owned his own
firm, Jim believed that his business was
stagnating, and the more he pressured the
others in the firm to produce, the more
both they and he became stressed. With
the downturn of the economy, fewer clients
were seeking the services of his firm, which
specialized in domestic relations. Jim told
the therapist that his goal in therapy was to
deal with the stress. Although he was very
verbal about expressing his stress, it was
later found that he had a great deal of difficulty talking about more personal issues.

Since "feeling stuck" and "stagnant" was
the client's presenting concern, the therapist began with the Drink the Water magic
trick and later introduced relaxation imagery along with small sensitive skin ther-
mometers to help him measure his progress

in managing stress (Biodot®, 2009). During the course of his therapy, he frequently commented to the therapist, upon entering the room, that he was *not* going to play in the sandtray. The therapist had never invited him to play in the sandtray, although doing so would, of course, have been acceptable. However, while discussing his work stress one session, the client began to play in the sandtray, which he so vehemently said he was not going to do. While talking to the therapist, the client put his hands in the tray. Suddenly, like an awakening from the sand, he brought out a Lego figure of a flatbed truck. The truck had barbed-wire sides and no back. He had placed a Lego man on the back of the truck with his arms entangled in the barbed wire. He excitedly exclaimed, "Look at this. This is me—this is what is going on with me!" Perplexed, the therapist asked him to explain.

Jim then told the therapist that he had been having an affair with a married woman for 5 years. He had just recently told his wife about the affair, and that he wanted a divorce. His wife promptly informed the husband of the other woman. Although this generated more stress in his life, he was not as concerned about that as the symbolism of the Lego truck. He informed the therapist that his wife thought the other woman had three children with her husband. She actually had two children in that marriage, and a 2-year-old as a result of the affair. He did not want to tell his wife about this child. He stated that since everyone involved knew about the affair, he and the other woman had moved into a condo together. It was then that he discovered, through living with this woman, that she was very much like his wife. He felt stuck in the new relationship because he felt a responsibility to the young child. It was then he said, holding the Lego truck up in the air, "See this—this is just like me! This guy could get out of this truck, but it would be very painful. That's just like me. I could get out of this relationship, but it would be very painful."

Although Jim was very verbal about his work stress, he had not been able to verbalize anything initially about this affair and the child. The symbolism from the sandtray had helped him to reveal and discuss this concern, and through in-depth exploration, to ascertain other unconscious material. As a result of that processing, the therapist sent the client on a scavenger hunt to ask six people what it is they find valuable in intimate relationships. Visual imagery was also used with Jim. He was asked to imagine an animal of one gender, then of the other gender, and then to create a story between the two of them. When he finished the imagery, he revealed to the therapist what he imagined. The imagery usually surfaces client expectations about intimate relationships. Jim's story was very different from what he had created in his own life.

In a subsequent session Jim was given the children's book *The Empty Pot* (Demi, 1999) to read. Although this book is intended for children, it is not very childlike in format. The theme of the book celebrates authenticity and was helpful to Jim in stimulating a discussion of that topic.

The Hinged House (Frey & Fitzharris, 1999a) play therapy technique was also used with Jim. In this technique the therapist creates a hinged house out of oak tag or other similar-weight paper. A house is cut with one side being hinged. (This could also be done with a manila folder.) The client is asked to draw something memorable from childhood on the front of the house; on the inside the client is asked to draw what happened in the house, and on the back, to draw "secrets" of the house. This technique is helpful to clients in ascertaining expectations of marriage, which come from their family of origin. Jim's drawings revealed a much more equalitarian relationship than either of his current relationships. These play therapy techniques helped Jim to do an autopsy of his failed relationships.

Although Jim initially presented with one aspect of stress, which he could talk about to some extent, the underlying stress was revealed through the sandtray. Sandplay helped in diagnosing the problem and other play therapy techniques were helpful in treatment. Play therapy helped Jim to transcend his communication barriers.

At Jim's last session he asked the therapist if she knew that Ohio would have new license plates in October. The state wanted the plates to read, "Ohio, birthplace of Superman" (Superman was created by two Cleveland teenage boys). The franchise owning the rights would not give permission for this, stating that everyone knows Superman was born in Krypton. This was not a joke, but he did follow this with a joke: What's the difference between Superman and an ordinary man? Superman wears his underwear over his pants. There are probably some embedded messages there! The plates now have the iconic Superman insignia with the words: Truth, Justice, and the American Way. Numerous calls have been received from people in other states, especially California, requesting to purchase the plates. However, only Ohio residents may purchase them.

Case 3

Eighty-five-year-old Louise approached the therapist at a meeting, stating that she needed to make an appointment with her. She stated that she had no friends and wanted to learn how to make friends. The therapist assumed that Louise meant that all her friends had died. Louise went on to say that all her life she had never had friends and that she "didn't want to die never having had any friends."

Louise presented in therapy as very psychologically unaware of why she had social skills deficits. She was also verbally deficient in being able to discuss her concerns to any degree. Louise reflected a common theme expressed by older adults, thinking of therapy as equivalent to revealing a weakness. She had an approach–avoidance way of dealing with therapy: She wanted to acquire coping skills, but she thought that

therapy was a reflection of her weakness. Louise was a retired judge, twice-divorced, and having an affair with a married man. In the first session she saw a picture on the wall, titled *A Skeptic's Look at Life* (Planick, 1978). The picture depicts a view of life's journey. Smiling people are shown entering a zigzag ladder, but as they traverse the ladder, they become more serious looking. As they approach the top of the ladder, their expressions are of astonishment and fear. At the top of the ladder all the people are falling off into a pile, deceased. Louise started to talk about how that picture depicted how she feels about life. This was a good example of the use of objects in play therapy. Discussing the picture enabled her to begin to experience self-disclosure.

The game Conversations to Go (Moonjar, 2005) was introduced to help her feel more comfortable with self-disclosure. Therapist and client take turns drawing a message strip from a box resembling a Chinese takeout box that includes strips resembling fortune cookie messages. Examples of the ones Louise drew are "Describe your perfect day," "What is the difference between wishing and realizing your dreams?", and "What is your definition of strong?" Louise's responses had a general theme of interacting positively with others and feeling pressured about running out of time in her life.

Louise was asked to respond to a page from the *Anti-Coloring Book for Adults Only* (Striker, 1983). She drew a response to a page with the stimulus value of "When you are old, what will your fondest memory be?" She drew a picture of herself as a judge. Video play therapy was also used with Louise. She was asked to view the film *Young @ Heart, You're Never Too Old to Rock* (George, 2008), and then the therapist processed it with her. In the sandtray she reenacted the ending she thought she might have for herself. Board games were also played with Louise. Through this game play Louise was able to become more verbally proficient at discussing her concerns and more psychologically aware of them. Since modeling is the best technique to use for social skills development, Louise was sent on a scavenger hunt to observe at least six people whom she determined had good social skills. When she returned to therapy her notes were reviewed. She also role-played several social situations. Through these play therapy techniques Louise was able to gain insight, improve her communication skills, reduce stress, and improve her self-esteem. At the end of therapy Louise felt more confident in her social skills. She had developed some new friends and felt more positive about the future.

Conclusion

It was in the early part of the 20th century that Carl Jung wrote about his own experience with play therapy as an adult playing in the sand to resolve his issues about leaving Freud's inner circle. In the 1970s Oaklander wrote about the effectiveness of using play therapy with adults (1978). Clearly the value of play therapy with adults has been noted for quite some time. More recently Schaefer (2003), L'Abate (2009), and Frey (1993, 1994) have discussed the value of play therapy with adults. Play therapy is an effective treatment modality to assist adults in assessment, stress release, mastery, communication, and insight development. It is an intervention that has no boundaries, embracing all ages, ethnicities, and gender. The numerous techniques available for this population have generated considerable interest for therapists.

George Bernard Shaw (1923) once said, "We don't stop playing because we grow old, we grow old because we stop playing." In a *New York Times* News Service (1992) article titled "Toys 'r' must for Boomers," it was reported that baby boomer adults were buying more and more toys for themselves as a method of escaping stress and developing effective coping mechanisms. Nearly 45% of 20,000 adults surveyed indicated

that they had purchased a toy or game for themselves or another adult in the past year. Perhaps, somewhat intuitively, adults are beginning to learn the value of play in their lives. It is hoped that more and more play therapists also will welcome this modality for adults.

What has been discussed about the value of play therapy for adults can best be summarized in this quotation by Dennis Marthaler (1991):

> When a child is born s/he is loving, lovable, intelligent, creative, energetic, powerful, gentle, sociable, and cooperative. We never lose these qualities because they are the essence of being human. Our bodies age, but the child within each of us remains the same. Each night the stars are shining, even though on some nights they can't be seen because of the clouds, which have accumulated along the way, to be cast off. And then the stars within us will shine with all their brilliance. (as cited in Frey, 1991, p. 58)

The process of play therapy with adults can be thought of as a way to help adults cast off the clouds that have accumulated for them and reveal again the child within them. It is then that adults can "shine with all their brilliance."

REFERENCES

Adatto, C. (1991). On play and the psychopathology of golf. *Journal of the American Psychoanalytic Association, 12,* 826–841.

American Association for Retired Persons. (1990). *Limbo.* Washington, DC: Author.

Answers in Motion. (1990). *Thumball.* Mapleshade, NJ: Author.

Bludworth, J. (2014). A successful aging group. In M. S. Corey, G., Corey, & C. Corey (Eds.), *Groups: Process and practice* (9th ed., p. 402). Independence, KY: Cengage Learning.

Brown, S. (2008, May). Play is more than just fun. *TED Talks.* Retrieved from *www.ted.can/talks.*

Brown, S., & Vaughn, C. (2009). *Play: How it shapes the brain, opens imagination, and invigorates the soul.* New York: Penguin.

Chance, P. (1979). *Learning through play: A sym-*

posium. New York: Johnson & Johnson Baby Products.

Dayton, T. (1991). *Drama games.* Deerfield Beach, FL: Health Communications.

Demi. (1991). *The empty pot.* New York: Holt.

Einstein, A. (1964). *The act of creation.* New York: Macmillan.

Elkind, D. (2007). *The power of play: How spontaneous, imaginative activities lead to happier, healthier children.* Cambridge, MA: Da Capo Press.

Enasco. (1994). *Chronic care challenges.* Chattanooga, TN: Author.

Frey, D. E. (1991). *100 inspirational quotations for enhancing self-esteem.* Dayton, OH: Educo Learning Systems.

Frey, D. E. (1993). I brought my own toys today!: Play therapy with adults. In T. Kottman & C. Schaefer (Eds.), *Play therapy in action: A casebook for practitioners* (pp. 589–606). New York: Jason Aronson.

Frey, D. E. (1994). The use of play with adults. In K. O'Conner & C. Schaefer (Eds.), *Handbook of play therapy: Vol. II. Advances and innovations* (pp. 189–205). New York: Wiley.

Frey, D. E., & Carlock, J. (1991). *Practical techniques for enhancing self-esteem.* Muncie, IN: Accelerated Development.

Frey, D. E., & Fitzharris, T. (1999a). Hinged house. In *Chart your course: Using play therapy to enhance emotional intelligence* (p. 84). Dayton, OH: Mandala.

Frey, D. E., & Fitzharris, T. (1999b). Three changes. In *Chart your course: Using play therapy to enhance emotional intelligence* (p. 55). Dayton, OH: Mandala.

Games Partnership. (1989). *Enchanted evening, an.* San Francisco: Author.

Garrett, M. (2013). Beyond play therapy: Using the sandtray as an expressive arts intervention in counselling adult clients. *Asia Pacific Journal of Counselling and Psychotherapy.* Retrieved from *www.tandfonline.com/doi/pdf/10.1080/21507686.2013.864319.*

George, (2008). *Young @ heart.* Beverly Hills, CA: Searchlight Pictures.

Glasser, W. (2001). *Counseling with choice theory.* New York: Harper.

Hesley, J. W., & Hesley J. G. (2001). *Rent two films and let's talk in the morning: Using popular movies in psychotherapy.* New York: Wiley.

Jung, C. (1981). *The collected works of C. G. Jung: Vol. 9i. The archetypes and the collective unconscious.* Princeton, NJ: Princeton University Press.

Kingsley, J. (1996). *Grief game.* London: Author.

Kristberg, W. (1980). *A quiet strength.* New York: Bantam Books.

L'Abate, L. (2009). *The Praeger handbook of play across the life cycle.* Santa Barbara, CA: ABL-CLIO.

Marthaler, D. (1985). *Picture me perfect.* Hollywood, CA: Newcastle Press.

Moonjar.com. (2005). *Conversations to go.* Beverly Hills, CA: Fox Searchlight Pictures.

Myrstad, B. (1988). *Freud toy.* New York: Freud Toy.

New York Times News Service. (1992). Toys 'r' must for boomers. *Dayton Daily News,* October 27, p. 11A.

Nin, A. (1977). *Good reads.* Retrieved from *www.goodreads.com/author/quotes/7190ana_s_nin.*

Oaklander, V. (1978). *Windows to our children.* Moab, UT: Real People Press.

Schaefer, C. (Ed.). (2003). *Play therapy with adults.* New York: Wiley.

Schaefer, C. (2011). *Foundations of play therapy* (2nd ed.). New York: Wiley.

Searkle, Y. (1996). *Grief game.* London: Jessica Kingsley.

Shaw, G. B. (1923). Brainyquote. Retrieved from *www.brainyquote.com/quotes/quotes/g/georgebern120971.html.*

Solomon, G. (Ed.). (1995). *Motion picture prescription: Watch this movie and call me in the morning.* Santa Rosa, CA: Asian Publishing

Stevens, J. (1991). *Awareness: Exploring, experimenting, and experiencing.* Moab, UT: Real People Press.

Striker, S. (1983). Anti-coloring book for adults only. New York: Holt, Rinehart & Winston.

Sutton-Smith, B. (1997). *The ambiguity of play.* Cambridge, MA: Harvard University Press.

Zakich, R. (1983). *Ungame card game.* Anaheim, CA: Ungame Company.

PART III

Research and Practice Guidelines in Play Therapy

INTRODUCTION

This volume is distinguished by its coverage of state-of-the-art play therapy research by Dee C. Ray, in Chapter 32, including findings not previously published. Dee Ray is one of the most highly respected researchers in the play therapy field from the University of North Texas. John W. Seymour and David A. Crenshaw in Chapter 33 delineate some of the essential internal disciplines of the reflective play therapist and/or play therapist supervisor. The chapter includes evocative reflective exercises to be used in self, individual, group, or peer supervision. Cultural issues so essential to the competent practice of play therapy are examined in Chapter 34 by Phyllis Post and Kathleen S. Tillman. An exceptionally critical coverage of ethical issues in play therapy practice is provided in Chapter 35 by Jeffrey S. Ashby and Kathleen McKinney Clark. The book ends with an extraordinary, must-read chapter on neuroscience and play therapy (Chapter 36) by Bonnie Badenoch and Theresa Kestly. The co-editors believe this chapter is not only unusually informative but reader friendly. What a way to finish this authoritative guide to theory, approaches, clinical applications, research, and practice guidelines in play therapy! We hope you've enjoyed the journey and found it enlightening as well as enlivening.

CHAPTER 32

Research in Play Therapy

EMPIRICAL SUPPORT FOR PRACTICE

Dee C. Ray

The review of play therapy research is a daunting task because play therapy has been conducted for such a long time period with so many populations. My goal in this chapter is to provide the reader with a brief review of historical play therapy research, examine research over the last decade in more detail, and summarize findings for the practicing play therapist. This chapter serves to offer specific details in support of using play therapy with children from specific backgrounds and with particular problem areas, as well as provide a comprehensive summary of play therapy outcomes.

Historical Play Therapy Research

In response to criticism that play therapy was not supported by sound scientific research, researchers in the last decade have reviewed, summarized, and analyzed play therapy studies conducted since their earliest publications dating back to the 1940s. Bratton and Ray (2000) conducted a thorough review of 82 play therapy studies published between 1940 and 2000. They

concluded that results were favorable and that research in play therapy showed promising results. Ray, Bratton, Rhine, and Jones (2001) conducted a preliminary meta-analysis of 94 experimental research studies in play therapy and concluded: "Play therapy appears to work in various settings, across modalities, age, and gender, clinical and nonclinical populations, and theoretical schools of thought" (pp. 93–94).

Using their initial findings to apply more rigorous design, Bratton, Ray, Rhine, and Jones (2005) included 93 play therapy studies published from 1942 to 2000 in their meta-analysis and reported an effect size (ES) of 0.80 (with an average age of study participants as 7.0 years). The researchers reported that parent participation was a significant predictor of positive outcome. They also noted moderate to large ESs for internalizing (ES = 0.81), externalizing (ES = 0.79), and combined problems (ES = 0.93). Both humanistic play therapy (ES = 0.92) and nonhumanistic or behavioral play therapy approaches (ES = 0.71) were considered to be effective. However, the effect size for humanistic play therapy was considered to be in the large effect category where the effect size for nonhumanistic interventions fell in the moderate category. Bratton and colleagues concluded that play therapy appeared effective across settings and presenting problems, but that future play therapy studies needed to adhere to rigorous design, analysis, and reporting guidelines in order for research to be considered evidence-based.

LeBlanc and Ritchie (2001) conducted a separate meta-analysis of 42 controlled play therapy studies and reported a moderate treatment ES of 0.66. Similar to findings of Bratton and colleagues, LeBlanc and Ritchie further reported that the average age of participants was 7.9 years and that duration of therapy and parent involvement were significant predictors of effectiveness. Consistent findings across meta-analyses indicate that play therapy is an effective intervention for younger children, especially when compared to mean ages reported in other meta-analyses and reviews (i.e., 10.3 years in Weisz, Jensen-Doss, & Hawley, 2005; 10.5 years in Weisz, Weiss, Han, Granger, & Morton, 1995). Bratton and Ray (2000) concluded that historical play therapy research demonstrated positive outcomes in the areas of self-concept/ locus of control, behavioral change, anxiety/fear reduction, cognitive ability, and social skills.

In subsequent attempts to critically review play therapy research, researchers have demonstrated further positive effects. Beelmann and Schneider (2003) conducted a meta-analysis of child therapy research conducted on German-language studies. Following the analysis of 47 treatment–control comparison design studies, they concluded that nondirective play therapy demonstrated sufficient treatment suitability for mixed groups. In a review of child-centered play therapy (CCPT) research, Ray (2011) presented results from 62 studies conducted from 1940 to 2010, finding an improvement in research rigor over time, a broad range of outcome variables, and substantial positive outcomes for CCPT. Historical research in

play therapy provides empirical support for the use of play therapy as an intervention. Researchers were nevertheless cautioned to improve the implementation and reporting of research designs in order to elevate the evidence base for play therapy in the future (Ray, 2006).

Research in the New Millennium

As researchers aggregated play therapy evidence, critiqued the research, and encouraged the application of rigor, individual studies increased over time. In order to identify play therapy studies published since 2000, I employed the following inclusion criteria: (1) Studies employed and reported descriptive information on intervention; (2) intervention was identified as play therapy; (3) play therapy intervention was child-focused; (4) participants were between the ages of 3 and 13 years old; (5) studies employed and reported quantitative measures to evaluate intervention; and (6) studies were published in peer-reviewed journals or books. Although I identified several studies published as dissertations or theses, I chose to exclude these manuscripts due to the number of concerns regarding quality of design, intervention, analyses, and interpretation of results. Yet, it should be noted that many play therapy studies can be found in dissertation form, and their existence stirs questions regarding the reason for lack of development to peer-reviewed publications.

After reviewing hundreds of potential studies for inclusion, 33 met criteria. Of the 33 studies, 17 used experimental group designs, 2 used quasi-experimental group designs, 3 had experimental single-case designs, and 10 were repeated measures of single-group designs. The majority of identified studies ($n = 26$) employed the exploration of CCPT; the remaining studies identified intervention as nondirective ($n = 1$), Gestalt ($n = 1$), sandtray ($n = 1$), cognitive-behavioral ($n = 1$), activity-based ($n = 2$), and unidentified ($n = 1$). In comparison, Bratton and Ray (2000) reviewed 82 studies meeting criteria for play therapy studies that were considered experimental designs and published from 1940 to 2000, over six decades. The number of studies conducted since 2000 represents a substantial increase from previous decades. Regarding modality, 7 studies employed group play therapy only, whereas 21 studies employed individual play therapy only. Two studies compared group play therapy to individual play therapy and the modality was unidentified in three studies. Table 32.1 provides a brief summary of each of the included studies.

The restriction of criteria to the use of the descriptor *play therapy* limited the inclusion of interventions that utilize games or materials but do not identify as play therapy. The Association for Play Therapy (APT; 2013) defines play therapy as "the systematic use of a theoretical model to establish an interpersonal process wherein trained play therapists use the therapeutic powers of play to help clients prevent or resolve psychosocial difficulties and achieve optimal growth and development." Because models of play therapy typically assert the "therapeutic powers of play" as a mechanism in the approach, research studies that used games and other materials but lacked identification with play therapy or explanation for use of materials were not considered for this review.

Surprisingly, cognitive-behavioral play therapy (CBPT) was identified in only one published experimental study (Mahmoudi-Gharaei, Bina, Yasami, Emami, & Naderi, 2006). Although cognitive-behavioral therapy (CBT) has earned a strong reputation in adolescent and adult therapy, the application of techniques to children is questionable. Dopheide (2006) concluded that children under 9 years may not have the verbal and cognitive processing skills to benefit from CBT. However, Knell (1993) presented a model of CBPT that integrates play with cognitive-behavioral techniques to meet the developmental needs of children. Knell and

Dasari (2011) cited 20 case studies of CBPT discussed in published literature. However, many of the case studies are lacking assessments to measure change. Furthermore, Knell and Dasari noted the lack of randomized, clinical intervention studies in CBPT.

The frequency of CCPT as the identified intervention marks an evolution in the study of play therapy. In previous reviews, Bratton and Ray (2000) and Ray (2006) found that nondirective play therapy was historically cited via a diversity of titles, such as *child-centered, nondirective, client-centered, self-directed,* and *relationship-oriented*. The movement toward using the title *CCPT* may indicate a unification of the person-centered approach to play therapy. Additionally, the development and publication of the CCPT manual (Ray, 2009, 2011) provided a clear identification of the process and protocol of CCPT for research exploration. The rise of CCPT research also coincides with the observed rise of person-centered research in the last decade (Elliott, Greenberg, Watson, Timulak, & Friere, 2013).

There was a noticeable absence of play therapy intervention studies from other theoretical orientations. Adlerian, Gestalt, Jungian, and existentially based play therapies, popularized through the works of Kottman (2003), Oaklander (1998), Allan (1988), and Moustakas (1997), respectively, have a limited research base but have a distinct presence in the literature and practice of counseling with children. Green (2011) observed that lack of Jungian research might be due to the approach's reliance on projective techniques and qualitative decision making in therapy. Both Green and Kottman (2011) noted lack of manualization for treatment protocol as a possible barrier to research on their respective approaches (Jungian and Adlerian). Kottman reported that an Adlerian manual had been developed for research purposes, and Green reported his development of a Jungian-based manual. These developments are likely to inspire research on a broadening range of play therapy approaches.

TABLE 32.1. Play Therapy Research Studies Since 2000

Study	Intervention/ No. of sessions/ Length of sessions	Design	Sample	Setting/ Country	Findings
Baggerly (2004)	Group CCPT 9–12 20 minutes	Repeated-measures single group	Children living in homeless shelter $N = 42$ Ages 5–11	Homeless shelter US	Results revealed significant improvement in self-concept, significance, competence, negative mood, and negative self-esteem related to depression and anxiety.
Baggerly & Jenkins (2009)	Individual CCPT 11–25 45 minutes	Repeated-measures single group	Children who were homeless $N = 36$ Ages 5–12	School for homeless children US	Children demonstrated statistically significant improvement on the developmental strand of internalization of controls and diagnostic profile of self-limiting features.
Bayat (2008)[a]	Nondirective play therapy 16	Repeated-measures single group	Preschoolers scoring high on behavioral problems measure	Iran	Results indicated a significant reduction of internalizing problems.
Blanco & Ray (2011)	Individual CCPT 16 30 minutes	Experimental pre–post control group	Academically at risk $N = 43$ 1st grade	School US	Children in the CCPT treatment group demonstrated significantly significant improvement on academic achievement composite score over children in control group.
Blanco, Ray, & Holliman (2012)	Individual CCPT 26 30 minutes	Repeated-measures single group Follow-up to Blanco & Ray (2011)	Academically at risk $N = 18$ 1st grade	School US	Children demonstrated statistically significant improvement on academic achievement composite over the full duration of the study.
Bratton et al. (2013)	Individual CCPT 17–21 30 minutes	Experimental pre–post active control group	Children with disruptive behaviors $N = 54$ 3–4 years old	Preschool US	Children in CCPT demonstrated statistically significant decreases in disruptive behaviors over children in active control group.
Danger & Landreth (2005)	Group CCPT 25 30 minutes	Experimental pre–post control group	Children who qualified for speech therapy $N = 21$ Ages 4–6	School US	Results revealed that children in CCPT demonstrated increased receptive language skills and expressive language skills with large practical significance over children in the control condition.

(continued)

TABLE 32.1. *(continued)*

Study	Intervention/ No. of sessions/ Length of sessions	Design	Sample	Setting/ Country	Findings
Dougherty & Ray (2007)	Individual CCPT 19–23 40–50 minutes	Archival repeated-measures within group	Children referred to counseling for behavioral problems *N* = 24 Ages 3–8	Clinic US	Children demonstrated statistically significant decreases in parent–child relationship stress with strong practical effects. Children in the concrete operations group experienced more change as a result of intervention than did children in the preoperational group.
Fall, Navelski, & Welch (2002)	Individual CCPT 6 30 minutes	Experimental pre–post control group	Children identified for special education *N* = 66 Ages 6–10	School US	Results demonstrated no difference between the groups in self-efficacy, but teacher ratings showed decreased problematic behavior and less social problems for the experimental group as compared to the control group.
Farahzadi, Bahramabadi, & Mohammadifar (2011)	Gestalt play therapy 10 90 minutes	Experimental pre–post control group	*N* = 12 4th grade	Girls' school Iran	Children in play therapy decreased scores of the diagnosing and severity factors of social phobia symptoms.
Flahive & Ray (2007)	Group sandtray therapy 10 45 minutes	Experimental pre–post control group	Children with behavioral difficulties *N* = 56 Ages 9–12	School US	Children in sandtray therapy group demonstrated statistically significant differences, as rated by teachers, in total, externalizing, and internalizing behaviors when compared to control group. Parents rated sandtray participants significantly different on externalizing behaviors.
Garofano-Brown (2010)	Individual CCPT 8 45 minutes	Single case	Children with developmental delays *N* = 3 Ages 3–5	Clinic US	Children increased in measured developmental age, reduced problematic behaviors related to developmental delays, and increased developmentally appropriate behaviors.
Garza & Bratton (2005)	Individual CCPT 15 30 minutes	Experimental pre-post comparison group	Children demonstrating behavioral problems *N* = 29 Ages 5–11	School US	Compared to comparison group, children receiving CCPT showed statistically significant decreases in externalizing behavior problems and moderate improvements in internalizing behavior problems as reported by parents.

(continued)

TABLE 32.1. *(continued)*

Study	Intervention/ No. of sessions/ Length of sessions	Design	Sample	Setting/ Country	Findings
Jalali & Molavi (2011)[a]	Group play therapy 6	Experimental pre–post control group	Children with separation anxiety $N = 30$	Clinic Iran	Children who participated in group play therapy demonstrated statistically significant reduction in separation anxiety as compared to no-treatment control group.
Jones & Landreth (2002)	Individual CCPT 12 30 minutes	Experimental pre–post control group	Children with diabetes $N = 30$ Ages 7–11	Diabetic summer camp US	Both groups improved anxiety scores; the experimental group showed a statistically significant increase in diabetes adaptation over the control group.
Mahmoudi-Gharaei, Bina, Yasami, Emami, & Naderi (2006)[a]	Group CBPT 12	Repeated-measures single group	Children who had experienced an earthquake in which they lost a family member $N = 13$ Ages 3–6	Iran	Children in play therapy demonstrated a statistically significant reduction in trauma-related symptoms and behavioral problems after participating in group play therapy.
Muro, Ray, Schottelkorb, Smith, & Blanco (2006)	Individual CCPT 32 30 minutes	Repeated-measures single group	Children with behavioral and emotional difficulties $N = 23$ Ages 4–11	School US	Ratings over 3 points of measure indicated statistically significant improvement on total behavioral problems, teacher–child relationship stress, and ADHD characteristics.
Naderi, Heidarie, Bouron, & Asgari (2010)	Activity-based play therapy 10 1 hour	Experimental pre–post control group	Children diagnosed with ADHD and anxiety $N = 80$ Ages 8–12	Clinic Iran	Children in therapy demonstrated statistically significant decreases in symptoms of ADHD and anxiety as compared to control group. Children in therapy demonstrated statistically significant improvement in social maturity as compared to control group.
Packman & Bratton (2003)	Humanistically based activity group therapy 12 60 minutes	Experimental pre–post control group	Children with learning disabilities and behavioral problems $N = 24$ 4th and 5th grades	School for learning disabilities US	Children in therapy demonstrated decreases in externalizing and internalizing problems with large effect sizes over the control group.

(continued)

TABLE 32.1. *(continued)*

Study	Intervention/ No. of sessions/ Length of sessions	Design	Sample	Setting/ Country	Findings
Ray (2007)	Individual CCPT 16 30 minutes	Experimental pre–post comparison groups 1. CCPT only 2. Person-centered teacher consultation (PCTC) 3. CCPT and PCTC	Children with emotional and behavioral difficulties N = 93 Ages 4–11	School US	Results demonstrated significant decreases in teacher–child relationship stress with large effects sizes in total stress for all three treatment groups.
Ray (2008)	Individual CCPT 1–19+ 40–50 minutes	Archival repeated-measures single group	Children referred for emotional and behavioral problems N = 202 Ages 2–13	Clinic US	CCPT demonstrated statistically significant effects for externalizing problems, combined externalizing/internalizing problems, and nonclinical problems. Results also indicated that CCPT effects increased with number of sessions, specifically reaching statistical significance at 11–18 sessions with large effect sizes.
Ray, Blanco, Sullivan, & Holliman (2009)	Individual CCPT 14 30 minutes	Quasi-experimental pre–post control group	Children demonstrating aggressive behaviors N = 41 Ages 4–11	School US	Children in CCPT showed a moderate decrease in aggressive behaviors over children in the control group according to teacher and parent report. Post hoc analysis revealed that children assigned to CCPT decreased aggressive behaviors to a statistically significant degree, and children assigned to control group demonstrated no statistically significant difference.
Ray, Henson, Schottelkorb, Brown, & Muro (2008)	Individual CCPT 16 30 minutes	Experimental pre–post comparison group 1. Short-term (16 sessions over 8 weeks) 2. Long-term (16 sessions over 16 weeks)	Children with emotional and behavioral difficulties N = 58 PreK–5th grades	School US	Results indicated that both intervention groups demonstrated significant improvement in teacher–student relationship stress. Post hoc analyses indicated that the short-term intensive intervention demonstrated statistical significance and larger effect sizes in overall total stress and in teacher and student characteristics.

(continued)

TABLE 32.1. *(continued)*

Study	Intervention/ No. of sessions/ Length of sessions	Design	Sample	Setting/ Country	Findings
Ray, Schottelkorb, & Tsai (2007)	Individual CCPT 16 30 minutes	Experimental pre–post active control group	Children with ADHD symptoms N = 60 Ages 5–11	School US	Results indicated that both conditions demonstrated statistically significant improvement on ADHD, student characteristics, anxiety, and learning disability. Children in CCPT demonstrated statistically significant improvement over active control children on student characteristics, emotional lability, and anxiety/withdrawal behaviors.
Ray, Stulmaker, Lee, & Silverman (2013)	Individual CCPT 12–16 sessions 30 minutes	Experimental pre–post control group	Children with clinical impairment N = 37 Ages 5–8	School US	CCPT group demonstrated decreased levels of impairment with medium effect size, whereas children in the delayed-start control group showed consistent or increased levels of impairment.
Schottelkorb, Doumas, & Garcia (2012)	Individual CCPT N = 17 30 minutes	Experimental pre–post comparison group 1. CCPT 2. Trauma-focused cognitive-behavioral therapy (TF-CBT)	Refugee children with trauma symptomology N = 26 Ages 6–13	School US	Results indicated that both CCPT and TF-CBT were effective in reducing trauma symptoms, according to child and parent reports.
Schottelkorb & Ray (2009)	Individual CCPT and person-centered teacher consultation (PCTC) 14–24 30 minutes	Single case	Children with ADHD symptoms N = 4 Ages 5–10	School US	Two children in CCPT demonstrated substantial reduction, and two students demonstrated questionable reduction in ADHD symptoms.
Schumann (2010)	Individual CCPT 12–15 30 minutes	Quasi-experimental pre–post comparison group 1. CCPT 2. Evidence-based guidance curriculum	Children demonstrating aggressive behaviors N = 37 Ages 5–12	School US	Participation in either CCPT or evidence-based guidance curriculum both resulted in significant decreases in aggressive behavior, internalizing problems, and externalizing problems.

(continued)

TABLE 32.1. (continued)

Study	Intervention/ No. of sessions/ Length of sessions	Design	Sample	Setting/ Country	Findings
Scott, Burlingame, Starling, Porter, & Lilly (2003)	Individual CCPT 7–13	Repeated-measures single group	Children referred for possible sexual abuse *N* = 26 Ages 3–9	Sexual abuse clinic US	Results indicated increased sense of competency over course of therapy.
Shen (2002)	Group CCPT 10 40 minutes	Experimental pre–post control group	Children at high risk for maladjustment following an earthquake *N* = 30 Ages 8–12	School Taiwan	CCPT group demonstrated a significant decrease in anxiety as well as a large treatment effect and significant decrease in suicide risk as compared to the control group.
Swan & Ray (2014)	Individual CCPT 15 30 minutes	Single case	Children with intellectual disabilities *N* = 2 Ages 6–7	School US	Results indicated that CCPT decreased hyperactivity and irritability behaviors following treatment intervention. For both participants, improvements in behaviors were maintained.
Tsai & Ray (2011)	Individual and group CCPT *N* = 28 40–45 minutes	Repeated-measures single group	Children referred to clinic for emotional and behavioral problems *N* = 82 Ages 3–10	School US	Results indicated statistically significant improvement on externalizing, internalizing, and total behavioral problems following participation in CCPT. Higher levels of internalizing and externalizing problem behaviors yielded greater gains from CCPT. Termination and family relationship concern variables were also found to be strong contributors to predicting greater improvement.
Tyndall-Lind, Landreth, & Giordano (2001)	Individual and group CCPT 12 45 minutes	Experimental pre–post comparison group 1. Sibling group CCPT 2. Individual CCPT 3. No-intervention control group	Children living in domestic violence shelter *N* = 32 Ages 4–10	Domestic violence shelter US	Children in sibling group play therapy demonstrated a significant reduction in total behavior, externalizing, and internalizing behavior problems, aggression, anxiety, and depression, and significant improvement in self-esteem. Results indicated that sibling group play therapy was equally effective to intensive individual play therapy.

[a]Details limited due to study published in language other than English. Information taken from abstract.

The greatest strength in play therapy research is the demonstration of its practicality in real-life settings. Many child intervention studies are criticized for being conducted in clinic laboratories and controlled university settings that lack applicability to clinical settings in the real world. Of the 33 studies reviewed in this chapter, settings included a homeless shelter, domestic violence shelter, sexual abuse center, diabetic camp, and counseling clinics. Notably, 22 of the studies were conducted in schools, mostly low-income, highly diverse schools, indicating that play therapy is effective with children in their natural settings. While generally accepted as evidence-based, verbally oriented child interventions struggle to produce strong positive findings in real-world settings with real-world clients (Weisz, Ugueto, Cheron, & Herren, 2013), yet play therapy studies are grounded in standard treatment settings.

Furthermore, play therapy studies are unique in their inclusion of children from multicultural backgrounds. Garza and Bratton (2005) conducted their study solely with Hispanic participants, whereas several other studies included a balanced percentage of Hispanic, African American, and European American participants. The substantial number of studies conducted in the real-world setting of schools most likely accounts for the diversity of the participants. In addition to the diversity within studies conducted in the United States, those conducted outside the United States point to promising findings that play therapy intervention is effective across international cultures. Bayat (2008); Farahzadi, Bahramabadi, and Mohammadifar (2011); and Naderi, Heidarie, Bouron, and Asgari (2010) in Iran and Shen (2002) in Taiwan demonstrated cross-cultural positive effects of play therapy. Additionally, a few studies from different countries were identified but were unavailable in English and therefore could not be included in this review.

The topics explored in play therapy research since 2000 highlight outcomes of interest currently in the mental health field overall. Table 32.2 categorizes the play therapy studies according to presenting problems or outcome of interest. These categories include externalizing/disruptive behaviors, internalizing problems, academic/language, relationships, trauma, self-concept/competency, development, and functional impairment. The most frequently researched sample population includes children who exhibit externalizing problem behaviors, such as aggression, attention-deficit/hyperactivity disorder (ADHD), and disruptive symptoms. Disruptive behavior problems are exhibited among many children and typically increase over time without intervention (Comer, Chow, Chan, Cooper-Vince, & Wilson, 2013; Studts & van Zyl, 2013). Fifteen play therapy studies reported positive impacts on externalizing problems, indicating that play therapy, most frequently in the form of CCPT, is effective in the reduction of externalizing behaviors.

Internalizing problems such as anxiety, mood disorders, and withdrawn behaviors were also heavily researched by play therapists. Most of the 13 studies examined both internalizing and externalizing problem behaviors and found improvements for both categories. Only four studies (i.e., Bayat, 2008; Farahzadi et al., 2011; Jalali & Molavi, 2011; Shen, 2002) explored internalizing problems exclusively, and all reported positive outcomes. Academic/language outcomes have been researched in historical play therapy studies and continue to be an area of interest. Although early research was concerned with intelligence, the five current studies in this category focused on academic achievement and language development, each resulting in positive outcomes for play therapy.

Emerging topics new to play therapy research include a focus on relationship—a focus that seems well aligned with treatment for children. Because relationships are fundamental to the growth and development of children, interventions designed

TABLE 32.2. Categories of Research Studies

Presenting problem/outcome variable	Individual studies
Externalizing/disruptive behaviors	Bratton et al. (2013); Fall et al. (2002); Flahive & Ray (2007); Garza & Bratton (2005); Muro et al. (2006); Naderi et al. (2010); Packman & Bratton (2003); Ray (2008); Ray et al. (2007, 2009); Schottelkorb & Ray (2009); Schumann (2010); Swan & Ray (2014); Tsai & Ray (2011); Tyndall-Lind et al. (2001)
Internalizing problems	Bayat (2008); Farahzadi et al. (2011); Flahive & Ray (2007); Garza & Bratton (2005); Jalali & Molavi (2011); Naderi et al. (2010); Packman & Bratton (2003); Ray (2008); Ray et al. (2007); Schumann (2010); Shen (2002); Tsai & Ray (2011); Tyndall-Lind et al. (2001)
Academic/language	Blanco & Ray (2011); Blanco et al. (2012); Danger & Landreth (2005); Packman & Bratton (2003); Swan & Ray (2014)
Relationships	Dougherty & Ray (2007); Muro et al. (2006); Ray (2007, 2008)
Trauma	Mahmoudi-Gharaei et al. (2006); Schottelkorb et al. (2012); Scott et al. (2003); Shen (2002); Tyndall-Lind et al. (2001)
Self-concept/competency	Baggerly (2004); Scott et al. (2003); Tyndall-Lind et al. (2001)
Development	Baggerly & Jenkins (2009); Dougherty & Ray (2007); Garofano-Brown (2010)
Functional impairment	Ray et al. (2013)

for children are commonly concerned with their relationships with caretakers, such as parents and teachers. Five studies demonstrated favorable effects of play therapy on the parent and teacher relationships of children participating in play therapy.

Another recent development in play therapy research is a focus on children who have been traumatized by either interpersonal trauma, violence, or natural disasters. Five studies, each with a different type of traumatized population, reported reduction in trauma symptoms or improvement in functioning for children in play therapy.

The study of self-concept, generally viewed as a variable of interest by play therapists, decreased in the last decade, resulting in only three studies examining the effect of play therapy on self-concept or personal competency. Researchers have noted the challenges and limitations of measuring the construct of self-esteem (Bracken & Lamprecht, 2003; Guindon, 2002) leading to mixed results when studied. This is one possible reason for a decrease in play therapy self-concept research. Nevertheless, the three studies listed in this review reported improvements in view of self and abilities.

The final two categories are development and functional impairment, variables of interest that encompass a greater holistic view of children. Two studies (Baggerly & Jenkins, 2009; Garofano-Brown, 2010) found that play therapy demonstrated positive effects on constructs related to development. Dougherty and Ray (2007) explored the effect of play therapy on children in different developmental stages, concluding that play therapy was effective with both younger and older children. Ray, Stulmaker, Lee, and Silverman (2013) noted that the construct of functional impairment is relevant to play therapy because of its broad inclusion of child functioning, including diminished ability to perform at developmentally expected levels, resulting in difficulties in daily life activities such as dysfunction or an absence of adaptation in social, emotional, psychological, or occupational/academic domains (Fabiano & Pelham, 2009). In their pilot study, Ray and colleagues (2013) found that participation in play therapy resulted in higher levels of functioning for children who had been identified with functional impairments.

Play-Based Interventions Involving Parents/Caretakers

The length of this chapter precludes a thorough review of play therapy interventions that focus on parents or parents in session with children. Several interventions focus on using play therapy skills or child's play to improve the parent–child relationship and/or address presenting problems. Most notably, the filial therapy model is an educational approach in which play therapists teach CCPT skills to parents for the purpose of holding weekly play sessions with their children. VanFleet (2011) reported that filial therapy is one of the most researched forms of play therapy and demonstrates improvements in child behavior and presenting problems, parental acceptance/empathy, parent skill and stress levels, and increased satisfaction with family life. Theraplay® is a structured form of play therapy that seeks to enhance parent–child attachments, self-esteem, and trust by guiding parents to become attuned and responsive to their children (Munns, 2011). Although research is cited to support the use of Theraplay, most studies have not been published in peer-reviewed venues,

limiting the ability to critically review outcomes. Dynamic play therapy (DPT), developed by Harvey (2008), is a family play intervention in which the therapist engages children and parents to become actively involved in play to address behavioral problems and family relationships. Preliminary study of DPT suggests that child behavior improved as a result of DPT and improvement was strongly correlated with positive relationships between parents and the therapist. Recently, researchers examining parent-focused interventions, such as parent–child interaction therapy (PCIT) and trauma-focused CBT (TF-CBT), have begun to identify their approaches as play therapy interventions. Both PCIT and TF-CBT are considered empirically supported interventions; however, the play components of these interventions have yet to be thoroughly explored in the research.

Using Research Findings in Clinical Practice

The purpose of intervention research is to provide empirical support for practices that will help support growth, improve functioning, and reduce problematic symptoms. Although an intervention may be well regarded in the world of academia, it will not be used unless practitioners embrace its utility and effectiveness. Rubin and Bellamy (2012) noted that evidence-based practice is "a process for making practice decisions in which practitioners integrate the best research evidence available with their practice expertise and with client attributes, values, preferences and circumstances" (p. 25). As noted previously, the purpose of this chapter is to provide the practicing play therapist with knowledge of historical and current outcome research in play therapy, as well as provide empirical information to help inform practice. The following overview may be useful to practitioners' understanding and communication of play therapy research.

- Play therapy research is over 70 years old, dating back to 1940, and includes over 100 studies supporting its effectiveness. Multiple research studies were conducted in each decade; the years 2000–2010 saw the greatest number of play therapy studies, indicating that play therapy is a current and relevant intervention.

- Play therapy is effective for multiple problems, multiple populations, and in multiple settings. Play therapists can refer to the tables in this chapter to identify research studies that support their areas of practice. Play therapists benefit from being able to cite research summaries such as meta-analyses as well as specific studies that provide evidence for the use of play therapy with their clientele.

- Individual and group modalities of play therapy demonstrate similar positive results. Individual studies employ different modalities based on population and outcomes of interest, but both modalities appear equally effective. The group modality used in play therapy research typically involves two to three children in each group.

- Parent participation in play therapy is associated with stronger positive outcomes. Play therapists who are able to engage parents in the play therapy process are likely to see better results. However, it should be noted that play therapy without parent involvement also demonstrates significant positive effects.

- Play therapy demonstrates positive impact in only a brief number of sessions. In studies conducted since 2000, the mean number of sessions was 16. In many studies, sessions were delivered in an intensive manner of two 30-minute sessions per week, resulting in effective results in 8 weeks or less. A notable number of studies found positive results following 8–10 sessions. These findings indicate that play therapy is competitive as a short-term intervention for children's presenting problems. However, it should be recognized that children with complicated issues and contexts benefit from lengthier therapeutic relationships.

- CCPT is, by far, the most researched approach to play therapy. Meta-analysis revealed that humanistic approaches to play therapy demonstrate strong effects. Individual CCPT studies consistently result in strong outcomes for the approach. Although mental health intervention heavily concentrates on cognitive-behavioral approaches, research strongly supports the person-centered model for working with children.

- Although many research studies may include practitioners who use games or play materials, there are few studies outside of CCPT embracing the power of therapeutic play as a rationale for intervention—a prerequisite for the play therapy designation. Although it seems logical that play therapy might be beneficially integrated with cognitive-behavioral or directive methods, there are few studies to support this supposition. More research needs to be conducted in this area.

- Play therapy research includes a cross-section of educational background, socioeconomic level, race, ethnicity, gender, and nationality. Play therapy incorporates the multicultural nature of mental health practice, thereby increasing its probability of success in real-life clinical settings.

- Play therapy research is most frequently conducted in real-world settings such as schools, counseling clinics, and social service agencies. The demonstration of positive impact on children who typically have complicated contextual environments lends credibility to the viability of play therapy as an everyday intervention.

- The evidence supporting the use of play therapy with multiple and various presenting problems or diagnoses is both a positive and negative outcome of summarizing play therapy research. Due to the complicated nature of working with children, combined with researchers' intentions to examine play therapy in real-life settings, presenting problems are widely arrayed, from separation anxiety to disruptive behaviors to parent–child relationships. The positive outcome of this approach to research is that there is some evidence to support the use of play therapy for many different areas of concern. Yet, critics might contend that play therapy research attempts to do too much for too many. The need for replication of studies with similar populations or outcomes of interest is crucial to elevate the evidence-based status of play therapy. Independent teams of researchers who replicate studies would provide strong empirical support for play therapy with specific childhood problems.

• Because play therapy research has focused on real-world settings, the collaboration between researcher and practitioner is necessary for the continued development of rigorous and evidence-based research. Researchers need the expertise of practitioners to design studies that meet the needs of clinical populations, and practitioners need researchers to conduct designs that are rigorous enough to provide credibility to play therapy intervention. Collaborative relationships between practitioners and researchers strengthen the field of play therapy.

REFERENCES

Allan, J. (1988). *Inscapes of the child's world: Jungian counseling in schools and clinics.* Dallas, TX: Spring.

Association for Play Therapy. (2013, August). Play therapy defined. Retrieved from *www.a4pt.org/ps.playtherapy.cfm?ID=1158.*

Baggerly, J. (2004). The effects of child-centered group play therapy on self-concept, depression, and anxiety of children who are homeless. *International Journal of Play Therapy, 13,* 31–51.

Baggerly, J., & Jenkins, W. (2009). The effectiveness of child-centered play therapy on developmental and diagnostic factors in children who are homeless. *International Journal of Play Therapy, 18,* 45–55.

Bayat, M. (2008). Nondirective play-therapy for children with internalized problems. *Journal of Iranian Psychologists, 4,* 267–276.

Beelmann, A., & Schneider, N. (2003). The effects of psychotherapy with children and adolescents: A review and meta-analysis of German-language research. *Zeitschrift fur Klinische Psychologie und Psychotherapie: Forschung und Praxis, 32,* 129–143.

Blanco, P., & Ray, D. (2011). Play therapy in the schools: A best practice for improving academic achievement. *Journal of Counseling and Development, 89,* 235–242.

Blanco, P., Ray, D., & Holliman, R. (2012). Long-term child centered play therapy and academic achievement of children: A follow-up study. *International Journal of Play Therapy, 21,* 1–13.

Bracken, B., & Lamprecht, S. (2003). Positive self-concept: An equal opportunity construct. *School Psychology Quarterly, 18,* 103–121.

Bratton, S., Ceballos, P., Sheely-Moore, A., Meany-Walen, K., Pronchenko, Y., & Jones, L. (2013). Head Start early mental health intervention: Effects of child-centered play therapy on disruptive behaviors. *International Journal of Play Therapy, 22,* 28–42.

Bratton, S., & Ray, D. (2000). What the research shows about play therapy. *International Journal of Play Therapy, 9,* 47–88.

Bratton, S., Ray, D., Rhine, T., & Jones, L. (2005). The efficacy of play therapy with children: A meta-analytic review of treatment outcome. *Professional Psychology: Research and Practice, 36*(4), 376–390.

Comer, J., Chow, C., Chan, P., Cooper-Vince, C., & Wilson, L. (2013). Psychosocial treatment efficacy for disruptive behavior problems in very young children: A meta-analytic examination. *Journal of the American Academy of Child and Adolescent Psychiatry, 52,* 26–36.

Danger, S., & Landreth, G. (2005). Child-centered group play therapy with children with speech difficulties. *International Journal of Play Therapy, 14,* 81–102.

Dopheide, J. A. (2006). Recognizing and treating depression in children and adolescents. *American Journal of Health-System Pharmacy, 63,* 233–243.

Dougherty, J., & Ray, D. (2007). Differential impact of play therapy on developmental levels of children. *International Journal of Play Therapy, 16,* 2–19.

Elliott, R., Greenberg, L., Watson, J., Timulak, L., & Friere, E. (2013). Research on humanistic–experiential psychotherapies. In M. Lambert (Ed.), *Bergin and Garfield's handbook of psychotherapy and behavior change* (pp. 495–538). Hoboken, NJ: Wiley.

Fabiano, G., & Pelham, W. (2009). Impairment in children. In S. Goldstein & J. Naglieri (Eds.), *Assessing impairment: From theory to practice* (pp. 105–119). New York: Springer.

Fall, M., Navelski, L., & Welch, K. (2002). Outcomes of a play intervention for children identified for special education services. *International Journal of Play Therapy, 11*, 91–106.

Farahzadi, M., Bahramabadi, M., & Mohammadifar, M. (2011). Effectiveness of Gestalt play therapy in decreasing social phobia. *Journal of Iranian Psychologists, 7*, 387–395.

Flahive, M., & Ray, D. (2007). Effect of group sandtray therapy with preadolescents in a school setting. *Journal for Specialists in Group Work, 32*, 362–382.

Garofano-Brown, A. (2010). Child centered play therapy and child development: A single-case analysis. In J. Baggerly, D. Ray, & S. Bratton (Eds.), *Child-centered play therapy research: The evidence base for effective practice* (pp. 231–248). Hoboken, NJ: Wiley.

Garza, Y., & Bratton, S. (2005). School-based child centered play therapy with Hispanic children: Outcomes and cultural considerations. *International Journal of Play Therapy, 14*, 51–80.

Green, E. (2011). Jungian analytical play therapy. In C. Schaefer (Ed.), *Foundations of play therapy* (2nd ed., pp. 61–84). Hoboken, NJ: Wiley.

Guindon, M. (2002). Toward accountability in the use of the self-esteem construct. *Journal of Counseling and Development, 80*, 204–214.

Harvey, S. (2008). An initial look at the outcomes for dynamic play therapy. *International Journal of Play Therapy, 17*, 86–101.

Jalali, S., & Molavi, H. (2011). The effect of play therapy on separation anxiety disorder in children. *Journal of Psychology, 14*, 370–382.

Jones, E., & Landreth, G. (2002). The efficacy of intensive individual play therapy for chronically ill children. *International Journal of Play Therapy, 11*, 117–140.

Knell, S. (1993). *Cognitive-behavioral play therapy.* Northvale, NJ: Aronson.

Knell, S. M., & Dasari, M. (2011). Cognitive-behavioral play therapy. In S. W. Russ & L. N.

Niec (Eds.), *Play in clinical practice: Evidence-based approaches* (pp. 236–263). New York: Guilford Press.

Kottman, T. (2003). *Partners in play: An Adlerian approach to play therapy* (2nd ed.). Alexandria, VA: American Counseling Association.

Kottman, T. (2011). Adlerian play therapy. In C. Schaefer (Ed.), *Foundations of play therapy* (2nd ed., pp. 87–104). Hoboken, NJ: Wiley.

LeBlanc, M., & Ritchie, M. (2001). A meta-analysis of play therapy outcomes. *Counseling Psychology Quarterly, 14*, 149–163.

Mahmoudi-Gharaei, J., Bina, M., Yasami, M., Emami, A., & Naderi, F. (2006). Group play therapy effect on Bam earthquake related emotional and behavioral symptoms in preschool children: A before–after trial. *Iranian Journal of Pediatrics, 16*, 137–142.

Moustakas, C. (1997). *Relationship play therapy.* Lanham, MD: Aronson.

Munns, E. (2011). Theraplay: Attachment-enhancing play therapy. In C. Schaefer (Ed.), *Foundations of play therapy* (2nd ed., pp. 275–296). Hoboken, NJ: Wiley.

Muro, J., Ray, D., Schottelkorb, A., Smith, M., & Blanco, P. (2006). Quantitative analysis of long-term child-centered play therapy. *International Journal of Play Therapy, 15*, 35–58.

Naderi, F., Heidarie, L., Bouron, L., & Asgari, P. (2010). The efficacy of play therapy on ADHD, anxiety and social maturity in 8 to 12 years aged clientele children of Ahwaz Metropolitan Counseling Clinics. *Journal of Applied Sciences, 10*, 189–195.

Oaklander, V. (1988). *Windows to our children.* Highland, NY: Gestalt Journal Press.

Packman, J., & Bratton, S. (2003). A school based play/activity therapy intervention with learning disabled preadolescents exhibiting behavior problems. *International Journal of Play Therapy, 12*(2), 7–29.

Ray, D. C. (2006). Evidence-based play therapy. In C. E. Schaefer & H. G. Kaduson (Eds.), *Contemporary play therapy: Theory, research, and practice* (pp. 136–157). New York: Guilford Press.

Ray, D. (2007). Two counseling interventions to reduce teacher–child relationship stress. *Professional School Counseling, 10*, 428–440.

Ray, D. (2008). Impact of play therapy on parent–child relationship stress at a mental health training setting. *British Journal of Guidance and Counselling, 36*, 165–187.

Ray, D. (2009). *Child centered play therapy treatment manual*. Royal Oak, MI: Self Esteem Shop.

Ray, D. (2011). *Advanced play therapy: Essential conditions, knowledge, and skills for child practice*. New York: Routledge.

Ray, D., Blanco, P., Sullivan, J., & Holliman, R. (2009). An exploratory study of child-centered play therapy with aggressive children. *International Journal of Play Therapy, 18*, 162–175.

Ray, D., Bratton, S., Rhine, T., & Jones, L. (2001). The effectiveness of play therapy: Responding to the critics. *International Journal of Play Therapy, 10*, 85–108.

Ray, D., Henson, R., Schottelkorb, A., Brown, A., & Muro, J. (2008). Impact of short-term and long-term play therapy services on teacher–child relationship stress. *Psychology in the Schools, 45*, 994–1009.

Ray, D., Schottelkorb, A., & Tsai, M. (2007). Play therapy with children exhibiting symptoms of attention deficit hyperactivity disorder. *International Journal of Play Therapy, 16*, 95–111.

Ray, D., Stulmaker, H., Lee, K., & Silverman, W. (2013). Child centered play therapy and impairment: Exploring relationships and constructs. *International Journal of Play Therapy, 22*, 13–27.

Rubin, A., & Bellamy, J. (2012). *Practitioner's guide to using research for evidence-based practice* (2nd ed.). Hoboken, NJ: Wiley.

Schottelkorb, A., Doumas, D., & Garcia, R. (2012). Treatment for childhood refugee trauma: A randomized, controlled trial. *International Journal of Play Therapy, 21*, 57–73.

Schottelkorb, A., & Ray, D. (2009). ADHD symptom reduction in elementary students: A single-case effectiveness design. *Professional School Counseling, 13*, 11–22.

Schumann, B. (2010). Effectiveness of child centered play therapy for children referred for aggression in elementary school. In J. Baggerly, D. Ray, & S. Bratton (Eds.), *Child-centered play therapy research: The evidence base for effective practice* (pp. 193–208). Hoboken, NJ: Wiley.

Scott, T., Burlingame, G., Starling, M., Porter, C., & Lilly, J. (2003). Effects of individual client-centered play therapy on sexually abused children's mood, self-concept, and social competence. *International Journal of Play Therapy, 12*, 7–30.

Shen, Y. (2002). Short-term group play therapy with Chinese earthquake victims: Effects on anxiety, depression, and adjustment. *International Journal of Play Therapy, 11*, 43–63.

Studts, C., & van Zyl, M. (2013). Identification of developmentally appropriate screening items for disruptive behavior problems in preschoolers. *Journal of Abnormal Child Psychology, 41*, 851–863.

Swan, K., & Ray, D. (2014). Effects of child-centered play therapy on irritability and hyperactivity behaviors of children with intellectual disabilities. *Journal of Humanistic Counseling, 53*, 120–133.

Tsai, M., & Ray, D. (2011). Play therapy outcome prediction: An exploratory study at a university-based clinic. *International Journal of Play Therapy, 20*(2), 94–108.

Tyndall-Lind, A., Landreth, G., & Giordano, M. (2001). Intensive group play therapy with child witnesses of domestic violence. *International Journal of Play Therapy, 10*, 53–83.

VanFleet, R. (2011). Filial therapy: Strengthening family relationships with the power of play. In C. Schaefer (Ed.), *Foundations of play therapy* (2nd ed., pp. 153–169). Hoboken, NJ: Wiley.

Weisz, J., Jensen-Doss, A., & Hawley, K. (2005). Youth psychotherapy outcome research: A review and critique of the evidence base. *Annual Review of Psychology, 56*, 337–363.

Weisz, J., Ugueto, A., Cheron, D., & Herren, J. (2013). Evidence-based youth psychotherapy in the mental health ecosystem. *Journal of Clinical Child and Adolescent Psychology, 42*, 274–286.

Weisz, J., Weiss, B., Han, S., Granger, D., & Morton, T. (1995). Effects of psychotherapy with children and adolescents revisited: A meta-analysis of treatment outcome studies. *Psychological Bulletin, 117*, 450–468.

CHAPTER 33

Reflective Practice in Play Therapy and Supervision

John W. Seymour
David A. Crenshaw

Be Reflective for a Moment

Pause for a moment and consider how reflective you are when doing play therapy or clinical supervision. Now, were you really able to pause? To be reflective? To reflect on your play therapy? To reflect on your clinical supervision? Were you able to respond to each part, make some connection of meaning, have some sort of thought or feeling in response to that meaning? Are you now sensing yourself becoming more engaged or less engaged in the meanings as you reflect? Are you finding your awareness shifting to every topic other than reflective practice? Next client? Broken copy machine? Achy muscles from a weekend of home repair work? Am I getting old? Next vacation? I'm bored! That sad client earlier today? What's for dinner? Why isn't someone answering the office phone?

Reflection is like that. It just happens. We live our lives as a constant combination of inner and outer dialogues. Sometimes reflection enriches us, sometimes it distracts us. As therapists, we may be quick to say that we are more often enriched by our reflections, and of course, enriching to

those around us. As therapists, let's hope that we would also be quick to say that we get more distracted than we care to admit by our reflections, affecting ourselves and those around us. Jeffrey Kottler (2010), in his book *On Being a Therapist*, gave readers an inside view of some of these distractions, and he has reported reader reactions ranging from understanding to indignation.

Active reflection is seen by many as a fundamental element of psychotherapy and clinical supervision, accepted as a given—sometimes without much reflection. Fortunately, in the last 30 years, there have been a number of positive contributions to our understanding of the role of active reflection in psychotherapy and clinical supervision. This chapter provides an overview of these research findings, including those addressing psychotherapy integration, common factors and therapeutic mechanisms, the therapeutic relationship, interpersonal neurobiology, and therapist development. Internal disciplines for the reflective play therapist are then described and illustrated for application in play therapy and clinical supervision.

Understanding Reflective Practice

Donald Schön (1983, 1987) studied psycho-therapists in training extensively to identify key skills needed to become a therapist and the experiences needed to develop those skills. He identified two characteristics of a reflective practitioner: He or she engages in "reflection-in-action" and "reflection-on-action," with each characteristic complementing the other. Schön defined *reflection-in-action* as the ability to think on one's feet and experiment as one works. It includes the abilities of looking at one's own experiences, connecting with one's own feelings, attending to the theories one uses, and handling the experience of surprise when faced with the unique or uncertain. *Reflection-on-action* occurs following the therapeutic session, as one is completing documentation, attending supervision, engaging in self-reflection, and engaging in self-supervision to identify patterns that would inform future therapeutic work.

Based on extensive research of developing therapists, Rønnestad and Skovholt (2013) suggest a model of *continuous reflection*, incorporating Schön's two characteristics into a seamless, interactive process. Rønnestad and Skovholt (2013) identified the primary catalyst for therapists' growth as having difficult or challenging experiences in their work, and if they are not having these experiences, then to seek them. However, these challenges would only lead to therapist growth if they were met with a response of continuous reflection, paired with the ability to develop personal strengths and the patience to bring the challenges to functional closure. Therapists faced with inadequate closure face the option of either developing the ability to continue in reflection until closure is gained, thereby promoting growth, or interrupting reflection, resulting in inadequate closure and exhaustion. Therapists with very limited ability for continuous reflection end up with premature closure and disengage-ment. Exhaustion and disengagement lead to stagnation in therapist growth and an eventual exit from the field. Maintaining a reflective practice is essential to both client and therapist well-being.

Psychotherapy Integration and Common Factors

The developmental history of play therapy has closely paralleled the history of psy-chotherapy research and practice (Drewes, 2011a, 2011b; Seymour, 2011). Much as in the broader field of psychotherapy, many of the early debates in play therapy focused on comparing the benefits of one particular model over another. As therapeutic models proliferated, there were early efforts at the-oretical integration and practical eclecti-cism. Early prescriptive models evolved into more fully integrative play therapy models (Drewes, Bratton, & Schaefer, 2011), just as they have in psychotherapy (Norcross & Goldfried, 2005; Prochaska & Norcross, 2014).

These integrative models represent a shift in understanding of the role of the therapist, from one who delivers a model-prescribed treatment to one who provides a relationship to facilitate client-based treat-ments. Continuous reflection provides the mechanism for this improvisation to ben-efit the client.

Recent research exploring the common factors of psychotherapy (Duncan, Miller, Wampold, & Hubble, 2010) and child psy-chotherapy (Kazdin, 2009; Shirk & Russell, 1996) has identified therapeutic mecha-nisms common to all therapy models and the effects of these mechanisms on thera-peutic outcomes. In the field of play therapy, Schaefer's (1993) earlier therapeutic mecha-nism research was recently updated, delin-eating 20 *therapeutic powers of play* (Schaefer & Drewes, 2014). Play therapists need con-tinuous reflection to maintain their aware-ness of client need and to cultivate options for implementing the therapeutic mechanisms imbedded in the functions of play.

The Therapeutic Relationship, Interpersonal Neurobiology, and Play

The therapeutic relationship is central in virtually all traditions of healing, whether Western or Eastern models of psychotherapy, or ancient or contemporary folk medicine (Frank & Frank, 1993). Recent research on common factors by Duncan and colleagues (2010) suggests that a strong therapeutic alliance and partnership are crucial for increasing the mechanisms of client participation and resource activation, identified in the research as the most significant factors in successful outcome. Siegel (2012) suggests that all therapeutic models should be experientially and relationally based, aimed toward promoting integration of body and brain through relationships. This integration first begins as children form attachments with caretakers through playful interactions, which over time develop into the play-based relational skills most evident in children.

Schore (2012) suggests that the work of psychotherapy "is not defined by what the therapist does for the patient, or says to the patient (left brain focus). Rather, the key mechanism is how to be with the patient, especially during affectively stressful moments (right brain focus)" (p. 44). Internal human development is mirrored in the interactions of children through their experiences and relationships, which are commonly mediated through relationships cultivated in natural play. Play is a natural interactional medium for healthy human development, providing the foundation for relationships and skills used throughout life (Brown, 2009; Russ, 2004). Play has a long history as a component of child psychotherapy (Drewes, 2006), as a developmentally informed way of cultivating an effective therapeutic relationship.

Therapist Development/Self of Therapist

Rønnestad and Skovholt (2013) summarized a number of findings from their extensive research on therapist development. Professional development for therapists is truly a lifetime process. Regardless of years of experience, cultivating continuous reflection is critical for maintaining good self-care of the therapist and positive therapeutic outcomes for the client. Optimal professional development involves an integration of one's personal self into a coherent professional self. The most impactful learning tends to occur in experiential, interpersonal learning (from clients, mentors, colleagues, and one's own life experiences) rather than in the impersonal learning of concepts.

Self-of-therapist work, incorporated with studies on integrative psychotherapy, can provide an important way to cultivate continuous reflection. Beitman and Soth (2006) have described the importance of self-observation as a core psychotherapy process, which includes an active scan of one's inner landscape, the ability for introspection, and a clear awareness of one's social and cultural environment. Supervision and training endeavors need to include methods for incorporating self-observation in all dimensions of providing psychotherapy. Aponte's (1982, 1994; Aponte & Carlsen, 2009; Aponte & Kissil, 2012) person-of-the-therapist (POTT) model, Anderson's (1997) as-if consultation, and Rober's (1999, 2005a, 2005b) inner conversation model can all be effectively used in self, individual, or group clinical supervision.

Internal Disciplines of the Reflective Play Therapist

Practice as a reflective play therapist requires internal discipline. It is hard work and demands a high priority of the busy practitioner, who often feels swamped with the rigors of providing high-quality work to child and family clients. In addition are the time-consuming and mostly ungratifying chores of filling out insurance forms or calling to get approval from health maintenance organizations (HMOs) for patient visits, along with phone calls to return and progress notes to do. Given these competing claims on the practitioner's time, it is easy to appreciate that the necessary internal disciplines of the reflective play therapist might get pushed aside or assigned a lower priority. These internal disciplines are indeed easy to forget, but, in our judgment, important to remember; they are easy to neglect but essential to practice. Although the following list of internal disciplines is not comprehensive and can be added to, we were reluctant to make the list longer because we are sensitive to the increasingly complex demands on the play therapist. The list is restricted to what we view as essential internal disciplines for the reflective play therapist:

- Discipline of empathy
- Discipline of wholeheartedness
- Discipline of vulnerability
- Discipline of genuineness
- Discipline of courage
- Discipline of self-care
- Discipline of humility
- Discipline of compassion

It is interesting to consider that the same dynamic forces that prevent our psychotherapy clients from fully communicating with us as therapists can block the self-reflection process called for with each of the internal disciplines. Two of the most potent of these forces operating in this dual process arena are denial and shame. Often like our clients, we masterfully push out of unawareness unpleasant realities, including our flaws and shortcomings. It is particularly distressing to acknowledge that limitations in the therapist may interfere with the committed efforts to help a troubled child.

Likewise our child clients are known for "reality blindness" when confronted with their part in an interpersonal encounter that has gone wrong. The high self-expectations of play therapists can lead to shame, which often then leads to silence and secrecy, just as it does when a child is unable to share a burdensome secret. A play therapist who no longer can approach this work wholeheartedly may be reluctant to share this fact with a supervisor or a colleague or perhaps even a therapist because he or she entered the field with such passion and commitment to helping children. In a parallel way to the helping process with child clients, the silence, secrecy, and shame curtail opportunities for confronting the barriers to wholeheartedness and for finding possible solutions or changes that would improve one's relation to the chosen work.

We want to make clear that we have no empirical data to back up our choices of these essential internal disciplines, nor do we doubt that the list can be improved on. Please read this section with that caveat in mind. What we offer is merely our experience of decades of work with children and families as well as supervision of play therapists. We value empirical research, and it greatly informs our work. We are grateful to those play therapists who work in research settings and contribute to the science behind our field. I (Crenshaw) never had the privilege of working in a research setting. I am a clinician at heart, and like other nonacademic play therapists I greatly admire and learn from, I still carry a full load of clinical cases that offers opportunities for rich learning and refinement of my clinical practice.

Discipline of Empathy

The research of Carl Rogers (1957) validated the essential role of empathy in psychotherapy outcome research. Empathy is one of the cornerstones of psychotherapy and encompasses a wide range of approaches in play therapy. The reflective practitioner will want to question whether empathy for child clients is a constant, a given, or does it vary based on a host of play therapist and child client factors or influences, positive and negative: the child's family and other circumstances that constitute the total context of the therapeutic work, such as cooperation with schools, social services, child protective services, courts, payment for therapy, and/or pressures from parents or other referring services. Since it is perilous for therapists, no matter how experienced or skilled, to claim immunity from heartbreaking failure, it likewise seems foolhardy to us that even the most admired play therapist would be exempt from empathy failures related to one of these many factors. If we were to simplify and focus on the ups and downs of a play therapist's life—which, at one time may include joyful events within one's family, at another time a serious illness in a family member, at another point of time recognition of one's accomplishments by play therapy colleagues, and at still another time sharp criticism of one's work by a highly respected play therapy colleague—it is hard to imagine that one's capacity for empathy might not be impacted in both positive and negative ways. What characterizes the reflective play therapist practitioner is the willingness to examine and learn from the fluctuations (Bager-Charleson, 2010). The internal discipline of empathy requires us to directly reflect on these variations in our capacities even as we extend empathy to ourselves. It is harmful to hold ourselves to expectations that we can only strive for but never meet. The same level of reflection is needed in relation to the many other variables of self, client, family, and community sources that can impact our empathic capacities in a particular case in either direction or possibly in mixed directions.

One cogent area of focus when considering the discipline of empathy is the variation in our capacity for empathy based on child client characteristics and/or presenting problem. A play therapist may easily experience empathy for a child who has been sexually abused, but the same play therapist may struggle to show empathy to a child who has sexually offended another child, even if that same child had previously been a victim of sexual abuse. Such disparity will be less problematic if the play therapist honestly examines this difficulty rather than allows it to become a blind spot by denying its existence. As a blind spot, the discordance in empathy doesn't disappear; it simply continues to operate outside of awareness and potentially creates havoc in work with clients who are sexually aggressive toward other children. A deeper exploration in one's own therapy, in supervision, or in discussions with colleagues would be needed to identify the underlying feelings creating the disparity and the blind spot. The extent and intensity of the affects underlying the discordance in empathy and its roots would determine whether this should be explored in personal therapy, supervision, or simply discussed with trusted colleagues. (Although the consideration of personal therapy, supervision, or consultation applies in the case of failure in any of the internal disciplines, we do not repeat this point.)

Discipline of Wholeheartedness

I (Crenshaw) was one of approximately 3,500 people sitting spellbound in a huge ballroom at the Omni Shoreham Hotel, Washington, DC, in the spring of 2009, listening to David Whyte, a British American poet, delivering a keynote address to the Psychotherapy Networker Symposium. Never have I seen a speaker hold an audience in such breathless focus as did this eloquent poet. One of his take-home points for me was his story about the burnout he experienced when he worked for a small nonprofit organization earlier in his career. In his eagerness to do the worthy work that nonprofit organizations almost always entail, he felt that he had lost his self. In the world of the nonprofit, he explained, there is almost always a compelling mission, with good-hearted people committed to doing all they can, but there are never enough people, resources, or money to do all this good work—and the end result is exhaustion. His message resonated with me, who at that point had been affiliated with worthy nonprofits for 38 years, as was the case for so many others in the audience. What was striking, however, was Whyte's answer to exhaustion. He met with a trusted, wise, long-time friend who told him that the antidote to exhaustion was not rest; rather, the answer was *wholeheartedness*. We don't burn out when we approach our work wholeheartedly.

Reflective play therapists will want to examine and consult with trusted others—a therapist, supervisor, or colleagues—about what has gone wrong that has caused them to lose their zest, if not self, in the worthy work of helping children and families. One doesn't have to work for a nonprofit to "hit the wall" in terms of loss of passion for one's vocation. It can easily happen in a private practice setting where the play therapist has to work increasing hours and see greater volumes of clients just to keep from losing income due to the unrelenting slide in reimbursement rates from managed care companies. Burnout can happen in for-profit agencies or academic or governmental organizations where the political undercurrents, policies, or regulations stifle the creativity of the play therapist or place inordinate demands of the kind that most play therapists find distasteful (e.g., committee work, time-consuming paperwork).

Self-reflection and honest sharing of the dilemma may lead to creative changes or new possibilities, circumventing the need to seek a new position. In some cases you may conclude in the self-examination that you have outgrown the challenges and opportunities available to you at present and you may need to begin the planning process to do something difficult for your own growth and well-being. It is as difficult for us, as well as our clients, to cross into new territory in our careers. Perhaps that level of change will be necessary for you to regain your love for the work, but it should not be done rashly or without careful reflection and consultation with trusted others. Sometimes our dissatisfaction in our vocation reflects other dissatisfactions in our life or losses that we have not fully grieved. Again, in parallel process to our clients, we may be tempted to move on rather than doing the hard internal work that is necessary for growth.

Discipline of Vulnerability

There is a steep price to be paid for trying to be a "super-therapist." Not only does the super-therapist function under impossibly high self-expectations, but his or her self-perceived invulnerability will be a barrier to forming healing relationships with child and family clients. Carl Rogers (1980) preceded many of our contemporary colleagues (Garry Landreth, J. P. Lilly, Eliana Gil, and Kenneth Hardy, to name a few) who talk about a therapeutic "way of being." *Doing*—which tends to be the fixation of young play therapists or play therapists early in the field—is the easy part. *Being* is much harder, and we are convinced that there is a prerequisite ripening of the play therapist before this makes any sense. Early in my career I (Crenshaw) also was preoccupied with learning every possible technique for every potential problem that might arise in a session so I would know what to *do*. I don't wish to devalue techniques; most of my earlier books were focused on techniques. There are situations where knowing "what to do" can improve results and avoid pitfalls.

A specific example in a case involving selective mutism taught me valuable lessons about technique (Crenshaw, 2007). I believe, however, that the main benefit of learning a wide array of techniques is that it helps us as therapists relax into the illusion that we know what to do. As a result, we can be present with children in a more unguarded, open way that is more healing. We are able to be more vulnerable and risk ourselves in the same way that we expect children in therapy to be vulnerable, unguarded, and share the feelings, thoughts, and events about which they are usually most reluctant to talk. This discipline of discovering and owning the multiple forms and shapes of our vulnerability is perhaps the most critical in terms of our being fully present in our therapeutic work. Daniel Stern (2004) has coined the term "moments of meeting" to capture the transformative power of the fully present therapist sensitively attuned in the present moment to the client, whether adult or child.

Discipline of Genuineness

Genuineness was one of the three factors that Rogers (1980) found in his research that increased the efficacy of the therapeutic relationship. Kazdin (2005) reviewed over 2,000 studies supporting the central importance of the therapeutic relationship in psychotherapy outcome research. In summarizing this research, Kazdin noted that the stronger the therapeutic relationship, the better the outcome. As an internal discipline of reflective practice, the genuineness extends not only to the client but also to oneself in the self-examination required for each of the named disciplines. Self-deception is not the sole province of our clients. Here is an example from my (Crenshaw) own struggles to be a reflective practitioner.

In consultation with a colleague, I decided it would be beneficial to me to write out my values, the beliefs that I stand for, what is important to me, and how I would like to live my life. I was excited about this undertaking because I viewed it as a wonderful way to stay focused on my priorities for my work life as well as my life outside of work. I vowed to put a short version of my values statement on my desktop and to review it at the beginning of each day so that the values that are the most important to

me would always be fresh in my mind. Yet I only practiced the discipline of reminding myself of those values for a relatively brief period. One day I noticed the short version of my values statement was no longer visible on my desktop. I looked into it and found out that if you don't click on the icon for 30 days, it is automatically removed from the desktop. It jolted me into thinking more deeply about how disingenuous I was with myself. A question that occurred to me was, if I am not genuine with *myself*, can I be trusted to be genuine with my clients?

Discipline of Courage

It takes considerable courage to do clinical work. As much as we might want to think that with dedication to our profession and a rigorous commitment to lifelong learning, we will eventually reach a time and place of total competence, this too is an illusion. After 45 years of postdoctoral experience, I (Crenshaw) still don't know if I will be equal to the challenge when the phone rings alerting me to a crisis. I have more faith in my skills and more importantly my way of being with children than I did during earlier points in my career, but when the new client comes through the door, who knows what new challenges may follow? I know of no textbook or graduate school text that prepares a play therapist to tell young children that their mother is dead, but I have had to do this with nine preschool children impacted by four separate tragedies in the past 2 years. I know of no empirical research I can draw on to inform me as to how to go into the play therapy room and tell these young children that their mother was murdered or died of a drug overdose. Any play therapist who works in the field long enough will encounter his or her share of these heartbreaking tragedies. In such situations when there are no guidebooks, no experts to call, we are forced to rely on self as the therapeutic instrument, on therapeutic presence, empathy, genuineness, and a large measure of courage.

Discipline of Self-Care

In 2008, I (Crenshaw) went to the Ackerman Institute for the Family in New York City to hear my friend and much-admired colleague, Kenneth Hardy, present on "Working with Low-Income Families." Although we have done some joint writing projects, our busy schedules seldom allow for opportunities to meet face-to-face. I met Ken on the stairs as I was walking into Ackerman, and we both looked tired and stressed. Ken commented, "The first thing that goes in our field when we are under stress is self-care." The wisdom of that comment has been shown repeatedly. I've noticed, for example, that even though I say that self-care is crucial, I've never made my own health a priority. I've been astonished that although I usually include self-care as am important item in presentations that I am invited to do, I frequently put it at the end and thus sometimes never get to it or rush through that section when time is running out. Self-care was highlighted in my values statement, but then I lost track of my values statement.

The reason I think self-care is an internal discipline to cultivate in the reflective play therapist is that without such a commitment, it likely will be ignored or neglected. Most play therapists recognize the value of good self-care. Our primary instrument in the work is our self, and it makes sense that we would value and take good care of that instrument. If I were fortunate enough to own a Stradivarius, I would probably polish it every day. If we don't exercise good self-care, it is likely that dynamic inner forces account for it. Reflective practice is a way of bringing into clear view those hidden, subtle influences that keep us from reaching more of our potential. Perhaps we don't give self-care a high priority because we don't value our self, our health, enough to give it compelling importance.

The late psychoanalyst Walter Bonime, MD, with whom I was privileged to study for 14 years, offered a related explanation. Bonime explained that individuals who enter our field tend to be giving, good-hearted people who are likely to put themselves in a secondary position. As a result they (we!) tend to make a practice of self-denial and placing the needs of others first. This is a recipe that doesn't work over a long period of time. Eventually, loss of self is the steep price to be paid.

Discipline of Humility

Clearly there is an overlap with disciplines of vulnerability and humility. The specific attitude of humility, however, is important in therapeutic work. I've (Crenshaw) learned that when I meet with parents and they share their concerns about their child, if I start to think "I've heard this story 500 times before," then I am in trouble. An attitude of humility will keep us listening carefully for the nuances and variations that make every child and family story unique. Such "deep listening" (Rogers, 1980) enables us to hear clues as to how to help this particular child.

Children again and again teach me valuable lessons in humility. The children I treat are, by far, my best teachers. We cannot continue to learn and grow absent an attitude of humility. An acclaimed family therapist, Olga Silverstein, taught me one of my cherished lessons in humility. In 1987, I attended a 2-day workshop on the "Art of Systems Family Therapy," with Olga as the sole presenter. She put on an amazing demonstration of clinical skill, keen insight, and understanding of families. At the end of the 2 days, people from all over the large ballroom at the Roosevelt Hotel stood up and praised her for such uncommon talents. What happened then was unforgettable to me. Olga became indignant. She explained that she had worked hard to refine her skills and that she recognized that she had a highly developed verbal facility, but then she pointed out that "I still have my share of heartbreaking failures." She further explained that she didn't want to be put on a pedestal. Olga adamantly stated, "Who needs it?"

This experience was a career changer for me, and I've shared this story with every intern and staff member I've supervised since. Up to that point, I was under the illusion that if I read enough books by the top people in the field, and went to enough workshops and presentations by the leaders in the family therapy and play therapy field, I would eventually reach a point where I would be immune to heartbreaking failures. Olga helped me to realize that we don't have that luxury in this field. We have to risk ourselves over and over, and sometimes things go wrong in spite of our best efforts, our training, our reading, our graduate school education, and our continuing supervision. Before Olga died in 2009, I had the opportunity to tell her what that experience meant to me, and how I will always be indebted to her for teaching me the value of the internal discipline of humility.

Discipline of Compassion

Here again is an overlap with the internal disciplines of empathy and compassion. There is a difference between the two, however, because empathy is expressed toward a particular person in a specific therapy process and relationship. Compassion is more general as an internal discipline. The term "compassion fatigue" was introduced in the literature by Charles Figley (1995) to describe the familiar feeling of "our tank being empty" and in need of refilling. The emotional work of play therapy with troubled or traumatized children can produce not only physical and emotional fatigue but, in some cases, secondary traumatization. The cultivation and practice of each of the preceding internal disciplines of reflective practice will help to keep the tank from sinking to empty. Self-care is certainly a key discipline to keep the play therapist energized, rested, and healthy, and wholeheartedness is pivotal as well. Part of the discipline of compassion is monitoring our caseloads, paying close attention to how many trauma cases we carry at any one time.

I (Crenshaw) remember clearly a Saturday morning many years ago when I arrived early at my office to meet a young man for the first time who had been driving a car when an accident occurred, killing his best friend. I remember vividly thinking, "I don't want to hear another horror story." I knew that I had to do something with regard to self-care, so I called a good friend and hiking partner and made a plan the next day to go hiking in the Catskill Mountains. Knowing that the plan was set, I was able to energize myself to meet the challenge of hearing the tragic story of this adolescent boy. I also decided not to take any more trauma cases in the near future. Clearly, it was my responsibility to do something so that my supply of compassion was not exhausted. It is not the responsibility of our patients to look after us, but that being said, widely acclaimed psychiatrist Robert Coles once said at a conference, "If your patient says to you, 'Doc, you look a little tired,'" Coles said, "Pay attention!"

Exercises in Reflection for Practice and Supervision

As is often the case, in our past presentations on "Reflective Practice in Play Therapy and Supervision" at the annual International Play Therapy Conference, we received feedback that the best part was the experiential exercises that demonstrated reflective practice in action. We share some of those exercises with our readers here for your own reflection and discussion in supervision.

Encounter with Younger Self

Pretend that you open the door to your waiting room and there you see a vaguely familiar-looking person whom you can't identify. As you get closer, you are jolted by the recognition that the person waiting to see you is a younger version of yourself—you, when you first entered the profession. Still in shock, you do your best to regain your composure and invite the younger person into your office. When this visitor, who is your younger self, is seated, you wait. Your younger self says, "I know you've been in the field now for _____ years, and undoubtedly you have gained considerable wisdom and insight from your experience. I am here as someone just starting out in the field and I am hoping you will share with me what you now know that you didn't know at the beginning. I know you can't tell me everything, but it would be so valuable if you could tell me the most important lessons, insights, and the most crucial understandings for someone just beginning the journey."

Depending on the context of self-reflection or individual or group supervision, you can either write out what you would tell your younger self or express it verbally in supervision. The key choice is to determine which format would be most beneficial to you. In a group or peer supervision the opportunities to be enriched by the insights and wisdom of others, in addition to your own sincere and honest self-reflections, make that alternative especially appealing. Of course, sufficient trust in the group would need to be established to enable the kind of open sharing needed to make the most of this evocative, reflective exercise.

Values Statement

I (Crenshaw) shared my own struggles with keeping my values statement fresh in my mind. Nevertheless, I find the exercise incredibly valuable and helpful for refocusing and reestablishing priorities. Write your own values statement as a play therapist and/or play therapy supervisor. State what is important to you. How do you want to conduct your practice of play therapy and/or supervision? What do you stand for? What do you believe with conviction? What ethical principles are particularly important to you? Write out your values statement and when finished, reflect on it to see if there is anything missing. You may wish to share

this "manifesto" in individual or group supervision. Supervisors may want to share it with other supervisors in peer supervision. When you are finished, reflect on what is there or not there that surprises you. Is self-care one of your values? Rank your values according to their priority. What rank does self-care receive? If sharing the values in a group setting, a peer may state a value that seems important to you but is not on your list. Reflect on why it is missing. How did that particular value get overlooked? This exercise has great dynamic potential for continual self-monitoring and reflection. Obviously, the values and priorities are likely to change, and the values statement will need to be reworked and refreshed. But it may be satisfying that the values and priorities change as a result of conscious reflection and self-examination rather than merely shifting out of awareness, as they often do. A plan to review the values statement at regular intervals can serve to guard against the unaware shifting of values and priorities that we all know from personal experience.

Adrift at Sea

Take a few minutes in the time you've set aside for self-reflection or in your supervisory sessions to draw a boat crossing the wide seas. Wherever you position the boat on the sea, draw a line that extends the trajectory of the boat to the far horizon. Now pretend that the course you've charted includes the hopes, dreams, expectations, and perhaps even illusions that you started with when you began your journey as a play therapist and/or supervisor. Now draw an X on the picture to mark where the boat is located at the present time. How far adrift, how off course are you? What are some of the forces, influences, and experiences that have caused you to go off-course, perhaps to become disillusioned or in some cases demoralized or even bitter? Often issues such as managed care, low reimbursement rates, government regulation, paperwork, and exhaustion come up. These dispiriting influences are familiar to most seasoned practitioners and supervisors.

It is also important to identify any strategies to help you get back on course or perhaps to charter a new course altogether. Reflect on and/or share in supervision whatever enlivens and reenergizes you. What helps you to revisit the original love and enthusiasm for play therapy that you experienced at the beginning of the journey? Could it be self-care? Could it be writing or presenting? Teaching? Changes in self-expectations? Changing the way you schedule yourself? Whatever reconnects you to the original passion is something to identify and to do more. Reflect on this and share with others as you see fit.

Your Unique Form of Genius

This particular reflective exercise was inspired by David Whyte (2009), the British-born, American poet, who discussed the unique genius that each of us brings to the conversation or encounter with another human being that can't be replicated by anyone else present, past, or future. Our particular form of genius is informed not only by our biology and genetic endowment, but by our parents, our extended family, the social environment and experiences that we've encountered along our life journey, and even the particular shape of the difficulties we've faced along the way. Our form of genius is one of a kind, and no one can do exactly what we do in exactly the same way. This is an important focus of serious self-reflection and discussion in supervision. There are a number of ways to approach this reflective exercise. One way is to write for 10 minutes without stopping about your particular form of genius. Another way is to simply try to name it. In workshops we sometimes ask play therapists and/or supervisors to pick a symbol that best captures their particular genius as a therapist or supervisor. After you have captured your unique genius in words or symbol, it is useful to reflect on how that genius serves you in play therapy, in supervision, with colleagues, and with the families

of your child clients. You may find it useful to reflect on whom you are indebted for this particular form of genius. Who in your life has been most influential in the shaping of your special shape and form of genius? We have sometimes found some skepticism among our colleagues attending our workshops as to the term *genius*. It is hard for some to view themselves in that light. That, too, is an important point on which to reflect in any dedicated self-examination or supervision, whether individual, group, or peer.

Charismatic Adults

Robert Brooks (2010) credits the late psychologist Julius Segal (1988) with introducing the concept of a "charismatic adult"—a person with whom resilient children can identify and from whom they gather strength (Segal, 1988, p. 3). This reflective exercise has been one of the more moving exercises that we use in our workshops. It can be approached from different angles. You can reflect on your childhood and identify someone in your developmental years with whom you identified and who gave you strength. Once the charismatic adult is identified, you are encouraged to write a note to that person (even if no longer living) expressing your feelings about the role or influence the person exercised in your life. It is important to recall whether you ever told that person what he or she meant to you. If the person is still alive, is this something that you wish to do? If this is important to you, make a plan to do it and make certain it happens. If you don't wish to share this with a person still available to you, this choice too can be a focus of reflection. If you do decide to tell the person, reflect on what took you so long.

This same reflective exercise can focus on possible charismatic adults encountered in your professional life. Who stands out in terms of their professional influence and impact on you? Who has inspired you to an unusual degree? It could be a standout teacher or an amazing supervisor or colleague from whom you learned so much. It can be quite interesting to reflect and discuss in supervision who your best, most inspiring teachers have been. Deeper reflection may lead you to wonder what it was about the particular individuals that so deeply influenced you. What does your choice say about them? What does it say about you? The same choices as to whether to share your feelings with your mentors can be reflected on and the reasons why or why not.

Finally, it is also important to reflect on this turnaround: For whom, among your child and family clients, colleagues, students, and supervisees, present and past, might *you* be a charismatic adult? If you have received feedback in keeping with the concept of a charismatic adult from a client, a student, a supervisee, why do you think you were the one who was able to play such a key, helpful role in this person's life? Most of the time, of course, we won't hear that we are a charismatic adult from someone along our professional path.

Conclusion

Freud spent 30 minutes at the end of each working day to examine his emotional reactions to patients he saw that day and to reflect on what was healthy, unhealthy, useful, and enlightening. Freud, of course, was particularly vigilant about the intrusion of unconscious forces into his work. In *Psychopathology of Everyday Life*, Freud (1914) tells the story of what prompted him to write the book. On a cold, wintry, and snowy night he received a call from a patient who urgently needed to see him. When he arrived at the office, he could not, after several attempts, get his key to work. Suddenly, he realized that he was trying to open his office with the key to his home—the warm, cozy place he wished to be. To be a reflective practitioner and/or supervisor of play therapy requires dedication to self-examination and a willingness to cultivate the internal disciplines described in this chapter: the

disciplines of empathy, wholeheartedness, vulnerability, genuineness, courage, self-care, humility, and compassion.

Reflective practice can be facilitated by various modes of supervision, including individual and group supervision, peer supervision groups, and personal self-reflection. The chapter ends with some of the more popular reflective exercises that we have used in our reflective practice workshops given frequently at the annual Association for Play Therapy conference. These exercises can be utilized in any form of self, individual, or group supervision.

REFERENCES

Anderson, H. (1997). *Conversation, language, and possibilities: A postmodern approach to therapy.* New York: Basic Books.

Aponte, H. J. (1982). The cornerstone of therapy: The person of the therapist. *Family Therapy Networker, 6*, 19–21.

Aponte, H. J. (1994). How personal can training get? *Journal of Marital and Family Therapy, 20*, 3–15.

Aponte, H. J., & Carlsen, J. C. (2009). An instrument for person-of-the-therapist supervision. *Journal of Marital and Family Therapy, 35*, 395–405.

Aponte, H. J. & Kissil, K. (2012). "If I can grapple with this I can truly be of use in the therapy room": Using the therapist's own emotional struggles to facilitate effective therapy. *Journal of Marital and Family Therapy.*

Bager-Charleson, S. (2010). *Reflective practice on counseling and psychotherapy.* London: Sage/Learning Matters.

Beitman, B. D., & Soth, A. M. (2006). Activation of self-observation: A core process among the psychotherapies. *Journal of Psychotherapy Integration, 16*, 873–397.

Brooks, R. (2010). Power of mind-sets: A personal journey to nurture dignity, hope, and resilience to children. In D. A. Crenshaw (Ed.), *Reverence in healing: Honoring strengths without trivializing suffering* (pp. 19–40). Lanham, MD: Aronson.

Brown, S. (2009). *Play: How it shapes the brain, opens the imagination, and invigorates the soul.* New York: Avery/Penguin.

Crenshaw, D. A. (2007). Play therapy with selective mutism: When Melissa speaks, everyone listens. *Play Therapy, 2*(2), 20–21.

Drewes, A. A. (2006). Play-based interventions. *Journal of Early Childhood and Infant Psychology, 2*, 139–156.

Drewes, A. A. (2011a). Integrating play therapy theories into practice. In A. A. Drewes, S. C. Bratton, & C. E. Schaefer (Eds.), *Integrative play therapy* (pp. 21–35). Hoboken, NJ: Wiley.

Drewes, A. A. (2011b). Integrative play therapy. In C. E. Schaefer (Ed.), *Foundations of play therapy* (2nd ed., pp. 349–364). Hoboken, NJ: Wiley.

Drewes, A. A., Bratton, S. C., & Schaefer, C. E. (Eds.). (2011). *Integrative play therapy.* New York: Wiley.

Duncan, B. L., Miller, S. D., Wampold, B. E., & Hubble, M. A. (Eds.). (2010). *The heart and soul of change: Delivering what works in therapy* (2nd ed.). Washington, DC: American Psychological Association Press.

Figley, C. R. (1995). *Compassion fatigue.* New York: Routledge.

Frank, J. D., & Frank, J. B. (1993). *Persuasion and healing* (3rd ed.). Baltimore: Johns Hopkins University Press.

Freud, S. (1914). *Psychopathology of everyday life* (A. A. Brill, Trans.). London: T. Fisher Unwin.

Kazdin, A. E. (2005). Treatment outcomes, common factors, and continued neglect of mechanisms of change. *Clinical Psychology: Science and Practice, 12*, 184–188.

Kazdin, A. E. (2009). Understanding how and why psychotherapy leads to change. *Psychotherapy Research, 19*, 418–428.

Kottler, J. A. (2010). *On being a therapist* (4th ed.). San Francisco: Jossey-Bass.

Norcross, J. C., & Goldfried, M. R. (Eds.). (2005). *Handbook of psychotherapy integration* (2nd ed.). New York: Oxford University Press.

Prochaska, J. O., & Norcross, J. C. (2014). *Systems of psychotherapy: A transtheoretical analysis* (8th ed.). Belmont, CA: Brooks/Cole.

Rober, P. (1999). The therapist's inner conversation in family therapy practice: Some ideas about the self of the therapist, therapeutic impasse, and the process of reflection. *Family Process, 38*, 209–228.

Rober, P. (2005a). Family therapy as a dialogue of living persons: A perspective inspired by Bakhtin, Voloshinov, and Shotter. *Journal of Marital and Family Therapy, 31*, 385–397.

Rober, P. (2005b). The therapist's self in dialogical family therapy: Some ideas about not-knowing and the therapist's inner conversation. *Family Process, 44*, 477–495.

Rogers, C. R. (1957). The necessary and sufficient conditions of therapeutic change. *Journal of Consulting Psychology, 21*, 95–103.

Rogers, C. R. (1980). *A way of being.* New York: Houghton-Mifflin.

Rønnestad, M. H., & Skovholt, T. M. (2013). *The developing practitioner: Growth and stagnation of therapists and counselors.* New York: Routledge/Taylor & Francis.

Russ, S. W. (2004). *Play in child development and psychotherapy: Toward empirically supported practice.* Mahwah, NJ: Erlbaum.

Schaefer, C. E. (Ed.). (1993). *The therapeutic powers of play.* Northvale, NJ: Aronson.

Schaefer, C. E., & Drewes (Eds.). (2014). *The therapeutic powers of play: 20 core agents of change* (2nd ed.). New York: Wiley.

Schön, D. A. (1983). *The reflective practitioner: How professionals think in action.* New York: Basic Books.

Schön, D. A. (1987). *Educating the reflective practitioner.* San Francisco: Jossey-Bass.

Schore, A. N. (2012). *The science of the art of psychotherapy.* New York: Norton.

Segal, J. (1988). Teachers have enormous power in affecting a child's self-esteem. *Brown University Child Behavior and Development Newsletter, 10*, 1–3.

Seymour, J. W. (2011). History of psychotherapy integration and related research. In A. A. Drewes, S. C. Bratton, & C. E. Schaefer (Eds.), *Integrative play therapy* (pp. 3–19). New York: Wiley.

Shirk, S. R., & Russell, R. L. (1996). *Change processes in child psychotherapy: Revitalizing treatment and research.* New York: Guilford Press.

Siegel, D. J. (2012). *The developing mind: How relationships and the brain interact to shape who we are* (2nd ed.). New York: Guilford Press.

Stern, D. (2004). *The present moment in psychotherapy and everyday life.* New York: Norton.

Whyte, D. (2009, March 27). *The edge of discovery.* Keynote address to the 32nd annual Psychotherapy Networker Symposium, Washington, DC.

CHAPTER 34

Cultural Issues in Play Therapy

Phyllis Post
Kathleen S. Tillman

> The principal problem is that children and their families are too often expected to fit around services, rather than provision being specifically designed for them.
> —Alan Glasper (2010, p. 1258)

Culture can be defined in a variety of ways. Most definitions of culture, or cultural groups, incorporate the belief that people from the same background have "shared knowledge and schemes created by a set of people for perceiving, interpreting, expressing, and responding to the social realities around them" (Lederach, 1995, p. 9). That is, groups of people have shared understandings of the ways they think about and interact with others and the world around them. These ways of identifying and interacting with themselves and others are usually rooted in how they have been raised, what they have been taught by key adults in their lives, and how they have been responded to by others who are (and are not) members of their identified cultural group(s). Although *culture* can be defined quite broadly and include many groups, in this chapter we focus on the influence of socioeconomic status, race and ethnicity, immigration status, and community type (i.e., rural, urban, suburban) when using play therapy with young children.

Culturally Related Factors

To be effective play therapists, we must be knowledgeable, aware, and responsive to each client's unique cultural needs and the changing demographics of children and families living in the United States. When conceptualizing culture, we often talk about the similarities that individuals within the same cultural group experience and how cultures differ from each other (Greenfield & Suzuki, 1998; Kim & Choi, 1994; Triandis, 1995). Although this perspective may be helpful in some clinical settings, it is also important to talk with the child and family about within-group differences and how their individual experiences may vary from the norms within the cultural groups to which they ascribe (Haidt, Koller, & Dias, 1993; Wainryb & Turiel, 1995). Culturally sensitive play therapists take such culturally related factors into account during the initial assessment stage and constantly reevaluate how these factors may be influencing the therapeutic relationship, engagement in treatment, and treatment outcomes in play therapy.

Socioeconomic Status

The socioeconomic status of the clients with whom we work affects their functioning on a daily basis, the struggles that they face, the concerns they may have about engaging in treatment, and the ways that clinicians conceptualize and intervene using play therapy. Abramsky (2012) reported that 16 million, or 22% of, children in the United States live in poverty. Recent poverty guidelines from the U.S. Department of Health and Human Services designate an income of $23,550 or less for a family of four as the poverty level (Assistant Secretary for Planning and Evaluation, 2013). This is consistent with a report almost 10 years ago that more than one in every four families with young children had annual earnings of less than $25,000 and families with two parents earning minimum wage earned only $21,400 per year (Sally, 2005). These data suggest that play therapists are likely to work with children who live in poverty at some point, so awareness of the culture of poverty is critical in our need to help this group of children.

Race and Ethnicity

In addition to paying attention to the socioeconomic status of clients, it is also important to understand how race and ethnicity may impact the process of our work with children. The U.S. Census Bureau (2010) reported that the demographic characteristics of people within the United States are quickly changing and predicted that diversity will continue to increase. As of 2010, 44% of children were deemed "minorities" (U.S. Census Bureau, 2010). It is predicted that by the year 2025, the number of children in this group will surpass the number of children in the current majority group, and by the year 2050, this percentage will increase to 62%. This change in U.S. demographics will impact the clientele that play therapists serve, and play therapists must be increasingly culturally responsive to the needs of this rapidly growing number of children of color (Chang, Ritter, & Hays, 2005; O'Connor, 2005; VanderGast, Post, & Kascsak-Miller, 2010).

In addition to this change in the demographics of the United States is our knowledge that minority group members often have great mistrust of health care professionals (U.S. Department of Health and Human Services, 2001). For example, African Americans sometimes view seeking help from therapists for their children as poor parenting, may hold a worldview that advocates maintaining privacy regarding their personal problems, and may believe that faith will solve their problems (Hinds, 2005). To best serve children in play therapy, we need to be sensitive to the varying worldviews of our clients around these crucial issues.

Immigration Status

In the United States today, the immigration status of children who need mental health services cannot be overlooked. Immigration trends in the United States changed because of legislation in the mid-1960s that reduced restrictions of non-European immigration (Suarez-Orozco & Suarez-Orozco, 2001). As a result, the United States has attracted more immigrants than any nation in the world, and these immigrants have been diverse in terms of their socioeconomic status, race, and national origin. In a study examining barriers faced by immigrant parents in schools, Turney and Kao (2009) found that compared to nonimmigrant parents, immigrant parents often feel unwelcomed in their children's schools, are not as involved in the school, and struggle with their English language proficiency. These families' experiences with the school system may influence their perception of therapy for their children. Play therapists must keep in mind the issues of immigrant status as they work with children from culturally diverse backgrounds. At times awareness could require that therapists collaborate not only with parents but also with other stakeholders in the schools, such as teachers and school counselors. In addition, translators may be required in sessions both with parents and with the children.

Community Type

Although the influence of community sometimes goes overlooked, children in urban, suburban, and rural areas grow up in significantly different ways. Eberhardt and Pamuk (2004) report that rural and urban areas are often more disadvantaged than are suburban areas. Children and families in urban areas who have limited resources typically have access to fewer and lower-quality educational, psychological, and medical services. Children in rural areas may grow up in towns that are homogeneous in terms of race, religion/spirituality, and political orientation and that offer only limited educational opportunities, little to no available health care services, and very few extracurricular activities. However, children in suburban areas, who are typically children of middle to upper socioeconomic status, have access to an array of educational opportunities, a variety of mental and physical health care resources, and opportunities for many extracurricular activities.

Interactions between Cultural Factors

There is a connection between the communities where children live and their socioeconomic status: One in five poor children lives in a rural area. Not only is the poverty rate for children in rural areas higher than the rates for urban children, but the gap has been growing over the past 20 years. These children are also more likely to be exposed to substance abuse and lack of health care. These differences often influence the worldview of not only the child, but also the family members, in terms of their perceptions of mental health, their help-seeking behaviors, engagement in treatment, and treatment outcomes. Play therapists must attend to the issues embedded in the communities where children live and to their socioeconomic status to design appropriate treatment programs that fit with the cultures of these children.

Demographics of Play Therapists

Despite the rapidly increasing racial and ethnic diversity in the country, approximately 92% of play therapists responding to a survey conducted by the Association for Play Therapy (APT; Ryan, Gomory, & Lacasse, 2002) were white/non-Hispanic, and approximately 90% were female. Ceballos, Parikh, and Post (2012) used a sample from APT to investigate social justice attitudes among play therapists ($N = 448$) and the relation of their attitudes to multicultural supervision and multicultural education. The demographics of respondents were similar to those found by Ryan and colleagues (2002), such that 93% of the respondents were females and 85% were white. Obviously, these percentages are not representative of the diversity of our clients, and as professionals in the field, we should actively seek to increase the diversity of the next generation of play therapists.

With regard to training in multicultural issues, Ritter and Chang (2002) found that 24% of APT members reported that they had not received formal coursework in multicultural counseling, and those who had received formal coursework thought that their training was less than adequate. More recently, Ceballos and colleagues (2012) found that whereas 46% of the children whom professionals served were members of a minority group, only 14% of therapists' time receiving supervision was related to multicultural issues. Such a finding highlights the need for specific supervision regarding issues of diversity and multiculturalism.

The statistics about play therapists, their training in multicultural issues, and their supervision regarding multicultural sensitivity indicate that play therapists may need support to provide the best possible services to clients. Additionally, it is concerning that most play therapists conceptualize and provide treatment to children based on their own cultural experiences rather than the cultural needs of their clients (Gil, 2005). As a profession, change is necessary. Our field needs more diversity among the clinicians providing services and more education and supervision around issues of multiculturalism and diversity. Clearly there is a need to address the issues of cultural knowledge, self-awareness, and appropriate skills in conducting play therapy with our increasingly diverse child clients.

Addressing Culture in Play Therapy

As play therapists who work with clients of different cultural groups, we have a responsibility to work not only to understand the worldview of the child, but also to understand his or her cultural context. Gil (2005) describes three levels of response to demonstrate cross-culture competence. The first level is to build sensitivity to cultural issues, which begins with increasing our awareness of our own personal biases and values. The second level is to acquire the knowledge and skills required to be helpful to clients. We can do this by recognizing our own limitations and biases, practicing within our area of competence, and consulting with other professionals. Gil suggests we "practice with accountability" (p. 9), which means that we should work with experienced colleagues and invite their feedback to improve our work. The final level, after awareness and knowledge are achieved, is using this information to change our own behavior.

Knowledge

Research indicates that African Americans, Latinos, and Asian Americans have lower rates of mental health treatment compared to nonminority clients and that they terminate prematurely (Chow, Jaffee, & Snowden, 2003). Although clinicians do not want to assume that all parents from minority groups would have this pattern, an awareness of and sensitivity to this issue is important when working with minority children. It is crucial for play therapists to understand the multiple complex cultural influences that shape the child and family. Hinman (2003) offers helpful guidance for play therapists as we continue learning and practicing in culturally competent ways: (1) Increase our knowledge and awareness of the specific cultural influences of the children with whom we work; (2) be aware of, and monitor, how culture plays a role in children's functioning, their approach to treatment, and the treatment process of the children with whom we work; (3) acknowledge the stressors that children and their families may experience as a result of racism and oppression; and (4) adapt our treatment approach to meet the unique cultural needs of each client. In addition to these four levels of awareness and skill, play therapists must practice in ways that acknowledge the role of childhood and, importantly, the ways in which children and play are perceived in each culture.

Self-Awareness

Issues of Power and Privilege

Play therapists should work toward increasing their personal awareness of the different ways that power and privilege influence relationships with clients and families, as well as the process of treatment during play therapy. This includes an awareness of the power inherent in the role of therapist. To reach all clients, especially those who have been traditionally underserved or marginalized, it is essential that play therapists increase their cultural knowledge and awareness by staying open to learning about the cultural experiences of our clients. When play therapists understand and are sensitive to the influence of culture on the counseling process, including the therapeutic relationship and the therapeutic approach, we can provide the best possible services for children and families with whom we work.

Values and Personal Biases

As culturally competent play therapists, we value diversity not only by assessing children's cultural beliefs and experiences, but also by recognizing, identifying, and challenging various cultural beliefs and stereotypes that we hold so that they do not turn into harmful client interactions. By challenging our preconceived notions, which may or may not match with clients' self-identified cultures, we can change the focus from our own understanding to that of developing an empathic understanding of clients' cultures, their experiences with culture, and how these experiences may affect their willingness to stay in treatment, the quality of the therapeutic relationship, and the therapeutic process itself. By being more open to clients' experiences, we can better include cultural components in our approaches to play therapy as we strive to help children and their families. We believe that play therapists should seek professional training and supervision in multicultural counseling and should reflect on their own values and beliefs to become more aware of how their own cultural backgrounds and experiences may influence their work with children and families.

Skills: Selecting an Approach to Play Therapy

All theoretical approaches to play therapy begin with the premise that play is universal, pleasurable, and natural for all children (Landreth, 2012). Play is an essential and fundamental part of their lives. However, although play is universal, the way it looks can be different across and within cultures. When it comes to culturally competent play therapy, there is not a one-size-fits-all approach. The varied cultural experiences of children and their families define how they perceive, approach, react, and engage in play therapy. Consequently, it is vitally important that as play therapists we seek to understand our clients' culture so that we can understand their beliefs and expectations of therapy, what they bring to the therapeutic relationship and the therapeutic process, and how we can best support children and families throughout the therapeutic process. In these ways we can respect the client's and family's values while integrating important cultural aspects into individualized play therapy approaches that best meet the needs of the client. For example, families whose culture is more collectivist may hesitate to have their children participate in individual play therapy. Such a family may prefer to include all members to reflect the way in which that family sees the family unit.

A Child-Centered Approach to Culturally Sensitive Play Therapy

Although there are many different theoretical models of play therapy, we selected the child-centered approach to play therapy for this case study. Not only has child-centered play therapy (CCPT) been demonstrated to be effective with diverse cultural groups (Baggerly & Parker, 2005; Post, McAllister, Sheely, Hess, & Flowers, 2004), but it has also been suggested that person-centered therapies are the treatment of choice for treating culturally diverse clients (Cochran, 1996; Garza & Bratton, 2005). Based on the theoretical constructs of person-centered therapy (Rogers, 1951), CCPT focuses on a "way of being with children rather than doing something to or for children" (Landreth & Sweeney, 1997, p. 17). Everything that children experience, both internally and externally, both consciously and unconsciously, provides information about how they experience their lives. Consequently, child-centered play therapists strive to understand and view the world through the eyes of children because they believe that the behavior of children is related to their view of themselves (Axline, 1969). This is the culturally sensitive rationale for not judging and evaluating children's behaviors. Instead, child-centered play therapists strive to create a safe and warm environment in the playroom with the goal of demonstrating understanding and care. Although it is the "being with" attitude of therapists that is most critical, child-centered play therapists also strive to respond to the feelings of children, return responsibility to children for their behaviors in the playroom, use esteem-building skills, and set necessary limits with children (Landreth, 2012).

This perspective can enable play therapists to learn about and demonstrate respect for the child's culture by entering into an attuned and responsive therapeutic relationship. The composition of the CCPT room follows the culturally inclusive suggestions of O'Connor (2005) that toys meet the needs of culturally diverse clients, including both culturally neutral and culturally specific toys. CCPT rooms typically include toys that represent various living spaces (e.g., single-family homes, townhomes, apartments), dolls that represent a full range of ethnicities, and a variety of religious or other cultural symbols. In this way, play therapists are intentional about providing materials in the playroom that represent the cultures of the children with whom they work, and the children have the freedom to use the toys in the ways that they choose.

Initial Meeting with Parents and Goal Setting

The first step in CCPT is meeting with parents to understand the child's strengths and weaknesses and to establish therapeutic goals. The literature indicates that collaborating with parents increases the likelihood of success with children (Cates, Paone, Packman, & Margolis, 2006; Shaw & Magnuson, 2006). The objectives for meeting with parents are to establish specific goals for children (Cates et al., 2006; McGuire & McGuire, 2001), to establish benchmarks for progress, and to create a basis for follow-up consultations. The child-centered theoretical orientation adheres to the broad objectives of helping children become (1) more self-reliant, (2) more accepting of themselves, (3) better problem solvers, and (4) better able to assume responsibility for their own behaviors (Landreth, 2012).

Clearly there is a danger that setting behavioral goals could lead child-centered play therapists to act in a certain way (Landreth & Sweeney, 1997). Awareness of this possibility is important and should be monitored through clinical supervision. However, we believe that a combination of broad objectives and specific behavioral goals is optimal for successful treatment. Focusing on the overarching objectives that can be observed in the playroom and in the child's life outside of the playroom helps monitor the broad-based changes discussed above. Focusing on more specific goals relating to the issues presented by children, families, and/or teachers ensures that there is also a focus on changes in those behaviors that will not be addressed directly in the playroom. Consequently, both the broad objectives and behavioral goals are useful in monitoring the effectiveness of play therapy interventions.

In the initial meeting with the parent(s), it is critical that the play therapist establish a positive relationship, identify concrete goals that reflect the cultural context of the family, and directly address how CCPT will help achieve these goals. Each family will have its own expectations and experiences with the meaning of seeking help, mental health, and play. Given the importance of preventing early termination of services, play therapists should help set appropriate goals that parents understand and accept, while also helping parents understand how CCPT will help achieve these goals. For example, in some cultures the demonstration of compliance is highly valued, whereas in other cultures it is not. If compliance is a goal for the child, in either the home or classroom setting, child-centered play therapists can relate how this approach to therapy will help the child learn to respond to clearly stated limits and control his or her behavior in the playroom. And as this happens in the playroom, it is likely to also be demonstrated in the home and school.

In addition to consulting with parents and talking with children to create goals, play therapists note significant behaviors observed during play therapy sessions with the child that might not have emerged as a goal in the initial parent consultation. For example, therapists might notice that the child persistently asks permission to play with toys, which could indicate a low level of confidence and an inability to act independently (Landreth, 2012). These clinical observations should be translated into additional behavioral goals for the child.

Assessing Progress through Ongoing Consultations

It is helpful to meet with the parents, without the child present, periodically. The purpose of ongoing parent consultations is threefold: (1) to maintain and foster a strong relationship with the parents; (2) to collaboratively assess the child's progress toward goals and to educate parents about child development and parenting skills; and (3) to provide parents with community resources that can be used to help the child. Most parents are eager to learn new approaches to discipline, and they highly value the skills of limit setting and choice giving that empower them as parents and that help their children feel safe and supported. Also, sharing the skills of

responding to the child and learning to help the child assume responsibility for his or her behaviors have been found to reduce parental stress and create a more positive environment in the home, which can influence the entire family system (Landreth & Bratton, 2006).

Before meeting with parents, it is helpful to review case notes and to prepare what to discuss. Although the specific behaviors of children are not shared with parents to protect the confidentiality of the children and the client–therapist relationship, play therapists can review established goals to assess progress, identify play themes to share with parents, and share any appropriate parenting skills with parents during the meeting. What to share in the meeting with the parents and how to share this information need to be considered in light of the cultural context of the child and the family.

Terminating

To honor the importance of the therapist–parent relationship and the pivotal role of parents in children's lives, the decision to terminate treatment is always done in collaboration with parents. Once there is a decision to terminate, therapists and parents decide collaboratively on a time frame for it. A clear, predictable termination process is particularly important for children who have been through major changes in their lives, such as changed living arrangements with parents because of separation of parents or trauma. That said, being open and direct about the termination process with the child is as essential as the communication that occurs with parents surrounding termination.

Clinical Case Example

The clinical case description that follows illustrates a culturally sensitive play therapy case that uses a child-centered approach to play therapy. The case is a composite of

4-year-old children in an urban preschool, and for the purposes of the chapter, the client is referred to as *Coby*. The general approach of working with a child and his or her parents is described prior to presenting the case.

Background Information

Once a week I (Post) worked in a preschool where I was able to conduct play therapy with children in a well-furnished playroom. The small, windowless room had toys and materials recommended for CCPT. The toys were in three categories: *real life* (e.g., baby-dolls, action figures, kitchen items, medical kit, cars, trucks, cell phone, ball, dress-up clothes, school supplies, blocks); *aggressive release* (e.g., handcuffs, punching bag, toy soldiers, puppets); and *creative* (e.g., crayons, paper, markers, paints, chalk, craft items, sand, water).

Coby was a 4-year-old African American male attending an urban preschool. He had lived in seven foster homes before he was adopted by his last foster care parents at 18 months of age. The concerned parents were African American high school graduates with a lower economic income. The parents had received minimal details about Coby's developmental and psychological history. When Coby was 2 years old, a newborn was adopted by the parents, creating a family with two children who were 2 years apart in age but who were adopted within 6 months of each other. The family lived in a small home with two bedrooms on the second floor. There was an attic on the third floor that was converted into Coby's bedroom when the family adopted their second child. Coby had had occasional sleep problems and nightmares since his adoption. At school, he was shy but very bright and able to interact moderately well with his peers. At times he would withdraw and show anxiety by putting his fingers in his mouth and wanting to stay close to his teachers.

A change occurred when Coby's preschool teacher introduced the idea that the following year the children would be leaving the preschool and entering kindergarten in a public school. His parents requested therapy for Coby because his nightmares increased in frequency and intensity. He began to express fears of losing his mother and wanted to be physically close with her all the time. He began going to his parents' bedroom every night. Coby's parents did not know how to help him. They valued both compliance and independence and tried using rewards to get him to stay in his own bedroom. They resorted to spanking him to force his compliance to return to his own bedroom.

At school, Coby's behavior also changed. He clung to his teachers and interacted with his peers less frequently. At times he would cry, say his stomach hurt, and ask for his mother. His engagement with peers, which had been reserved, became more uncomfortable for him. For example, on the playground, he no longer showed any interest in playing with his peers, and he often stood close to one of the adults. He also had a hard time transitioning between different activities in the classroom, especially if it involved a change in the teacher; this is another time that he would put his fingers in his mouth to self-soothe.

Teacher Consultation and Initial Meeting with Coby's Parents

Before meeting with Coby's parents, I consulted with Coby's lead teacher and observed him in the classroom and on the playground. His teacher shared that Coby's behaviors had changed greatly since she began talking about the transition to another school; he now wanted to stay close to her and to interact less with his peers. The teacher also noted that Coby had difficulty making decisions about what to do during free time in the classroom.

I met with Coby's parents before meeting with Coby. The goals of the meeting were twofold. First, I wanted to develop a genuine, respectful, and warm relationship with them. Second, I wanted to understand their concerns about Coby, including the cultural context and his life experiences, to develop realistic outcome goals that we could assess regularly to determine progress and to instill hope that CCPT would help Coby.

I shared with Coby's parents both the goals of CCPT and what I would be doing with Coby in the playroom. Specifically, I told them that I would not be talking directly with Coby about his problems; rather, I would make every effort to create a safe and warm environment in the playroom where I would show Coby that I cared and understood his emotional world. I would allow Coby to decide what he would do in the playroom. I shared that, when necessary, I would set limits with Coby if he was going to hurt himself, hurt me, destroy materials, or do any inappropriate activities, such as taking off his clothes. Coby's parents expressed some doubt about the effectiveness of such a nondirective approach. They came to see me with the expectation that I would focus on Coby's nightmares and talk with him about his progress. In spite of their reservations, they seemed interested in this approach; they knew that their focus on his behaviors had not helped him and so were open to trying something different.

After listening to Coby's parents, consulting with his teachers, and observing him, his parents and I collaboratively developed the following broad objective and specific goals for play therapy:

Broad Objective

1. Increase Coby's ability to assume responsibility for his own decisions about what to do in the classroom or on the playground.

Specific Goals

1. Increase the number of nights that Coby could sleep each week without nightmares (to 4 nights each week from the current baseline of 1 night per week).

2. Increase the number of nights that Coby could sleep in his own bed (to 4 nights each week from the current baseline of 1 night per week).
3. Increase the number of days that Coby went without asking if he were going to lose his mother (from 2 days each week to 6 days each week).
4. Increase the number of days that Coby played with his peers, rather than standing with his teachers, during recess (from 0 days per week to 4 days per week).
5. Increase the number of days that Coby could transition between activities in the classroom (to 5 times a day from once a day).

In addition to identifying these goals for Coby, the parents committed to returning to see me in 4 weeks to talk about how Coby was doing at home and to hear about how he was doing at school.

To ensure that these goals did not interfere with my way of being with Coby in the playroom, I sought supervision that focused on my ability to relate to Coby without focusing on "problems" and "goals."

Play Therapy Sessions

Parent Session 1

I met with Coby's parents prior to meeting with him to discuss their concerns, goals for counseling, and CCPT. The mother helped to prepare Coby by reading him *A Child's First Book about Play Therapy* (Nemiroff & Annunziata, 1990), which describes play therapy in language appropriate for 4-year-olds. They also told him about me and that I would be seeing him to help him feel more comfortable and less worried at home and at school.

Child Session 1

On the morning of our first session, Coby's mother and teachers told him that I would be coming to get him and take him to our "special playroom." I went to Coby's classroom to get him for our first session. I saw him and went over to him. He was standing playing at the water table. I leaned down to his level and said, "Hi, Coby. My name is Phyllis. It is time for us to go to the playroom now." Coby stood up, looked at the floor, put his fingers in his mouth, and did not move. Then he walked over to one of his teachers and stood beside her without speaking. The teacher warmly encouraged him to go with me, and he complied. He walked silently with me out of his classroom and down the hall to the playroom. I introduced him to the playroom, saying, "Coby, this is our playroom, and you can play with the toys in a lot of the ways you would like to." Then I sat in my chair and watched as Coby stood in the middle of the room without looking around for several minutes. I responded to his behavior by voicing my thoughts about how Coby might be feeling (i.e., unsure, uneasy). He asked me what to play with, and I responded that he could decide. Then he noticed the dress-up clothes hanging on the Peg-Board and the other clothes and masks in a box below. Coby found a scary mask and threw it over the Peg-Board. Then he played with each of the puppets with great imagination. He buried almost all of the animal families in the sand. He played without ever facing me during that session. He was eager to return to his classroom when our time was up, but he did run to his teacher and tell him what he did in the playroom.

Child Session 2

Coby was eager to come to playroom for the second play therapy session. Again, I engaged Coby using a child-centered way of being with him. I invited him to play with the toys in the ways that he wanted, I reflected his feelings, I encouraged him to assume responsibility for his decisions in the playroom, and I noted times he was genuinely working hard to do what he was trying to do. It was clear that Coby had been thinking about what to do because when he entered the playroom, he immediately started playing with the same toys he had used the previous week and in many of the same ways. Again, he began the session with finding the same scary mask and throwing it over the Peg-Board. His commitment to his work was strong. He was neat with the materials and put everything he played with away after he was finished with it. During this session, Coby created a game for himself and worked extremely hard to accomplish his goals. He talked about himself with me, sharing some activities he liked and didn't like in his classroom and talking about his little brother. Our session lasted about 45 minutes. When I took him back to his classroom, Coby was excited to share with his teacher what he had done in the playroom.

Child Session 3

Coby began his session by throwing the scary mask over the Peg-Board yet again. In the first two sessions, Coby buried a variety of toys in the sand, paying particular attention to totally covering the items. Today, he began that activity but quickly stopped and played with the yo-yo, dart gun, and paddle-ball. With each of these toys, Coby worked hard, learned from his mistakes, and did not enjoy much success. Coby painted a picture for his brother. At this point, the pattern of behavior of throwing the mask over the Peg-Board and the themes of diligence and persistence were emerging.

Child Session 4

Again, Coby began his session with throwing the scary mask over the Peg-Board. As in earlier sessions, he did not say a word when he did this. After burying animal families in the sand, Coby explored more of the arts and crafts materials in this session. He created a Popsicle sculpture for his father and for himself. He was excited and confident during the session today. Again, I observed that Coby's level of persistence is high and he is highly motivated without getting discouraged when his efforts do not immediately produce the effects he would wish.

Parent Session 2

Following child session 4, I made an appointment to see Coby's parents to touch base with them and to assess progress toward the original goals established. Before this meeting I reviewed the initial goals that we'd established, consulted with Coby's teachers, observed Coby in the classroom and during recess, and reviewed my case notes to conceptualize themes to share with the parents. The teachers reported that Coby continued to cling to them and still struggled with making decisions for himself in the classroom. From the review of my case notes and thoughts about our time together in the playroom, I decided to check in with the parents about their comfort level with using a nondirective approach and to share my perceptions regarding Coby's increasing level of comfort in the sessions, his increasing ability to make decisions for himself in the playroom, and his commitment to task.

Coby's mother came to meet with me. I began the parent session by asking her a general question about how things were going with Coby. When I inquired about her comfort using CCPT, she told me that they felt less hesitant because Coby told them how much he enjoyed his time in the playroom and that his stress level at home seemed to be diminishing some. His mother told me that changes were minor in terms of his nightmares but that he was able to stay in his bedroom more nights each week, presumably when he did not have a nightmare. She shared that they were tired and that their patience was sometimes low. They felt bad about how stern they were when sending him back to his own bed. As she talked, I responded to her with empa-

thy. Then I reviewed the other goals they established during our first meeting, and I shared some strategies for setting limits and using choice giving with Coby. Based on her interest, I loaned her a copy of the DVD *Cookies, Choices, and Kids* (Landreth, 2008), which presents a concrete strategy for helping parents use choice-giving alternatives with their children. It provides some challenging and amusing examples to make the process clear.

Child Sessions 5–12

During child sessions 5–12, I strived to maintain a safe, judgment-free environment for Coby, who continued to throw the scary mask over the Peg-Board to begin each session. Maintaining similar patterns of play, Coby worked hard burying animal families, and then blocks, in the sand. Some days he would bury them completely. Some days he would work hard not to bury them completely. One day he buried only one block and said, "I'm burying you because you've been bad." Coby was consistent in his willingness to come to the playroom. Around session 10, other children in the classroom would approach me when I came to get Coby or return him to the classroom and beg to come with him. Coby would tell them, with a smile on his face, that he got to come by himself. His joy was clear, and his commitment to working in the playroom was strong.

Child Session 13

For the first time, Coby did not look for the scary mask. He entered the playroom and ran to play with the animal families. His play during this session was similar to past sessions in terms of his selection of toys and his task commitment.

Parent Session 3

One week following Session 13, I met with Coby's mother for the third time. I prepared for the parent meeting in the same way I had for the previous meetings. I began the session with asking how things were going with Coby. His mother reported that quite suddenly, about 2 weeks ago, Coby's nightmares had ended, and he was sleeping in his own bed most nights in a week. Although he had talked at home about his fears of going to another school, she could not remember when he'd last expressed fear of losing her. She also shared that the DVD on choice giving had been helpful in teaching her some ways to provide choices to both Coby and his brother. She expressed her surprise and satisfaction that a nondirective approach to working with Coby had resulted in changes in his behaviors. I shared that many factors impact change in children so young, and that a child-centered approach to play therapy could have been one of them. I expressed my appreciation for her willingness to reflect on changes in her own behaviors and noted that I had observed changes in the way that teachers were responding to Coby. I shared my observation of Coby in his classroom and the teacher's report about his increased comfort interacting with peers, ability to transition in the classroom, and more independence when making decisions.

It seemed that the goals of the play therapy intervention had been achieved. Coby's mother and I determined together that it was time to end the play therapy with Coby. We spoke about the importance of clarity, especially for a child who struggled with change and transitions, and decided together that I would introduce termination during the next session and then have two more sessions with Coby.

Child Session 16

I began our last session by reminding Coby that this was his last session with me. Coby did not acknowledge my statement and immediately engaged in play. He diligently tried to use the paddleball and the yo-yo. He said they were "hard," but he put a tre-

mendous amount of effort into his play with them, and he commented on how much he loved the yo-yo. For the first time, Coby used the Jenga blocks. He built a high tower that required a lot of balancing of the blocks. After it was built, he knocked the tower over by throwing the football at it. Then he took the blocks to the sand. Just like the pattern in his first sessions, he worked hard to bury all the blocks he put in the sand. He said, "This is a house." After burying the "house" completely, he said that he needed "to get the people out" and he "found" the blocks. He repeated this play sequence several times. He hit the Bop Bag for the first time, and he hit it very hard for about 15 minutes. When our time was over, Coby and I left the playroom . . . without a word about the end of our relationship together. Coby ran into his classroom and immediately got involved with a small group of children at the water table. He was smiling.

Summary and Highlights

With Coby's early, and unknown, history of multiple foster care homes, his fears around change and transitions were not unexpected. The goal of CCPT with Coby was to provide a safe, calm, and nonjudgmental relationship where he could work through his anxiety about the upcoming changes in his life in his own way on his own time. His pattern with the scary mask emerged in the first session and was the first thing he did for 12 sessions. Although I never discussed this pattern with him, the behavior ended at the same time that his nightmares ended. A change in patterns of behavior linked with changes in children's lives outside of the playroom happens frequently with CCPT.

Cultural Issues

Coby's parents entered the relationship with some doubt about the effectiveness of a nondirective approach to play therapy. They had expected a more direct, problem-solving approach. However, they appreciated the specific goals we set during our first sessions together. In addition, they were open to this approach and were willing to attend regular meetings with me. They seemed to value my work with Coby more over time because they began to see changes in his behaviors at home and because he liked his sessions.

Conclusion

The chapter began by focusing on the influence of socioeconomic status, race and ethnicity, immigration status, and community type on the cultural experiences of children and families. Additionally, we discussed the importance of play therapists' knowledge of specific cultures as well as individual differences and self-awareness with regard to their own cultural experiences, their power and privilege, and their beliefs about different cultures. We introduced CCPT and discussed the ways that it is culturally sensitive and responsive to the needs of children and parents. The chapter concluded with a case presentation that illustrated how CCPT respects culture, and how the child-centered play therapist responds to the family's culture and beliefs, and works collaboratively with parents to provide the best possible services for children.

As play therapists, it is vitally important that we understand the multitude of cultural factors that influence children and families. In order to provide culturally sensitive and culturally responsive treatment to children and families, play therapists need to learn about the unique needs of specific cultures while also talking to families about their individual experiences and needs. Culturally sensitive play therapists must collaborate with parents and seek to understand and repeatedly assess how culture and culturally related issues (e.g., racism, oppression) affect the child's functioning, the family's approach to treatment, and the treatment process. After exploring these foundational issues, play therapists utilize culturally appropriate treatment interventions or adapt the chosen treatment approaches to meet the unique cultural needs of the clients, and continue to discuss progress with parents.

Timely and important guidance—the National Standards for Culturally and Linguistically Appropriate Services (CLAS)—has been released from the Office of Minority Health (U.S. Department of Health and Human Services, 2011). The CLAS document provides 15 standards for addressing cultural disparities in health care and will help government departments, health and human service agencies, and education and training programs across all disciplines improve the health outcomes for all children and families seeking health care by reducing inequalities in access and treatment. Play therapists who serve young children must strive to promote social justice in mental health care for all children by advocating for, and working with, traditionally underserved populations.

REFERENCES

Abramsky, S. (2012). The other America 2012. *Nation, 294*(20), 11–18.

Assistant Secretary for Planning and Evaluation. (2013). 2013 Poverty guidelines. Office of the Assistant Secretary for Planning and Evaluation. Retrieved from *http://aspe.hhs.gov/poverty/13poverty.cfm*.

Axline, V. M. (1969). *Play therapy*. New York: Ballantine Books.

Baggerly, J., & Parker, M. (2005). Child-centered group play therapy with African American boys at the elementary school level. *Journal of Counseling and Development, 83*, 387–396.

Cates, J., Paone, T. R., Packman, J., & Margolis, D. (2006). Effective parent consultation in play therapy. *International Journal of Play Therapy, 15*, 87–100.

Ceballos, P. L., Parikh, S., & Post, P. B. (2012). Examining the relationship between multicultural education, multicultural focus of supervision as related to social justice advocacy attitudes among members of Association for Play Therapy. *International Journal of Play Therapy, 21,* 232–243.

Chang, C. Y., Ritter, K. B., & Hays, D. G. (2005). Multicultural trends and toys in play therapy. *International Journal of Play Therapy, 14,* 69–85.

Chow, J. C.-C., Jaffee, K., & Snowden, L. (2003). Racial/ethnic disparities in the use of mental health services in poverty areas. *American Journal of Public Health, 93,* 792–797.

Cochran, J. (1996). Using play and art therapy to help culturally diverse students overcome barriers to school success. *The School Counselor, 43,* 287–298.

Eberhardt, M. S., & Pamuk, E. R. (2004). The importance of place of residence: Examining health in rural and non-rural areas. *American Journal of Public Health, 94,* 1682–1686.

Garza, Y., & Bratton, S. (2005). School-based child-centered play therapy with Hispanic children: Outcomes and cultural considerations. *International Journal of Play Therapy, 14,* 51–79.

Gil, E. (2005). From sensitivity to competence in working across cultures. In E. Gil & A. A. Drewes (Eds.), *Cultural issues in play therapy* (pp. 3–25). New York: Guilford Press.

Glasper, A. (2010). Achieving a culture of equity and excellence for children in the NHS. *British Journal of Nursing, 19,* 1258–1259.

Greenfield, P. M., & Suzuki, L. K. (1998). Culture and human development: Implications for parenting, education, pediatrics, and mental health. In W. Damon (Series Ed.), I. E. Sigel & K. A. Renninger (Eds.), *Handbook of child psychology: Vol. 4. Child psychology in practice* (5th ed., pp. 1059–1109). New York: Wiley.

Haidt, J., Koller, S. H., & Dias, M. G. (1993). Affect, culture, and morality, or is it wrong to eat your dog? *Journal of Personality and Social Psychology, 65,* 613–628.

Hinds, S. (2005). Play therapy in the African American village. In E. Gil & A. A. Drewes (Eds.), *Cultural issues in play therapy* (pp. 115–147). New York: Guilford Press.

Hinman, C. (2003). Multicultural considerations in the delivery of play therapy services. *International Journal of Play Therapy, 12,* 107–122.

Kim, U., & Choi. S. (1994). Individualism, collectivism, and child development: A Korean perspective. In P. Greenfield & R. Cocking (Eds.), *Cross-cultural roots of minority child development* (pp. 227–258). Hillsdale, NJ: Erlbaum.

Landreth, G. L. (2008). *Cookies, choices, and kids: A creative approach to discipline.* Denton, TX: University of North Texas, Center for Play Therapy.

Landreth, G. L. (2012). *Play therapy: The art of the relationship* (3rd ed.). New York: Routledge.

Landreth, G., & Bratton, S. (2006). *Child parent relationship therapy (CPRT): A 10-session filial therapy model.* New York: Routledge/Taylor & Francis Group.

Landreth, G. L., & Sweeney, D. (1997). Child-centered play therapy. In K. V. O'Connor & L. Mages (Eds.), *Play therapy theory and practice: A comparative presentation* (pp. 17–43). New York: Wiley

Lederach, J. P. (1995). *Preparing for peace: Conflict transformation across cultures.* Syracuse, NY: Syracuse University Press.

McGuire, D. K., & McGuire, D. E. (2001). *Linking parents to play therapy: A practical guide with applications, interventions, and case studies.* Philadelphia: Brunner-Routledge.

Nemiroff, M. A., & Annunziata, J. (1990). *A child's first book about play therapy.* Washington, DC: American Psychological Association.

O'Connor, K. (2005). Assessing diversity issues in play therapy. *Professional Psychology: Research and Practice, 36,* 566–573.

Post, P., McAllister, M., Sheely, A., Hess, B., & Flowers, C. (2004). Child-centered kinder training for teachers of at-risk pre-school children. *International Journal of Play Therapy, 13,* 53–74.

Ritter, K. B., & Chang, C. Y. (2002). Play therapists' self-perceived multicultural competence and adequacy of training. *International Journal of Play Therapy, 11,* 103–113.

Rogers, C. R. (1951). *Client-centered therapy.* Boston: Houghton Mifflin.

Ryan, S. D., Gomory, T., & Lacasse, J. R. (2002). Who are we?: Examining the results of the Association for Play Therapy Membership Survey. *International Journal for Play Therapy, 11,* 11–41.

Sally R. (2005). Eye on Washington. *Journal of Child and Adolescent Psychiatric Nursing, 18,* 36–37.

Shaw, H., & Magnuson, S. (2006). Enhancing play therapy with parent consultation: A behavioral/solution-focused approach. In C. E.

Schaefer & H. G. Kaduson (Eds.), *Short-term play therapy for children* (2nd ed., pp. 216–241). New York: Guilford Press.

Suarez-Orozco, C., & Suarez-Orozco, M. (2001). *Children of immigration*. Cambridge, MA: Harvard University Press.

Triandis, H. C. (1995). *Individualism and collectivism*. Boulder, CO: Westview Press.

Turney, K., & Kao, G. (2009). Barriers to school involvement: Are immigrant parents disadvantaged? *Journal of Educational Research, 102*, 257–271.

U.S. Census Bureau. (2010). Poverty: 2008 and 2009—American community survey briefs. Retrieved from *www.census.gov/prod/2010pubs/acsbr09-1.pdf.*

U.S. Department of Health and Human Services. (2001). *Mental health: Culture, race, and ethnicity (A supplement to mental health: A report of the Surgeon General)*. Rockville, MD: Author.

U.S. Department of Health and Human Services. (2011). HHS action plan to reduce racial and ethnic health disparities: A nation free of disparities in health and health care. Retrieved from *http://minorityhealth.hhs.gov/npa/files/Plans/HHS/HHS_Plan_complete.pdf.*

VanderGast, T. S., Post, P. B., & Kascsak-Miller, T. (2010). Graduate training in child–parent relationship therapy with a multicultural immersion experience: Giving away the skills. *International Journal of Play Therapy, 19*, 198–208.

Wainryb, C., & Turiel, E. (1995). Diversity in social development: Between or within cultures. In M. Killen & D. Hart (Eds.), *Morality in everyday lives* (pp. 283–313). New York: Cambridge University Press.

CHAPTER 35

Ethics in Play Therapy

Jeffrey S. Ashby
Kathleen McKinney Clark

Always do right. This will gratify some people
and astonish the rest.
—MARK TWAIN

Play therapy ethics, as the ethics of all helping professions, are based on the primary tenet of promoting the welfare of the client. Although this seems straightforward, the application of these tenets to the practice of play therapy can raise a number of questions and complexities. For instance, in the practice of play therapy the question "Who is the client?" is an essential question to answer that may not come up in other types of counseling. The question is essential because the play therapist must ultimately determine to whom he or she owes a professional obligation. The play therapist certainly owes a professional obligation to the child client. Does the play therapist also owe an obligation to the client's parents/guardians? Are there other entities? What about society? The school? Other systems? Asking "Who is the client?" is just one example of some of the unique applications of ethics to the practice of play therapy.

The purpose of this chapter is to illustrate the application of professional ethics to the practice of play therapy. We consider the application of several primary ethical issues—competence, informed consent, confidentiality, and multiple relationships—to the practice of play therapy and discuss ethical decision-making models. Although this list of issues is certainly not exhaustive, it does represent several key areas of ethics within play therapy. Play therapists and aspirational play therapists will be familiar with these ethical constructs from the ethical codes of their primary professions. Additionally, we attempt to highlight the particular thorny issues unique to play therapy that are likely to arise. At the conclusion of the chapter, we review ethical decision-making models that can guide the play therapist through ethical decisions that may arise.

Play Therapy as a Secondary Profession

Play therapy is generally understood as being the secondary profession or secondary identity of the play therapist. Play therapists have a primary identity, and usually a professional license or certification related to that identity, as an umbrella profession under which they practice play therapy. Play therapists can have a primary profession of social worker, counselor, psychologist, marriage and family therapist, or other mental health professional. As a result, play therapists have a primary obligation to endorse and uphold the ethical codes of their primary profession. Although the codes of these professions are generally consistent with one another, each may have specific principles or applications that are relevant to mental health professionals who have secondary identities as play therapists. Consistent with the counsel of numerous authors (e.g., Doverspike, 1999), we recommend that play therapists regularly review the ethical codes and practice guidelines of their primary professional organization. Note that many professionals review their ethical codes as a ritual consistent with renewing their license, paying professional dues, etc.—much like the old advice to change the batteries in your smoke alarms when you change your clocks for daylight savings time. This regular review can help play therapists assure themselves that they are mindful of their professional obligations and the ethical mandates of their primary identity.

While there are no ethical guidelines specific to play therapy, the Association for Play Therapy (APT; 2009) has published practice guidelines. These guidelines are aspirational and indicate some of the overlap and extension of the tenets of the ethical codes of primary identities to the field of play therapy. We would commend these to you as an excellent reference to act as an addendum to the ethical codes of your primary profession.

Competence: What Can the Play Therapist Ethically Do?

Julie is a licensed mental health professional and a registered play therapist with 12 years of experience in a variety of clinical settings. She was recently referred a 9-year-old private practice client diagnosed by a psychiatrist with obsessive–compulsive disorder and major depression. The client's parents are seeking a play therapist for their child and were referred to Julie. Julie has openings in her private practice caseload and is a member of the insurance panel the client's parents anticipate using. Upon hearing this referral information, Julie decides to . . .

At the root of Julie's decision-making process of whether to accept this play therapy referral is the issue of competence. Fairburn and Cooper (2011) defined competence as "the extent to which a therapist has the knowledge and skill required to deliver a treatment to the standard needed for it to achieve its expected effects" (p. 375). The ethical codes of all mental health professions are clear about the mandate to practice only within the boundaries of one's competence. For instance, the Code of Ethics for the American Counseling Association (ACA) states, "Counselors practice only within the boundaries of their competence, based on their education, training, supervised experience, state and national professional credentials, and appropriate professional experience" (2005, C.2.a, p. 9).

In deciding whether or not to see the referred client in play therapy, Julie must assess her own competence in a number of potentially overlapping areas. One important consideration is that therapist competence is largely self-determined and self-monitored. Although a professional credential (e.g., licensure, certification) may create broad boundaries of potential competence (e.g., therapy, assessment, consultation, prescription privileges), simply holding the credential does not substantiate a specific therapist as competent to perform all of the tasks, or see all of the clients, that the license might allow. The burden is typically on the play therapist to self-define the boundaries of his or her competence.

Although there are no clear criteria for determining professional competence in most mental health professions, the generally accepted evidence for the establishment of competence is formal academic training, professional training, and supervised experience (Pope & Vasquez, 2010). Showing that a professional knows *about* a particular treatment, population, and/or presenting problem (through formal instruction and training on these topics) and knows *how* to deliver a particular treatment and/or treat a client with a particular issue and from a particular cultural or age group (through supervised experience) clearly indicates competence in a particular area.

A first question Julie might consider in her decision-making process of whether or not to accept this referral is whether she is competent (has the appropriate training, experience, etc.) to treat children. Play therapists have often been trained as generalists and, as a result, may have completed most of their study and supervised experience with older adolescents and adults. Although much of the knowledge and skills developed in this training is applicable, specialized training (e.g., in child development, child psychopathology) and supervised experience treating children might be considered necessary in establishing competence in treating children.

There are a number of effective treatment modalities for counseling children. Since the referral Julie is considering is specifically for a play therapist, a second question Julie might ask is, "Am I competent to do play therapy?" Play therapy is considered a "limited-domain intervention" (Barber, Sharpless, Klostermann, & McCarthy, 2007) and, as such, requires a competence within this specialty area. As a result, not all clinicians competent to treat children are competent to conduct play therapy. However, since most training in play therapy addresses its application with children, most clinicians who are competent to conduct play therapy are likely competent to see children (e.g., not all child therapists

are play therapists but most play therapists are child therapists, even if they apply the specialty to other groups at times).

In this case example, Julie is a registered play therapist (RPT). Meeting the requirements to be an RPT (see *www.a4pt.org/ps.training.cfm*) is one way "licensed mental health professionals might demonstrate and promote their specialized play therapy knowledge and training." However, APT is careful to note that, "The designation as a RPT or RPT-S does not certify, imply, or affirm the knowledge or competency of such individual but only confirms that the education and training requirements identified herein have been satisfied." Julie's RPT credential is a well-established way for her to document evidence of play therapy competence, in that the RPT criteria include specific formal training in various aspects of play therapy and supervised play therapy practice. Training and experience in play therapy include, but are not limited to, theories of play therapy, techniques or methods of play therapy, and applications of play therapy to special settings or populations (Carmichael, 2006). Although holding the RPT credential does not officially certify competence in play therapy, it does provide evidence of Julie's having completed the training and supervised experience that lead to competence.

In some ways a more difficult question for Julie to answer in considering this referral is, "Am I competent to see a client with these diagnoses from this particular cultural background?" Although the case scenario does not describe the cultural backgrounds of Julie or the client, Sue, Arrendondo, and McDavis (1992) have noted that all therapy and counseling dyads are cross-cultural. Even in the case of play therapist and client sharing a particular cultural identity (e.g., both African American), there are likely also cultural differences (e.g., religious/spiritual background or identity). The National Association of Social Workers (NASW) ethical code (2008) indicates that "social workers should have a knowledge base of their clients' cultures and be able to demonstrate competence in the provision of services that are sensitive to clients' cultures and to differences among people and cultural groups" (1.05-B). In order to ethically take this referral, Julie will need to self-assess and determine that she has the adequate knowledge, skills, and attitudes (Sue et al., 1992) to competently work with this particular client in play therapy.

An additional question for Julie when considering the appropriateness of taking this referral is whether she is competent clinically to address the presenting problem or diagnoses of the client. Specifically, she would need to ask herself, "Do I have adequate training and supervised experience to provide competent care as the primary clinician assisting the client in addressing this presenting problem?" The concern regarding this question is easily apparent in certain presenting problems and diagnoses. For instance, in the case of restricting eating disorders (e.g., anorexia nervosa), less than competent care could result in the persistence of the disorder and significant physical health problems—even, in some cases, death (see Arcelus, Mitchell, Wales, & Nielsen, 2011). As a result, specialized training in the treatment of eating disorders is typically understood as the standard in establishing competence (Thompson-Brenner, Satir, Franko, & Herzog, 2012). However, for many other presenting problems there is no accepted standard of what constitutes competence. Julie will need to determine whether she has adequate training and experience to render her competent in addressing the presenting problem of this particular client.

Julie will have to self-assess to determine if she has the appropriate formal didactic training and supervised experience to treat the client's presenting problems of obsessive–compulsive disorder and depression. She will need to consider a number of questions, including the following: Am I aware of clinical considerations in the treatment of obsessive–compulsive disorder and/or depression in children? Do I have adequate training and supervised experience to be competent in treating those disorders as comorbid conditions? How serious or debilitating are the conditions (e.g., dysthymia vs. major depression with strong suicidal ideation) and do I have adequate experience and training to treat these presenting problems at this level of severity? Is play therapy an appropriate intervention for these disorders? How does my theoretical approach to play therapy work with these disorders?

One final consideration in the discussion of competence is the important distinction between clinical supervision and consultation (Knoff, 1988). A competent play therapist should actively consult with other play therapists with the goal of maintaining the highest standards of care with clients. However, the assumption in consultation is that the competent play therapist is consulting with other competent play therapists to consider options, test hypotheses, ask relevant questions, etc. Play therapists often consult when they are providing competent care but would like to be more expert. In contrast, play therapists seek clinical supervision when they are working outside the boundaries of their competence. In these cases, the play therapist is working under the supervision of a competent play therapist supervisor. The supervisor is advising, coaching, and guiding the play therapist supervisee's work and taking responsibility for the play therapy the supervisee is conducting. If Julie decides that she is competent to take this referral, she might regularly consult with another competent play therapist who also has experience with these issues. In contrast, if Julie decides she is not competent to take the referral, she might seek supervision from a competent supervisor and take the referral under the supervision of the play therapist supervisor, who will take responsibility for the competent care of the client.

Informed Consent:
What Do Clients Need to Know?

Julie decides to see the client for play therapy. In advance of treating the client, there is a lot that Julie would like for the client and client's family to know. For instance, she wants the client and the client's family to understand the process of play therapy and what it will likely entail. She wants to create a safe and therapeutic relationship with the child. She wants to keep parents informed about the client's progress and any concerns she has about her. She plans to go on vacation for a month in summer. She regularly bills clients if they fail to show up for appointments. She does not socialize with clients or their families. She does not accept social media friend or connection requests from clients or their families. She charges for phone consultations beyond simple rescheduling calls. How much of this information (and what other information) should Julie share with the client and the client's family before play therapy begins? How should she share this information? When should she share it?

Informed consent is the cornerstone of professional ethics, and once again, each discipline's code of ethics addresses it. For instance, the code of ethics of the American Mental Health Counselors Association (AMHCA) states: "Mental health counselors are responsible for making their services readily accessible to clients in a manner that facilitates the clients' abilities to make an informed choice when selecting a provider" (2010, B.2, p. 4). Informed consent may be best understood as a process during which the play therapist "makes readily accessible" the information a client and client's family would need to adequately support their ability to make a choice about treatment options that are in their best interest (Beahrs & Gutheil, 2001). Said another way, the intent of informed consent is to inform the client of what to expect during the process of therapy, and other treatment options, so that the client can make a

free and informed choice about whether or not to enter into the therapeutic contract. The goal is to avoid the situation where the client consents to treatment but would not have consented if all relevant information had been disclosed.

The three traditional elements basic to informed consent are capacity, comprehension, and voluntariness (Corey, Corey, & Callanan, 2011). *Capacity* refers to the client's ability to make rational decisions. In the case of play therapy, because the client is typically a minor, the child client does not have the capacity to make decisions about his or her own care. Therefore, legal consent is required from a parent or legal guardian. When working with a child of divorced or unmarried parents, the play therapist would be well advised to consider state laws regarding custody and the rights of parents. It is often the case in divorce that one parent has medical decision-making rights, which means that the therapist must obtain consent from that parent. Other states allow either parent to consent to treatment regardless of custody. The play therapist may even be confronted with a situation in which the parent bringing the child for therapy does not know the legal details of the custody arrangement. In those sticky situations it is prudent to have the parent bring a copy of the custody arrangement in order to be certain that consent is given by the appropriate party.

Although a minor child cannot give legal consent to participate in play therapy, the client can assent (Welfel, 2010). Welfel (2010) defined *assent* as the involvement of children in decisions about their own care in the agreement of whether or not to participate in counseling. She is careful to point out that this assent is supplemental to parental consent. Since Julie has decided to accept the play therapy referral, she will need to obtain informed consent from the client's parent or legal guardian and assent from the client before beginning treatment. Obtaining assent from the child contributes to the therapeutic alliance and to engaging the child in the therapeutic process.

The second element of informed consent is comprehension (Corey et al., 2011). *Comprehension* of informed consent implies that clients have received adequate information, communicated in ways they can understand, to make an informed choice about therapy. For instance, to provide adequate information, play therapists would outline their background and training and the services in which they are competent (e.g., graduate degrees, relevant license, RPT status, competence or expertise in the treatment of presenting problems and concerns). Similarly, play therapists inform prospective clients about issues including, but not limited to, other treatment options, the limits of confidentiality, dual relationships, and fee structures and payment. The key feature to keep in mind about comprehension is that the information must be conveyed to clients in such a way that they understand the contract involved in the therapeutic agreement.

In informed consent, the play therapist is mandated to provide prospective clients and their families with adequate information to make an informed choice about engaging in play therapy. Extensive and somewhat varied lists of the information that should be included are available. For example, Pope and Vasquez (2010) suggest that the therapist can evaluate the adequacy of informed consent if, after consent has been attained, the prospective client understands the following information: who is providing the service and the clinician's qualifications, as well as the nature, extent, and possible consequences of the services the clinician is offering. The prospective client would also understand the degree to which there may be alternatives to the services provided by the clinician, the actual or potential limitations to the services, and the ways services could be terminated. Finally, for informed consent to be adequate, the client would understand all fee policies and procedures, the implications of missed or canceled appointments, all policies and procedures concerning access to the therapist, and the limits and exceptions to confidentiality, privilege, and privacy. Although this list seems extensive, it doesn't include a discussion of the implications of formal psychiatric diagnosis, dealing with managed care, and a number of other potentially important issues that many people believe ought to be included in informed consent. As in most ethical situations, the burden is on the play therapist to decide what information is adequate to ensure that potential clients and their families have what they need to truly consent to services.

One helpful consideration in the process of informed consent is to frame it as an ongoing process rather than a one-time event (Fisher & Oransky, 2008). Although it is generally considered the standard of care to have a written informed consent statement that the client can read, sign, and take a copy for future reference, it is also helpful to think of the informed consent process as ongoing (Pope & Vasquez, 2010).

As an established play therapist, Julie likely has a document explaining how she conducts therapy, how she can be reached, the process for making and cancelling appointments, payment procedures, confidentiality, and more. It is also likely that Julie's goal in the document is to provide potential clients with all the information they would need to make an informed choice about whether to begin play therapy. Consistent with the ethical code of the American Psychological Association (APA), Julie will need to take care that the information conveyed is in a form that is "reasonably understandable" (2010, 3.10, p. 6). However, simply having adequate information clearly communicated in a document that is signed by the client may not truly represent comprehension. For instance, when locating appropriate services, the parents of play therapy clients are not at their best because they are concerned about their children. As a result, they may not fully comprehend all of the information presented in a document or a one-time conversation with a play therapist. The best way to confirm that parents have comprehended the information is to revisit important points throughout the process of play therapy. Reviewing information in the service of informed consent can be a natural part of the process with play therapy approaches that include parental consultation as an ongoing part of therapy (Kottman, 2011), but may need to be more intentional for play therapists using approaches with less emphasis on ongoing parental consultation.

The third component of informed consent is voluntariness (Corey et al., 2010). *Voluntariness* means that the person who has given consent has done so freely and without compulsion or deception. Voluntariness also implies that the person giving consent understands that he or she is free to withdraw consent to play therapy at any time. When considering formal informed consent, the issue of voluntariness in play therapy is relatively straightforward. However, cases of court-mandated play therapy add a level of complexity and raise issues of voluntariness, as parents may be responding to the directive of the court rather than being self-directed.

An additional complicating issue is the role of voluntariness in the assent of the child play therapy client. If the parents of the child have given informed consent, some compulsion seems inherent in the client's being asked to give assent for the treatment. Parekh (2007) noted that "a child can consent to treatment but usually in practice is unable to refuse it" (p. 78). As a result, play therapists should take particular care in eliciting the voluntary assent of the child client in addition to the voluntary consent of the parent/guardian.

Confidentiality: What, If Anything, Do I Tell to Whom . . . and When?

Julie has developed a good relationship with Charisse, her play therapy client, who has been a willing participant in therapy and engaged in the process. Charisse's parents have been pleased with the therapy and believe that she is doing well. However, recently the parents have pressed Julie to know exactly what Charisse has said about their family, etc. Julie has tried to speak generally about the themes of the client's play and to remind the parents of how helpful to the process of play therapy it is to respect Charisse's privacy and the confidential nature of their work together. However, the parents continue to press for detail.

No discussion of play therapy ethics is complete without a consideration of confidentiality—a fundamental maxim of ethical therapy identified and discussed in all of the major mental health ethical codes (e.g., ACA, 2005; APA, 2010; NASW, 2008) as well as the practice guidelines for play therapy (APT, 2009). In mental health settings *confidentiality* refers to the rules and standards that protect clients from disclosure of private information gathered in the clinical setting (Smith-Bell & Winslade, 1994). Confidentiality is foundational in mental health and play therapy ethics because it is a "hallmark of the therapeutic relationship, a sine qua non for successful therapy, and the cornerstone of therapeutic trust" (Parsi, Winslade, & Coracoran, 1995, p. 78).

Parsi and colleagues (1995) noted that there are three elements to confidentiality in therapy. These include (1) information that is private to the client, (2) disclosure of information from the client to a therapist, and (3) expectation of nondisclosure by the therapist to a third party. As we have discussed earlier, the application of more straightforward ethical tenets to work with adult clients in counseling or psychotherapy become much more complex in the application to play therapy practice. As Sweeney (2001) concisely put it, "Confidentiality with children can be challenging" (p. 67).

One of the challenging aspects of confidentiality with child play therapy clients is the question of obligation. The obligation of confidentiality typically implies that the therapist owes the obligation to the person or persons who have given informed consent to therapy. As we noted when we discussed informed consent, there are limits to confidentiality in the practice of play therapy. For instance, play therapists, as licensed or otherwise credentialed professionals, usually have a legal obligation to disclose the reasonable suspicion of child abuse. There are typically other limits to confidentiality (e.g., disclosure to insurance companies and third-party payers) that the therapist will make clear to the client so that the client can make an informed decision about whether to begin therapy and disclose private information. This explanation of confidentiality and its limits is made to the person or persons who are considering giving consent to therapy. This situation is obviously made more complex in the application to play therapy where the client receiving the therapy gives assent, rather than consent, and those who give consent are not the ones actually participating in play therapy and disclosing private information.

In our example, Julie, after accepting the play therapy referral, has received informed consent from the client's parents and informed assent from the child client to proceed in therapy. In the informed consent process, Julie has explained and documented that the private information gathered from the client and her family is confidential within certain boundaries (e.g., disclosures that are required or permitted by law). Julie also explained that information she gathers directly from the child client in play therapy is confidential (e.g., will not be disclosed to third parties except in cases where it is permitted or required by law). Finally, in the informed assent process, Julie has explained to the child client that the private information the child discloses in play therapy will not be disclosed to others outside her family. This raises a potential tension in confidentiality with play therapy clients and their parents. Is all of the information disclosed by the child client in play therapy always available to the parent(s) who has given legal consent for treatment?

In considering this tension around confidentiality and treating child clients, Lawrence and Robinson-Kurpius (2000) noted, "The basic dilemma with respect to confidentiality is who is the client, the parent or the child?" (p. 131). In many cases, the law identifies the parents as the client, in that the obligation of confidentiality is to the parents. Since the parents of the client are empowered to give informed consent for treatment of the child, they also have a legal right to all information gathered in play therapy sessions. Although this is the generally accepted status of most play therapy clients, play therapists who are school counselors may have the additional complication that their state laws may protect the confidentiality of the student seeing a counselor. As a result, school counselors must be familiar with local statutes in determining the boundaries of confidentiality to understand where their obligation of confidentiality rests: with the child or with the parents (Mitchell, Disque, & Robertson, 2002).

Whereas the law may mandate that confidentiality is owed to the parents alone, there are a number of additional considerations for the play therapist in protecting the privacy of the client. These include questions of how to best ensure a safe and therapeutic setting for the child to engage in play therapy, respecting the client's privacy, while still honoring the role of parents and their care and concern for their child. Goldberg (1997) suggested that confidentiality be discussed in the first session of therapy with the parents and the child together. At this time, the play therapist can highlight the importance of creating a safe and trusting atmosphere for the child in therapy, encourage the parents to respect the child's need for privacy, and reassure the parents that the play therapist will inform them of progress, concerns, and other pertinent information as developmentally appropriate.

This discussion highlights the integral connection between confidentiality and informed consent. Clarifying the obligation, boundaries, and exceptions of confidentiality is critical at the outset of therapy and is an excellent example of the kind of information that is best reintroduced throughout the course of play therapy. In addition, both parents and child clients need to be informed when and how confidentiality will be broken, either because of client permission (e.g., disclosure to insurance company) or mandated by law (e.g., mandatory reporting of the reasonable suspicion of child abuse). In either case, informed consent helps clients and their families anticipate how the play therapist will protect their confidentiality.

Multiple Relationships: Can't We All Just Be Friends?

Julie's play therapy with Charisse is going well. Charisse's parents have been responsive in parental consultation and have communicated that they are very pleased with Julie's work with Charisse, adding that Julie has also been helpful to them as parents. At the conclusion of a recent play therapy consultation with Charisse's parents, they give Julie a written invitation to a party they are giving to celebrate Charisse's birthday. They indicate that there will be numerous adults and children there, and that they are inviting people who are important in Charisse's life. They add that they have thought carefully about this and want to communicate, through the invitation, how valuable they think Julie has been to Charisse this year. Should Julie attend?

Even though Julie's invitation to the party is because of her role as Charisse's play therapist, to attend the party could be reasonably considered as the establishment of another relationship (e.g., more personal than professional) with the client. If Julie decides to attend, she might be described as having multiple relationships with the client. Julie's primary professional identity (e.g., psychologist, counselor, social worker) is of particular import in this situation as there are some subtle differences in how the ethical codes of different professional organizations address multiple relationships.

The ethical code of the APA states that a multiple relationship occurs when a clinician has a professional role with a client at the same time as he or she has another relationship with the person, or a person closely associated or related to the client, or when he or she has promised to enter into another relationship with the client or client's relative at some time in the future (APA, 2010). The code goes on to clarify that a clinician "refrains from entering into a multiple relationship if the multiple relationship could reasonably be expected to impair the psychologist's objectivity, competence, or effectiveness in performing his or her functions as a psychologist, or otherwise risks exploitation or harm to the person with whom the professional relationship exists. Multiple relationships that would not reasonably be expected to cause impairment or risk exploitation or harm are not unethical" (3.05, p. 6). Similarly, the NASW ethical code indicates that "social workers should not engage in dual or multiple relationships with clients or former clients in which there is a risk of exploitation or potential harm to the client" (1.06c, p. 3). The ethical code of the American Association of Marriage and Family Therapy (AAMFT) also addresses multiple relationships: "Therapists, therefore, make every effort to avoid conditions and multiple relationships with clients that could impair professional judgment or increase the risk of exploitation" (2012, 1.3, p. 2).

Kitchener (1988) identified three potential factors in multiple relationships that might result in harm to clients: (1) the incompatibility of expectations between the roles associated with each relationship, (2) the divergence of the obligations associated with the roles, and (3) the potential impact of the power and prestige of the mental health professional. If Julie were a psychologist, social worker, or marriage and family therapist, she could evaluate the implications of accepting this invitation based on Kitchener's factors to determine if there was the potential for impairment, exploitation, or harm. She could then decide whether or not to attend.

The ethical code of the ACA offers a somewhat different perspective on multiple relationships. According to the ACA code, "Counselor–client nonprofessional relationships with clients, former clients, their romantic partners, or their family members should be avoided, except when the interaction is potentially beneficial to the client" (2005, A.5.c, p. 5). The code goes on to say that if a counselor decides to engage in a potentially beneficial relationship, he or she must document in case records prior to the interaction, the rationale for the interaction and potential benefits and consequences of the dual relationship. If Julie were a counselor, she would need to evaluate the potential consequences and benefits of accepting the invitation. If she determined that accepting the invitation was potentially beneficial to the client, and that potential benefit outweighed potential risks of impairment, exploitation, or harm, she would need to document her rationale for accepting the invitation and the potential benefits and consequences in advance of attending.

Although all of the ethical codes are clear about prohibiting current and future sexual relationships with clients, there is less clarity around other potential relationships and roles. Herlihy and Corey (2006) noted that possible dual relationships between clinicians and clients range from those that have little potential for harm to those that are potentially extremely harmful. The play therapist needs to examine the potential benefits and potential harm to the child client and the parents in all decision-making processes regarding multiple relationships. One of the key consid-

erations here is "potential harm," as we can never fully predict or consider all the possible consequences of decisions related to multiple roles. Through the process of informed consent, as discussed earlier, play therapists can help children and parents understand the professional role of the play therapist and the limitations that places on other potential roles.

Ethical Decision Making: How Do I Decide?

Ethical codes published by professional organizations generally provide clear guidelines for mental health service providers. However, it is impossible to address all possible ethical scenarios. As a result, clinicians are regularly faced with circumstances not directly addressed in ethical codes. Therapists may encounter situations in which ethical standards appear to conflict with one another, with laws, or with organizational policies. In recent years, there has been much discussion of ethical decision-making models to guide professionals through an informed process so that they can make clear and intentional decisions. There are many ethical decision models to help facilitate a balanced ethical decision-making process (e.g., Koocher & Keith-Spiegel, 2008; Wilcoxon, Remley, & Gladding, 2013).

Based on their analysis of several ethical decision-making models, Corey and colleagues (2011, pp. 21–23) developed a model for ethical decision making for mental health clinicians. The eight steps of their model are:

1. Identify the problem or dilemma.
2. Identify the potential issues involved.
3. Review the relevant ethical guidelines.
4. Know the applicable laws and regulations.
5. Obtain consultation.
6. Consider possible and probable courses of action.

7. Enumerate consequences of various courses of action.
8. Decide on what appears to be the best course of action.

This integrative model is largely consistent with other models in the mental health field and, like other models, suggests a careful consideration of the ethical guidelines of a clinician's primary professional identity (e.g., counselor, psychologist, social worker, marriage and family therapist). Play therapists can apply this model (or other general ethical decision-making models) to the practice of play therapy in conjunction with a review of APT's practice guidelines (2009) to help address the issues and concerns specific to the practice of play therapy.

Although models such as Corey and colleagues' (2011) can be applied to play therapy settings, a number of authors (e.g., Jackson, 1998; Jackson, Puddy, & Lazicki-Puddy, 2001; Sweeney, 2001) have called for an ethical decision-making model specific to play therapy. Seymour and Rubin (2006) proposed an ethical decision-making model for play therapists from all disciplines, allowing them to apply their more generic ethical code to specific dilemmas faced in play therapy. Recognizing that many of the decision-making models are linear in design and that ethical questions faced by play therapists do not often fit a linear model, the authors designed a model that is more dynamically driven. Their model, called the *Principles, Principals, Process Model* (P³ Model), "combines the historical ethics codes (*Principles*) of the professional disciplines providing play therapy with the contemporary voices of all the persons (*Principals*) involved in the ethics circumstance through dialogue (*Process*)" (p. 106). The P³ Model is based on the conceptualization of psychotherapy (to include play therapy) that is fundamentally relational and acknowledges that consideration of social context is critical in ethical decision making. The model is designed to consider the a priori principles that apply to a situation as well as the contextual factors.

In applying the P³ Model to address a potential ethical dilemma in our example above, Julie would first identify and consider all of the relevant principles. These would include the historical principles of autonomy, nonmalfeasance, beneficence, fidelity, and justice. These principles would serve as a starting point for Julie as she also considers relevant guidelines from the ethical codes of her discipline, any relevant laws or instructive case law, and any other guidelines such as clinic or school policies.

Once Julie has carefully considered all of the principles relevant to the situation, she would then identify all of the principals involved. Julie would consider herself, as therapist; Charisse, the child client; Charisse's parents; and what Seymour and Rubin (2006) call *collateral voices* (e.g., family members, teachers, medical professionals) and the community. After identifying these principals, Julie would review the earlier identified principles from the perspective of each of these principals, getting input directly whenever possible. The P³ Model places special emphasis on the consideration of the client's voice because it highlights the power differential between the child and the play therapist. Finally, the perspective of the community is of particular importance because it would add to Julie's understanding of how cultural influences may impact the therapeutic relationship and frame any ethical decision.

In the final step of the P³ Model, Julie would begin the process of engaging the principles and principals in dialogue. In this process, "the therapist facilitates a recursive dialogue concerning the principles, with the principals, to develop a shared understanding that will inform an ethical decision" (Seymour & Rubin, 2006, p. 110). Using this P³ Model, Julie would arrive at a course of ethical action that considers both the historical and ethical principles guiding her primary mental health identity, the context of the particular situation, and the specific practice of play therapy.

Conclusion

This chapter has provided a brief overview of four important issues relevant to play therapy: establishing competence, providing informed consent, protecting confidentiality, and evaluating multiple relationships. The above discussion is not comprehensive, nor is this a complete list of ethical issues relevant to the practice of play therapy. Instead, we hoped to explore the treatment of these four issues in a way that could guide play therapists in their consideration of other relevant issues and related areas that were not discussed. The chapter also provided examples of a general model and a model specific to play therapy specific for ethical decision making as a means of illustrating how play therapists can best arrive at ethical decisions.

Ultimately, play therapists are committed to helping children. Using children's natural medium of communication, play therapists attempt to facilitate the welfare and well-being of their young clients. As Sweeney (2001) noted, practicing play therapy in an ethical manner is a natural extension of the practice of play therapy, and ultimately guides the play therapist to act in the best interest of children. By considering the issues raised in this chapter and the careful use of an ethical decision-making model, we hope you will continue to successfully promote the best interests of children.

REFERENCES

American Association of Marriage and Family Therapy. (2012). *AAMFT code of ethics*. Alexandria, VA: Author.

American Counseling Association. (2005). *ACA code of ethics and standards of practice*. Alexandria, VA: Author.

American Mental Health Counselors. (2010). *Principles for AMHCA code of ethics*. Alexandria, VA: Author.

American Psychological Association. (2010). *Ethical principles of psychologists and code of conduct*. Washington, DC: Author.

Arcelus, J., Mitchell, A. J., Wales, J., & Nielsen, S. (2011). Mortality rates in patients with anorexia nervosa and other eating disorders: A meta-analysis of 36 studies. *Archives of General Psychiatry, 68*, 724–731.

Association for Play Therapy. (2009). *Play therapy best practices*. Fresno, CA: Author.

Barber J. P., Sharpless B. A., Klostermann S., & McCarthy, K. S. (2007). Assessing intervention competence and its relation to therapy outcome: A selected review derived from the outcome literature. *Professional Psychology: Research and Practice, 38*, 493–500.

Beahrs, J. O., & Gutheil, T. G. (2001). Informed consent in psychotherapy. *American Journal of Psychiatry, 158*, 4–10.

Carmichael, K. D. (2006). Legal and ethical issues in play therapy. *International Journal of Play Therapy, 15*(2), 83–99.

Corey, G., Corey, M. S., & Callanan, P. (2011). *Issues and ethics in the helping professions* (8th ed.). Belmont, CA: Brooks/Cole.

Doverspike, W. F. (1999). *Ethical risk management: Guidelines for practice*. Sarasota, FL: Professional Resource Press.

Fairburn, C. G., & Cooper, Z. (2011). Therapist competence, therapy quality, and therapist training. *Behaviour Research and Therapy, 49*(6–7), 373–378.

Fisher, C. B., & Oransky, M. (2008). Informed consent to psychotherapy: Protecting the dignity and respecting the autonomy of patients. *Journal of Clinical Psychology, 64*, 576–588.

Goldberg, R. (1997). Ethical dilemmas in working with children and adolescents. In D. T. Marsh & R. Magee (Eds.), *Ethical and legal issues in professional practice with families* (pp. 97–111). Toronto: Wiley.

Herlihy, B., & Corey, G. (2006). *ACA ethical standards casebook* (6th ed.). Alexandria, VA: American Counseling Association.

Jackson, Y. (1998). Applying APA ethical guidelines to individual play therapy with children. *International Journal of Play Therapy, 7*, 1–15.

Jackson, Y., Puddy, R., & Lazicki-Puddy, T. (2001). Ethical practices reported by play therapists: An outcome study. *International Journal of Play Therapy, 10*, 31–51.

Kitchener, K. S. (1988). Dual role relationships: What makes them so problematic? *Journal of Counseling and Development, 67,* 217–221.

Knoff, H. M. (1988). Clinical supervision, consultation, and counseling: A comparative analysis for supervisors and other educational leaders. *Journal of Curriculum and Supervision, 3,* 240–252.

Koocher, G. P., & Keith-Spiegel, P. (2008). *Ethics in psychology and the mental health professions: Standards and cases* (3rd ed.). New York: Oxford University Press.

Kottman, T. (2011). *Play therapy: Basics and beyond* (2nd ed.). Alexandria, VA: American Counseling Association.

Lawrence, G., & Robinson-Kurpius, S. E. (2000). Legal and ethical issues involved when counseling minors in nonschool settings. *Journal of Counseling and Development, 78,* 130–137.

Mitchell, C. W., Disque, J. G., & Robertson, P. (2002). When parents want to know: Responding to parental demands for confidential information. *Professional School Counseling, 6,* 151–161.

National Association of Social Workers (NASW). (2008). *Code of ethics.* Washington, DC: Author.

Parekh, S. A. (2007). Child consent and the law: An insight and discussion into the law relating to consent and competence. *Child: Care, Health, and Development, 33,* 78–82.

Parsi, K. P., Winslade, W. J., & Coracoran, K. (1995). Does confidentiality have a future?: The computer-based patient record and managed mental health care. *Trends in Health Care Law Ethics, 10*(1–2), 78–82.

Pope, K. S., & Vasquez, M. J. T. (2010). *Ethics in psychotherapy and counseling: A practical guide.* San Francisco: Jossey-Bass.

Seymour, J. W., & Rubin, L. (2006). Principles, principals, and process (P³): A model for play therapy ethics problem solving. *International Journal of Play Therapy, 15,* 101–123.

Smith-Bell, M., & Winslade, W. (1994). Privacy, confidentiality, and privilege in psychotherapeutic relationships. *American Journal of Orthopsychiatry, 64,* 180–183.

Sue, D. W., Arrendondo, P., & McDavis, R. J. (1992). Multicultural counseling competencies and standards: A call to the profession. *Journal of Counseling and Development, 70,* 477–486.

Sweeney, D. (2001). Legal and ethical issues in play therapy. In G. Landreth (Ed.), *Innovations in play therapy: Issues, process, and special populations* (pp. 65–81). New York: Brunner-Routledge.

Thompson-Brenner, H., Satif, D. A., Franko, D. L., & Herzog, D. B. (2012). Clinician reactions to patients with eating disorders: A review of the literature. *Psychiatric Services, 63,* 73–78).

Welfel, E. R. (2010). *Ethics in counseling and psychotherapy: Standards, research and emerging issues* (4th ed.). Pacific Grove, CA: Brooks/Cole.

Wilcoxin, S. A., Remley, T. P., Jr., & Gladding, S. T. (2013). *Ethical, legal, and professional issues in the practice of marriage and family therapy* (5th ed.). Upper Saddle River, NJ: Pearson.

CHAPTER 36

Exploring the Neuroscience of Healing Play at Every Age

Bonnie Badenoch
Theresa Kestly

The image of 5-year-old Julia[1] peeking out from behind her mother's skirt fit perfectly with the way her parents described her when we met a week earlier to talk about their highly anxious daughter. Mrs. McKeen was worried that something was terribly wrong with Julia, and she felt guilty because she believed that somehow her own serious bout with cancer had affected her daughter. In addition to being concerned about his daughter, Mr. McKeen felt that Julia's anxious and clinging behaviors were adding an unbearable burden to his wife's fragile recovery. They both made it clear to me that they would do whatever was necessary to help Julia change her behavior. They had already pursued a number of avenues, including parenting classes and educating themselves on child development, but they felt stuck. The father said, "Nothing seems to work. We need some professional expertise, and we came to you because a close friend told us that play therapy might help."

When Julia came with her mother for her first play therapy session, we talked for a few minutes in the consultation room until I (Kestly) could sense that Julia might be willing to go with me to see the playroom. When I asked her if she wanted to see it, she glanced at me, and then quickly looked away. As we entered the playroom, however, I could see her body relax slightly, and then stiffen again when I said, "This is a place where you and I can spend some special time together. Is there anything here that looks interesting to you?" She looked at me again, a little longer this time, and I could feel her searching my face for presence, as if to say, "Will you stay with me? Do you notice that I am scared and hurting?"

Having Julia look deeply at my face that way, and sensing her parents' urgent need for her to feel more secure so that she could move out into the world with confidence and joy, I was aware of a slight tension arising in my body. I really wanted to get this right. I took a slightly longer breath and reminded myself that I could count on several principles that we are beginning to understand from the field of relational neuroscience. Julia's SEEKING and PLAY circuits[2] (two of the seven emotional–motivational circuits identified by neuroscientist Jaak Panksepp [Panksepp & Biven, 2012]) were already present within her system, and they would be available for healing purposes if I could provide the safe presence of CARE, another emotional system identified by Panksepp, that allows us to connect deeply with one another. With the natural interweaving of these subcortical systems at Julia's growing edge, I believed that my support in our relational play could help her express and then coregulate her painful implicit memories of the early sense of abandonment she experienced due to her mother's illness, in collaboration with her brain's natural push toward wholeness (Siegel, 2012). These relationally supported changes would gradually make room for a more permanent shift in her behavior, whereas simply addressing the behaviors would leave these underlying implicit memories in place to arise in times of stress. As I settled into this perspective, my body relaxed, an easy smile came to my face, and with her next glance, Julia's body was able to follow mine in forming an initial connection between us.

Why Study Neuroscience?

It might seem like the rigors of learning about relational neuroscience and the free-flowing joy of play therapy have little to do with each other. However, as we begin to understand that in the midst of play, neurotransmitters move toward balance, belly brains relax, heart brains learn something wonderful about relationships, autonomic nervous systems find easy access to the branch that allows us to connect with one another, and old memories of trauma and loss can surface and be reworked, then we can begin to confidently settle into supporting people of all ages in this most joyous of all manifestations of mental health. Cultivating a felt sense of the neurobiology that underlies play can give us the confidence to talk with parents and teachers about the value of play therapy as an optimal means for children to find their way back to a healthy developmental path, even when there has been trauma or other forms

of challenge. A secure foundation here can also help us recognize and support the emergence of playfulness in our work with clients of every age. It may even be possible that these discoveries about how our brains and minds are continually being modified in our connection to one another in play can become a solid scientific base for including this way of being together in all areas of our therapeutic work.

With these intentions in the background, let's explore some of the main strands of relational neuroscience that illuminate play therapy. We're going to begin with some basic principles and then look at how play makes the most of what we know about how the developing brain heals. We consider how the growing awareness of the following areas can support our playful work with children and adults: (1) the brain as a system that is always moving toward greater integration; (2) the nature of implicit memory and how it can change; (3) how presence itself is the foundation on which all else rests; (4) the role of the autonomic nervous system in providing safety; and (5) the neural circuitry of play itself, buried deep in the roots of our brains.

Relational Foundations of Healing Play

Let's begin with the first few moments with Julia. When she glanced up at me, looked away, and then looked back for a little longer, what might she have been seeking? Most likely, her nervous system was rapidly assessing whether this could be a safe place or not. For we humans, safety is supported when we can connect with someone who is present without judgments or expectations, someone who can receive us just as we are. We can check this out for ourselves by running quickly through our last several encounters with others and sensing what happened in our bodies. We might notice that when we felt the other person had an agenda, our bodies—perhaps beginning with our bellies—began to tighten and withdraw from vulnerability. When we felt open curiosity and warm acceptance, relaxation may have begun to move through our system and we more easily stepped into our own vulnerability within the shelter of safe relatedness. Since Julia was not familiar with me, it was especially important for her to feel my welcoming and warm presence. As part of our flexible and adaptive natures, all of us are continually seeking the warmest attachments we can imagine (based on both our previous experiences and our genetically based propensity to move toward safe proximity with each other), so in a way, Julia's system was primed to be both cautious *and* available for connection at the same time. These bonds begin with a very rapid conversation below the level of conscious awareness between my state of being and hers.

Two states of mind can help create the foundation for offering this kind of presence: a felt sense that, regardless of current behaviors, everyone is adapting as best they can, given their neurobiological makeup and the kind of support they are receiving; and that letting go of an agenda for change actually creates space for change to happen. Even coming from a paradigm that is often identified with goals and treatment plans, Semple, Lee, Williams, and Teasdale, authors of *Mindfulness-Based Cognitive Therapy for Anxious Children* (2011), write, "The most difficult component of MBCT-C (Mindfulness-Based Cognitive Therapy for Children) for a conventionally trained therapist may be to abandon the desire for change. Letting go of the desire to change may in itself catalyze significant changes" (p. 3). Our systems know how to find their way when they are given space, time, and abundant support, and often tighten down when there is a sense that the other person needs us to be a certain way. This is one reason that therapy centering on behavior change rather than relationship can have mixed long-term results.

Complex Systems and Constraints

What would relational neuroscience have to say about these two foundational states of mind? It tells us that our brains are complex systems that are self-organizing, always on the move toward greater integration and coherence within the limits of whatever constraints are on the system (Siegel, 2012). This integrating process is something we can trust. *Constraints* are encoded prior experiences that guide our perceptions and expectations in a particular direction. If we have had a warm, secure entry into this life, these constraints will guide us toward continuing to find similar relational experiences as we move down our developmental path. On the other hand, if our early days were marked by various kinds of pain and fear within our relationships, those constraints will color our current experiences with a similar felt sense, will likely leave us hypersensitive to anything that resembles our embodied memories, and will guide our behaviors in response to these engrained patterns. As we develop greater trust that the complex brains of our clients of all ages will integrate as these constraints change—with the support of a safe, accepting relationship—it can become easier to release our agendas to make room for each person's system to unfold with the guidance of its own wisdom.

Julia's earliest life was marked by her mother's continuing illness, which meant long separations and care by many others, who, although meaning well, were not able to focus on her legitimate emotional need for continuity, proximity, understanding, and reassurance. These continually shifting connections frightened her in the midst of dealing with the grief of separation from her beloved mother. Now her system was constrained in such a way that she was continually on the lookout for the next relational loss, leading to clinging, crying, and sometimes anger at home. As she looked toward me, she needed to sense that I could accept her in this moment just as she is. If she saw in my face any need for her to be different or any sense that she is broken or defective, our connection would lack the nurturing soil it needed to begin to take root. If instead she could see welcome and openness to who she is *right now*, she might begin to hope that this could be different. Given the magnitude of her earlier experience, it might take some time for her system to begin to *expect* that this relationship could be stable and consistent; however, if she encountered the same receptivity visit after visit, deep within her most core implicit structure, shifts would be possible.

In addition to awareness of these constraints, I could also feel her parents' urgent need for Julia to feel more secure and less clingy, springing from their love for her, but knew if I embodied that same urgency in our play therapy, Julia would feel it, perhaps below the level of conscious awareness, and would begin to tighten in protection. We have more to say about this autonomic nervous system process later on, but for the moment, we can likely each feel our embodied response to urgency within our own systems. Another's anxious need for us to change communicates that something is wrong, and that felt sense activates our nervous system. If instead we sense that the other person understands the protective wisdom in the way our systems have adapted to circumstance, our bodies have room to relax into greater openness. With Julia, it was easy for me to feel the appropriateness of her anxious expectation of loss, so, trusting her system's ability to find its way, I could let go of urgency. Within our growing connection, her constraints could shift at their own pace, and her brain and body could begin to find a way toward greater integration. I was confident that as this implicit foundation changed, her behaviors would start to change as well to align with her greater sense of security. When we feel connected and safe, the need to cling recedes (Panksepp & Biven, 2012).

Implicit Memory and the Core Process of Change

Our understanding of how we shape one another's brains and minds from before birth until our last breath is the focus of *interpersonal* neurobiology (IPNB; Schore, 2012; Siegel, 2012), a scientifically grounded paradigm of how change is possible within secure relationships. This paradigm focuses on what unfolds in the space between people, and lets us know about the power of being present, while our clients of any age follow the guidance of their naturally integrating brains toward health, well-being, and the emerging capacity for warm relationships. In the micro-second interactions between us, there is the possibility that our systems will come into resonance with our clients' in a way that they will feel seen and heard at a depth that allows their embodied memories of pain and fear to come into the room—one essential step on the way to transformation (Schore, 2012). At that point, if we meet them with what they needed, but didn't receive, at the time of the original experience, the circuitry holding that old implicit memory can open to receive new energy and information, changing the felt sense of that memory, even though the explicit memory doesn't change (Ecker, Ticic, Hulley, & Neimeyer, 2012).

The Relationship between Implicit Memory and Behavior

Let's explore this core pattern of change more fully. Our first question might concern what actually needs to shift within our play therapy clients for them to move into new patterns of experiencing and behavior. The struggles that manifest themselves as ways of behaving (clinging and anger, in Julia's case) are rooted in the implicit patterns that accumulate as we move through our lives. Implicit memory is embodied memory, made up of the *bodily sensations, emotional surges, behavioral impulses, percep-*

tions, and *sensory fragments* that are encoded as part of all our experiences (Badenoch, 2011). When our brains are new in this world, the neurons in the limbic region and neocortex are largely undifferentiated. This means that they are not connected to each other; the experience of our earliest relationships is needed to create these connections and the patterns they will hold. We certainly arrive here with genetic and epigenetic predispositions and temperament, which then encounter the relational world. For the first 12–18 months of life, the only kind of memories we make are implicit ones (Siegel, 2012), anchored in the limbic region, and receiving input from the belly and heart brains, as well as the subcortical regions that hold our primary emotions (Panksepp & Biven, 2012). These embodied implicit memories, when repeated often enough, become what we might call *embodied anticipations* about how life will unfold for us (Badenoch, 2013).

For Julia, the pattern of "my mother's here–my mother's gone" was repeated many times in her first 3 years, often with a sense of emergency because her mother was so ill. Because everyone was legitimately caught up in this stressful situation, Julia's frightening and grief-filled experiences were not met with sustained acknowledgment, understanding, and comfort. Trauma arises not from what happens to us, but from no one being truly present with us to help us integrate the experience (Dobbs, 2012). As a result, Julia's implicit memory of these repeated losses became wired in as an embodied anticipation that all relationships are dangerous and painful sometimes, but also wonderful and nurturing at other times, and that loss can happen unexpectedly at any moment. We can each perhaps sense anxiety in the form of hypervigilance in our own bodies as we feel into her experience.

Unlike explicit memory (our narrative recall that something happened in the past and has a beginning, middle, and end), implicit memory, when it is reawakened, is never experienced as being in the past. Instead, it comes up in our bodies as though it were happening right this minute. We can test this right now by taking a few moments to remember something pleasant that happened in the last couple of weeks. If we sit with this memory for a few moments, we may notice that we *know* this event happened a while ago, and that *our bodies* are having the same sensations as though it were happening now. For Julia, any sense that her mother (or anyone) is turning away might activate her implicit memory stream and feel to her as if loss were imminent. Simple daily activities, such as her mother leaving her room at bedtime or dropping her off at school, could invoke the fear and grief that had accumulated in her implicit memories over the course of her early life. Crying and clinging are our natural, healthy responses to fear of loss, as we shall see from Panksepp's work (Panksepp & Biven, 2012).

All of us are continually making new implicit memories with every experience. Unlike explicit memory, which requires conscious attention to encode, implicit memories are neurally engrained without our attention, likely meaning that we are always making more implicit memories than explicit ones, just by being alive within the environment. Also, even if our child or adult clients had fairly secure beginnings, trauma and other challenges later in life can still create implicit streams that can be touched and reawakened by daily events.

What Needs to Change—and How Change Happens

Given all of this, it would seem that what most needs to change is the *embodied subjective sense within the implicit memory,* since that is what continues to come into the present, bringing perceptions, feelings, and behaviors with it. Until recently, we didn't have the science to understand how this kind of change can happen; however, work on memory reconsolidation is providing us with some clues (for a review of the research, see Ecker et al., 2012). It appears that the neural nets holding implicit memory open to new information when two conditions are met: The implicit memory is alive in the body and it is met with what is called a *disconfirming experience*. That is, the implicit memory is met with an embodied experience of what was missing and needed at the time of the original event. If we are frightened, we need safety and protection; if we feel humiliated, we long for acceptance; if we are grief-stricken, our systems yearn for comfort.

In the context of a play therapy relationship that is intent on being alive to the present moment, it is possible for these disconfirming experiences to unfold in the moment-to-moment relational interchange surrounding the arising of these implicit memories. Even in the first moment of meeting with Julia, her glances told me her implicit world was coming alive as I saw both fear and the need for reassurance in her eyes. If I could be a consistent presence for her, both acknowledging the validity of her fear and providing a calm, safe, consistent space, the upwelling of the earlier implicit experiences could be met, over and over, by disconfirmation until they began to settle into a new pattern of security. New neural pathways between her limbic region and prefrontal cortex, particularly in the right hemisphere, would hold this new pattern. As these connections strengthened, a number of capacities would begin to appear in Julia: the ability to pause long enough to choose between possible responses; greater regulation of both her autonomic nervous system and her emotions; a decrease in her felt sense of fear because of the increasing flow of the soothing neurotransmitter gamma-aminobutyric acid (GABA); and a greater capacity to "read" the reassuring messages in the faces of others (Siegel, 2012).

We could ask why this wasn't happening at home since her mother's illness had resolved by the time Julia was 4 years old. I spent time with her parents before and dur-

ing the time I was seeing Julia on her own, and they shared how guilty and sad they both felt that she'd had such a rough start. They both felt so anxious for her to feel safe now, even though they were both still feeling some understandable fear about the possible return of mother's illness. Part of the struggle was that this ongoing fear was alive in the family system and so continuing to touch everyone, even though it wasn't verbalized in Julia's presence. We have such powerful resonance systems that whatever is unfolding in the nervous system of parents is experienced also by the children—and the less it is talked about, the more children inherit the felt sense patterns without being able to understand them.

In addition, daily life often brought the need for Julia and her mother to come together and part—going to school and even going to bed—so the conditions for the activation of her implicit memories were alive in the environment every day and with the very people with whom the original memories had formed. Without an understanding of how implicit memories work, her parents then became upset by Julia's realistic upset—she really couldn't know if her mom would be there in the morning. As a result, they weren't able to provide the calmness and ongoing, repeated reassurance that her system needed to rewire a sense of security.

In our parent meetings, we not only talked about implicit memory, but we also worked with their continuing activation around Mrs. McKeen's illness, so they developed a strong felt sense about how tender these areas of memory continued to be for everyone in the family. I taught them some mindfulness practices for staying in the moment rather than running into the feared future—something our minds tend to do adaptively to prepare us for what may come, but since we can't know the future, may actually undermine our ability to stay present to life now. We also did some sandtray work that allowed both parents to express and release some of the intensity they were still carrying in their bodies, out of conscious awareness, from those 4 years of life-or-death struggle. Mr. and Mrs. McKeen took to the sand and miniatures with ease once they understood that so much of what is encoded in our implicit memories can't be expressed in words. As they placed their hands in the sand, they felt some of the anxiety release into this soothing medium. Choosing the objects by their felt resonance, the themes of these most difficult years gradually unfolded so they could be silently held by the three of us. Sometimes a story in words would also emerge; sometimes the processing was mainly through the free flow of emotions. As the painful experiences became more integrated and settled, their capacity for calmness was restored. Their ability to hold one another soon expanded to their beloved daughter, and we gradually became a supportive team on Julia's behalf.

Healing Play as an Optimal Means for Supporting Change

If the subjective sense of implicit, embodied memories is what needs to change in order for us to have more settled and fulfilling lives, how might play offer optimal conditions for this to happen? Because these memories come up mostly without words, in the present moment, as bodily sensations, emotions, behaviors, and perceptions, what better way for them to come alive than turning a child or adult loose with sand and miniatures or toys of every kind so their systems can have the opportunity to bring the painful and frightening experiences into the play therapy room in a living way—within the embrace of a safe, accepting relationship, which is the essential support. Just catching sight of the resources for play begins to touch the parts of our brain, mostly in the right hemisphere, that hold our unresolved painful or frightening experiences: times when we had big or small traumatic events and no one was

available to see what was happening and to provide witness and comfort.

With the support provided in a secure relationship, children and adults will move naturally toward expressing what is awakening within, using their bodies and whatever play resources are available to share the unseen and heretofore unknown story. Since implicit memories are embodied, mostly below the level of conscious awareness, and without words, the possibility of moving toward them is greatest when the environment provides ways for those memories to "speak" through symbols and actions. Let's turn to an exploration of the neural circuitry of safety and play to broaden our foundation for understanding how play therapy can facilitate these changes.

The Primary Foundation: Safety

As we have already seen, Julia's first need was to find out whether I was going to be a safe companion for her. The work of Stephen Porges (2011) (building on the legacy of Paul MacLean, 1990) illuminates the tripartite autonomic nervous system (ANS) and its role in the experience of safety. Traditionally, the ANS was thought to be composed of two branches: the sympathetic branch, as the accelerator, and the parasympathetic branch, as the brakes. From this perspective, the goal was to keep the two in balance. Instead, Porges's research tells us that the ANS has three branches that are hierarchically arranged so that with increasing "neuroception" of danger, one branch goes offline in favor of the next to ensure our survival. The word *neuroception* was coined by Stephen Porges (2003) to talk about how our ANS, along with several other circuits, can detect danger and safety without our conscious awareness. Before we perceive safe/not safe, a conscious state, our system can "neuroceive" the signal and act on it. The ANS does not operate alone, but works in conjunction with circuits that recognize faces, assess intention, rapidly assess threat, and carry emotionally relevant information from the body to the limbic region—in short, those circuits that alert us to how safe we are with others and the environment (Adolphs, 2002; Critchley, 2005; Morris, Ohman, & Dolan, 1999; Winston, Strange, O'Doherty, & Dolan, 2002).

The Social Engagement System

For we human beings, our nervous system's preferred way of finding and maintaining safety is via connection with others (Beckes & Coan, 2011). Porges (2011) tells us that the first and most preferred system in the ANS hierarchy is the *ventral vagal parasympathetic*, or the social engagement system, a circuit that allows us to settle into relationship with one another—a central requirement for both secure attachment and implicit memory change. This circuit slows the heart (the vagal brake), decreases our fight–flight–freeze response, and reduces cortisol, a stress hormone (Porges, 2011). In short, it prevents the sympathetic branch from taking over. Interestingly, this circuit also reduces inflammation and puts us in a state of growth and restoration.

One person in this state can support regulation for another, even in stressful situations, largely because in the course of mammalian evolution, the ventral vagus became integrated with the circuits that control the muscles of the face and head. These neural pathways regulate eye gaze, prosody, ability to listen, and facial expression—many of the nonverbal ways through which we communicate our connection with each other (Porges, 2011). A calmly beating heart and relaxed yet animated face signals our readiness to engage. Julia's initial glances at my face and eyes were her adaptive way of finding out if this new relationship could possibly provide the safety she needed to allow her inner world to open. She wouldn't consciously have that thought, but if we remember that our complex systems are always seeking greater integration, which is neurobiology's way of understanding healing, we can imagine how her system was look-

ing for the conditions that would make it possible for her earlier traumas to join the stream of integration.

The Neuroception of Danger and Sympathetic Arousal

Julia's life experiences had left her with tenuous access to this state of security and connection. Instead, her nervous system easily moved to a neuroception of danger any time her mother or anyone else left her view. At those moments, her body reflected this shift to activation of the *sympathetic nervous system* with her heart rate increasing, the chemicals needed for protection coming into her system, and the behaviors of crying and clinging appearing as signals of relational distress and calls for help (Panksepp & Biven, 2012; Porges, 2011). In the interests of survival, her rising fear caused the circuits that connected her to her parents to go offline so that she could focus on the perceived threat, and, at the same time, her capacity to take in new information was dramatically reduced. This meant that any attempt by her parents to explain to her that she was safe now could literally not be heard and taken in. Since their nervous systems were similarly activated, it was not possible for Julia to find a safe haven to return to a ventral vagal state that allows soothing connection to emerge.

As her parents and I worked together, they began to see her legitimate cries for help as her implicit memories coming alive rather than as a manifestation of irrational fear, and they became much more able to provide the wordless comfort and connection that her system was seeking for as long as she needed. As they comforted her whenever her fears arose, they found that she could become calm and connected more quickly and easily as time passed and her brain registered the repeated support of disconfirming experiences. In this way, Julia could integrate the old fears, allowing her to begin to have the embodied experience that life is different now.

Helplessness and Dorsal Vagal Collapse

The ANS has a third branch as well. Under dire circumstances, as our neuroception shifts from safety or danger to a felt sense of all-out life threat, brought on by feelings of helplessness, the sympathetic circuit turns off in favor of the second branch of the parasympathetic: the *dorsal vagal*. This branch dramatically reduces heart rate and shuts down other metabolic systems to move into death-feigning behavior—a collapsed state that may be marked by dissociation or a movement into stillness (Porges, 2011). Julia's parents told me that on rare occasions she would move from crying to screaming, and then suddenly fall silent and become what they called "distant." This behavior had bewildered and frightened them, so that they weren't able to use their own ventral vagal state to help her come back into connection. Together, we recognized that at these moments, she moved into a dorsal state as a form of protection from the intolerable anguish of the implicit memories of being separated from her mother—memories that were likely encoded when she was quite small. With this new understanding, they were able to intervene in her distress long before this dissociated collapse became an adaptive necessity for her.

Supporting Connection through Play: Widening the Window of Tolerance

In the playroom, Julia and I had the opportunity to coregulate each other, with my ventral vagal state acting as anchor for our experiences together. One way to picture her ongoing struggle is to say that her earlier life experiences had left her with a narrow *window of tolerance* (Siegel, 2012) for strong emotions, meaning that what might seem like small nudges—her mother turning her back to cook at the stove—could lead to a cascade of large physical and emotional responses. Our window's size reflects the degree of integration between the limbic region of the brain, where our sensitivity to potentially fearful situations is centered, and areas of our prefrontal cortex, particularly the orbitofrontal cortex, that help with calming fear.

By genetic design, these two parts of the brain begin to integrate at about 24 months; however, even in the first few months of life, the foundations for this integration take place in the relationship between a baby and her mothering person. If the mother's brain is well integrated—meaning that she is able to be warmly attuned and responsive to her little one much of the time and to repair ruptures when they inevitably occur—the baby's prefrontal circuitry begins to be prewired for a smooth integration experience toward the end of the second year of life. Because of numerous caregivers she experienced and an ongoing sense of emergency in the home, this didn't happen for Julia, so the connections between these two key brain areas were tenuous and easily ruptured by reminders of loss and abandonment in her current experience. Here in the playroom, we had the opportunity to strengthen those connections just by the way we played together—attuned, responsive, coregulated, leading to an expanding window of tolerance.

"Just Playing" and the Seven Emotional–Motivational Systems

The beauty of "just playing" is that it makes room to recruit the energies of the sympathetic nervous system without leaving the ventral vagal state of safety in connection. Instead of her regular movement into fear and sympathetic arousal, Julia's experience of repeated abandonment could emerge in play and be held within our connected relationship until it found its way to resolution. By our third session, her play was centering around themes of parting. The teddy bear mother left her cub in the snow, or all the hunters on the sandtray shelves took the mother lion and buried her in the sand. I could sense agitation rising in her body, and as I quietly tracked her experience and reflected her play to her, the anxious wave would calm enough to stay within our joined windows of tolerance, so the implicit experience could be met and held within our ventral vagal connection. Through the influence of our resonance circuitry, Julia could use my ANS to calm her own and continue her healing play. She would frequently look up at me as though to say, "We're just playing, right?" She could see my agreement—"Yes, we are just playing"— in my face and eyes, as well as hear it in the sound of my voice, those all-important nonverbal ways we communicate safety to one another (Porges, 2011; Schore, 2012).

Because we were staying in connection, the circuitry of play could remain online and serve as a means to be with these implicit memories in a different way than when Julia was triggered and pulled into sympathetic arousal because of fear. To explore the neural circuitry of play, we can turn to the work of Jaak Panksepp (Panksepp & Biven, 2012), which has illuminated seven primary emotional–motivational systems buried deep in the evolutionary history of the midbrain: SEEKING, CARE/BONDING, PLAY, LUST (arising in adolescence), RAGE, FEAR, and PANIC/GRIEF/SEPARATION DISTRESS. When we feel disconnected from those around us, we will likely feel distress, which generates a need to cling until we feel connected again—a wise adaptive strategy to try to keep the one we need from leaving us. Our SEEKING system uses its resources to find a way back to a safe haven through signaling our pain. If our grief-filled face doesn't bring someone to us, then our fear escalates, and if this isn't enough to draw in the help we need, the frustration of SEEKING with no result generates RAGE. When parents can begin to see these signals—grief and clinging, fear, and rage—as cries for help rather than as bad behavior, they can begin to come toward their children in these moments and provide the all-important disconfirming ex-

periences for which their children's systems are yearning.

Many of the parents who bring their children for play therapy are encountering these signals on a daily basis and want the behavior to change so the suffering will stop. If we begin with correcting the behavior instead of addressing the underlying need for connection, the improvement is likely to be temporary, lasting only until the stresses of disconnection build again and their child's system adaptively calls out for help once more. This expanded perspective can be life-altering information for families.

Connection, Safety, and Play

In the playroom we immediately have the resource of ourselves to begin to meet an upset child's need for connection. Once that relational experience is established, the SEEKING system no longer has to devote its resources to finding a safe haven and can begin to explore what matters most in that child's world at that moment. Once in a felt sense of relationship, the inborn PLAY system comes online to help these little ones (and adults as well) in that creative exploration. If we play therapists have developed some trust that the brain is always moving toward integration, we may be able to relax and be responsive to this person's emerging experience in the certainty that he or she knows just what to do—with support. In working with families from different cultural backgrounds, we may find that the outward norms for playing and relating in general may be different, while also knowing that the underlying systems for play and attachment are similar in all people. Respecting and moving with the outer differences while holding the overall foundational picture can honor both aspects of our systems.

For Julia, repeated experiences of entering these embodied implicit memories within safety and play, and being met with sustained presence and reflection, built those all-important connections between the limbic region and prefrontal cortex that were gradually expanding her window of tolerance, as reflected in her greater capacity for self-regulation. At the same time, she was accumulating a storehouse of disconfirming experiences as my embodied capacity to stay present when she felt abandoned provided what she had needed at the time of the original experience. Because we internalize one another (Badenoch, 2011; Iacoboni, 2009), she was also taking me in as an ongoing inner companion who could help her return to calmness when the old fears might arise. At home, she could count on her parents' support when her implicit memories came to the surface, too. As Julia's implicit fears were gradually transforming, allowing security to emerge, her natural playfulness and cooperative nature began to appear where it counted most: with her family.

Speaking for the Value of Play at Every Age

Many of us may have found that it is difficult to justify the use of play, particularly child-guided play, as a means of healing and learning. A society that is often restricting or removing recess from the school day doesn't have ears to easily hear the value of play. In spite of evidence that recess improves focus, cognition, retention, and relational capacity in our children, our fear of academic failure and the mandated need to provide certain test scores drives us toward the very decisions that undermine these most desired outcomes (Pellegrini & Bohn, 2005; Ramstetter, Murray, & Garner, 2010; Ridgway, Northrup, Pellegrini, LaRue, & Hightsoe, 2003; Sibley & Etnier, 2003). Similarly, the emphasis on using evidence-based approaches and treatment planning in the therapeutic community can lead us away from what neuroscience suggests about child-guided play: that an accepting relationship that follows the child's impulse

opens the royal road to changing the behaviors that arise out of implicit pain and fear (Wipfler, 2006).

If it is difficult to "sell" play for children, how much more challenging might it be to bring play into our work with adults? Yet our play circuitry remains central to who we are throughout our lives. Although most play scholars agree that play is necessary in the neurobiological development of children, Brown (Brown & Vaughn, 2009) draws from research and clinical observations to suggest that play is equally important for the well-being of adults. Theresa Kestly (2014) cites recent corroborating research:

> Similarly, in a formal study of adult development conducted at Harvard Medical School, Vaillant (2002) concluded that playfulness and creativity were among some of the important factors that determine a retiree's sense of well-being and happiness. Knowing how to play, which often overlaps with being creative, made all the difference, according to the Harvard study, in whether retirees ended up in a sad-sick or a happy-well category.

With this research in mind, we may want to explore ways of bringing playfulness into our work with adult clients.

Actually, the playfulness is already potentially present since the circuitry is inborn. However, these neural pathways begin to be shaped by experience very early in life, and if play was not encouraged then, we may protect ourselves from the pain of feeling that loss of an essential aspect of childhood by thinking of play as silly, a waste of time, or not serious enough for the struggles of adult life. The nature of our current society and our immersion in its need for success can also undermine the possibility of play being seen as profitable. Providing serious left-hemisphere explanations for the value of certain kinds of play may loosen the constraints a bit and begin to enlist the protective parts of our adults into the cause. If play can be understood as a powerful way into the inner world, then perhaps it might be all right to experiment a bit.

Preparing a Space for Adults to Play

I (Badenoch) provide enticements for my adult clients in the form of shelves of miniatures, delicious kinds of sand, and abundant art supplies, along with a few stuffed animals and an exceptionally soft blanket.[3] This is bait for the right hemisphere's need to express itself in the nonverbal and embodied way that is its natural medium, as well as an offer of potential experiences of comfort for tattered attachment systems. While their senses begin to get engaged with miniatures and crayons and fur, we talk about how we store painful and frightening experiences in our bodies in the form of implicit memories that are mostly out of conscious awareness but that nonetheless provide the templates that guide our lives—and especially our relationships. With whatever degree of detail seems to fit the particular person, we explore the neural circuitry of accessing and healing these memories and the relational and behavioral changes that can follow from this healing. Rather than use the word *play*, I talk about having experiences together that can modify the felt sense that is so troubling for them. This is usually enough to open the possibility of drawing or doing a tray, just to see what might emerge. What unfolds from there is often so deep and so startlingly accurate that further engagement in this way becomes easy.

Marshall

Some people adapt to the play environment right away, and others take more time to find their way in. Pacing and patience often win the day. Marshall, a stockbroker, entered my office for the first time, glanced around, and commented that he felt like he was in his grandmother's house because of all the knickknacks on my shelves. This impression was mildly annoying for him, but he was particularly appalled by the large black teddy bear sitting on the couch. He sat as far away from it as possible. He

shared a history of poverty and abuse, and his ongoing pursuit of financial security at all costs. What brought him to me was the sense that whenever he wasn't busy, there was an encroaching sense of meaninglessness that made him think about dying. He drank to drive it away and then found himself in an altered state on his motorcycle in the middle of the night. After he had a nightmare of killing a child on one of these drunken drives, he knew he needed help. He had come to me because he heard I was familiar with the new neuroscience, so he thought I would provide intelligent advice. Imagine his shock and discomfort as he walked into what he later called my "toy store." To his credit, he stayed put long enough for me to hear his history and for us to begin to explore ways to alleviate his loss of meaning.

I knew better than to jump right in with encouragement to play. Instead, I listened without judgment to his bewilderment about why his very good life was so unfulfilling. He pushed me to give advice, and I asked what it would be like for him that I wasn't going to do that. When he asked why not, the door was open to begin to explore the neuroscience of change, of implicit memories, of disconfirming experiences. This talk helped his left hemisphere make sense of our process and likely allowed his intellect to calm a bit, it seemed, because he began to drift toward more contact with his earlier life experiences.

One day, as he shared his mother's fear of his father and how alone he felt in the chaos, his hand drifted toward the black teddy bear and began to caress the soft fur. I breathed a little deeper to calm my excitement, to not disturb what I believed was his child's hand seeking comfort. After about 30 seconds of this contact, he glanced over at his hand and yanked it back onto his thigh, saying, "What the hell am I doing?" He was clearly frightened and somewhat disgusted by this emerging gesture. I wondered with him when he learned he was not allowed to seek comfort—and that began our descent into the implicit depths. The safety of our relationship and the invitation offered by the environment to express these deeper needs had gotten the attention of his integrating brain, making room for the quiet appearance of this small child.

Marshall began to notice these impulses to touch the bear or the blanket, and as we began to more consciously encounter the child inside who had been utterly bereft of such comforts, his history of play started to emerge. He had engaged in structured play—baseball and other sports, learning chess at a young age because his father would do that with him, but had not had many opportunities to just romp around in free play or explore creatively with no particular purpose in mind. Now, watching children run around in the local park near his home made him acutely uncomfortable. Supported again by my sharing neuroscience information about the importance of play, he was able to grieve with and for the small boy inside him. This releasing process seemed to open a door to the sand and miniatures. Over a 2-year period, he did 38 trays, sharing a saga of chaos and terror without words, and gradually finding the joy inside the playing. As we moved into our second year together, we laughed more, told dumb jokes, and had some verbal sparring matches with the sparkling eyes that characterize adults with their play circuitry flourishing. Near the end of our time together, he told me that the turning point had been his hand moving, without his knowledge or permission, toward Montgomery Big Bear (with whom he was now on a first-name basis). He shared a most tender story of how his father removed both his teddy bear and his blanket the day he went to preschool. He said something had broken inside him that day that we had now repaired.

Play Will Find a Way

Marshall's reluctance to play was an adaptive protection against all the losses he had suffered, and I have found this to be the case with most of my adult clients. Play is natural at every stage in life, so it takes considerable relational wounding to blunt this circuitry. Once we can establish an environment that is rich in safety, opportunity, curiosity, and acceptance, play will find a way—if we are comfortable with playing ourselves. If we aren't, then our hesitation will resonate with whatever reluctance our adult clients may bring and make it difficult for us to truly hold the door open while they find their path toward healing. Exploring our own history with play, with support, can help us gain a felt sense of how our early lives shaped our circuitry, and open those neural pathways to joyous expression and engagement now.

We have personally found it worthwhile to spend the time and energy to learn enough about interpersonal neurobiology and the science of play to offer bits and pieces of this wisdom at the right empathic moments to young ones, teens, adults, parents, teachers, and anyone else who will listen. Our society has grown so inhospitable to free, interpersonally engaged play that it needs wise voices to continue to create a potential space for this essential activity to flourish. One additional benefit may be the creation of a perspective and foundation that support our ability to be more present with our clients of all ages because we have a deepening sense of what is unfolding inside them. Although neuroscience is in its infancy, dedicated scientists such as Jaak Panksepp and Stephen Porges and seminal theoreticians such as Daniel Siegel and Allan Schore have devoted decades to uncovering the pathways of safety and play as well as building systems of understanding from the science. They have opened windows to help us appreciate why play offers such an optimal environment for change. As we are able to picture these pathways of healing more clearly, our systems can relax into presence, openness, and care—the essential relational supports for the people who come to us.

Kevin

Let's finish as we began—with a story. Scott, one of our colleagues, told us about Kevin, a 16-year-old young man who had been setting fires for the last 2 years, being dragged into his playroom by the boy's terrified mother. She had selected Scott as the counselor because he had a reputation for being unfazed by resistant teens. Kevin was not much interested in talking about what he had done or anything else, but he became seriously intrigued when Scott began to share his understanding of what is happening in the dynamic and sometimes challenging adolescent brain. Kevin, who had also been in trouble for his colorful and profane graffiti creations, grabbed the large paper and markers to begin drawing his own embodied brain. Interestingly enough, most of the drawings included flames—some in the region near his limbic system, some emerging from his hands and feet, and some jetting out in front of him toward an unknown target. He rarely spoke more than a few words, but filled the hours with the wordless narrative of his art, the expressions on his face, the movements of his body, and the increasingly full space between him and Scott—who watched, reflected, and held the process with respect for this young man whom he saw working so hard.

Kevin occasionally looked at the sandtray figures, something Scott noted but didn't speak to. Then one day, Kevin said, "You know, it's really stupid to have these toys in here." Having declared his adversarial position, he got up and took a single figure, a man made entirely of flames, from the shelf and placed it in the sand. They contemplated his creation in silence together for a full 5 minutes. Then Kevin retrieved the fire extinguisher and placed it next to the fiery man. He sat down, saying, "Really stupid, man." He never set a fire again. Even in the face of apparent resistance, play can often find a way. Scott and Kevin continued together for 2 more years, moving, often

wordlessly, through his early history with a violent, abusive father and terrified, impotent mother. Throughout their process, Kevin's words maintained his sarcastic, protective stance, while his body found a way to express and heal the pain and fear. Such is the power of play.

NOTES

1. Julia is a composite case drawn from several young ones cared for by Theresa Kestly.

2. Jaak Panksepp capitalizes these words to indicate that they have a special meaning in regard to the emotional–motivational circuitry of the brain in both mammals and that special subclass, humans.

3. In this section, Bonnie Badenoch talks about her work with adults, combining several people she has seen in therapy in her stories.

REFERENCES

Adolphs, R. (2002). Trust in the brain. *Nature Neuroscience, 5*, 192–193.

Badenoch, B. (2011). *The brain-savvy therapist's workbook*. New York: Norton.

Badenoch, B. (2013). A transformational learning group: Inviting the implicit. In S. P. Gantt & B. Badenoch (Eds.), *The interpersonal neurobiology of group psychotherapy and group process* (pp. 189–201). London: Karnac.

Beckes, L., & Coan, J. A. (2011). Social baseline theory: The role of social proximity in emotion and economy of action. *Social and Personality Psychology, 5*(12), 976–988.

Brown, S., & Vaughan, C. (2009). *Play: How it shapes the brain, opens the imagination, and invigorates the soul*. New York: Avery.

Critchley, H. D. (2005). Neural mechanisms of autonomic, affective, and cognitive integration. *Comparative Neurology, 493*, 154–166.

Dobbs, D. (2012, December 24). A new focus on the "post" in post-traumatic stress. *New York Times*. Retrieved from *www.nytimes.com/2012/12/25/science/understanding-the-effects-of-social-environment-on-trauma-victims.html?pagewanted=all&_r=0*.

Ecker, B., Ticic, R., Hulley, L., & Neimeyer, R. A. (2012). *Unlocking the emotional brain: Eliminat-*

ing symptoms at their roots using memory reconsolidation. New York: Routledge.

Iacoboni, M. (2009). Imitation, empathy, and mirror neurons. *Annual Review of Psychology, 60,* 653–670.

Kestly, T. (2014). *The interpersonal neurobiology of play: Brain-building interventions for emotional well-being.* New York: Norton.

MacLean, P. D. (1990). *The triune brain in evolution: Role in paleocerebral functions.* New York: Plenum Press.

Morris, J. S., Ohman, A., & Dolan, R. J. (1999). A subcortical pathway to the right amygdala mediating "unseen" fear. *Proceedings of the National Academy of Science, USA, 96,* 1680–1685.

Panksepp, J., & Biven, L. (2012). *The archaeology of mind: Neuroevolutionary origins of human emotions.* New York: Norton.

Pellgrini, A., & Bohn, C. (2005). The role of recess in children's cognitive performance and school adjustment. *Educational Research for Policy and Practice, 34*(1), 13–19.

Porges, S. W. (2003). The polyvagal theory: Phylogenetic contributions to social behavior. *Physiology and Behavior, 79*(3), 503–513.

Porges, S. W. (2011). *The polyvagal theory: Neurophysiological foundations of emotions, attachment, communication, and self-regulation.* New York: Norton.

Ramstetter, C. L., Murray, R., & Garner, A. S. (2010). The crucial role of recess in schools. *Journal of School Health, 80*(11), 517–526.

Ridgway, A., Northrup, J., Pellegrin, A., LaRue, R., & Hightsoe, A. (2003). Effects of recess on the classroom behavior of children with and without attention-deficit hyperactivity disorder. *School Psychology Quarterly, 18*(3), 253–268.

Schore, A. N. (2012). *The science of the art of psychotherapy.* New York: Norton.

Semple, R., Lee, J., Williams, M., & Teasdale J. D. (2011). *Mindfulness-based cognitive therapy for anxious children: A manual for treating childhood anxiety.* Oakland, CA: New Harbinger.

Sibley, B., & Etnier, J. (2003). The relationship between physical activity and cognition in children: A meta-analysis. *Pediatric Exercise Science, 15,* 243–256.

Siegel, D. J. (2012). *The developing mind: How relationships and the brain interact to shape who we are* (2nd ed.). New York: Guilford Press.

Vaillant, G. E. (2002). *Aging well.* Boston: Little, Brown.

Winston, J. S., Strange, B. A., O'Doherty, J., & Dolan, R. J. (2002). Automatic and intentional brain responses during evaluation of trustworthiness of faces. *Nature Neuroscience, 5,* 277–283.

Wipfler, P. (2006). *How children's emotions work.* Palo Alto, CA: Hand in Hand.

Index

Page numbers followed by *f* indicate figure; *n*, note; and *t*, table.